Pulmonary Fibrosis: Mechanisms, Diagnosis and Treatment

Pulmonary Fibrosis: Mechanisms, Diagnosis and Treatment

Editor: Liam Lawrence

AMERICAN
MEDICAL PUBLISHERS
www.americanmedicalpublishers.com

AMERICAN
MEDICAL PUBLISHERS
www.americanmedicalpublishers.com

Cataloging-in-Publication Data

Pulmonary fibrosis : mechanisms, diagnosis and treatment / edited by Liam Lawrence.
p. cm.
Includes bibliographical references and index.
ISBN 979-8-88740-581-0
1. Pulmonary fibrosis. 2. Pulmonary fibrosis--Diagnosis. 3. Pulmonary fibrosis--Treatment.
4. Lungs--Diseases. I. Lawrence, Liam.
RC776.F5 P85 2023
616.24--dc23

American Medical Publishers,
41 Flatbush Avenue,
1st Floor, New York,
NY 11217, USA

ISBN 979-8-88740-581-0 (Hardback)

Contents

Preface

Pulmonary fibrosis refers to a medical condition that causes scarring in the lungs over time. The scarring in the lungs thickens with passage of time and makes it difficult for the person to breathe. Dry cough, weight loss, shortness of breath, fatigue, and aching joints and muscles are a few signs and symptoms of pulmonary fibrosis. The risk factors associated with this medical condition include, smoking, cancer therapies, aging and genetic factors. Respiratory failure, high blood pressure, lung cancer and right-sided heart failure are some of the complications linked with pulmonary fibrosis. The diagnosis of this disease can be done by performing lung function tests, medical imaging and lung biopsy. There is no cure for this disease and medicines can aid in maintaining lung function and slow the progression of scarring. Staying active and receiving oxygen therapy may help to alleviate symptoms. This book strives to provide a fair idea about pulmonary fibrosis and to help develop a better understanding of the latest advances in its clinical management. It will serve as a reference to a broad spectrum of readers. Different evaluations and advanced studies on the mechanisms and diagnosis of pulmonary fibrosis have been included in this book.

This book is a result of research of several months to collate the most relevant data in the field.

When I was approached with the idea of this book and the proposal to edit it, I was overwhelmed. It gave me an opportunity to reach out to all those who share a common interest with me in this field. I had 3 main parameters for editing this text:

1. Accuracy - The data and information provided in this book should be up-to-date and valuable to the readers.

2. Structure - The data must be presented in a structured format for easy understanding and better grasping of the readers.

3. Universal Approach - This book not only targets students but also experts and innovators in the field, thus my aim was to present topics which are of use to all.

Thus, it took me a couple of months to finish the editing of this book.

I would like to make a special mention of my publisher who considered me worthy of this opportunity and also supported me throughout the editing process. I would also like to thank the editing team at the back-end who extended their help whenever required.

Editor

1

The Epithelial-Immune Crosstalk in Pulmonary Fibrosis

Thomas Planté-Bordeneuve[1], *Charles Pilette*[1,2] *and Antoine Froidure*[1,2*]

[1] Pôle de pneumologie, O.R.L. et dermatologie, Institut de Recherche Expérimentale et Clinique, Université catholique de Louvain, Bruxelles, Belgium, [2] *Service de pneumologie, Cliniques universitaires Saint-Luc, Bruxelles, Belgium*

***Correspondence:**
Antoine Froidure
antoine.froidure@uclouvain.be

Interactions between the lung epithelium and the immune system involve a tight regulation to prevent inappropriate reactions and have been connected to several pulmonary diseases. Although the distal lung epithelium and local immunity have been implicated in the pathogenesis and disease course of idiopathic pulmonary fibrosis (IPF), consequences of their abnormal interplay remain less well known. Recent data suggests a two-way process, as illustrated by the influence of epithelial-derived periplakin on the immune landscape or the effect of macrophage-derived IL-17B on epithelial cells. Additionally, damage associated molecular patterns (DAMPs), released by damaged or dying (epithelial) cells, are augmented in IPF. Next to "sterile inflammation", pathogen-associated molecular patterns (PAMPs) are increased in IPF and have been linked with lung fibrosis, while outer membrane vesicles from bacteria are able to influence epithelial-macrophage crosstalk. Finally, the advent of high-throughput technologies such as microbiome-sequencing has allowed for the identification of a disease-specific microbial environment. In this review, we propose to discuss how the interplays between the altered distal airway and alveolar epithelium, the lung microbiome and immune cells may shape a pro-fibrotic environment. More specifically, it will highlight DAMPs-PAMPs pathways and the specificities of the IPF lung microbiome while discussing recent elements suggesting abnormal mucosal immunity in pulmonary fibrosis.

Keywords: lung fibrosis, mucosal immunity, epithelium, mucus, innate immunity

INTRODUCTION

The role of the immune system in the development and disease course of idiopathic pulmonary fibrosis (IPF) has been a matter of heated debate over the last decades. Initial observations of increased neutrophil counts in the broncho-alveolar lavage (BAL) (1, 2) alongside the histologic presence of neutrophils, lymphocytes and macrophages in the proximity of fibrotic areas (1) led to the hypothesis that IPF starts as an inflammatory alveolitis and progresses to alveolar septal fibrosis over time. These observations formed the basis for the use of immunosuppressive therapies, in particular corticosteroids, in IPF. Although randomized controlled trials evaluating the role of steroids were missing (3, 4), observational data suggested a heterogeneous response in patients (5). In the early 2000s, the influence of immunity and immunomodulatory medication in IPF began to be questioned, with the emergence of alveolar epithelial dysfunction as one of the main contributors to pathogenesis (6) and the observations that, with further refinement of disease classification criteria (7), better characterized patients with a usual interstitial pneumonia pattern (UIP) displayed only mild inflammation (8). Finally, a milestone study assessing the effect of N-acetylcysteine, azathioprine, and prednisone in IPF reported a deleterious effect of this combination therapy (9) further weakening the "inflammatory hypothesis" in IPF. The emergence of high-throughput technologies, such as single-cell RNA sequencing, have allowed for the discovery of fibrosis-specific cell populations and fueled a renewed interest for the immune system in this disease. Thus, the place of immunity and inflammation in the course of this pathology has evolved, from causal to modulating (10) and unravelling the subtleties underlying this influence could help discover new targets and understand why immunosuppressive interventions have failed in the past.

The distal lung epithelium forms a continuous layer of cells responsible for gas transport and exchange as well as host defense. A complete overview of pulmonary cell composition can be found in (11, 12). Briefly, whereas in proximal conducting airways, it is principally composed of ciliated, secretory and basal stem cells, monostratified type-1 and type-2 alveolar epithelial cells (AEC) are present in the alveoli (11) (**Figure 1**). As the lung lays at the interface between host and environment, constantly exposed to external stimulation, a tight regulation of inflammatory mechanisms is required to preclude inadequate immune reactions. Lung epithelial cells participate in this equilibrium through several mechanisms. While the contribution of myeloid cells to lung immune mechanisms and secondary fibrosis in IPF has been extensively studied, the participation of the epithelium remains to be fully determined. Although *ex vivo* epithelial cultures are a tedious process, notably hampered by the rapid dedifferentiation of, for example, monocultured alveolar type-2 epithelial cells (AEC2) (13), both *in vivo* and *in vitro* evidence point towards the implication of the epithelium in the aforementioned processes. In this review, we will summarize how epithelial cells' biology and their crosstalk with immune cells and microbes may, under some circumstances, conduct to aberrant, pro-fibrotic signaling in the lung. We will discuss how epithelial cells form a physical barrier through their secretion and removal of mucus, while forming a continuous cell layer, and how alterations in these mechanisms can fuel pro-fibrotic mechanisms. Furthermore, we will review the data regarding their ability to sense and react to danger and pathogen associated molecules and the existing links between alterations in those mechanisms and lung fibrosis. Finally, we will address the epithelial capacity to modulate lung immune responses, notably through the secretion of several soluble mediators (14, 15), and to trigger the recruitment, polarization and activation of pro-fibrotic myeloid cells.

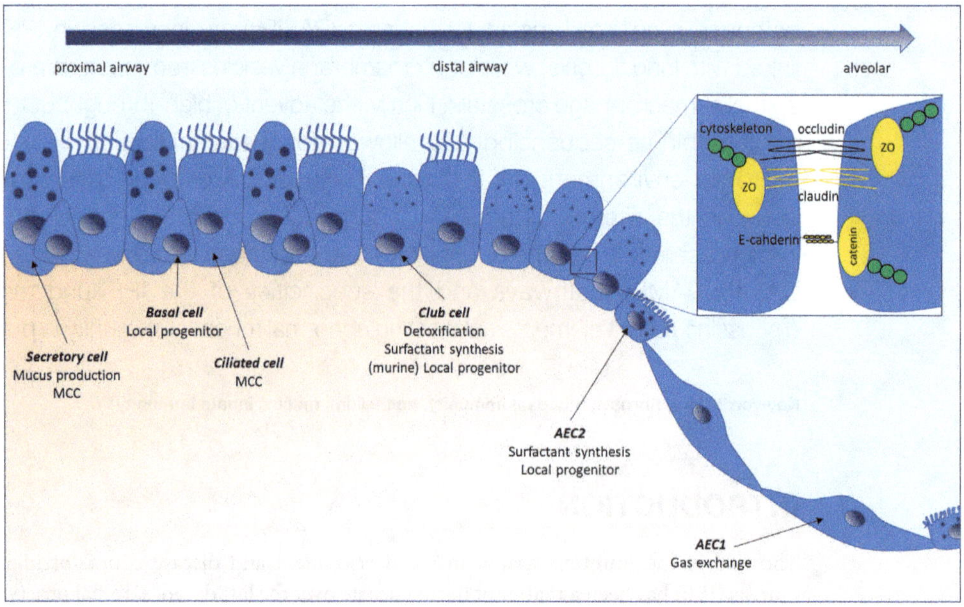

FIGURE 1 | The normal lung epithelium composition changes along the respiratory tree from proximal airways to alveolar areas. Secretory cells produce the mucus lining the airways, which is moved upstream by the ciliated beats originating from ciliated cells. Basal cells have a local progenitor function, possessing the ability to differentiate into several cell types, including secretory and ciliated cells. In small airways, basal and secretory cells are progressively replaced by club (ex-Clara) cells, which can serve as local facultative progenitors (besides basal cells), secrete components of the bronchiolar lining fluid, and play a detoxifying role through their expression of cytochrome p450. In the alveoli, alveolar type-1 epithelial cells (AEC1) are responsible for gas exchange, while alveolar type-2 epithelial cells (AEC2) produce surfactant and serve as local progenitors. Epithelial cells are connected by tight- and adherens junctions, forming a continuous layer separating the intra-luminal content from the submucosal environment and regulating intercellular permeability. Tight junctions are composed of integral membrane proteins like claudins and occludins, which are linked to the cytoskeleton through cytosolic protein complexes such as Zonula Occludens (ZO). Adherens junctions, formed by E-cadherin proteins, linked to the cytoskeleton by catenins are responsible for the maintenance of cell-cell adhesion while being involved in many intracellular signaling and transcriptional pathways. MCC, mucociliary clearance.

THE EPITHELIUM AS A PHYSICAL BARRIER

Mucins and Mucociliary Clearance

The mucus layer covering the respiratory tract epithelium is able to trap and remove noxious stimuli thanks to mucociliary clearance and cough, forming the lung's first line of defense in the airways (16). Mucins are glycosylated proteins that help constitute this visco-elastic layer, isolating the underlying structures from the outer world. The human lung expresses 16 different types of mucins, which can be separated into two families, namely secreted (predominantly MUC5AC and MUC5B) and membrane-bound mucins (mainly MUC1, MUC4 and MUC16) (17). Mucins fulfill multiple roles, forming a mesh hampering epithelial access to noxious stimuli, acting as lubricant as well as (decoy) receptors for pathogens, associating with several cytokines and growth factors, and, for membrane bound mucins, influencing intracellular signaling pathways such as NFκB or β-catenin (18–22). Mucin expression is regulated by numerous signals, including cytokines such as TNF-α, IL-1β, IL-6, IL-13 or IL-17, growth factors like EGF, Damage-Associated Molecular Patterns, bacterial and viral products or proteases (23–28). Of note, membrane-bound mucins consist of 2 non-covalently linked α- and β-chains, which, when exposed to physical stress, inflammatory mediators or changes in their ionic environment, can separate, causing the release of the α-chain (29).

Mucins seem to play a favoring role in the development of lung fibrosis and its subsequent course. Indeed, the most important genetic risk factor associated with IPF is the single nucleotide polymorphism (SNP) rs35705950 in the promoter region of *MUC5B* (30). This common allelic variant, present in 38% of IPF patients and 9% of controls (30), is both predictive and prognostic in lung fibrosis (31), as it is associated with a significant increase in the risk of having pulmonary fibrosis in the Framingham Heart Study population (32) and decreased mortality in 2 IPF cohorts (33). This polymorphism is linked with an increased expression of *MUC5B* (30) and its homonymous mucin protein (34). Furthermore, independently of their genetic background, IPF patients display increased levels of MUC5B in the distal airways (35, 36) and MUC5B is the main mucin present in honeycomb cysts (36). How MUC5B accumulation influences lung fibrosis is still not completely determined but could involve decreased mucociliary clearance with local inflammation or abnormal epithelialization. Supporting the former, a recent link between C3, a component of the complement cascade, the MUC5B polymorphism and IPF has been described (37). Additionally, distal overexpression of MUC5B in mice leads to a thickened mucus layer, impaired mucociliary clearance, augmented honeycomb cyst size and increased fibrosis after bleomycin challenge (38, 39). *In vivo* data indicates a crucial role for MUC5B in the maintenance of healthy interactions between the host and bacteria, as *Muc5b*$^{-/-}$ but not *Muc5ac*$^{-/-}$ animals display impaired survival related to respiratory infections (40). Impaired mucociliary clearance, present in both *Muc5b*$^{-/-}$ and Muc5b overexpressing animals could result in suboptimal clearance of organisms and increased epithelial-bacterial contact. Besides, although currently no causal relationship can be established, IPF subjects with increased bacterial loads display worse survival (41) while the presence of the rs35705950 SNP is associated with lower bacterial burden (41) and improved outcomes (33). Much less is known about the potential implication of MUC5AC in IPF. Recently, a single nucleotide variant in *MUC5AC* was described (42), but the exact effects on protein expression and clinical outcome remain to be determined. Independently from this observation and similarly to MUC5B, MUC5AC expression is increased in the distal IPF lung (36) and is expressed within HC, albeit at a much lower level (35, 36). Similarly to their secreted counterparts, the expression of MUC1 and MUC4 is increased in IPF lungs (43, 44). These mucins are involved in lung fibrosis through their α- and β-chain. In fact, the MUC1 and MUC16 extracellular domains contain the KL-6 and CA125 epitopes respectively, which have been linked with disease progression (45, 46). Furthermore, KL-6 can promote fibroblast proliferation and migration while exerting anti-apoptotic activities (47, 48) and was implicated in an *in vivo* experimental model of lung fibrosis (49). Finally, implication of the cytoplasmic tails of both MUC1 and MUC4 is suggested by the fact that their genetic and pharmacologic modulation is sufficient to protect bleomycin treated mice and by their role in TGF-β1-induced EMT or myofibroblast differentiation (43, 44).

Intercellular Junctions

Tight junctions (TJ) and adherens junctions (AJ) act as apical junctional complexes, connecting adjacent cells, regulating the transport of solutes, allowing cell polarity and permitting the separation of the airway lumen and the underlying mucosa through a physical barrier (50, 51). Briefly, TJ are composed of integral membrane proteins, such as claudins and occludins and cytosolic protein complexes comprising Zonula Occludens proteins (ZO-1, 2, 3) (52) linked to actin binding proteins and the cytoskeleton (**Figure 1**) (51, 53). Claudin expression varies in function of the tissue (54) and these proteins can be divided in two groups based on their permeability properties, with claudins-2, -7, -10, -15 and -16 promoting paracellular flux, while claudins-1, -4, -5, -8, -11, -14 and -18 have a sealing function (55, 56). Within the human lung, claudin expression is variable, the main bronchiolar claudins being claudin-1, -2, -3, -4, -5 and -7, while alveolar cells are positive for claudin-3, -4, -7 and -18 (57–59), suggesting tailored expression in function of the localization. AJ are especially important for the maintenance of cell-cell adhesion but are also involved in many intracellular signaling and transcriptional pathways. In the alveolar epithelium, the hallmark structure of AJ consists of a complex formed by the E-cadherin cell adhesion molecules linked to the actin cytoskeleton thanks to catenins (**Figure 1**) (51). β-catenin, in particular, serves important signaling functions, linking structural junctions with the Wnt pathway. At last, desmosomes, specialized membrane complexes, help maintain the mechanical integrity of tissues and are particularly represented in tissues undergoing high mechanical stress, such as the lungs (60). They are composed by desmosomal cadherins, Armadillo proteins and plakins, and are present throughout the bronchial and alveolar epithelium (61). Lungs of patients affected by IPF present several signs of epithelial integrity disruption, with basement membrane denudation (62) and downregulation of several junctional proteins, suggesting that alterations in one, or several, of these structures are present.

Tight junctions are altered in IPF, with immunohistochemical observations showing an increased expression of occludin, claudin-1, -2, -3 and -7 and a downregulation of claudin-18 within regions of abnormal epithelialization (57–59). Discrepant results exist for claudin-4, with reports of increased (58, 59) or decreased expression (57) but this can at least partly be explained by differences in epithelial classification between studies, since alveolar and bronchiolar zones were not always separated. Measures of lung epithelial permeability through 99m-labelled diethylenetriamine penta-acetic acid (^{99m}Tc-DTPA) measurement, although quite non-specific, shows that patients have faster clearance than control subjects, suggesting increased epithelial permeability (63). Similarly, intraperitoneal bleomycin injections, resulting in lung fibrosis, lead to decreased pulmonary expression of claudin-5 and -18 as well as occludins (64) while claudin-4 is upregulated after experimental acute lung injury (65). The mechanisms underlying these alterations are unclear; however, TGF-β1, one of the main profibrotic cytokines involved in IPF, is capable of inducing TJ disassembly (64), increases claudin-4 (66) and decreases claudin-18 expression (67). Interestingly, genetic deletion of *cldn18* results in (pathologic) epithelial regeneration efforts with alveolar enlargement, impaired barrier function, alveolar type-1 epithelial cell (AEC1) injury, AEC2 expansion and YAP activation, a proliferation/differentiation protein activated in IPF alveolar cells (68–70). Furthermore, preserved epithelial barrier integrity and polarization permit modulation of the interaction between growth factors or cytokines and their receptors, further implicating TJ in innate immune processes and epithelialization. For instance, expression of heregulin, a Human Epidermal growth Receptor (HER) ligand, is normally restricted to the apical surface of the lung epithelium, separated from its coreceptor HER2/3 at the basal level by intact TJ (71). Upon disruption of TJ integrity, the ligand is able to gain access to its receptor, prompting downstream signaling implicated in experimental pulmonary fibrosis (72). Although these lines of evidence point towards a role for TJ dysfunction in lung fibrosis, it is still uncertain whether TJ alterations can directly influence this process or are mere bystanders of abnormal epithelialization, necessitating further mechanistic studies before definitive conclusions can be drawn.

Loss of E-cadherin and gain of N-cadherin is a salient feature of epithelial-mesenchymal transition (EMT), a process by which epithelial cells gain mesenchymal characteristics, as observed in IPF. Accordingly, the IPF lung epithelium displays alterations in the expression of these AJ proteins, with decreased basal cell expression of E-cadherin and co-expression of E-cadherin and N-cadherin in hyperplasic pneumocytes (73). Additionally, treatment with bleomycin, either in experimental models of lung fibrosis or on an alveolar epithelial cell-line reduces E-cadherin expression (74, 75). Similarly to TJ, TGF-β1 seems to be one of the main mediators of AJ alteration, as it has the ability to downregulate E-cadherin (76, 77). A complete overview of the role of EMT in IPF is proposed by Salton et al. (78). Finally, lung-specific deletion of E-cadherin in mice results in loss of airway epithelial cells, epithelial denudation, and increased presence of α-smooth muscle actin (α-SMA) expressing cells alongside increased alveolar diameters (79).

Periplakin and desmoplakin, two plakins linking the desmosomal plaque with intermediate filaments have also been implicated in lung fibrosis. Recently, variants of *DSP*, the gene coding for desmoplakin, were associated with IPF while mRNA levels are elevated in diseased lungs (80). Periplakin was initially identified as a potential contributor to pulmonary fibrosis due to the presence of anti-periplakin antibodies in the serum of 40% of IPF patients, and alterations in its alveolar expression (61). Further mechanistic insights show that these antibodies impact epithelial migration and wound closure while BAL of IPF patients downregulates *Ppl* mRNA in murine alveolar cells (61, 81). Furthermore, *Ppl*$^{-/-}$ animals are protected from experimental lung fibrosis, display altered downstream signaling in pro-fibrotic pathway synchronously to an anti-inflammatory alveolar environment and decreased, pro-fibrotic, alternatively activated macrophages (81). No alterations of other cell junctional components could be observed, arguing against a loss of epithelial integrity and for a direct role of periplakin as modulator of its immune milieu and downstream profibrotic signals.

THE LUNG EPITHELIUM SENSES AND REACTS TO DANGER SIGNALS

Aside from disrupting the physical barrier separating the basal membrane and submucosal tissue from the luminal content, epithelial injury also leads to the release of danger signals, so called Damage-Associated Molecular Patterns (DAMPs). This results in the activation of inflammatory pathways and the promotion of damaged structures clearance in a process of "sterile inflammation" (82). A wide variety of proteins can act as DAMPs, sharing the feature of being either mislocalized or altered. High Motility Group Box 1 (HMGB1) is the first described DAMP following the "danger theory" (83) and is normally spatially restricted to the nucleus, where it regulates DNA organization and transcription, but can act as a strong pro-inflammatory stimulus when passively released in the surrounding milieu by necro(pto)tic cells (83). Next to passive release, HMGB1 can also be actively secreted by non-necrotic cells of the immune system and intestinal epithelial cells after immune stimulation (84, 85). Similarly, the production of hyaluronan fragments from extracellular matrix high-molecular weight (HMW) hyaluronan can trigger inflammatory pathways (86). Furthermore, disruption of physical defense mechanisms will also lead to increased contact with bacterial and viral products named Pathogen-Associated

Molecular Patterns (PAMPs), such as lipopolysaccharides, ds/ssRNA or unmethylated CpG DNA (87). Both DAMPs and PAMPs downstream signaling is mediated through Pattern Recognition Receptors (PRR), intracytoplasmic and membrane receptors consisting of 4 classes, Toll-Like Receptors (TLR), NOD-Like Receptors (NLR), C-type Lectin Receptors (CLR) and RIG-I-Like receptors (RLR) (88). These receptors are present on cells from the immune system, but also expressed by lung epithelial cells (15) and can trigger a wide array of effects, resulting in activation of NFκB, MAPK and interferon pathways.

The Epithelium as Source and Target of DAMPs in IPF

Although DAMPs primarily serve an inflammatory function, they are increased in IPF and, based on experimental results, seem to be involved in fibrogenesis. As stated previously, DAMPs can originate from necro(pto)tic cells, and increased levels of RIPK3, a regulator of necroptosis have been observed in IPF lungs and in experimental, bleomycin-induced pulmonary fibrosis, particularly within alveolar epithelial cells (89). Further implication comes from the observation that HMGB1, uric acid or extracellular ATP (eATP), all recognized DAMPs, are increased in both human BAL as well as *in vivo* and *in vitro* experimental conditions (89–93). Although the origin of these signals is multiple, distal lung epithelial cells contribute to this altered environment as they show staining for HMGB1 and bleomycin-stimulated alveolar cells produce high levels of HMGB1 and eATP (90, 93). Additionally, inhibition of HMGB1 by a neutralizing antibody, of uric acid levels by a xanthine-oxidase inhibitor and interference with eATP signaling all decrease bleomycin-induced lung fibrosis (90, 92, 93). The exact mechanisms implicating DAMPs in fibrosis are currently incompletely elucidated but include direct interactions with fibroblasts as well as epithelial cells and promotion of IL-1β production, a cytokine involved in lung fibrosis (94). Indeed, addition of HMGB1 to fibroblasts promotes cell viability and myofibroblast differentiation (90, 95) while decreased IL-1β levels are observed in bleomycin instilled mice treated with anti-HMGB1 antibodies (90). HMGB1 also influences epithelial behavior, as it enhances scratch-wound closure by AECs through the production of IL-1β and activation of TGF-β1 (96), potentially fueling frustrated repair mechanisms in the alveoli, and promotes epithelial-mesenchymal transition in bronchial cells (97). Finally, HMGB1 can shape the immune contribution to fibrosis as it prompts macrophages to produce high levels of IL-1β, which could influence collagen deposition (98) and triggers the release of chemokines such as MCP-1/CCL2 by lung epithelial cells (99), a molecule known to enhance fibrocyte recruitment (100). Additionally, epithelial cells exposed to this molecule produce higher levels of TNF-α, which has been linked with TJ disassembly (101), fibroblast apoptosis (102) and EMT (103, 104). The latter pro- and anti-fibrotic effect are mirrored by *in vivo* data, reporting both protective and promoting roles of this cytokine in lung fibrosis (105, 106). Likewise, extracellular application of ATP is able to provoke an upregulation of TGF-β1, collagen and fibronectin mRNA in cultured fibroblasts (107), increases fibroblast migration and proliferation (108) while $P2X_7^{-/-}$ mice, a knock-out model for a receptor of eATP, are protected from fibrosis and show lower IL-1β levels than control animals (93).

PAMPs and the Lung Epithelium

PAMPs are similarly capable of influencing cell behavior and ultimately fibrosis. Lipopolysaccharides (LPS), membrane components of gram-negative bacteria, recognized by the membrane receptor TLR4, have been involved in experimental lung fibrosis (109, 110), are capable of promoting fibroblast proliferation *in vitro* (111) and induce the early secretion of IL-1β, MCP-1/CCL2 or IL-8 by AEC2 (112, 113). Additionally, bacterial and viral DNA contains hypomethylated CpG zones, and treatment of UIP lung fibroblasts and healthy peripheral monocytes with CpG oligodeoxyribonucleotides (ODN), results in increased myofibroblast as well as fibrocyte differentiation respectively (114, 115). Moreover, fibroblasts from rapidly progressive IPF patients show an enhanced susceptibility to CpG stimulation, probably due to an increased expression of its cytosolic receptor TLR9 in these subjects (115). Epithelial cells are also capable of sensing and responding to CpG, with most experiments linking CpG, lung epithelium and fibrosis conducted in the alveolar A549 cell-line. Both TLR9-dependent and -independent mechanisms could be implicated. Indeed, the induction of EMT observed after CpG treatment of alveolar cells is absent after TLR9 silencing (115) but their upregulation of CCN1, a matricellular protein with pleiotropic functions implicated in IPF and experimental lung fibrosis (116), is predominantly linked to CpG-induced endoplasmic reticulum-(ER) stress (117). Interestingly, integrin αVβ6, an epithelial cell surface receptor implicated in the activation of latent TGF-β, is simultaneously upregulated, potentially linking this with increased TGF-β1 signaling. Conversely, experiments in mice showed that addition of CpG after bleomycin instillations reduced fibrosis (118), possibly reflecting immunological species differences.

Implication of TLR in Lung Fibrosis

Additional evidence implicating these pathways and epithelial cells arise from clinical, *in vivo*, and *in vitro* studies showing alterations of PRR in lung fibrosis. Firstly, polymorphisms affecting PRR, more specifically, TLR have been associated with IPF. In 2013, the L412F *TLR3* polymorphism was linked with respiratory decline and mortality in IPF and shown to influence fibroblast proliferation (119). The same year, SNPs in the *TOLLIP* genetic locus, resulting in lower *TOLLIP* expression levels, were associated with IPF susceptibility and for one of them disease course and mortality (120). *TOLLIP* codes for the Toll-interacting protein (TOLLIP), an inhibitory adaptor protein of downstream TLR2/4 signaling, hampering NF-κB activation (121). In addition, epithelial expression of TOLLIP is associated with resistance to *in vitro* bleomycin induced apoptosis and is locally increased in an aberrant basaloid cell population in IPF (122). Furthermore, TLR2/4 expression is increased at the epithelial level in patients with an UIP pattern

(123). Secondly, evidence from knock-out experiments show differential effects in experimental lung fibrosis. TLR2 and -4 are membrane PRR recognizing DAMPs (for example HMGB1 or hyaluronan fragments) and PAMPs from Gram-positive (lipoproteins) and -negative bacteria (LPS) respectively (124). They have seemingly paradoxical effects as TLR2 alteration exerts a protective, and TLR4 alteration a promoting effect on lung fibrosis. In fact, TLR2 deficiency is associated with improved survival and decreased fibrosis in an experimental model, attenuating the pro-fibrotic T_H2 environment (125), altering immune cell recruitment (125, 126) and diminishing IL-17 production through epithelial IL-27 production (126). TLR2 is expressed by both epithelial and immune cells, and further involvement of lung epithelial cells was shown by chimeric experiments revealing that epithelial TLR2 expression is probably the main contributor to these findings (126). Conversely, $TLR4^{-/-}$ animals show augmented deposition of collagen in the lungs when challenged with different fibrotic stimuli (127), and display a shift towards a T_H2 immune milieu as well as decreased autophagy, potentially impacting collagen degradation (127). Illustrating the complexity and the interplay between these different mechanisms, hyaluronan low molecular weight fragments are responsible for the production of chemokine by macrophages and redundantly signal through TLR2 and 4 whereas high molecular weight hyaluronan only need TLR4 to promote AEC regeneration and renewal (128, 129). Contradictory results, suggesting a protective role of TLR4 inhibition have also been published (110) and further studies are sorely needed to evaluate the exact contribution of each component of these complex systems.

MODIFIED LUNG BACTERIAL LANDSCAPE COULD INFLUENCE EPITHELIAL BIOLOGY

Fueled by negative results of culture-based assessments, the lungs were until recently considered as a sterile environment. The advent of high throughput bacterial sequencing has allowed the identification of a diversified bacterial flora in healthy human lungs which showed modifications in chronic respiratory diseases (130). Current techniques are based on the sequencing of highly conserved genes, such as the 16S ribosomal RNA gene, to identify and quantify bacterial communities and cluster them into operational taxonomic units (OTU) (131, 132). In the healthy lung, bacterial composition resembles the oropharyngeal flora and its structure is regulated through three mechanisms, namely the amount of bacterial immigration, the rate of elimination and the reproduction rate of local bacteria (133). Architectural changes and disruption of these homeostatic pathways in disease cause the genesis of niches permitting the emergence of select bacterial populations, resulting in changes in composition and diversity of airway bacteria (134–137). The epithelium from the respiratory tract can influence the two last determinants through mucus production, mucociliary clearance, secretion of inflammatory mediators as well as alterations of the local micro-environment (133, 138).

Airway bacterial composition is altered in IPF, with patients displaying increased bacterial loads and decreased diversity (41, 139). Additionally, patients with the highest bacterial burden have a markedly worse prognosis than those with lower loads, further supporting a link between bacteria and IPF (41, 140). Of note, this correlation could not be found in a recent study evaluating chronic hypersensitivity pneumonitis patients, suggesting disease specific features (139). Prior observations had identified *Streptococcus* sp., *Prevotella* sp., and *Veillonella* sp. as the most identified bacteria in IPF lungs, questioning the association between bacterial composition and disease. Several studies have suggested a relation between certain genera and OTUs, host defense pathways (140, 141), fibroblast behavior (141) or clinical outcomes (139, 142, 143). Although descriptive, these data suggest that changes in the local bacterial landscape could lead to epithelial injury as well as influence the fibrotic and immune response. Further implication of the bacterial landscape in lung fibrosis development can be gathered from animal studies in which the flora can be controlled to express no or selected bacteria. Indeed, germ-free animals instilled with bleomycin display lower mortality (140, 144) and indices of fibrosis (144). Although this data suggests a potential role of bacteria in the development of fibrosis, studies demonstrating a causal link are scarce. In one study, macrophages exposed to outer membrane vesicles from gram-negative bacteria released IL-17B through TLR2/4 sensing, subsequently inducing the secretion of chemokines and growth factor by alveolar epithelial cells, resulting in the development of pulmonary fibrosis (144). Next to influencing immune-epithelial crosstalk, certain bacteria could directly harm the epithelium by secreting cytotoxic compounds. Indeed, streptolysin (a pore-forming cytotoxin) producing *Streptococcus* and corisin (a recently discovered cytotoxic compound) secreting *Staphylococcus* had direct effects on experimental lung fibrosis, increasing AEC2 apoptosis (145) and hampering anti-fibrotic mechanisms (146). The interactions between the microbiome, the epithelium and the immune system have just started to be unraveled and form an exciting prospect for research in the coming years. Understanding the mechanisms underlying these interactions could help to identify prognostic or therapeutic targets, especially in patients developing acute exacerbations of the disease.

THE EPITHELIUM AS A MODULATOR OF LUNG IMMUNITY

Epithelial Injury can Promote a T_H2 Polarized Environment

T-helper 2 (T_H2) lymphocytes, type 2 innate lymphoid cells (ILC2) and alternatively active macrophages (M2) shape a type 2 immune landscape and form the basis of complex crosstalk networks between epithelial, mesenchymal, innate, and adaptive immunity cells. Studies conducted in typical type 2 pathology such as asthma, have revealed a major role for the airway epithelium in the genesis and maintenance of this immune milieu (147), through the recruitment, polarization and activation of myeloid cells. This environment has been involved in mechanisms of tissue repair through TGF-β1-dependent and -independent pathways. Furthermore, studies initially conducted in *S. mansoni* infected mice allowed to show that the development of fibrosis was linked with a T_H2 environment, involving cytokines like IL-4 and IL-13 (148). These cytokines are mainly produced by T_H2 lymphocytes, ILC2 and macrophages. In IPF, IL-4 as well as IL-13, are elevated in the BAL of patients (149), suggesting a role in lung fibrotic processes. Congruently, overexpression of GATA3, a transcription factor implicated in T_H2 differentiation leads to augmented lung collagen deposition (150) while animals in which IL-4 and IL-13 has been modulated, are protected from bleomycin-induced lung fibrosis (151, 152). Nonetheless, IL-13 seems to be the main fibrotic driver as on the one hand overexpression of IL-13 but not IL-4 induces spontaneous lung fibrosis (153, 154) and on the other hand *IL-13*$^{-/-}$ mice but not *IL4*$^{-/-}$ are protected from FITC-related fibrosis (155). Furthermore, IL-13 promotes fibrosis by enhancing TGF-β production by macrophages and epithelial cells, influencing TGF-β activation (154), and directly impacting myofibroblast differentiation (156). Although the bases of epithelial cell implication in type 2 immunity have been extensively studied in asthma, several links can also be established in the distal lung with regards to IPF and lung fibrosis.

First of all, epithelial cells can recruit immune cells partaking in type 2 immunity and by extension IL-13 secretion. Indeed, they can secrete chemokines such as CCL17 and CCL22, acting on T_H2 cells and ILC2, next to the eotaxins CCL11, CCL24 and CCL26 (147). Both CCL17 and CCL22 are increased in the BAL of IPF patients as well as bleomycin treated mice and are expressed by hyperplasic (alveolar) epithelial cells (157–159). Intriguingly, CCL17 but not CCL22 inhibition leads to decreased lung collagen deposition even though they both share the same receptor, CCR4 (159). The implication of eotaxins in lung fibrosis are poorly understood, nonetheless, CCL11 is increased in experimental lung fibrosis while CCL11 deficient mice are protected and both CCL11, CCL24 and CCL26 are able to influence fibroblast behavior (160–162).

Secondly, the epithelium can influence the behavior of surrounding immune cells through the secretion of IL-25, Thymic Stromal Lymphopoietin (TSLP) or IL-33, several type-2 promoting components. IL-25 can be released by different cell types, including AEC and bronchial epithelial cells (163, 164). T-cells and ILC2, are some of the targets of this cytokine and respond by expansion and secretion of type 2 cytokines like IL-4 and IL-13 (163, 165). Its potential role in disease is suggested by the fact that IPF subjects have higher IL-25 levels in their BAL compared to controls (166). This cytokine can be involved in fibrosis by both its direct effects on fibroblasts as well as its indirect influence on IL-13-dependent fibrosis. Indeed, *in vitro* data shows a direct influence on fibroblast differentiation, cytokine and growth factor secretion (167, 168). Moreover, IL-25 overexpression is associated with perivascular fibrosis in an IL-4 and IL-13 dependent manner (169) and *IL-25*$^{-/-}$ animals are protected from *S. Mansoni* and bleomycin-induced lung fibrosis due to ILC2 related IL-13 production (166), emphasizing its upstream role in type 2 immunity mediated fibrosis.

Similarly, TSLP can be produced by a wide range of cells, including epithelial and mesenchymal cells, similarly promoting a pro-T_H2 environment (170, 171). Staining for TSLP in IPF lungs reveals the presence of this protein in alveolar epithelial cells and fibroblasts within fibroblastic foci (172). Additionally, its concentration in the BAL of patients is significantly elevated, showing an upregulation in this disease (173). Bleomycin instillation induces the expression of TSLP in bronchial and alveolar epithelial cells, but contradictory results have been published regarding the protective character of TSLP deletion in mice (174, 175). Furthermore, stimulation of primary human fibroblasts with this cytokine results in the secretion of CCL2 and chemotaxis of monocytes to the site of injury (172) while AEC undergo EMT (176). The role of TSLP thus seems complex with seemingly contradictory *in vivo* observation and further studies are needed to evaluate its exact role in the fibrotic cascade.

After injury or necrosis, epithelial full-length IL-33 (flIL-33) will be released from the cell nucleus in the surrounding environment, where neutrophil and mast cell proteases will cleave it to its modified form (mIL-33) (177). mIL-33 binds to cells expressing its receptor, ST2, such as ILC2, T_H2 lymphocytes, macrophages, dendritic cells or mast cells, and promotes a pro-T_H2 environment (178). Similarly to IL-25 or TSLP, IL-33 can be found in increased concentrations in the BAL and lung tissue of IPF patients (173, 179) and is upregulated in experimental lung fibrosis (179). Both full-length and the modified form seem to be involved as addition of either recombinant protein enhances collagen deposition after bleomycin challenge (179, 180). The processes underlying this effect are ill-defined but seem to be both ST2 dependent and independent. On the one hand, flIL-33 affects lung fibrosis by modulating the innate immune landscape, directly or indirectly increasing the presence of MCP-1/CCL2, IL-6, TGF-β1 and DAMPs such as HSP70, independently of ST2, IL4 or IL-13 (179). On the other hand, mIL-33 provokes the polarization of lung macrophages, ILC2 expansion and subsequent IL-13 secretion, relying on ST2 to do so (180). Interestingly, peripheral recruitment of ST2 positive cells by IL-33 seems to be one of the prevalent factors driving this observation, as selective bone-marrow ST2 deficiency was sufficient to protect mice from bleomycin lung fibrosis (181).

Next to these cytokines, other DAMPs like HMGB1 or uric acid can promote the formation of a T_H2 driven environment. Indeed, addition of HMGB1 enhances the expression of GATA3 by T_H2 cells and increases the levels of IL-4 and IL-13 (182) and uric acid is implicated in the release of IL-33 and TSLP by airway epithelial cells and the production of IL-13 after respiratory syncytial virus infection (183).

Finally, a T_H2 environment can in turn affect epithelial cell biology. Indeed, continuous exposure of bronchial cells to IL-13 results in an increase in MUC5AC production and induces collagen deposition by fibroblasts in a co-culture model (184). Additionally, IL-13 alters the integrity of the bronchial epithelial barrier by downregulating TJ (185). In the distal lung, AEC2 serve a progenitor function in the alveolar epithelium and are capable of renewing AEC1. Exposure of these cells to IL-13 results in impaired AEC1 differentiation and development of a bronchiolar transcriptomic phenotype (186) aside from increased *in vitro* apoptosis (187), potentially affecting the development of lung fibrosis.

This suggests that the lung epithelium is capable of actively and passively altering its immune environment towards a type-2 polarization and thus exert a pro-fibrotic influence through an additional mechanism. Despite the fact that overwhelming evidence exists regarding the role of type 2 immunity in lung fibrosis, these findings should be contrasted with the disappointing results of therapeutic trials of IL-13 and dual IL-4/IL-13 inhibition in IPF, which both failed to meet their therapeutic endpoints (188, 189). Arguably, these results could be explained by the fact that IL-4/IL-13 are mediators of an upstream fibrotic process of which type 2 inflammation is only one of the (redundant) aspects, resulting in the observed lack of efficacy. This is illustrated by the fact that pirfenidone, one of the two currently validated treatments of IPF with broad anti-fibrotic effects, decreases IL-4 and IL-13 concentrations in the BAL of ovalbumin challenged mice (190).

Epithelial Cells Are Implicated in Alveolar Homeostasis and Pathologic Monocyte/ Macrophage Recruitment

Alveolar macrophages (AM) are a self-renewing population of the distal lung, maintaining lung homeostasis through their role in surfactant recycling, repair following injury and tightly controlled inflammatory processes (191). To exert their many functions, macrophages can notably polarize into different subsets, namely classically activated macrophages (M1) and alternatively activated macrophages (M2). Although historically, they have been divided into two subtypes, macrophage polarization should be approached as a reversible continuum rather than a definitive dichotomic classification. Briefly, M1 macrophages are induced by LPS, IFN-γ and TNF-α, produce pro-inflammatory cytokines such as IL-1β, TNF-α, IL-12, IL-23 and promote a T_H1 response, displaying enhanced pathogenicidal properties. M2 macrophages are promoted by TGF-β, IL-4, IL-13 and secrete pro-fibrotic chemo- or cytokines like TGF-β, PDGF, or CCL18, promoting tissue repair and immunomodulation (192, 193). Damaged AEC can release a range of signals promoting the recruitment and activation of macrophages to the site of injury, fueling a pro-inflammatory environment. In a normal response, this phase would be subsequently followed by a self-limited anti-inflammatory repair stage, characterized by M2 polarization and the production of TGF-β1 or PDGF (194). Pathologic perpetuation of these processes leads to an aberrant wound response with excessive collagen deposition and ultimately organ function impairment. AEC2 dysfunction is one of the hallmark features of IPF and *in vivo* experimental data has shown that AEC2 injury is sufficient to trigger lung fibrosis (195). Furthermore, this triggers the influx of monocyte-derived macrophages (Mo-MA) possessing a pro-fibrotic phenotype *via* an interaction with CCR2, the MCP-1 receptor (196). Accordingly, *in vivo* models have subsequently demonstrated the importance of alveolar epithelial cells MCP-1/CCL2 secretion in lung fibrosis (197, 198). MCP-1/CCL2 is a chemotactic factor for myeloid cells such as monocytes, macrophages and fibrocytes (198, 199), which can also influence fibrocyte as well as fibroblast migration, proliferation, and differentiation *in vitro* (200–202). The exact link between epithelial injury and CCL2 secretion are not fully determined, but stimulation with TGF-β1 or tunicamycin (mimicking ER-stress), 2 components implicated in AEC2 dysfunction in IPF, directly upregulate CCL2 secretion by isolated AEC2 (197). Mo-MAs can replace the native AM after depletion of this compartment, for example after bleomycin administration (203), and are one of the drivers of experimental lung fibrosis (203). In line with their monocytic origin, they express high levels of *Ccr2* mRNA (204), suggesting that CCL2 (partly) mediates the recruitment of these cells. Evidence reinforcing this interaction comes from a model in which AEC-specific deletion of CCL12 (the murine equivalent of CCL2) was able to ablate the recruitment of these cells after bleomycin challenge (197). It is unclear if this mechanism similarly mediates the recruitment of a recently discovered macrophage subpopulation in IPF (205). Of note, monocytic myeloid-derived suppressor cells (M-MDSC), a population of immunosuppressive, pro-fibrotic cells also express CCR2 (206) and emerging evidence points towards their implication in IPF (207). Furthermore, IPF patients display increased concentrations of CCL2 in their BAL (208) and immunostainings have shown a partly epithelial origin for this chemokine (209). Based on overwhelming evidence implicating CCL2/CCR2 in (experimental) pulmonary fibrosis, a trial with carlumab, an anti-CCL2 antibody was conducted in IPF. Unfortunately, no effect of this treatment could be observed, and the study was halted prematurely (210). Of note, free CCL2 levels rose in the treatment, but not the placebo group (210), suggesting the activation of compensatory mechanisms.

CONCLUDING REMARKS

Alveolar epithelial dysfunction due to repetitive injury in susceptible/ageing lungs forms the current paradigm of IPF pathogenesis. Experimental evidence supports the involvement of the immune system in (pathologic) repair attempts and collagen deposition. The pulmonary epithelium, laying at the forefront of mucosal immunity plays a crucial role in lung homeostasis, inflammation, and subsequent repair mechanisms. It is thus capable of sensing and reacting to danger stimuli to ultimately regulate lung responses at the level of both structural and immune (myeloid) cells (**Figure 2** and **Table 1**). Aberrant alveolar epithelial biology represents a hallmark of IPF, also potentially impacting immune mechanisms. Determining the exact contribution of these mechanisms remains a challenge, as they are at the cross-point of multiple regulatory networks also involving myeloid and mesenchymal cells. For example, whether differential expression of co-stimulatory molecules such as B7 complex (including PD-L1) may interfere with the crosstalk between epithelium and immune cells remains elusive. Importantly, trials evaluating immunosuppressive medications have yielded disappointing results until now, questioning our understanding of the mechanisms at stake. Nonetheless, in-depth understanding of the epithelial contribution to the immune-fibrotic paradigm should

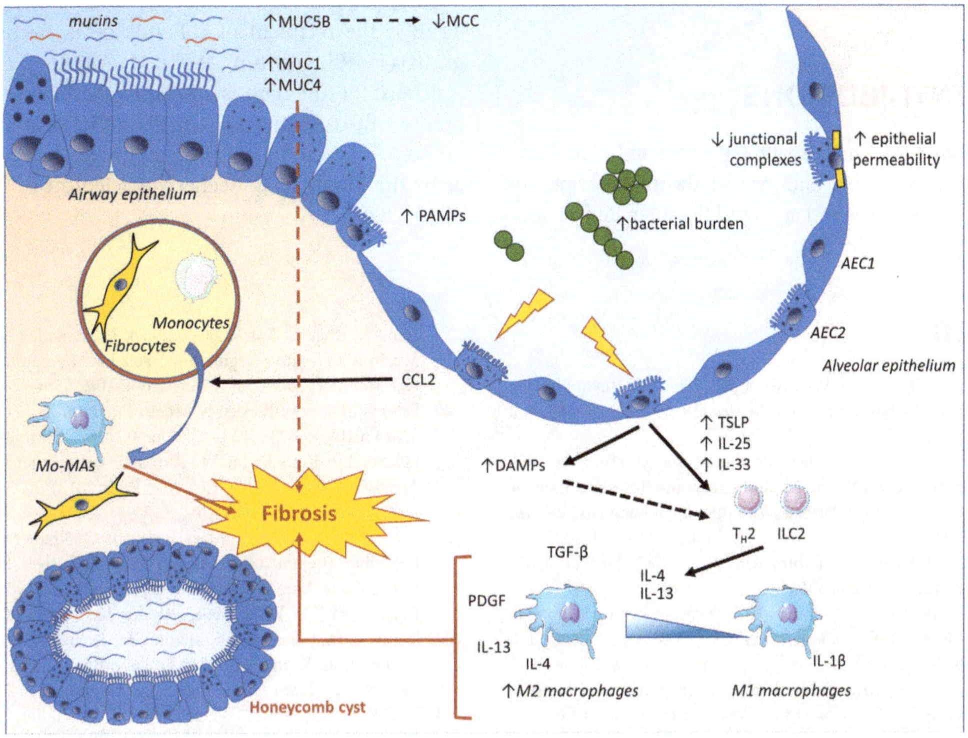

FIGURE 2 | The IPF lung epithelium displays increased concentrations of secreted and membrane-bound mucins, as well as altered junctional complexes, potentially influencing local barrier mechanisms and fibrosis through impaired mucociliary clearance (MCC), promotion of epithelial to mesenchymal transition (EMT) and increased epithelial permeability. Lung epithelial cells are also confronted to an increased bacterial burden and pathogen-associated molecular patterns (PAMPs). Furthermore, epithelial damage will result in the production of damage-associated molecular patterns (DAMPs), triggering pro-inflammatory pathways and T_H2 polarizing cytokines. These cytokines exert a pro-fibrotic influence by directly affecting mesenchymal cells and polarizing macrophages towards an alternatively activated phenotype (M2). Finally, epithelial dysfunction will result in the release of CCL2, a chemokine directly affecting fibroblasts as well as fibrocyte recruitment and differentiation while mediating the recruitment of monocytes to the site of injury. The latter will differentiate into monocyte-derived macrophages (Mo-MA), which have been implicated in lung fibrosis. AEC1, alveolar type-1 epithelial cell; AEC2, alveolar type-2 epithelial cell; Mo-MA, monocyte-derived macrophage; MCC, mucociliary clearance; ILC2, type 2 innate lymphoid cell; T_H2, type 2 helper T-cell.

TABLE 1 | Summary of the epithelial-immune interactions in IPF.

	Observations in IPF	Putative mechanisms (experimental data)
Physical barrier properties		
- **Mucus production**	↑MUC5B (35, 36) ↑MUC1 (43) ↑MUC4 (44)	MUC5B: ↓MCC (38) MUC1/4: TGF-β1 signaling, fibroblast differentiation, EMT (43, 44)
- **Intercellular junctions**	↑claudin-1, -2, -3, -7 (57–59) ↓claudin-18 (57) ↓E-cadherin (73)	↑epithelial dysfunction (69, 70) ↑polarized receptor-ligand interactions (71) ↑epithelial denudation (79)
Environmental sensing		
- **PRR**	↑TLR2 ↑TLR4 ↑TLR9 (123, 211)	$TLR2^{-/-}$: ↓fibrosis, ↓T_H2 environment, altered immune cell recruitment, ↓IL-17 production (125, 126) $TLR4^{-/-}$: ↓↑fibrosis, ↑T_H2 environment, ↓autophagy ↓AEC2 proliferation (110, 127, 128) TLR9: ↑EMT ↑myofibroblast differentiation (114, 115)
- **DAMPs**	↑HMGB1 ↑eATP ↑uric acid ↑HA (90–93, 212)	↑EMT ↑IL-1β ↑CCL2 ↑fibroblast proliferation and differentiation (90, 95, 97–99, 108)
- **Bacterial PAMPs**	↑Bacterial load ↓diversity (41)	LPS: ↑fibroblast proliferation (111) ↑IL-1β ↑CCL2 (112)
Modulation of the immune environment		
- **T_H2 environment promotion**	↑CCL17 ↑CCL22 ↑IL25 ↑TSLP ↑IL-33 (158, 166, 173)	↑Recruitment of T_H2 and ILC2, ↑fibroblast proliferation, differentiation and collagen synthesis, ↑EMT (167, 176, 180)
- **Recruitment of myeloid cells**	↑CCL2 (208)	↑Recruitment of Mo-AM (197)

MCC, mucociliary clearance; EMT, epithelial-mesenchymal transition; eATP, extracellular ATP; HA, hyaluronan; LPS, lipopolysaccharide; TSLP, Thymic Stromal Lymphopoietin; Mo-AM, monocyte-derived alveolar macrophages.

help to appreciate the reasons underlying these clinical failures and design more targeted and effective therapies.

AUTHOR CONTRIBUTIONS

TP-B designed and wrote the manuscript. CP wrote and revised the manuscript. AF designed, wrote and revised the manuscript. All authors contributed to the article and approved the submitted version.

FUNDING

TP-B is the recipient of a Fonds de la Recherche Scientifique grant (FNRS grant n°ASP/DM A814). CP is postdoctoral specialist of the Fonds de la Recherche Scientifique (FNRS grants 1.R016.16 and 1.R016.18). AF is supported by the Fonds de Recherche Clinique, Cliniques universitaires Saint-Luc, as well as by the Fonds de la Recherche Scientifique (FNRS CDR grant n° J007820).

REFERENCES

1. Crystal RG, Fulmer JD, Roberts WC, Moss ML, Line BR, Reynolds HY. Idiopathic Pulmonary Fibrosis. *Ann Internal Med* (1976) 85(6):769–88. doi: 10.7326/0003-4819-85-6-769
2. Hunninghake GW, Kawanami O, Ferrans VJ, Young RC, Roberts WC, Crystal RG. Characterization of the Inflammatory and Immune Effector Cells in the Lung Parenchyma of Patients With Interstitial Lung Disease. *Am Rev Respir Dis* (1981) 123(4):407–12. doi: 10.1164/arrd.1981.123.4.407
3. Noble PW, Homer RJ. Back to the Future. *Am J Respir Cell Mol Biol* (2005) 33(2):113–20. doi: 10.1165/rcmb.F301
4. Richeldi L, Davies HR, Ferrara G, Franco F. Corticosteroids for Idiopathic Pulmonary Fibrosis. *Cochrane Database syst Rev* (2003) 3:Cd002880. doi: 10.1002/14651858.CD002880
5. Turner-Warwick M, Burrows B, Johnson A. Cryptogenic Fibrosing Alveolitis: Response to Corticosteroid Treatment and its Effect on Survival. *Thorax* (1980) 35(8):593–9. doi: 10.1136/thx.35.8.593
6. Selman M, King TE, Pardo A. Idiopathic Pulmonary Fibrosis: Prevailing and Evolving Hypotheses About Its Pathogenesis and Implications for Therapy. *Ann Internal Med* (2001) 134(2):136–51. doi: 10.7326/0003-4819-134-2-200101160-00015
7. American Thoracic Society and European Respiratory Society. American Thoracic Society/European Respiratory Society International Multidisciplinary Consensus Classification of the Idiopathic Interstitial Pneumonias. *Am J Respir Crit Care Med* (2002) 165(2):277–304. doi: 10.1164/ajrccm.165.2.ats01
8. Katzenstein A-LA, Myers JL. Idiopathic Pulmonary Fibrosis. *Am J Respir Crit Care Med* (1998) 157(4):1301–15. doi: 10.1164/ajrccm.157.4.9707039
9. Idiopathic Pulmonary Fibrosis Clinical Research N, Raghu G, Anstrom KJ, King TE Jr, Lasky JA, Martinez FJ. Prednisone, Azathioprine, and N-acetylcysteine for Pulmonary Fibrosis. *New Engl J Med* (2012) 366 (21):1968–77. doi: 10.1056/NEJMoa1113354
10. Desai O, Winkler J, Minasyan M, Herzog EL. The Role of Immune and Inflammatory Cells in Idiopathic Pulmonary Fibrosis. *Front Med* (2018) 5:43. doi: 10.3389/fmed.2018.00043
11. Rackley CR, Stripp BR. Building and Maintaining the Epithelium of the Lung. *J Clin Invest* (2012) 122(8):2724–30. doi: 10.1172/JCI60519
12. Tata PR, Rajagopal J. Plasticity in the Lung: Making and Breaking Cell Identity. *Development* (2017) 144(5):755. doi: 10.1242/dev.143784
13. Jacob A, Morley M, Hawkins F, McCauley KB, Jean JC, Heins H, et al. Differentiation of Human Pluripotent Stem Cells Into Functional Lung Alveolar Epithelial Cells. *Cell Stem Cell* (2017) 21(4):472–88.e10. doi: 10.1016/j.stem.2017.08.014
14. Whitsett JA, Alenghat T. Respiratory Epithelial Cells Orchestrate Pulmonary Innate Immunity. *Nat Immunol* (2015) 16(1):27–35. doi: 10.1038/ni.3045
15. Leiva-Juárez MM, Kolls JK, Evans SE. Lung Epithelial Cells: Therapeutically Inducible Effectors of Antimicrobial Defense. *Mucosal Immunol* (2018) 11 (1):21–34. doi: 10.1038/mi.2017.71
16. Denneny E, Sahota J, Beatson R, Thornton D, Burchell J, Porter J. Mucins and Their Receptors in Chronic Lung Disease. *Clin Trans Immunol* (2020) 9 (3):e01120. doi: 10.1002/cti2.1120
17. Ballester B, Milara J, Cortijo J. Mucins as a New Frontier in Pulmonary Fibrosis. *J Clin Med* (2019) 8(9):1447. doi: 10.3390/jcm8091447
18. Kim KC, Lillehoj EP. Muc1 Mucin. *Am J Respir Cell Mol Biol* (2008) 39 (6):644–7. doi: 10.1165/rcmb.2008-0169TR
19. Ueno K, Koga T, Kato K, Golenbock DT, Gendler SJ, Kai H, et al. MUC1 Mucin is a Negative Regulator of Toll-Like Receptor Signaling. *Am J Respir Cell Mol Biol* (2008) 38(3):263–8. doi: 10.1165/rcmb.2007-0336RC
20. Fahy JV, Dickey BF. Airway Mucus Function and Dysfunction. *New Engl J Med* (2010) 363(23):2233–47. doi: 10.1056/NEJMra0910061
21. Lillehoj EP, Kato K, Lu W, Kim KC. Cellular and Molecular Biology of Airway Mucins. *Int Rev Cell Mol Biol* (2013) 303:139–202. doi: 10.1016/B978-0-12-407697-6.00004-0
22. Cebo C, Dambrouck T, Maes E, Laden C, Strecker G, Michalski JC, et al. Recombinant Human Interleukins IL-1alpha, IL-1beta, IL-4, Il-6, and IL-7 Show Different and Specific Calcium-Independent Carbohydrate-Binding Properties. *J Biol Chem* (2001) 276(8):5685–91. doi: 10.1074/jbc.M008662200
23. Symmes BA, Stefanski AL, Magin CM, Evans CM. Role of Mucins in Lung Homeostasis: Regulated Expression and Biosynthesis in Health and Disease. *Biochem Soc Trans* (2018) 46(3):707–19. doi: 10.1042/BST20170455
24. Thai P, Loukoianov A, Wachi S, Wu R. Regulation of Airway Mucin Gene Expression. *Annu Rev Physiol* (2008) 70:405–29. doi: 10.1146/annurev.physiol.70.113006.100441
25. Kummarapurugu AB, Zheng S, Ledford J, Karandashova S, Voynow JA. High-Mobility Group Box 1 Upregulates MUC5AC and MUC5B Expression in Primary Airway Epithelial Cells. *Am J Respir Cell Mol Biol* (2018) 58 (1):126–8. doi: 10.1165/rcmb.2017-0250LE
26. Chen Y, Thai P, Zhao YH, Ho YS, DeSouza MM, Wu R. Stimulation of Airway Mucin Gene Expression by Interleukin (IL)-17 Through IL-6 Paracrine/Autocrine Loop. *J Biol Chem* (2003) 278(19):17036–43. doi: 10.1074/jbc.M210429200
27. Inoue D, Yamaya M, Kubo H, Sasaki T, Hosoda M, Numasaki M, et al. Mechanisms of Mucin Production by Rhinovirus Infection in Cultured Human Airway Epithelial Cells. *Respir Physiol Neurobiol* (2006) 154(3):484–99. doi: 10.1016/j.resp.2005.11.006
28. Smirnova MG, Guo L, Birchall JP, Pearson JP. LPS Up-Regulates Mucin and Cytokine mRNA Expression and Stimulates Mucin and Cytokine Secretion in Goblet Cells. *Cell Immunol* (2003) 221(1):42–9. doi: 10.1016/S0008-8749 (03)00059-5
29. van Putten JPM, Strijbis K. Transmembrane Mucins: Signaling Receptors at the Intersection of Inflammation and Cancer. *J Innate Immun* (2017) 9 (3):281–99. doi: 10.1159/000453594
30. Seibold MA, Wise AL, Speer MC, Steele MP, Brown KK, Loyd JE, et al. A Common Muc5b Promoter Polymorphism and Pulmonary Fibrosis. *New Engl J Med* (2011) 364(16):1503–12. doi: 10.1056/NEJMoa1013660
31. Yang IV, Fingerlin TE, Evans CM, Schwarz MI, Schwartz DA. MUC5B and Idiopathic Pulmonary Fibrosis. *Ann Am Thoracic Soc* (2015) 12(Suppl 2): S193–S9. doi: 10.1513/AnnalsATS.201503-110AW
32. Hunninghake GM, Hatabu H, Okajima Y, Gao W, Dupuis J, Latourelle JC, et al. MUC5B Promoter Polymorphism and Interstitial Lung Abnormalities. *New Engl J Med* (2013) 368(23):2192–200. doi: 10.1056/NEJMoa1216076
33. Peljto AL, Zhang Y, Fingerlin TE, Ma S-F, Garcia JGN, Richards TJ, et al. Association Between the MUC5B Promoter Polymorphism and Survival in Patients With Idiopathic Pulmonary Fibrosis. *JAMA* (2013) 309(21):2232–9. doi: 10.1001/jama.2013.5827
34. Nakano Y, Yang IV, Walts AD, Watson AM, Helling BA, Fletcher AA, et al. Muc5b Promoter Variant Rs35705950 Affects Muc5b Expression in the Distal Airways in Idiopathic Pulmonary Fibrosis. *Am J Respir Crit Care Med* (2016) 193(4):464–6. doi: 10.1164/rccm.201509-1872LE

35. Conti C, Montero-Fernandez A, Borg E, Osadolor T, Viola P, De Lauretis A, et al. Mucins MUC5B and MUC5AC in Distal Airways and Honeycomb Spaces: Comparison Among Idiopathic Pulmonary Fibrosis/Usual Interstitial Pneumonia, Fibrotic Nonspecific Interstitial Pneumonitis, and Control Lungs. *Am J Respir Crit Care Med* (2016) 193(4):462–4. doi: 10.1164/rccm.201507-1322LE
36. Seibold MA, Smith RW, Urbanek C, Groshong SD, Cosgrove GP, Brown KK, et al. The Idiopathic Pulmonary Fibrosis Honeycomb Cyst Contains a Mucocilary Pseudostratified Epithelium. *PloS One* (2013) 8(3):e58658. doi: 10.1371/journal.pone.0058658
37. Okamoto T, Mathai SK, Hennessy CE, Hancock LA, Walts AD, Stefanski AL, et al. The Relationship Between Complement C3 Expression and the MUC5B Genotype in Pulmonary Fibrosis. *Am J Physiology-Lung Cell Mol Physiol* (2018) 315(1):L1–L10. doi: 10.1152/ajplung.00395.2017
38. Hancock LA, Hennessy CE, Solomon GM, Dobrinskikh E, Estrella A, Hara N, et al. Muc5b Overexpression Causes Mucociliary Dysfunction and Enhances Lung Fibrosis in Mice. *Nat Commun* (2018) 9(1):5363–. doi: 10.1038/s41467-018-07768-9
39. Kurche JS, Dobrinskikh E, Hennessy CE, Huber J, Estrella A, Hancock LA, et al. Muc5b Enhances Murine Honeycomb-like Cyst Formation. *Am J Respir Cell Mol Biol* (2019) 61(4):544–6. doi: 10.1165/rcmb.2019-0138LE
40. Roy MG, Livraghi-Butrico A, Fletcher AA, McElwee MM, Evans SE, Boerner RM, et al. Muc5b is Required for Airway Defence. *Nature* (2014) 505 (7483):412–6. doi: 10.1038/nature12807
41. Molyneaux PL, Cox MJ, Willis-Owen SAG, Mallia P, Russell KE, Russell A-M, et al. The Role of Bacteria in the Pathogenesis and Progression of Idiopathic Pulmonary Fibrosis. *Am J Respir Crit Care Med* (2014) 190 (8):906–13. doi: 10.1164/rccm.201403-0541OC
42. Lorenzo-Salazar JM, Ma S-F, Jou J, Hou P-C, Guillen-Guio B, Allen RJ, et al. Novel Idiopathic Pulmonary Fibrosis Susceptibility Variants Revealed by Deep Sequencing. *ERJ Open Res* (2019) 5(2):00071–2019. doi: 10.1183/23120541.00071-2019
43. Milara J, Ballester B, Montero P, Escriva J, Artigues E, Alós M, et al. MUC1 Intracellular Bioactivation Mediates Lung Fibrosis. *Thorax* (2020) 75(2):132. doi: 10.1136/thoraxjnl-2018-212735
44. Milara J, Ballester B, Safont MJ, Artigues E, Escrivá J, Morcillo E, et al. MUC4 is Overexpressed in Idiopathic Pulmonary Fibrosis and Collaborates With Transforming Growth Factor β Inducing Fibrotic Responses.. *Mucosal Immunol* (2020) 14(2):377–88. doi: 10.1038/s41385-020-00343-w
45. Maher TM, Oballa E, Simpson JK, Porte J, Habgood A, Fahy WA, et al. An Epithelial Biomarker Signature for Idiopathic Pulmonary Fibrosis: An Analysis From the Multicentre PROFILE Cohort Study. *Lancet Respir Med* (2017) 5(12):946–55. doi: 10.1016/S2213-2600(17)30430-7
46. Chiba H, Otsuka M, Takahashi H. Significance of Molecular Biomarkers in Idiopathic Pulmonary Fibrosis: A Mini Review. *Respir Invest* (2018) 56 (5):384–91. doi: 10.1016/j.resinv.2018.06.001
47. Hirasawa Y, Kohno N, Yokoyama A, Inoue Y, Abe M, Hiwada K. Kl-6, a Human MUC1 Mucin, is Chemotactic for Human Fibroblasts. *Am J Respir Cell Mol Biol* (1997) 17(4):501–7. doi: 10.1165/ajrcmb.17.4.2253
48. Ohshimo S, Yokoyama A, Hattori N, Ishikawa N, Hirasawa Y, Kohno N. Kl-6, a Human MUC1 Mucin, Promotes Proliferation and Survival of Lung Fibroblasts. *Biochem Biophys Res Commun* (2005) 338(4):1845–52. doi: 10.1016/j.bbrc.2005.10.144
49. Xu L, Yang D, Zhu S, Gu J, Ding F, Bian W, et al. Bleomycin-Induced Pulmonary Fibrosis is Attenuated by an Antibody Against KL-6. *Exp Lung Res* (2013) 39(6):241–8. doi: 10.3109/01902148.2013.798056
50. Brune K, Frank J, Schwingshackl A, Finigan J, Sidhaye VK. Pulmonary Epithelial Barrier Function: Some New Players and Mechanisms. *Am J Physiol Lung Cell Mol Physiol* (2015) 308(8):L731–L45. doi: 10.1152/ajplung.00309.2014
51. Georas SN, Rezaee F. Epithelial Barrier Function: at the Front Line of Asthma Immunology and Allergic Airway Inflammation. *J Allergy Clin Immunol* (2014) 134(3):509–20. doi: 10.1016/j.jaci.2014.05.049
52. Van Itallie CM, Anderson JM. Architecture of Tight Junctions and Principles of Molecular Composition. *Semin Cell Dev Biol* (2014) 36:157–65. doi: 10.1016/j.semcdb.2014.08.011
53. Rezaee F, Georas SN. Breaking Barriers. New Insights Into Airway Epithelial Barrier Function in Health and Disease. *Am J Respir Cell Mol Biol* (2014) 50 (5):857–69. doi: 10.1165/rcmb.2013-0541RT
54. Krause G, Winkler L, Mueller SL, Haseloff RF, Piontek J, Blasig IE. Structure and Function of Claudins. *Biochim Biophys Acta (BBA) - Biomembranes* (2008) 1778(3):631–45. doi: 10.1016/j.bbamem.2007.10.018
55. Soini Y. Claudins in Lung Diseases. *Respir Res* (2011) 12(1):70–. doi: 10.1186/1465-9921-12-70
56. Li G, Flodby P, Luo J, Kage H, Sipos A, Gao D, et al. Knockout Mice Reveal Key Roles for Claudin 18 in Alveolar Barrier Properties and Fluid Homeostasis. *Am J Respir Cell Mol Biol* (2014) 51(2):210–22. doi: 10.1165/rcmb.2013-0353OC
57. Zou J, Li Y, Yu J, Dong L, Husain AN, Shen L, et al. Idiopathic Pulmonary Fibrosis is Associated With Tight Junction Protein Alterations. *Biochim Biophys Acta (BBA) - Biomembranes* (2020) 1862(5):183205. doi: 10.1016/j.bbamem.2020.183205
58. Lappi-Blanco E, Lehtonen ST, Sormunen R, Merikallio HM, Soini Y, Kaarteenaho RL. Divergence of Tight and Adherens Junction Factors in Alveolar Epithelium in Pulmonary Fibrosis. *Hum Pathol* (2013) 44(5):895–907. doi: 10.1016/j.humpath.2012.08.016
59. Kaarteenaho-Wiik R, Soini Y. Claudin-1, -2, -3, -4, -5, and -7 in Usual Interstitial Pneumonia and Sarcoidosis. *J Histochem Cytochem* (2009) 57 (3):187–95. doi: 10.1369/jhc.2008.951566
60. Kowalczyk AP, Green KJ. Structure, Function, and Regulation of Desmosomes. *Prog Mol Biol Trans Sci* (2013) 116:95–118. doi: 10.1016/B978-0-12-394311-8.00005-4
61. Taillé C, Grootenboer-Mignot S, Boursier C, Michel L, Debray M-P, Fagart J, et al. Identification of Periplakin as a New Target for Autoreactivity in Idiopathic Pulmonary Fibrosis. *Am J Respir Crit Care Med* (2011) 183 (6):759–66. doi: 10.1164/rccm.201001-0076OC
62. Selman M, Pardo A. Idiopathic Pulmonary Fibrosis: An Epithelial/Fibroblastic Cross-Talk Disorder. *Respir Res* (2001) 3(1):3. doi: 10.1186/rr198
63. Mogulkoc N, Brutsche MH, Bishop PW, Murby B, Greaves MS, Horrocks AW, et al. Pulmonary Tc-DTPA Aerosol Clearance and Survival in Usual Interstitial Pneumonia (UIP). *Thorax* (2001) 56(12):916. doi: 10.1136/thorax.56.12.916
64. Ohta H, Chiba S, Ebina M, Furuse M, Nukiwa T. Altered Expression of Tight Junction Molecules in Alveolar Septa in Lung Injury and Fibrosis. *Am J Physiol Lung Cell Mol Physiol* (2012) 302(2):L193–205. doi: 10.1152/ajplung.00349.2010
65. Wray C, Mao Y, Pan J, Chandrasena A, Piasta F, Frank JA. Claudin-4 Augments Alveolar Epithelial Barrier Function and is Induced in Acute Lung Injury.. *Am J Physiology-Lung Cell Mol Physiol* (2009) 297(2):L219–L27. doi: 10.1152/ajplung.00043.2009
66. Rachakonda G, Vu T, Jin L, Samanta D, Datta PK. Role of TGF-β-Induced Claudin-4 Expression Through c-Jun Signaling in non-Small Cell Lung Cancer. *Cell Signal* (2016) 28(10):1537–44. doi: 10.1016/j.cellsig.2016.07.006
67. Overgaard CE, Schlingmann B, Dorsainvil White S, Ward C, Fan X, Swarnakar S, et al. The Relative Balance of GM-CSF and TGF-β1 Regulates Lung Epithelial Barrier Function.. *Am J Physiol Lung Cell Mol Physiol* (2015) 308(12):L1212–L23. doi: 10.1152/ajplung.00042.2014
68. Gokey JJ, Sridharan A, Xu Y, Green J, Carraro G, Stripp BR, et al. Active Epithelial Hippo Signaling in Idiopathic Pulmonary Fibrosis. *JCI Insight* (2018) 3(6):e98738. doi: 10.1172/jci.insight.98738
69. Zhou B, Flodby P, Luo J, Castillo DR, Liu Y, Yu F-X, et al. Claudin-18–Mediated YAP Activity Regulates Lung Stem and Progenitor Cell Homeostasis and Tumorigenesis. *J Clin Invest* (2018) 128(3):970–84. doi: 10.1172/JCI90429
70. LaFemina MJ, Sutherland KM, Bentley T, Gonzales LW, Allen L, Chapin CJ, et al. Claudin-18 Deficiency Results in Alveolar Barrier Dysfunction and Impaired Alveologenesis in Mice. *Am J Respir Cell Mol Biol* (2014) 51 (4):550–8. doi: 10.1165/rcmb.2013-0456OC
71. Vermeer PD, Einwalter LA, Moninger TO, Rokhlina T, Kern JA, Zabner J, et al. Segregation of Receptor and Ligand Regulates Activation of Epithelial Growth Factor Receptor. *Nature* (2003) 422(6929):322–6. doi: 10.1038/nature01440
72. Faress JA, Nethery DE, Kern EF, Eisenberg R, Jacono FJ, Allen CL, et al. Bleomycin-Induced Pulmonary Fibrosis is Attenuated by a Monoclonal Antibody Targeting HER2. *J Appl Physiol (Bethesda Md 1985)* (2007) 103 (6):2077–83. doi: 10.1152/japplphysiol.00239.2007
73. Morbini P, Inghilleri S, Campo I, Oggionni T, Zorzetto M, Luisetti M. Incomplete Expression of Epithelial-Mesenchymal Transition Markers in

Idiopathic Pulmonary Fibrosis. *Pathol Res Pract* (2011) 207(9):559–67. doi: 10.1016/j.prp.2011.06.006
74. Tian R, Zhu Y, Yao J, Meng X, Wang J, Xie H, et al. NLRP3 Participates in the Regulation of EMT in Bleomycin-Induced Pulmonary Fibrosis. *Exp Cell Res* (2017) 357(2):328–34. doi: 10.1016/j.yexcr.2017.05.028
75. Lin L, Han Q, Xiong Y, Li T, Liu Z, Xu H, et al. Krüpple-Like-Factor 4 Attenuates Lung Fibrosis Via Inhibiting Epithelial-Mesenchymal Transition. *Sci Rep* (2017) 7(1):15847. doi: 10.1038/s41598-017-14602-7
76. Xu J, Lamouille S, Derynck R. Tgf-β-Induced Epithelial to Mesenchymal Transition. *Cell Res* (2009) 19(2):156–72. doi: 10.1038/cr.2009.5
77. Tanjore H, Xu XC, Polosukhin VV, Degryse AL, Li B, Han W, et al. Contribution of Epithelial-Derived Fibroblasts to Bleomycin-Induced Lung Fibrosis. *Am J Respir Crit Care Med* (2009) 180(7):657–65. doi: 10.1164/rccm.200903-0322OC
78. Salton F, Volpe MC, Confalonieri M. Epithelial–Mesenchymal Transition in the Pathogenesis of Idiopathic Pulmonary Fibrosis. *Med (Kaunas Lithuania)* (2019) 55(4). doi: 10.3390/medicina55040083
79. Post S, Heijink IH, Hesse L, Koo HK, Shaheen F, Fouadi M, et al. Characterization of a Lung Epithelium Specific E-cadherin Knock-Out Model: Implications for Obstructive Lung Pathology. *Sci Rep* (2018) 8 (1):13275. doi: 10.1038/s41598-018-31500-8
80. Mathai SK, Pedersen BS, Smith K, Russell P, Schwarz MI, Brown KK, et al. Desmoplakin Variants are Associated With Idiopathic Pulmonary Fibrosis. *Am J Respir Crit Care Med* (2016) 193(10):1151–60. doi: 10.1164/rccm.201509-1863OC
81. Besnard V, Dagher R, Madjer T, Joannes A, Jaillet M, Kolb M, et al. Identification of Periplakin as a Major Regulator of Lung Injury and Repair in Mice. *JCI Insight* (2018) 3(5). doi: 10.1172/jci.insight.90163
82. Zindel J, Kubes P. Damps, PAMPs, and LAMPs in Immunity and Sterile Inflammation. *Annu Rev Pathol: Mech Dis* (2020) 15(1):493–518. doi: 10.1146/annurev-pathmechdis-012419-032847
83. Scaffidi P, Misteli T, Bianchi ME. Release of Chromatin Protein HMGB1 by Necrotic Cells Triggers Inflammation. *Nature* (2002) 418(6894):191–5. doi: 10.1038/nature00858
84. Liu S, Stolz DB, Sappington PL, Macias CA, Killeen ME, Tenhunen JJ, et al. HMGB1 is Secreted by Immunostimulated Enterocytes and Contributes to Cytomix-Induced Hyperpermeability of Caco-2 Monolayers. *Am J Physiol Cell Physiol* (2006) 290(4):C990–9. doi: 10.1152/ajpcell.00308.2005
85. Gardella S, Andrei C, Ferrera D, Lotti LV, Torrisi MR, Bianchi ME, et al. The Nuclear Protein HMGB1 is Secreted by Monocytes Via a non-Classical, Vesicle-Mediated Secretory Pathway. *EMBO Rep* (2002) 3(10):995–1001. doi: 10.1093/embo-reports/kvf198
86. Jiang D, Liang J, Noble PW. Hyaluronan as an Immune Regulator in Human Diseases. *Physiol Rev* (2011) 91(1):221–64. doi: 10.1152/physrev.00052.2009
87. Hiemstra PS, McCray PBJr., Bals R. The Innate Immune Function of Airway Epithelial Cells in Inflammatory Lung Disease. *Eur Respir J* (2015) 45 (4):1150–62. doi: 10.1183/09031936.00141514
88. Takeuchi O, Akira S. Pattern Recognition Receptors and Inflammation. *Cell* (2010) 140(6):805–20. doi: 10.1016/j.cell.2010.01.022
89. Lee J-M, Yoshida M, Kim M-S, Lee J-H, Baek A-R, Jang AS, et al. Involvement of Alveolar Epithelial Cell Necroptosis in Idiopathic Pulmonary Fibrosis Pathogenesis. *Am J Respir Cell Mol Biol* (2018) 59 (2):215–24. doi: 10.1165/rcmb.2017-0034OC
90. Hamada N, Maeyama T, Kawaguchi T, Yoshimi M, Fukumoto J, Yamada M, et al. The Role of High Mobility Group Box1 in Pulmonary Fibrosis. *Am J Respir Cell Mol Biol* (2008) 39(4):440–7. doi: 10.1165/rcmb.2007-0330OC
91. Markart P, Luboeinski T, Korfei M, Schmidt R, Wygrecka M, Mahavadi P, et al. Alveolar Oxidative Stress is Associated With Elevated Levels of Nonenzymatic Low-Molecular-Weight Antioxidants in Patients With Different Forms of Chronic Fibrosing Interstitial Lung Diseases. *Antioxidants Redox Signaling* (2009) 11(2):227–40. doi: 10.1089/ars.2008.2105
92. Gasse P, Riteau N, Charron S, Girre S, Fick L, Pétrilli V, et al. Uric Acid is a Danger Signal Activating Nalp3 Inflammasome in Lung Injury Inflammation and Fibrosis. *Am J Respir Crit Care Med* (2009) 179 (10):903–13. doi: 10.1164/rccm.200808-1274OC
93. Riteau N, Gasse P, Fauconnier L, Gombault A, Couegnat M, Fick L, et al. Extracellular ATP is a Danger Signal Activating P2x7 Receptor in Lung Inflammation and Fibrosis. *Am J Respir Crit Care Med* (2010) 182(6):774–83. doi: 10.1164/rccm.201003-0359OC
94. Borthwick LA. The IL-1 Cytokine Family and its Role in Inflammation and Fibrosis in the Lung. *Semin immunopathol* (2016) 38(4):517–34. doi: 10.1007/s00281-016-0559-z
95. Lee C-C, Wang C-N, Lee Y-L, Tsai Y-R, Liu J-J. High Mobility Group Box 1 Induced Human Lung Myofibroblasts Differentiation and Enhanced Migration by Activation of MMP-9. *PloS One* (2015) 10(2):e0116393. doi: 10.1371/journal.pone.0116393
96. Pittet JF, Koh H, Fang X, Iles K, Christiaans S, Anjun N, et al. HMGB1 Accelerates Alveolar Epithelial Repair Via an IL-1β- and αvβ6 Integrin-Dependent Activation of TGF-β1. *PloS One* (2013) 8(5):e63907. doi: 10.1371/journal.pone.0063907
97. Chen Y-C, Statt S, Wu R, Chang H-T, Liao J-W, Wang C-N, et al. High Mobility Group Box 1-Induced Epithelial Mesenchymal Transition in Human Airway Epithelial Cells. *Sci Rep* (2016) 6(1):18815. doi: 10.1038/srep18815
98. Yang H, Hreggvidsdottir HS, Palmblad K, Wang H, Ochani M, Li J, et al. A Critical Cysteine is Required for HMGB1 Binding to Toll-like Receptor 4 and Activation of Macrophage Cytokine Release. *Proc Natl Acad Sci USA* (2010) 107(26):11942–7. doi: 10.1073/pnas.1003893107
99. Wu X, Mi Y, Yang H, Hu A, Zhang Q, Shang C. The Activation of HMGB1 as a Progression Factor on Inflammation Response in Normal Human Bronchial Epithelial Cells Through RAGE/JNK/NF-κb Pathway. *Mol Cell Biochem* (2013) 380(1):249–57. doi: 10.1007/s11010-013-1680-0
100. Moore BB, Kolodsick JE, Thannickal VJ, Cooke K, Moore TA, Hogaboam C, et al. Ccr2-Mediated Recruitment of Fibrocytes to the Alveolar Space After Fibrotic Injury. *Am J Pathol* (2005) 166(3):675–84. doi: 10.1016/S0002-9440(10)62289-4
101. Petecchia L, Sabatini F, Usai C, Caci E, Varesio L, Rossi GA. Cytokines Induce Tight Junction Disassembly in Airway Cells Via an EGFR-dependent MAPK/ERK1/2-Pathway. *Lab Invest* (2012) 92(8):1140–8. doi: 10.1038/labinvest.2012.67
102. Redente EF, Chakraborty S, Sajuthi S, Black BP, Edelman BL, Seibold MA, et al. Loss of Fas Signaling in Fibroblasts Impairs Homeostatic Fibrosis Resolution and Promotes Persistent Pulmonary Fibrosis. *JCI Insight* (2020) 6 (1):e141618. doi: 10.1172/jci.insight.141618
103. Câmara J, Jarai G. Epithelial-Mesenchymal Transition in Primary Human Bronchial Epithelial Cells is Smad-dependent and Enhanced by Fibronectin and TNF-Alpha. *Fibrogenesis Tissue Repair* (2010) 3(1):2–. doi: 10.1186/1755-1536-3-2
104. Yamauchi Y, Kohyama T, Takizawa H, Kamitani S, Desaki M, Takami K, et al. Tumor Necrosis Factor-α Enhances Both Epithelial-Mesenchymal Transition and Cell Contraction Induced in A549 Human Alveolar Epithelial Cells by Transforming Growth Factor-β1. *Exp Lung Res* (2010) 36(1):12–24. doi: 10.3109/01902140903042589
105. Redente EF, Keith RC, Janssen W, Henson PM, Ortiz LA, Downey GP, et al. Tumor Necrosis Factor-α Accelerates the Resolution of Established Pulmonary Fibrosis in Mice by Targeting Profibrotic Lung Macrophages. *Am J Respir Cell Mol Biol* (2014) 50(4):825–37. doi: 10.1165/rcmb.2013-0386OC
106. Oikonomou N, Harokopos V, Zalevsky J, Valavanis C, Kotanidou A, Szymkowski DE, et al. Soluble TNF Mediates the Transition From Pulmonary Inflammation to Fibrosis. *PloS One* (2006) 1(1):e108–e. doi: 10.1371/journal.pone.0000108
107. Janssen LJ, Farkas L, Rahman T, Kolb MR. ATP Stimulates Ca(2+)-waves and Gene Expression in Cultured Human Pulmonary Fibroblasts. *Int J Biochem Cell Biol* (2009) 41(12):2477–84. doi: 10.1016/j.biocel.2009.08.004
108. Müller T, Fay S, Vieira RP, Karmouty-Quintana H, Cicko S, Ayata K, et al. The Purinergic Receptor Subtype P2Y2 Mediates Chemotaxis of Neutrophils and Fibroblasts in Fibrotic Lung Disease. *Oncotarget* (2017) 8(22):35962–72. doi: 10.18632/oncotarget.16414
109. de Souza Xavier Costa N, Ribeiro Júnior G, dos Santos Alemany AA, Belotti L, Zati DH, Frota Cavalcante M, et al. Early and Late Pulmonary Effects of Nebulized LPS in Mice: An Acute Lung Injury Model. *PloS One* (2017) 12(9): e0185474. doi: 10.1371/journal.pone.0185474
110. He Z, Zhu Y, Jiang H. Inhibiting Toll-Like Receptor 4 Signaling Ameliorates Pulmonary Fibrosis During Acute Lung Injury Induced by

Lipopolysaccharide: An Experimental Study. *Respir Res* (2009) 10(1):126. doi: 10.1186/1465-9921-10-126
111. He Z, Gao Y, Deng Y, Li W, Chen Y, Xing S, et al. Lipopolysaccharide Induces Lung Fibroblast Proliferation Through Toll-like Receptor 4 Signaling and the Phosphoinositide3-kinase-Akt Pathway. *PloS One* (2012) 7(4):e35926–e. doi: 10.1371/journal.pone.0035926
112. Thorley AJ, Ford PA, Giembycz MA, Goldstraw P, Young A, Tetley TD. Differential Regulation of Cytokine Release and Leukocyte Migration by Lipopolysaccharide-Stimulated Primary Human Lung Alveolar Type II Epithelial Cells and Macrophages. *J Immunol* (2007) 178(1):463. doi: 10.4049/jimmunol.178.1.463
113. Thorley AJ, Grandolfo D, Lim E, Goldstraw P, Young A, Tetley TD. Innate Immune Responses to Bacterial Ligands in the Peripheral Human Lung – Role of Alveolar Epithelial TLR Expression and Signalling. *PloS One* (2011) 6 (7):e21827. doi: 10.1371/journal.pone.0021827
114. Meneghin A, Choi ES, Evanoff HL, Kunkel SL, Martinez FJ, Flaherty KR, et al. TLR9 is Expressed in Idiopathic Interstitial Pneumonia and its Activation Promotes In Vitro Myofibroblast Differentiation. *Histochem Cell Biol* (2008) 130(5):979–92. doi: 10.1007/s00418-008-0466-z
115. Trujillo G, Meneghin A, Flaherty KR, Sholl LM, Myers JL, Kazerooni EA, et al. TLR9 Differentiates Rapidly From Slowly Progressing Forms of Idiopathic Pulmonary Fibrosis. . *Sci Trans Med* (2010) 2(57):57ra82–2. doi: 10.1126/scitranslmed.3001510
116. Kurundkar AR, Kurundkar D, Rangarajan S, Locy ML, Zhou Y, Liu R-M, et al. The Matricellular Protein CCN1 Enhances TGF-β1/SMAD3-Dependent Profibrotic Signaling in Fibroblasts and Contributes to Fibrogenic Responses to Lung Injury. *FASEB J* (2016) 30(6):2135–50. doi: 10.1096/fj.201500173
117. Moon HG, Qin Z, Quan T, Xie L, Dela Cruz CS, Jin Y. Matrix Protein CCN1 Induced by Bacterial DNA and CpG ODN Limits Lung Inflammation and Contributes to Innate Immune Homeostasis. *Mucosal Immunol* (2015) 8 (2):243–53. doi: 10.1038/mi.2014.62
118. Luckhardt TR, Coomes SM, Trujillo G, Stoolman JS, Vannella KM, Bhan U, et al. TLR9-Induced Interferon β is Associated With Protection From Gammaherpesvirus-Induced Exacerbation of Lung Fibrosis. *Fibrogenesis Tissue Repair* (2011) 4:18–. doi: 10.1186/1755-1536-4-18
119. O'Dwyer DN, Armstrong ME, Trujillo G, Cooke G, Keane MP, Fallon PG, et al. The Toll-like Receptor 3 L412F Polymorphism and Disease Progression in Idiopathic Pulmonary Fibrosis. *Am J Respir Crit Care Med* (2013) 188 (12):1442–50. doi: 10.1164/rccm.201304-0760OC
120. Noth I, Zhang Y, Ma S-F, Flores C, Barber M, Huang Y, et al. Genetic Variants Associated With Idiopathic Pulmonary Fibrosis Susceptibility and Mortality: A Genome-Wide Association Study. *Lancet Respir Med* (2013) 1 (4):309–17. doi: 10.1016/S2213-2600(13)70045-6
121. Zhang G, Ghosh S. Negative Regulation of Toll-Like Receptor-Mediated Signaling by Tollip. *J Biol Chem* (2002) 277(9):7059–65. doi: 10.1074/jbc.M109537200
122. Li X, Kim SE, Chen T-Y, Wang J, Yang X, Tabib T, et al. Toll Interacting Protein Protects Bronchial Epithelial Cells From Bleomycin-Induced Apoptosis. *FASEB J* (2020) 34(8):9884–98. doi: 10.1096/fj.201902636RR
123. Go H, Koh J, Kim HS, Jeon YK, Chung DH. Expression of Toll-Like Receptor 2 and 4 is Increased in the Respiratory Epithelial Cells of Chronic Idiopathic Interstitial Pneumonia Patients. *Respir Med* (2014) 108(5):783–92. doi: 10.1016/j.rmed.2013.12.007
124. Karampitsakos T, Woolard T, Bouros D, Tzouvelekis A. Toll-Like Receptors in the Pathogenesis of Pulmonary Fibrosis. *Eur J Pharmacol* (2017) 808:35–43. doi: 10.1016/j.ejphar.2016.06.045
125. Yang H-Z, Cui B, Liu H-Z, Chen Z-R, Yan H-M, Hua F, et al. Targeting TLR2 Attenuates Pulmonary Inflammation and Fibrosis by Reversion of Suppressive Immune Microenvironment. *J Immunol* (2009) 182(1):692. doi: 10.4049/jimmunol.182.1.692
126. Kim HS, Go H, Akira S, Chung DH. Tlr2-Mediated Production of IL-27 and Chemokines by Respiratory Epithelial Cells Promotes Bleomycin-Induced Pulmonary Fibrosis in Mice. *J Immunol* (2011) 187(8):4007. doi: 10.4049/jimmunol.1101654
127. Yang H-Z, Wang J-P, Mi S, Liu H-Z, Cui B, Yan H-M, et al. Tlr4 Activity is Required in the Resolution of Pulmonary Inflammation and Fibrosis After Acute and Chronic Lung Injury. *Am J Pathol* (2012) 180(1):275–92. doi: 10.1016/j.ajpath.2011.09.019
128. Liang J, Zhang Y, Xie T, Liu N, Chen H, Geng Y, et al. Hyaluronan and TLR4 Promote surfactant-protein-C-positive Alveolar Progenitor Cell Renewal and Prevent Severe Pulmonary Fibrosis in Mice. *Nat Med* (2016) 22 (11):1285–93. doi: 10.1038/nm.4192
129. Jiang D, Liang J, Fan J, Yu S, Chen S, Luo Y, et al. Regulation of Lung Injury and Repair by Toll-like Receptors and Hyaluronan. *Nat Med* (2005) 11 (11):1173–9. doi: 10.1038/nm1315
130. Budden KF, Shukla SD, Rehman SF, Bowerman KL, Keely S, Hugenholtz P, et al. Functional Effects of the Microbiota in Chronic Respiratory Disease. *Lancet Respir Med* (2019) 7(10):907–20. doi: 10.1016/S2213-2600(18)30510-1
131. Spagnolo P, Molyneaux PL, Bernardinello N, Cocconcelli E, Biondini D, Fracasso F, et al. The Role of the Lung's Microbiome in the Pathogenesis and Progression of Idiopathic Pulmonary Fibrosis. *Int J Mol Sci* (2019) 20 (22):5618. doi: 10.3390/ijms20225618
132. Moffatt MF, Cookson WO. The Lung Microbiome in Health and Disease. *Clin Med (London England)* (2017) 17(6):525–9. doi: 10.7861/clinmedicine.17-6-525
133. Huffnagle GB, Dickson RP, Lukacs NW. The Respiratory Tract Microbiome and Lung Inflammation: A Two-Way Street. *Mucosal Immunol* (2017) 10 (2):299–306. doi: 10.1038/mi.2016.108
134. Hilty M, Burke C, Pedro H, Cardenas P, Bush A, Bossley C, et al. Disordered Microbial Communities in Asthmatic Airways. *PloS One* (2010) 5(1):e8578. doi: 10.1371/journal.pone.0008578
135. Garcia-Nuñez M, Millares L, Pomares X, Ferrari R, Pérez-Brocal V, Gallego M, et al. Severity-Related Changes of Bronchial Microbiome in Chronic Obstructive Pulmonary Disease. *J Clin Microbiol* (2014) 52(12):4217–23. doi: 10.1128/JCM.01967-14
136. Einarsson GG, Comer DM, McIlreavey L, Parkhill J, Ennis M, Tunney MM, et al. Community Dynamics and the Lower Airway Microbiota in Stable Chronic Obstructive Pulmonary Disease, Smokers and Healthy non-Smokers. *Thorax* (2016) 71(9):795–803. doi: 10.1136/thoraxjnl-2015-207235
137. Whelan FJ, Heirali AA, Rossi L, Rabin HR, Parkins MD, Surette MG. Longitudinal Sampling of the Lung Microbiota in Individuals With Cystic Fibrosis. *PloS One* (2017) 12(3):e0172811–e. doi: 10.1371/journal.pone.0172811
138. Invernizzi R, Lloyd CM, Molyneaux PL. Respiratory Microbiome and Epithelial Interactions Shape Immunity in the Lungs. *Immunology* (2020) 160(2):171–82. doi: 10.1111/imm.13195
139. Invernizzi R, Wu BG, Barnett J, Ghai P, Kingston S, Hewitt RJ, et al. RespiratoryMicrobiome in Chronic Hypersensitivity Pneumonitis is Distinct From That of Idiopathic Pulmonary Fibrosis. . *Am J Respir Crit Care Med* (2020) 203(3):339–47. doi: 10.1164/rccm.202002-0460OC
140. O'Dwyer DN, Ashley SL, Gurczynski SJ, Xia M, Wilke C, Falkowski NR, et al. Lung Microbiota Contribute to Pulmonary Inflammation and Disease Progression in Pulmonary Fibrosis. *Am J Respir Crit Care Med* (2019) 199 (9):1127–38. doi: 10.1164/rccm.201809-1650OC
141. Huang Y, Ma S-F, Espindola MS, Vij R, Oldham JM, Huffnagle GB, et al. Microbes Are Associated With Host Innate Immune Response in Idiopathic Pulmonary Fibrosis. *Am J Respir Crit Care Med* (2017) 196(2):208–19. doi: 10.1164/rccm.201607-1525OC
142. Han MK, Zhou Y, Murray S, Tayob N, Noth I, Lama VN, et al. Lung Microbiome and Disease Progression in Idiopathic Pulmonary Fibrosis: An Analysis of the COMET Study. *Lancet Respir Med* (2014) 2(7):548–56. doi: 10.1016/S2213-2600(14)70069-4
143. Takahashi Y, Saito A, Chiba H, Kuronuma K, Ikeda K, Kobayashi T, et al. Impaired Diversity of the Lung Microbiome Predicts Progression of Idiopathic Pulmonary Fibrosis. *Respir Res* (2018) 19(1):34. doi: 10.1186/s12931-018-0736-9
144. Yang D, Chen X, Wang J, Lou Q, Lou Y, Li L, et al. Dysregulated Lung Commensal Bacteria Drive Interleukin-17B Production to Promote Pulmonary Fibrosis Through Their Outer Membrane Vesicles. *Immunity* (2019) 50(3):692–706:e7. doi: 10.1016/j.immuni.2019.02.001
145. D'Alessandro-Gabazza CN, Kobayashi T, Yasuma T, Toda M, Kim H, Fujimoto H, et al. A Staphylococcus Pro-Apoptotic Peptide Induces Acute Exacerbation of Pulmonary Fibrosis. *Nat Commun* (2020) 11(1):1539. doi: 10.1038/s41467-020-15344-3
146. Knippenberg S, Ueberberg B, Maus R, Bohling J, Ding N, Tort Tarres M, et al. Streptococcus pneumoniae triggers progression of pulmonary fibrosis

through pneumolysin. *Thorax* (2015) 70(7):636. doi: 10.1136/thoraxjnl-2014-206420

147. Hammad H, Lambrecht BN. Barrier Epithelial Cells and the Control of Type 2 Immunity. *Immunity* (2015) 43(1):29–40. doi: 10.1016/j.immuni.2015.07.007
148. Wynn TA. Fibrotic Disease and the TH1/TH2 Paradigm. *Nat Rev Immunol* (2004) 4:583. doi: 10.1038/nri1412
149. Park SW, Ahn MH, Jang HK, Jang AS, Kim DJ, Koh ES, et al. Interleukin-13 and its Receptors in Idiopathic Interstitial Pneumonia: Clinical Implications for Lung Function. *J Korean Med Sci* (2009) 24(4):614–20. doi: 10.3346/jkms.2009.24.4.614
150. Kimura T, Ishii Y, Yoh K, Morishima Y, Iizuka T, Kiwamoto T, et al. Overexpression of the Transcription Factor GATA-3 Enhances the Development of Pulmonary Fibrosis. *Am J Pathol* (2006) 169(1):96–104. doi: 10.2353/ajpath.2006.051160
151. Huaux F, Liu T, McGarry B, Ullenbruch M, Phan SH. Dual Roles of IL-4 in Lung Injury and Fibrosis. *J Immunol* (2003) 170(4):2083. doi: 10.4049/jimmunol.170.4.2083
152. Belperio JA, Dy M, Burdick MD, Xue YY, Li K, Elias JA, et al. Interaction of IL-13 and C10 in the Pathogenesis of Bleomycin-Induced Pulmonary Fibrosis. *Am J Respir Cell Mol Biol* (2002) 27(4):419–27. doi: 10.1165/rcmb.2002-0009OC
153. Izbicki G, Or R, Christensen TG, Segel MJ, Fine A, Goldstein RH, et al. Bleomycin-Induced Lung Fibrosis in IL-4-overexpressing and Knockout Mice. *Am J Physiology-Lung Cell Mol Physiol* (2002) 283(5):L1110–6. doi: 10.1152/ajplung.00107.2002
154. Lee CG, Homer RJ, Zhu Z, Lanone S, Wang X, Koteliansky V, et al. Interleukin-13 Induces Tissue Fibrosis by Selectively Stimulating and Activating Transforming Growth Factor Beta(1). *J Exp Med* (2001) 194 (6):809–21. doi: 10.1084/jem.194.6.809
155. Kolodsick JE, Toews GB, Jakubzick C, Hogaboam C, Moore TA, McKenzie A, et al. Protection From Fluorescein Isothiocyanate-Induced Fibrosis in IL-13-deficient, But Not IL-4-deficient, Mice Results From Impaired Collagen Synthesis by Fibroblasts. *J Immunol (Baltimore Md 1950)* (2004) 172 (7):4068–76. doi: 10.4049/jimmunol.172.7.4068
156. Guo J, Yao H, Lin X, Xu H, Dean D, Zhu Z, et al. Il-13 Induces YY1 Through the AKT Pathway in Lung Fibroblasts. *PloS One* (2015) 10(3):e0119039. doi: 10.1371/journal.pone.0119039
157. Marchal-Sommé J, Uzunhan Y, Marchand-Adam S, Kambouchner M, Valeyre D, Crestani B, et al. Dendritic Cells Accumulate in Human Fibrotic Interstitial Lung Disease. *Am J Respir Crit Care Med* (2007) 176 (10):1007–14. doi: 10.1164/rccm.200609-1347OC
158. Yogo Y, Fujishima S, Inoue T, Saito F, Shiomi T, Yamaguchi K, et al. Macrophage Derived Chemokine (CCL22), Thymus and Activation-Regulated Chemokine (CCL17), and CCR4 in Idiopathic Pulmonary Fibrosis. *Respir Res* (2009) 10(1):80. doi: 10.1186/1465-9921-10-80
159. Belperio JA, Dy M, Murray L, Burdick MD, Xue YY, Strieter RM, et al. The Role of the Th2 CC Chemokine Ligand CCL17 in Pulmonary Fibrosis. *J Immunol* (2004) 173(7):4692–8. doi: 10.4049/jimmunol.173.7.4692
160. Huaux F, Gharaee-Kermani M, Liu T, Morel V, McGarry B, Ullenbruch M, et al. Role of Eotaxin-1 (CCL11) and CC Chemokine Receptor 3 (CCR3) in Bleomycin-Induced Lung Injury and Fibrosis. *Am J Pathol* (2005) 167 (6):1485–96. doi: 10.1016/S0002-9440(10)61235-7
161. Puxeddu I, Bader R, Piliponsky AM, Reich R, Levi-Schaffer F, Berkman N. The CC Chemokine Eotaxin/CCL11 has a Selective Profibrogenic Effect on Human Lung Fibroblasts. *J Allergy Clin Immunol* (2006) 117(1):103–10. doi: 10.1016/j.jaci.2005.08.057
162. Kohan M, Puxeddu I, Reich R, Levi-Schaffer F, Berkman N. Eotaxin-2/CCL24 and eotaxin-3/CCL26 Exert Differential Profibrogenic Effects on Human Lung Fibroblasts. *Ann allergy Asthma Immunol* (2010) 104(1):66–72. doi: 10.1016/j.anai.2009.11.003
163. Angkasekwinai P, Park H, Wang Y-H, Wang Y-H, Chang SH, Corry DB, et al. Interleukin 25 Promotes the Initiation of Proallergic Type 2 Responses. *J Exp Med* (2007) 204(7):1509–17. doi: 10.1084/jem.20061675
164. Kouzaki H, Tojima I, Kita H, Shimizu T. Transcription of interleukin-25 and Extracellular Release of the Protein is Regulated by Allergen Proteases in Airway Epithelial Cells. *Am J Respir Cell Mol Biol* (2013) 49(5):741–50. doi: 10.1165/rcmb.2012-0304OC
165. Barlow JL, Bellosi A, Hardman CS, Drynan LF, Wong SH, Cruickshank JP, et al. Innate IL-13–producing Nuocytes Arise During Allergic Lung Inflammation and Contribute to Airways Hyperreactivity. *J Allergy Clin Immunol* (2012) 129(1):191–8:e4. doi: 10.1016/j.jaci.2011.09.041
166. Hams E, Armstrong ME, Barlow JL, Saunders SP, Schwartz C, Cooke G, et al. Il-25 and Type 2 Innate Lymphoid Cells Induce Pulmonary Fibrosis. *Proc Natl Acad Sci USA* (2014) 111(1):367–72. doi: 10.1073/pnas.1315854111
167. Park S-K, Jin Y-D, Park Y-K, Yeon S-H, Xu J, Han R-N, et al. Il-25-induced Activation of Nasal Fibroblast and its Association With the Remodeling of Chronic Rhinosinusitis With Nasal Polyposis. *PloS One* (2017) 12(8): e0181806–e. doi: 10.1371/journal.pone.0181806
168. Létuvé S, Lajoie-Kadoch S, Audusseau S, Rothenberg ME, Fiset PO, Ludwig MS, et al. Il-17E Upregulates the Expression of Proinflammatory Cytokines in Lung Fibroblasts. *J Allergy Clin Immunol* (2006) 117(3):590–6. doi: 10.1016/j.jaci.2005.10.025
169. Fort MM, Cheung J, Yen D, Li J, Zurawski SM, Lo S, et al. Il-25 Induces Il-4, IL-5, and IL-13 and Th2-Associated Pathologies In Vivo. *Immunity* (2001) 15(6):985–95. doi: 10.1016/S1074-7613(01)00243-6
170. Kitajima M, Lee H-C, Nakayama T, Ziegler SF. TSLP Enhances the Function of Helper Type 2 Cells. *Eur J Immunol* (2011) 41(7):1862–71. doi: 10.1002/eji.201041195
171. Soumelis V, Reche PA, Kanzler H, Yuan W, Edward G, Homey B, et al. Human Epithelial Cells Trigger Dendritic Cell Mediated Allergic Inflammation by Producing TSLP. *Nat Immunol* (2002) 3(7):673–80. doi: 10.1038/ni805
172. Datta A, Alexander R, Sulikowski MG, Nicholson AG, Maher TM, Scotton CJ, et al. Evidence for a Functional Thymic Stromal Lymphopoietin Signaling Axis in Fibrotic Lung Disease. *J Immunol (Baltimore Md 1950)* (2013) 191(9):4867–79. doi: 10.4049/jimmunol.1300588
173. Lee J-U, Chang HS, Lee HJ, Jung CA, Bae DJ, Song HJ, et al. Upregulation of interleukin-33 and Thymic Stromal Lymphopoietin Levels in the Lungs of Idiopathic Pulmonary Fibrosis. *BMC pulm Med* (2017) 17(1):39–. doi: 10.1186/s12890-017-0380-z
174. Herro R, Da Silva Antunes R, Aguilera AR, Tamada K, Croft M. Tumor Necrosis Factor Superfamily 14 (LIGHT) Controls Thymic Stromal Lymphopoietin to Drive Pulmonary Fibrosis. *J Allergy Clin Immunol* (2015) 136(3):757–68. doi: 10.1016/j.jaci.2014.12.1936
175. Shubin NJ, Clauson M, Niino K, Kasprzak V, Tsuha A, Guga E, et al. Thymic Stromal Lymphopoietin Protects in a Model of Airway Damage and Inflammation Via Regulation of Caspase-1 Activity and Apoptosis Inhibition. *Mucosal Immunol* (2020) 13(4):584–94. doi: 10.1038/s41385-020-0271-0
176. Li G, Jin F, Du J, He Q, Yang B, Luo P. Macrophage-Secreted TSLP and MMP9 Promote Bleomycin-Induced Pulmonary Fibrosis. *Toxicol Appl Pharmacol* (2019) 366:10–6. doi: 10.1016/j.taap.2019.01.011
177. Liew FY, Girard J-P, Turnquist HR. Interleukin-33 in Health and Disease. *Nat Rev Immunol* (2016) 16(11):676–89. doi: 10.1038/nri.2016.95
178. Drake LY, Kita H. Il-33: Biological Properties, Functions, and Roles in Airway Disease. *Immunol Rev* (2017) 278(1):173–84. doi: 10.1111/imr.12552
179. Luzina IG, Kopach P, Lockatell V, Kang PH, Nagarsekar A, Burke AP, et al. Interleukin-33 Potentiates Bleomycin-Induced Lung Injury. *Am J Respir Cell Mol Biol* (2013) 49(6):999–1008. doi: 10.1165/rcmb.2013-0093OC
180. Li D, Guabiraba R, Besnard A-G, Komai-Koma M, Jabir MS, Zhang L, et al. Il-33 Promotes ST2-dependent Lung Fibrosis by the Induction of Alternatively Activated Macrophages and Innate Lymphoid Cells in Mice. *J Allergy Clin Immunol* (2014) 134(6):1422–32:e11. doi: 10.1016/j.jaci.2014.05.011
181. Zhao Y, De Los Santos FG, Wu Z, Liu T, Phan SH. An ST2-dependent Role of Bone Marrow-Derived Group 2 Innate Lymphoid Cells in Pulmonary Fibrosis. *J Pathol* (2018) 245(4):399–409. doi: 10.1002/path.5092
182. Ma L, Zeng J, Mo B, Wang C, Huang J, Sun Y, et al. High Mobility Group Box 1: A Novel Mediator of Th2-type Response-Induced Airway Inflammation of Acute Allergic Asthma. *J thoracic Dis* (2015) 7(10):1732–41. doi: 10.3978/j.issn.2072-1439.2015.10.18
183. Fonseca W, Malinczak C-A, Schuler CF, Best SKK, Rasky AJ, Morris SB, et al. Uric Acid Pathway Activation During Respiratory Virus Infection Promotes Th2 Immune Response Via Innate Cytokine Production and ILC2 Accumulation. *Mucosal Immunol* (2020) 13(4):691–701. doi: 10.1038/s41385-020-0264-z

184. Malavia NK, Mih JD, Raub CB, Dinh BT, George SC. Il-13 Induces a Bronchial Epithelial Phenotype That is Profibrotic. *Respir Res* (2008) 9(1):27. doi: 10.1186/1465-9921-9-27
185. Sugita K, Steer CA, Martinez-Gonzalez I, Altunbulakli C, Morita H, Castro-Giner F, et al. Type 2 Innate Lymphoid Cells Disrupt Bronchial Epithelial Barrier Integrity by Targeting Tight Junctions Through IL-13 in Asthmatic Patients. *J Allergy Clin Immunol* (2018) 141(1):300–10:e11. doi: 10.1016/j.jaci.2017.02.038
186. Glisinski KM, Schlobohm AJ, Paramore SV, Birukova A, Moseley MA, Foster MW, et al. Interleukin-13 Disrupts Type 2 Pneumocyte Stem Cell Activity. *JCI Insight* (2020) 5(1). doi: 10.1172/jci.insight.131232
187. Borowski A, Kuepper M, Horn U, Knüpfer U, Zissel G, Höhne K, et al. Interleukin-13 Acts as an Apoptotic Effector on Lung Epithelial Cells and Induces Pro-Fibrotic Gene Expression in Lung Fibroblasts. *Clin Exp Allergy* (2008) 38(4):619–28. doi: 10.1111/j.1365-2222.2008.02944.x
188. Parker JM, Glaspole IN, Lancaster LH, Haddad TJ, She D, Roseti SL, et al. A Phase 2 Randomized Controlled Study of Tralokinumab in Subjects With Idiopathic Pulmonary Fibrosis. *Am J Respir Crit Care Med* (2018) 197(1):94–103. doi: 10.1164/rccm.201704-0784OC
189. Raghu G, Richeldi L, Crestani B, Wung P, Bejuit R, Esperet C, et al. SAR156597 in Idiopathic Pulmonary Fibrosis: A Phase 2 Placebo-Controlled Study (DRI11772). *Eur Respir J* (2018) 52(6):1801130. doi: 10.1183/13993003.01130-2018
190. Hirano A, Kanehiro A, Ono K, Ito W, Yoshida A, Okada C, et al. Pirfenidone Modulates Airway Responsiveness, Inflammation, and Remodeling After Repeated Challenge. *Am J Respir Cell Mol Biol* (2006) 35(3):366–77. doi: 10.1165/rcmb.2005-0452OC
191. Byrne AJ, Mathie SA, Gregory LG, Lloyd CM. Pulmonary Macrophages: Key Players in the Innate Defence of the Airways. *Thorax* (2015) 70(12):1189. doi: 10.1136/thoraxjnl-2015-207020
192. Zhang L, Wang Y, Wu G, Xiong W, Gu W, Wang C-Y. Macrophages: Friend or Foe in Idiopathic Pulmonary Fibrosis? *Respir Res* (2018) 19(1):170. doi: 10.1186/s12931-018-0864-2
193. Prasse A, Pechkovsky DV, Toews GB, Jungraithmayr W, Kollert F, Goldmann T, et al. A Vicious Circle of Alveolar Macrophages and Fibroblasts Perpetuates Pulmonary Fibrosis Via CCL18. *Am J Respir Crit Care Med* (2006) 173(7):781–92. doi: 10.1164/rccm.200509-1518OC
194. Murray PJ, Wynn TA. Protective and Pathogenic Functions of Macrophage Subsets. *Nat Rev Immunol* (2011) 11(11):723–37. doi: 10.1038/nri3073
195. Sisson TH, Mendez M, Choi K, Subbotina N, Courey A, Cunningham A, et al. Targeted Injury of Type Ii Alveolar Epithelial Cells Induces Pulmonary Fibrosis. *Am J Respir Crit Care Med* (2010) 181(3):254–63. doi: 10.1164/rccm.200810-1615OC
196. Osterholzer JJ, Olszewski MA, Murdock BJ, Chen GH, Erb-Downward JR, Subbotina N, et al. Implicating Exudate Macrophages and Ly-6C(high) Monocytes in CCR2-dependent Lung Fibrosis Following Gene-Targeted Alveolar Injury. *J Immunol (Baltimore Md 1950)* (2013) 190(7):3447–57. doi: 10.4049/jimmunol.1200604
197. Yang J, Agarwal M, Ling S, Teitz-Tennenbaum S, Zemans RL, Osterholzer JJ, et al. Diverse Injury Pathways Induce Alveolar Epithelial Cell CCL2/12, Which Promotes Lung Fibrosis. *Am J Respir Cell Mol Biol* (2020) 62(5):622–32. doi: 10.1165/rcmb.2019-0297OC
198. Young LR, Gulleman PM, Short CW, Tanjore H, Sherrill T, Qi A, et al. Epithelial-Macrophage Interactions Determine Pulmonary Fibrosis Susceptibility in Hermansky-Pudlak Syndrome. *JCI Insight* (2016) 1(17). doi: 10.1172/jci.insight.88947
199. Gschwandtner M, Derler R, Midwood KS. More Than Just Attractive: How CCL2 Influences Myeloid Cell Behavior Beyond Chemotaxis. *Front Immunol* (2019) 10:2759–. doi: 10.3389/fimmu.2019.02759
200. Moore BB, Kolodsick JE, Thannickal VJ, Cooke K, Moore TA, Hogaboam C, et al. CCR2-Mediated Recruitment of Fibrocytes to the Alveolar Space After Fibrotic Injury. *Am J Pathol* (2005) 166(3):675–84. doi: 10.1016/S0002-9440(10)62289-4
201. Moore BB, Peters-Golden M, Christensen PJ, Lama V, Kuziel WA, Paine R, et al. Alveolar Epithelial Cell Inhibition of Fibroblast Proliferation is Regulated by MCP-1/CCR2 and Mediated by PGE2. *Am J Physiol Lung Cell Mol Physiol* (2003) 284(2):L342–9. doi: 10.1152/ajplung.00168.2002
202. Ekert JE, Murray LA, Das AM, Sheng H, Giles-Komar J, Rycyzyn MA. Chemokine (C-C Motif) Ligand 2 Mediates Direct and Indirect Fibrotic Responses in Human and Murine Cultured Fibrocytes. *Fibrogenesis Tissue Repair* (2011) 4(1):23. doi: 10.1186/1755-1536-4-23
203. Misharin AV, Morales-Nebreda L, Reyfman PA, Cuda CM, Walter JM, McQuattie-Pimentel AC, et al. Monocyte-Derived Alveolar Macrophages Drive Lung Fibrosis and Persist in the Lung Over the Life Span. *J Exp Med* (2017) 214(8):2387. doi: 10.1084/jem.20162152
204. Aran D, Looney AP, Liu L, Wu E, Fong V, Hsu A, et al. Reference-Based Analysis of Lung Single-Cell Sequencing Reveals a Transitional Profibrotic Macrophage. *Nat Immunol* (2019) 20(2):163–72. doi: 10.1038/s41590-018-0276-y
205. Reyfman PA, Walter JM, Joshi N, Anekalla KR, McQuattie-Pimentel AC, Chiu S, et al. Single-Cell Transcriptomic Analysis of Human Lung Provides Insights Into the Pathobiology of Pulmonary Fibrosis. . *Am J Respir Crit Care Med* (2018) 199(12):1517–36. doi: 10.1164/rccm.201712-2410OC
206. Kumar V, Patel S, Tcyganov E, Gabrilovich DI. The Nature of Myeloid-Derived Suppressor Cells in the Tumor Microenvironment. *Trends Immunol* (2016) 37(3):208–20. doi: 10.1016/j.it.2016.01.004
207. Fernandez IE, Greiffo FR, Frankenberger M, Bandres J, Heinzelmann K, Neurohr C, et al. Peripheral Blood Myeloid-Derived Suppressor Cells Reflect Disease Status in Idiopathic Pulmonary Fibrosis. *Eur Respir J* (2016) 48(4):1171. doi: 10.1183/13993003.01826-2015
208. Suga M, Iyonaga K, Ichiyasu H, Saita N, Yamasaki H, Ando M. Clinical Significance of MCP-1 Levels in BALF and Serum in Patients With Interstitial Lung Diseases. *Eur Respir J* (1999) 14(2):376–82. doi: 10.1034/j.1399-3003.1999.14b23.x
209. Mercer PF, Johns RH, Scotton CJ, Krupiczojc MA, Königshoff M, Howell DC, et al. Pulmonary Epithelium is a Prominent Source of Proteinase-Activated Receptor-1-Inducible CCL2 in Pulmonary Fibrosis. *Am J Respir Crit Care Med* (2009) 179(5):414–25. doi: 10.1164/rccm.200712-1827OC
210. Raghu G, Martinez FJ, Brown KK, Costabel U, Cottin V, Wells AU, et al. CC-Chemokine Ligand 2 Inhibition in Idiopathic Pulmonary Fibrosis: A Phase 2 Trial of Carlumab. *Eur Respir J* (2015) 46(6):1740–50. doi: 10.1183/13993003.01558-2014
211. Samara KD, Antoniou KM, Karagiannis K, Margaritopoulos G, Lasithiotaki I, Koutala E, et al. Expression Profiles of Toll-like Receptors in non-Small Cell Lung Cancer and Idiopathic Pulmonary Fibrosis. *Int J Oncol* (2012) 40(5):1397–404. doi: 10.3892/ijo.2012.1374
212. Bjermer L, Lundgren R, Hällgren R. Hyaluronan and Type III Procollagen Peptide Concentrations in Bronchoalveolar Lavage Fluid in Idiopathic Pulmonary Fibrosis. *Thorax* (1989) 44(2):126–31. doi: 10.1136/thx.44.2.126

2

Mesenchymal Stem Cells for the Treatment of Idiopathic Pulmonary Fibrosis

Argyrios Tzouvelekis [1,2†], *Rebecca Toonkel* [3†], *Theodoros Karampitsakos* [1†], *Kantha Medapalli* [3,4], *Ioanna Ninou* [2], *Vasilis Aidinis* [2,4], *Demosthenes Bouros* [1] and *Marilyn K. Glassberg* [4,5*]

[1] First Academic Respiratory Department, Sotiria General Hospital for Thoracic Diseases, University of Athens, Athens, Greece, [2] Division of Immunology, Alexander Fleming Biomedical Sciences Research Center, Athens, Greece, [3] Department of Medicine, Florida International University Herbert Wertheim College of Medicine, Miami, FL, United States, [4] Department of Surgery, University of Miami Miller School of Medicine, Miami, FL, United States, [5] Department of Medicine, University of Miami Miller School of Medicine, Miami, FL, United States

***Correspondence:**
Marilyn K. Glassberg
mglassbe@med.miami.edu

† These authors have contributed equally to this work.

Idiopathic pulmonary fibrosis (IPF) is an inexorably progressive lung disease of unknown origin. Prognosis is poor, with limited treatment options available, and the median survival remains just 3–5 years. Despite the use of pirfenidone and nintedanib for the treatment of IPF, curative therapies remain elusive and mortality remains high. Regenerative medicine and the use of cell-based therapies has recently emerged as a potential option for various diseases. Promising results of preclinical studies using mesenchymal stem cells (MSCs) suggest that they may represent a potential therapeutic option for the treatment of chronic lung diseases including IPF. Encouraging results of Phase 1 studies of MSCs various have reduced safety concerns. Nonetheless, there is still a pressing need for exploratory biomarkers and interval end-points in the context of MSCs investigation. This review intends to summarize the current state of knowledge for stem cells in the experimental and clinical setting of IPF, present important safety and efficacy issues, highlight future challenges and address the need for large, multicenter clinical trials coupled with realistic end-points, including biomarkers, to assess treatment efficacy.

Keywords: idiopathic pulmonary fibrosis, mesenchymal stem cells, treatment, safety, efficacy

INTRODUCTION

Idiopathic Pulmonary Fibrosis (IPF) is a progressive debilitating lung disease of unknown etiology (1–4). The disease is characterized by a combination of histological changes including extracellular matrix (ECM) deposition, phenotypic changes of fibroblasts and alveolar epithelial cells, formation of fibroblastic foci, and scattered areas of aberrant wound healing interspersed with normal lung parenchyma (1, 5–14).

Current evidence suggests that the areas of fibrosis seen in lungs of patients with IPF share many features with normal aging lung, such as genomic instability, telomere attrition, mitochondrial dysfunction, cellular senescence, and immune dysregulation (10, 15, 16). Due to the inefficacy of immunomodulatory and immunosuppressive agents in the past, the role of the immune system in the pathogenesis of IPF remains poorly understood (17–22). However, highly activated and proliferative CD4+ cells and functional impairment of T regulatory cells (Tregs) in patients with IPF, suggest a link between immunity and pulmonary fibrosis (10, 23, 24).

There are two approved compounds for the treatment of IPF: pirfenidone and nintedanib. Pirfenidone is an antifibrotic compound with an unclear mechanism of action targeting several molecules including transforming growth factor-β (TGF-β), tumor necrosis factor-α (TNF-α), and interleukin 6 (25). Nintedanib is a tyrosine-kinase inhibitor, targeting vascular endothelial growth factor receptor (VEGFR), fibroblast growth factor receptor (FGFR), and platelet derived growth factor receptor (PDGFR) (22).While the use of pirfenidone and nintedanib have been shown to slow the progression of IPF (26–28), both compounds have significant side effects and neither is curative (28–30). Morbidity and mortality from IPF remains high and thus there is a pressing need for alternative therapeutic options for this complex disease (7, 31–33). The US National Institutes of Health database lists 493 complete or ongoing clinical trials of MSCs (34). Toward this end, regeneration and cell therapies such as the use of mesenchymal stem cells (MSCs) have emerged as a potential option.

MSCs are multipotent cells able to differentiate into a number of different cell lines and exert immunomodulatory, anti-proliferative, and anti-inflammatory effects. Their multipotency, migratory ability, and immunoprivileged state has led to extensive research efforts for therapeutic applications in several diseases including cardiac ischemia (35–39), ischemic acute renal failure (37), sepsis (40), autoimmune disorders (41), severe graft-vs. -host disease (42), pancreatic islet and renal glomerular repair in diabetes (43), fulminant hepatic failure (44), chronic lung diseases (45–48), and acute lung injury (49–53) (**Table 2**).

MSCs are easily harvested from many tissues (peripheral blood, adipose tissue, bone marrow, and umbilical cord) and may be expanded *in vitro* with minimal modifications. MSCs represent the most extensively studied stem cell population (54). Research supports the immunomodulatory, anti-inflammatory, and potentially anti-fibrotic properties of MSCs (49, 55, 56). Importantly, MSCs are "immune privileged," lacking expression of class II major histocompatibility complex (MHC-II). Therefore, allogeneic use of MSCs is possible (57).

PRECLINICAL STUDIES

Recent studies on the pathophysiology of IPF suggest that early alveolar injury activates abnormal alveolar epithelial cells and stimulates the release of mediators including matrix metalloproteinases and TGF beta-1 (2, 58–61). These mediators activate cytokines and chemokines including IL-1 and IL-13 leading to the phenotype of abnormal wound healing (62–65). Therefore, IPF is considered a complex and multifactorial disease characterized by alveolar epithelial injury and alveolar collapse, fewer alveolar epithelial type II cells, alveolar stem cell exhaustion, and myofibroblast deregulation due to living on a fibrotic matrix (66, 67).

Several experimental studies have been conducted in order to investigate the effect of MSCs from various organs, mainly from bone marrow with a dosage ranging between 0.1×10^6 and 4×10^6 cells, in pathways associated with lung injury and pulmonary fibrosis and several end-points had been set (68, 69) (**Table 1**). The majority of studies recorded substantial improvement in histopathology (56, 64, 70–82), decrease to Ashcroft score (70–72, 77, 79, 80, 83) and lung collagen content (56, 70–81), reduced pulmonary transforming growth factor-b (TGFb) levels (56, 70–81, 84) and decreased BAL neutrophil count (76, 77, 80, 81, 85) following to MSCs administration. Importantly, both bone marrow and amnion-derived MSCs reduced TGFb levels (84). However, to this end, data are still conflicting regarding levels of tumor necrosis factor-a (TNF-a) (56, 71, 83–85), interleukins IL-1, IL-6 (71, 77, 81, 84, 86) and metalloproteinases MMP-2, MMP-9, MMP-13 (56, 71, 83, 84) following administration of MSCs (4, 87–89).

The majority of studies investigating the effect of donor MSCs on BLM-induced pulmonary fibrosis have used young male mouse models (90, 91). Young mice, however, undergo spontaneous resolution of BLM-induced pulmonary fibrosis in some studies (69, 90, 91). Although IPF is primarily a disease of individuals over the age of 50, most studies have also utilized young female mice to evaluate the molecular patterns and potential therapeutic targets for patients with IPF (92–94). Interestingly, in one study of bleomycin induced fibrosis in mice, MSCs were found to improve survival when compared with pirfenidone (64). This study also reported downregulation of IL-2, IL-1b, TNF-α, and TGFβ leading to a reduction in inflammation (64). In addition, downregulation of MMPs was noted with a reduction in collagen deposition and fibrosis (64).

Collectively, MSCs seem to exert pleiotropic effects in the site of lung injury including anti-inflammatory, immunomodulatory, antifibrotic effects (65), engagement in paracrine signaling (95), activation of resident stem cells, and differentiation into local cell types (56, 65, 74, 77, 79, 83, 85, 96–98). Preclinical studies have shown MSCs to be efficacious in the treatment and prevention of lung fibrosis (65, 69). Nonetheless, concerns remain regarding the activity of MSCs within a pro-fibrotic microenvironment (99–102). While some preclinical studies suggest that MSCs might promote fibrosis, to date, no human studies have found a similar pro-fibrotic effect (37, 42, 91, 100, 101, 103–112).

TABLE 1 | Main results of preclinical studies of mesenchymal stem cell therapy in experimental pulmonary fibrosis based on end-points set.

End-point	Outcome	Studies
Histopathology	Significant improvement	(56, 64, 70–82)
Ashcroft score	Decrease	(70–72, 77, 79, 80, 83)
Lung collagen content	Decrease	(56, 70–81)
TGF-b	Decrease	(56, 70–81, 84)
BAL neutrophil count	Decrease	(76, 77, 80, 81, 85)
TNF-a	Conflicting	(56, 71, 83–85)
IL-1, IL-6	Conflicting	(71, 77, 81, 84, 86)
MMP-2, MMP-9, MMP-13	Conflicting	(56, 71, 83, 84)
Survival compared with pirfenidone	Improved	(64)

BAL, bronchoalveolar lavage, IL, interleukin, MMP, metalloproteinases, TGF-b, transforming growth factor-beta, TNF-a, tumor necrosis factor-a.

TABLE 2 | Results of clinical human studies of mesenchymal stem cell therapy.

Study	Disease model	Cell type	Delivery and dose	Safety results	Efficacy results
(42)	Acute graft versus host disease	Allogeneic BM-MSCs; HLA matched and mismatched	IV, 1.4 × 10^6 cells/kg	No adverse effects reported	Complete response in 30 of 55 patients. Partial response in 9 of 55 patients
(37)	Myocardial infarction	Allogeneic BM-MSCs; Non-HLA matched	IV, 0.5, 1.6, or 5.0 × 10^6 cells/kg	No difference in adverse events compared with placebo	Decreased arrhythmic events. Decreased PVCs. Improved post-event ejection fraction. Improved overall clinical status. Improved FEV_1 percent predicted
(41)	Refractory lupus	Allogeneic BM-MSCs; Non-HLA matched family members	IV, 1 × 10^6 cells/kg	No adverse events reported	Improved SLE disease activity index score. Improved 24-h proteinuria
(112)	Ischemic cardiomyopathy	Allogeneic vs. autologous BM-MSCs; Non-HLA matched (allogeneic)	Endocardial, 20, 100, or 200 × 10^6 cells	One patient in each arm hospitalized for heart failure. No statistically significant difference in adverse events between arms	Improvement in 6MWT and QOL index with autologous MSCs. CT evidence of reverse LV remodeling in both arms. Improved LV and diastolic volumes with allogeneic MSCs
(110)	COPD	Allogeneic BM-MSCs; Non-HLA matched	IV, 100 × 10^6 cells/ infusion Four monthly infusions	No difference in adverse events compared with placebo	No effect seen on frequency of COPD exacerbation or PFTs. Decreased circulating C-reactive protein in patients with high baseline levels
(103)	IPF	ADSCs-SVF	Endobronchial, 0.5 × 10^6 cells/kg of body weight in 10cc; 3 dosages over 3 months	No difference in adverse events compared with placebo. No ectopic tissue formation	Cell-treated patients did not deteriorate in both functional parameters and indicators of quality of life
(109)	IPF	Allogeneic placental MSCs	IV, 1 & 2 × 10^6 cells/kg; one dose	Minor and transient acute adverse events	Stable lung function. No evidence of worsening fibrosis
(53)	ARDS	Allogeneic BM-MSC	IV, 1, 5, or 10 × 10^6 cells/kg; 3 patients per dosage arm	No adverse events Serious adverse events after infusion (3 patients), non-MSC related	None
(105)	IPF	Allogeneic BM-MSC	IV, one dose: 20 × 106 (n = 3) 100 × 106 (n = 3) and 200 × 106 cells (n = 3)	No treatment-emergent serious adverse events. Two non-treatment related deaths due to progression of IPF	(Exploratory results): 3.0% mean decline in % predicted FVC and 5.4% mean decline in % predicted DLCO
(113)	IPF	ADSCs-SVF	Endobronchial, 0.5 × 10^6 cells/kg of body weight in 10cc; 3 dosages over 3 months	No difference in adverse events compared with placebo. No ectopic tissue formation	Median overall progression-free survival 26 months. Median overall survival 32 months. All patients alive for at least 2 years after first administration

ADSCs-SVF, autologous adipose derived stromal cells-stromal vascular fraction; BM-hMSCs, human bone marrow-derived mesenchymal stem cells; IPF, Idiopathic pulmonary fibrosis; PD-MSCs, placenta-derived mesenchymal stem cells.

CLINICAL TRIALS

Early clinical studies of MSCs in patients with IPF have shown promising safety profiles (30, 103, 114). Phase 1 clinical trials have been conducted for safety of MSC therapy. A phase Ib study of endobronchially administered autologous adipose-derived MSCs showed not only acceptable safety outcomes, but also improvements in quality of life parameters (103). The recently published longitudinal outcomes of this study also demonstrated an acceptable safety profile, 100% survival rate 2 years after first administration and a median overall progression-free survival of 26 months (113). Furthermore, studies of intravenously administered placental derived MSCs (105, 109) found that administration of up to 2 × 10^6 cells per kilogram was safe in subjects with moderately severe IPF (109). Importantly, the authors reported only minor and transient alterations in peri-infusion hemodynamics and gas exchange, reducing the concerns for embolization of stem cells to an already compromised pulmonary vasculature. Subjects were followed for six months with no observed decline in forced vital capacity (FVC), diffusing lung capacity for carbon monoxide (DLCO), six-minute walk test (6MWT), or CT fibrosis score (90). The AETHER trial also showed favorable safety outcomes for the intravenous delivery of a single dose of allogeneic MSCs in patients with IPF up to 2 × 10^8 cells (105). Although this was an underpowered study for the detection of significant changes in functional indices, the mean decline in % predicted FVC and DLCO were below the thresholds for disease progression (1, 115). ReCell, an FDA approved phase 1b multidose, randomized, double-blind trial of 10 × 10^6 cells delivered intravenously to patients with IPF, has not yet begun enrollment.

OUTSTANDING CHALLENGES

While it now appears that it is safe to use MSCs in patients with IPF, many questions and challenges remain. In the preclinical realm, there is a need for animal models more representative of chronic IPF (91, 116) for the continued study of how MSCs exert their effects. Bleomycin induced pulmonary fibrosis is still considered the best available animal model for preclinical testing (91, 117). However, there is increasing criticism that potential therapies usually administered the first 7 days following bleomycin exposure may act mainly through prevention of the inflammatory cascade rather than reversal of fibrosis, thus limiting their applicability to human IPF (69). First, improved animal models will enable the identification of biomarkers that may be useful as measures of disease activity and/or treatment effect. Second, the timing of treatment for best effect needs to be better elucidated. Furthermore, the most efficacious source of MSCs and the role of age need to be more fully explored. One report suggesting that adipose-derived MSCs from young, but not old, mice prevent bleomycin induced lung fibrosis in an aged mouse model (118) highlights the need for further research in this area.

Several challenges in the clinical setting also remain to be addressed. The optimal source of MSCs, the best route of administration, the number and timing of administrations, and the appropriate dosing interval. Thus, allogeneic human bone marrow-derived and autologous adipose derived MSCs have been the most studied in the context of IPF. There are limited studies on endogenous stem cells from the lungs of patients with IPF and concerns remain surrounding the risk of biopsy and the potential for intervention-induced IPF exacerbation and the possibility of detrimental effects on lung function from biopsy. Lung tissue obtained at the time of lung transplant remains the best tool for study.

It is also critical to characterize appropriate endpoints to assess treatment effectiveness in these patients (100, 119–129). Molecular biomarkers would be the optimal choice for the assessment of cell based therapies. Finally, well-designed and meticulously conducted multicenter randomized clinical trials of MSCs for the treatment of IPF are needed to assess efficacy.

MOVING FORWARD

While preclinical trials suggest that MSCs may be effective in the treatment of IPF, and early clinical trials suggest that they are likely to be safe in the population, insufficient data exists at this time to definitely state that the use of MSCs for the treatment of IPF is either safe or efficacious. Despite this lack of evidence, cell based therapies are being aggressively marketed to this vulnerable patient population. A recent study found that as of August of 2016, there were at least 351 stem cell related businesses registered in the United States. These sites offer unproven, experimental treatments for a wide variety of conditions (130, 131). In the case of IPF, desperate patients and their physicians continue to succumb to an onslaught of marketing and branding of as yet unproven "stem cell" treatments. Unfortunately, these businesses are also almost wholly unregulated (132). Publication of case reports of harm arising from the misuse of unproven treatments support increased government oversight in the interest of patient safety.

CONCLUSION

Idiopathic Pulmonary Fibrosis (IPF) is a debilitating lung disease characterized by a progressive decline in lung function ultimately resulting in death. The lack of curative treatments for this disease has created an urgency for other potential therapeutic options. Preclinical studies suggest that because MSCs have immunomodulatory, anti-inflammatory, and potentially anti-fibrotic properties, they may be efficacious in the treatment of IPF. Early clinical trials have shown that MSCs may be safely administered to patients with IPF, but large multicenter randomized trials still need to be performed.

AUTHOR CONTRIBUTIONS

AT, RT and TK wrote the initial manuscript. The manuscript was supervised and significantly modified by MG, AT, DB. KM, IN, VA offered significant intellectual contribution. All authors approved the final form of the manuscript.

REFERENCES

1. Raghu G, Collard HR, Egan JJ, Martinez FJ, Behr J, Brown KK, et al. An official ATS/ERS/JRS/ALAT statement: idiopathic pulmonary fibrosis: evidence-based guidelines for diagnosis and management. *Am J Respir Crit Care Med.* (2011) **183**:788–824. doi: 10.1164/rccm.2009-040GL
2. Raghu G, Weycker D, Edelsberg J, Bradford WZ, Oster G. Incidence and prevalence of idiopathic pulmonary fibrosis. *Am J Respir Crit Care Med.* (2006) **174**:810–6. doi: 10.1164/rccm.200602-163OC
3. Tzilas V, Valeyre D, Tzouvelekis A, Bouros D. Taking a giant step in the diagnosis of idiopathic pulmonary fibrosis. *Lancet Respir Med.* (2017) **6**:82–4. doi: 10.1016/S2213-2600(17)30443-5
4. Geiger S, Hirsch D, Hermann FG. Cell therapy for lung disease. *Eur Respir Rev.* (2017) **26**:170044. doi: 10.1183/16000617.0044-2017
5. Ryu C, Sun H, Gulati M, Herazo-Maya JD, Chen Y, Osafo-Addo A, et al. Extracellular mitochondrial DNA is generated by fibroblasts and predicts death in idiopathic pulmonary fibrosis. *Am J Respir Crit Care Med.* (2017) **196**:1571–81. doi: 10.1164/rccm.201612-2480OC
6. Tomos IP, Tzouvelekis A, Aidinis V, Manali ED, Bouros E, Bouros D, et al. Extracellular matrix remodeling in idiopathic pulmonary fibrosis. It is the 'bed' that counts and not 'the sleepers'. *Expert Rev Respir Med.* (2017) **11**:299–309. doi: 10.1080/17476348.2017.1300533
7. Spagnolo P, Sverzellati N, Rossi G, Cavazza A, Tzouvelekis A, Crestani B, et al. Idiopathic pulmonary fibrosis: an update. *Ann Med.* (2015) **47**:15–27. doi: 10.3109/07853890.2014.982165
8. Spagnolo P, Cottin V. Genetics of idiopathic pulmonary fibrosis: from mechanistic pathways to personalised medicine. *J Med Genet.* (2017) **54**:93–9. doi: 10.1136/jmedgenet-2016-103973
9. Tzouvelekis A, Kaminski N. Epigenetics in idiopathic pulmonary fibrosis. *Biochem Cell Biol.* (2015) **93**:159–70. doi: 10.1139/bcb-2014-0126
10. Karampitsakos T, Woolard T, Bouros D, Tzouvelekis A. Toll-like receptors in the pathogenesis of pulmonary fibrosis. *Eur J Pharmacol.* (2017) **808**:35–43. doi: 10.1016/j.ejphar.2016.06.045

11. Travis WD, Costabel U, Hansell DM, King TE, Lynch DA, Nicholson AG, et al. An official American Thoracic Society/European Respiratory Society statement: Update of the international multidisciplinary classification of the idiopathic interstitial pneumonias. *Am J Respir Crit Care Med.* (2013) **188**:733–48. doi: 10.1164/rccm.201308-1483ST
12. Tzouvelekis A, Yu G, Lino Cardenas CL, Herazo-Maya JD, Wang R, Woolard T, et al. SH2 domain-containing phosphatase-2 is a novel antifibrotic regulator in pulmonary fibrosis. *Am J Respir Crit Care Med.* (2017) **195**:500–14. doi: 10.1164/rccm.201602-0329OC
13. Selman M, Pardo A. Revealing the pathogenic and aging-related mechanisms of the enigmatic idiopathic pulmonary fibrosis. an integral model. *Am J Respir Crit Care Med.* (2014) **189**:1161–72. doi: 10.1164/rccm.201312-2221PP
14. Bouros D, Tzouvelekis A. Idiopathic pulmonary fibrosis: on the move. *Lancet Respir Med.* (2014) **2**:17–9. doi: 10.1016/S2213-2600(13)70240-6
15. Karampitsakos T, Tzilas V, Tringidou R, Steiropoulos P, Aidinis V, Papiris SA, et al. Lung cancer in patients with idiopathic pulmonary fibrosis. *Pulm Pharmacol Ther.* (2017) **45**:1–10. doi: 10.1016/j.pupt.2017.03.016
16. Yu G, Tzouvelekis A, Wang R, Herazo-Maya JD, Ibarra GH, Srivastava A, et al. Thyroid hormone inhibits lung fibrosis in mice by improving epithelial mitochondrial function. *Nat Med.* (2018) **24**:39–49. doi: 10.1038/nm.4447
17. Herazo-Maya JD, Sun J, Molyneaux PL, Li Q, Villalba JA, Tzouvelekis A, et al. Validation of a 52-gene risk profile for outcome prediction in patients with idiopathic pulmonary fibrosis: an international, multicentre, cohort study. *Lancet Respir Med.* (2017) **5**:857–68. doi: 10.1016/S2213-2600(17)30349-1
18. Luzina IG, Todd NW, Iacono AT, Atamas SP. Roles of T lymphocytes in pulmonary fibrosis. *J Leukoc Biol.* (2008) **83**:237–44. doi: 10.1189/jlb.0707504
19. Idiopathic Pulmonary Fibrosis Clinical Research N, Raghu G, Anstrom KJ, King TE Jr, Lasky JA, Martinez FJ. Prednisone, azathioprine, and N-acetylcysteine for pulmonary fibrosis. *N Engl J Med.* (2012) **366**:1968–77. doi: 10.1056/NEJMoa1113354
20. Antoniou KM, Nicholson AG, Dimadi M, Malagari K, Latsi P, Rapti A, et al. Long-term clinical effects of interferon gamma-1b and colchicine in idiopathic pulmonary fibrosis. *Eur Respir J.* (2006) **28**:496–504. doi: 10.1183/09031936.06.00032605
21. Raghu G, Brown KK, Bradford WZ, Starko K, Noble PW, Schwartz DA, et al. A placebo-controlled trial of interferon gamma-1b in patients with idiopathic pulmonary fibrosis. *N Engl J Med.* (2004) **350**:125–133. doi: 10.1056/NEJMoa030511
22. Fletcher S, Jones MG, Spinks K, Sgalla G, Marshall BG, Limbrey R, et al. The safety of new drug treatments for idiopathic pulmonary fibrosis. *Expert Opin Drug Saf.* (2016) **15**:1483–9. doi: 10.1080/14740338.2016.1218470
23. Richeldi L, Costabel U, Selman M, Kim DS, Hansell DM, Nicholson AG, et al. Efficacy of a tyrosine kinase inhibitor in idiopathic pulmonary fibrosis. *N Engl J Med.* (2011) **365**:1079–87. doi: 10.1056/NEJMoa1103690
24. Wuyts WA, Agostini C, Antoniou KM, Bouros D, Chambers RC, Cottin V, et al. The pathogenesis of pulmonary fibrosis: a moving target. *Eur Respir J.* (2013) **41**:1207–18. doi: 10.1183/09031936.00073012
25. Kolb M, Bonella F, Wollin L. Therapeutic targets in idiopathic pulmonary fibrosis. *Respir Med.* (2017) **131**:49–57. doi: 10.1016/j.rmed.2017.07.062
26. King TE, Bradford WZ, Castro-Bernardini S, Fagan EA, Glaspole I, Glassberg MK, et al. phase 3 trial of pirfenidone in patients with idiopathic pulmonary fibrosis. *N Engl J Med.* (2014) **370**:2083–92. doi: 10.1056/NEJMoa14 02582
27. Richeldi L, du Bois RM, Raghu G, Azuma A, Brown KK, Costabel U, et al. Efficacy and safety of nintedanib in idiopathic pulmonary fibrosis. *N Engl J Med.* (2014) **370**:2071–82. doi: 10.1056/NEJMoa1402584
28. Tzouvelekis A, Karampitsakos T, Kontou M, Granitsas A, Malliou I, Anagnostopoulos A, et al. Safety and efficacy of nintedanib in idiopathic pulmonary fibrosis: a real-life observational study. *Pulm Pharmacol Ther.* (2018) **49**:61–6. doi: 10.1016/j.pupt.2018.01.006
29. Tzouvelekis A, Karampitsakos T, Ntolios P, et al. Longitudinal "real-world" outcomes of pirfenidone in idiopathic pulmonary fibrosis in Greece. *Front Med.* (2017) **4**:213. doi: 10.3389/fmed.2017.00213
30. Tzouvelekis A, Ntolios P, Karampitsakos T, Tzilas V, Anevlavis S, Bouros E, et al. Safety and efficacy of pirfenidone in severe Idiopathic Pulmonary Fibrosis: a real-world observational study. *Pulm Pharmacol Ther.* (2017) **46**:48–53. doi: 10.1016/j.pupt.2017.08.011
31. Tzouvelekis A, Bonella F, Spagnolo P. Update on therapeutic management of idiopathic pulmonary fibrosis. *Ther Clin Risk Manag.* (2015) **11**:359–370. doi: 10.2147/TCRM.S69716
32. Tzouvelekis A, Spagnolo P, Bonella F, Vancheri C, Tzilas V, Crestani B, et al. Patients with IPF and lung cancer: diagnosis and management. *Lancet Respir Med.* (2017) **6**:86–8. doi: 10.1016/S2213-2600(17)30478-2
33. Tzouvelekis A, Spagnolo P, Bonella F, Vancheri C, Tzilas V, Crestani B, et al. Combination therapy: the future of management for idiopathic pulmonary fibrosis? *Lancet Respir Med.* (2014) **2**:933–42. doi: 10.1016/S2213-2600(14)70232-2
34. Turner L. ClinicalTrials.gov, stem cells and 'pay-to-participate' clinical studies. *Regen Med.* (2017) **12**:705–19. doi: 10.2217/rme-2017-0015
35. Schuleri KH, Feigenbaum GS, Centola M, Weiss ES, Zimmet JM, Turney J, et al. Autologous mesenchymal stem cells produce reverse remodelling in chronic ischaemic cardiomyopathy. *Eur Heart J.* (2009) **30**:2722–32. doi: 10.1093/eurheartj/ehp265
36. Miyahara Y, Nagaya N, Kataoka M, Yanagawa B, Tanaka K, Hao H, et al. Monolayered mesenchymal stem cells repair scarred myocardium after myocardial infarction. *Nat Med.* (2006) **12**:459–65. doi: 10.1038/nm1391
37. Hare JM, Traverse JH, Henry TD, Dib N, Strumpf RK, Schulman SP, et al. A randomized, double-blind, placebo-controlled, dose-escalation study of intravenous adult human mesenchymal stem cells (prochymal) after acute myocardial infarction. *J Am Coll Cardiol.* (2009) **54**:2277–86. doi: 10.1016/j.jacc.2009.06.055
38. Heldman AW, DiFede DL, Fishman JE, Zambrano JP, Trachtenberg BH, Karantalis V, et al. Transendocardial mesenchymal stem cells and mononuclear bone marrow cells for ischemic cardiomyopathy: the TAC-HFT randomized trial. *JAMA* (2014) **311**:62–73. doi: 10.1001/jama.2013.282909
39. Ramireddy A, Brodt CR, Mendizabal AM, DiFede DL, Healy C, Goyal V, et al. Effects of transendocardial stem cell injection on ventricular proarrhythmia in patients with ischemic cardiomyopathy: results from the POSEIDON and TAC-HFT trials. *Stem Cells Transl Med.* (2017) **6**:1366–72. doi: 10.1002/sctm.16-0328
40. Németh K, Leelahavanichkul A, Yuen PS, Mayer B, Parmelee A, Doi K, et al. Bone marrow stromal cells attenuate sepsis via prostaglandin E(2)-dependent reprogramming of host macrophages to increase their interleukin-10 production. *Nat Med.* (2009) **15**:42–9. doi: 10.1038/nm.1905
41. Liang J, Zhang H, Hua B, Wang H, Lu L, Shi S, et al. Allogenic mesenchymal stem cells transplantation in refractory systemic lupus erythematosus: a pilot clinical study. *Ann Rheum Dis.* (2010) **69**:1423–29. doi: 10.1136/ard.2009.123463
42. Le Blanc K, Frassoni F, Ball L, Locatelli F, Roelofs H, Lewis I, et al. Mesenchymal stem cells for treatment of steroid-resistant, severe, acute graft-versus-host disease: a phase II study. *Lancet* (2008) **371**:1579–86. doi: 10.1016/S0140-6736(08)60690-X
43. Lee RH, Seo MJ, Reger RL, Spees JL, Pulin AA, Olson SD, et al. Multipotent stromal cells from human marrow home to and promote repair of pancreatic islets and renal glomeruli in diabetic NOD/scid mice. *Proc Natl Acad Sci USA.* (2006) **103**:17438–43. doi: 10.1073/pnas.0608249103
44. Parekkadan B, van Poll D, Suganuma K, Carter EA, Berthiaume F, Tilles AW, et al. Mesenchymal stem cell-derived molecules reverse fulminant hepatic failure. *PLoS ONE* (2007) **2**:e941. doi: 10.1371/journal.pone.0000941
45. Ishizawa K, Kubo H, Yamada M, Kobayashi S, Numasaki M, Ueda S, et al. Bone marrow-derived cells contribute to lung regeneration after elastase-induced pulmonary emphysema. *FEBS Lett.* (2004) **556**:249–52. doi: 10.1016/S0014-5793(03)01399-1
46. Spees JL, Pociask DA, Sullivan DE, Whitney MJ, Lasky JA, Prockop DJ, et al. Engraftment of bone marrow progenitor cells in a rat model of asbestos-induced pulmonary fibrosis. *Am J Respir Crit Care Med.* (2007) **176**:385–94. doi: 10.1164/rccm.200607-1004OC
47. Spees JL, Whitney MJ, Sullivan DE, Lasky JA, Laboy M, Ylostalo J, et al. Bone marrow progenitor cells contribute to repair and remodeling of the lung and heart in a rat model of progressive pulmonary hypertension. *FASEB J.* (2008) **22**:1226–36. doi: 10.1096/fj.07-8076com
48. Bonfield TL, Koloze M, Lennon DP, Zuchowski B, Yang SE, Caplan AI. Human mesenchymal stem cells suppress chronic airway inflammation in

the murine ovalbumin asthma model. *Am J Physiol Lung Cell Mol Physiol.* (2010) **299**:L760–70. doi: 10.1152/ajplung.00182.2009

49. Rojas M, Xu J, Woods CR, Mora AL, Spears W, Roman J, et al. Bone marrow-derived mesenchymal stem cells in repair of the injured lung. *Am J Respir Cell Mol Biol.* (2005) **33**:145–52. doi: 10.1165/rcmb.2004-0330OC
50. Matthay MA, Thompson BT, Read EJ, McKenna DH, Liu KD, Calfee CS, et al. Therapeutic potential of mesenchymal stem cells for severe acute lung injury. *Chest* (2010) **138**:965–972. doi: 10.1378/chest.10-0518
51. Lim R, Milton P, Murphy SV, Dickinson H, Chan ST, Jenkin G. Human mesenchymal stem cells reduce lung injury in immunocompromised mice but not in immunocompetent mice. *Respiration* (2013) **85**:332–41. doi: 10.1159/000343078
52. Lee JW, Fang X, Gupta N, Serikov V, Matthay MA. Allogeneic human mesenchymal stem cells for treatment of *E. coli* endotoxin-induced acute lung injury in the ex vivo perfused human lung. *Proc Natl Acad Sci USA.* (2009) **106**:16357–62. doi: 10.1073/pnas.0907996106
53. Wilson JG, Liu KD, Zhuo H, Caballero L, McMillan M, Fang X, et al. Mesenchymal stem (stromal) cells for treatment of ARDS: a phase 1 clinical trial. *Lancet Respir Med.* (2015) **3**:24–32. doi: 10.1016/S2213-2600(14)70291-7
54. Bourin P, Bunnell BA, Casteilla L, Dominici M, Katz AJ, March KL, et al. Stromal cells from the adipose tissue-derived stromal vascular fraction and culture expanded adipose tissue-derived stromal/stem cells: a joint statement of the International Federation for Adipose Therapeutics and Science (IFATS) and the International Society for Cellular Therapy (ISCT). *Cytotherapy* (2013) **15**:641–8. doi: 10.1016/j.jcyt.2013.02.006
55. Shigemura N, Okumura M, Mizuno S, Imanishi Y, Nakamura T, Sawa Y. Autologous transplantation of adipose tissue-derived stromal cells ameliorates pulmonary emphysema. *Am J Transplant.* (2006) **6**:2592–600. doi: 10.1111/j.1600-6143.2006.01522.x
56. Ortiz LA, Gambelli F, McBride C, Gaupp D, Baddoo M, Kaminski N, et al. Mesenchymal stem cell engraftment in lung is enhanced in response to bleomycin exposure and ameliorates its fibrotic effects. *Proc Natl Acad Sci USA.* (2003) **100**:8407–11. doi: 10.1073/pnas.1432929100
57. Loebinger MR, Janes SM. Stem cells as vectors for antitumour therapy. *Thorax* (2010) **65**:362–9. doi: 10.1136/thx.2009.128025
58. Selman M, King TE, Pardo A. Idiopathic pulmonary fibrosis: prevailing and evolving hypotheses about its pathogenesis and implications for therapy. *Ann Intern Med.* (2001) **134**:136–51. doi: 10.7326/0003-4819-134-2-200101160-00015
59. Michaelson JE, Aguayo SM, Roman J. Idiopathic pulmonary fibrosis: a practical approach for diagnosis and management. *Chest* (2000) **118**:788–94. doi: 10.1378/chest.118.3.788
60. Karampitsakos T, Tzouvelekis A, Chrysikos S, Bouros D, Tsangaris I, Fares WH. Pulmonary hypertension in patients with interstitial lung disease. *Pulm Pharmacol Ther.* (2018) **50**:38–46. doi: 10.1016/j.pupt.2018.03.002
61. Papaioannou O, Karampitsakos T, Barbayianni I, Chrysikos S, Xylourgidis N, Tzilas V, et al. Metabolic disorders in chronic lung diseases. *Front Med.* (2017) **4**:246. doi: 10.3389/fmed.2017.00246
62. Bagnato G, Harari S. Cellular interactions in the pathogenesis of interstitial lung diseases. *Eur Respir Rev.* (2015) **24**:102–14. doi: 10.1183/09059180.00003214
63. Wolters PJ, Collard HR, Jones KD. Pathogenesis of idiopathic pulmonary fibrosis. *Annu Rev Pathol.* (2014) **9**:157–79. doi: 10.1146/annurev-pathol-012513-104706
64. Reddy M, Fonseca L, Gowda S, Chougule B, Hari A, Totey S. Human adipose-derived mesenchymal stem cells attenuate early stage of bleomycin induced pulmonary fibrosis: comparison with pirfenidone. *Int J Stem Cells* (2016) **9**:192–206. doi: 10.15283/ijsc16041
65. Toonkel RL, Hare JM, Matthay MA, Glassberg MK. Mesenchymal stem cells and idiopathic pulmonary fibrosis. Potential for clinical testing. *Am J Respir Crit Care Med.* (2013) **188**:133–40. doi: 10.1164/rccm.201207-1204PP
66. Liang J, Zhang Y, Xie T, Liu N, Chen H, Geng Y, et al. Hyaluronan and TLR4 promote surfactant-protein-C-positive alveolar progenitor cell renewal and prevent severe pulmonary fibrosis in mice. *Nat Med.* (2016) **22**:1285–93. doi: 10.1038/nm.4192
67. Allen RJ, Porte J, Braybrooke R, Flores C, Fingerlin TE, Oldham JM, et al. Genetic variants associated with susceptibility to idiopathic pulmonary fibrosis in people of European ancestry: a genome-wide association study. *Lancet Respir Med.* (2017) **5**:869–80. doi: 10.1016/S2213-2600(17)30387-9
68. Gupta N, Su X, Popov B, Lee JW, Serikov V, Matthay MA. Intrapulmonary delivery of bone marrow-derived mesenchymal stem cells improves survival and attenuates endotoxin-induced acute lung injury in mice. *J Immunol.* (2007) **179**:1855–63. doi: 10.4049/jimmunol.179.3.1855
69. Srour N, Thebaud B. Mesenchymal stromal cells in animal bleomycin pulmonary fibrosis models: a systematic review. *Stem Cells Transl Med.* (2015) **4**:1500–10. doi: 10.5966/sctm.2015-0121
70. Gazdhar A, Susuri N, Hostettler K, Gugger M, Knudsen L, Roth M, et al. HGF expressing stem cells in usual interstitial pneumonia originate from the bone marrow and are antifibrotic. *PLoS ONE* (2013) **8**:e65453. doi: 10.1371/journal.pone.0065453
71. Moodley Y, Atienza D, Manuelpillai U, Samuel CS, Tchongue J, Ilancheran S, et al. Human umbilical cord mesenchymal stem cells reduce fibrosis of bleomycin-induced lung injury. *Am J Pathol.* (2009) **175**:303–13. doi: 10.2353/ajpath.2009.080629
72. Aguilar S, Scotton CJ, McNulty K, Nye E, Stamp G, Laurent G, et al. Bone marrow stem cells expressing keratinocyte growth factor via an inducible lentivirus protects against bleomycin-induced pulmonary fibrosis. *PLoS ONE* (2009) **4**:e8013. doi: 10.1371/journal.pone.0008013
73. Cargnoni A, Gibelli L, Tosini A, Signoroni PB, Nassuato C, Arienti D, et al. Transplantation of allogeneic and xenogeneic placenta-derived cells reduces bleomycin-induced lung fibrosis. *Cell Transplant* (2009) **18**:405–22. doi: 10.3727/096368909788809857
74. Ono M, Ohkouchi S, Kanehira M, Tode N, Kobayashi M, Ebina M, et al. Mesenchymal stem cells correct inappropriate epithelial-mesenchyme relation in pulmonary fibrosis using stanniocalcin-1. *Mol Ther.* (2015) **23**:549–60. doi: 10.1038/mt.2014.217
75. Zhao F, Zhang YF, Liu YG, Zhou JJ, Li ZK, Wu CG, et al. Therapeutic effects of bone marrow-derived mesenchymal stem cells engraftment on bleomycin-induced lung injury in rats. *Transplant Proc.* (2008) **40**:1700–5. doi: 10.1016/j.transproceed.2008.01.080
76. Lee SH, Lee EJ, Lee SY, Kim JH, Shim JJ, Shin C, et al. The effect of adipose stem cell therapy on pulmonary fibrosis induced by repetitive intratracheal bleomycin in mice. *Exp Lung Res.* (2014) **40**:117–25. doi: 10.3109/01902148.2014.881930
77. Garcia O, Carraro G, Turcatel G, Hall M, Sedrakyan S, Roche T, et al. Amniotic fluid stem cells inhibit the progression of bleomycin-induced pulmonary fibrosis via CCL2 modulation in bronchoalveolar lavage. *PLoS ONE* (2013) **8**:e71679. doi: 10.1371/journal.pone.0071679
78. Huang K, Kang X, Wang X, Wu S, Xiao J, Li Z, et al. Conversion of bone marrow mesenchymal stem cells into type II alveolar epithelial cells reduces pulmonary fibrosis by decreasing oxidative stress in rats. *Mol Med Rep.* (2015) **11**:1685–92. doi: 10.3892/mmr.2014.2981
79. Jun D, Garat C, West J, Thorn N, Chow K, Cleaver T, et al. The pathology of bleomycin-induced fibrosis is associated with loss of resident lung mesenchymal stem cells that regulate effector T-cell proliferation. *Stem Cells* (2011) **29**:725–35. doi: 10.1002/stem.604
80. Kumamoto M, Nishiwaki T, Matsuo N, Kimura H, Matsushima K. Minimally cultured bone marrow mesenchymal stem cells ameliorate fibrotic lung injury. *Eur Respir J.* (2009) **34**:740–48. doi: 10.1183/09031936.00128508
81. Lee SH, Jang AS, Kim YE, Cha JY, Kim TH, Jung S, et al. Modulation of cytokine and nitric oxide by mesenchymal stem cell transfer in lung injury/fibrosis. *Respir Res.* (2010) **11**:16. doi: 10.1186/1465-9921-11-16
82. Perez JR, Lee S, Ybarra N, Maria O, Serban M, Jeyaseelan K, et al. A comparative analysis of longitudinal computed tomography and histopathology for evaluating the potential of mesenchymal stem cells in mitigating radiation-induced pulmonary fibrosis. *Sci Rep.* (2017) **7**:9056. doi: 10.1038/s41598-017-09021-7
83. Min F, Gao F, Li Q, Liu Z. Therapeutic effect of human umbilical cord mesenchymal stem cells modified by angiotensin-converting enzyme 2 gene on bleomycin-induced lung fibrosis injury. *Mol Med Rep.* (2015) **11**:2387–96. doi: 10.3892/mmr.2014.3025
84. Moodley Y, Vaghjiani V, Chan J, Baltic S, Ryan M, Tchongue J, et al. Anti-inflammatory effects of adult stem cells in sustained lung injury: a comparative study. *PLoS ONE* (2013) **8**:e69299. doi: 10.1371/journal.pone.0069299

85. Gao F, Li Q, Hou L, Li Z, Min F, Liu Z. Mesenchymal stem cell-based angiotensin-converting enzyme 2 in treatment of acute lung injury rat induced by bleomycin. *Exp Lung Res.* (2014) **40**:392–403. doi: 10.3109/01902148.2014.938200
86. Min JH, Lee HY, Lim H, Ahn MJ, Park K, Chung MP, et al. Drug-induced interstitial lung disease in tyrosine kinase inhibitor therapy for non-small cell lung cancer: a review on current insight. *Cancer Chemother Pharmacol.* (2011) **68**:1099–109. doi: 10.1007/s00280-011-1737-2
87. Li F, Han F, Li H, Zhang J, Qiao X, Shi J, et al. Human placental mesenchymal stem cells of fetal origins-alleviated inflammation and fibrosis by attenuating MyD88 signaling in bleomycin-induced pulmonary fibrosis mice. *Mol Immunol.* (2017) **90**:11–21. doi: 10.1016/j.molimm.2017.06.032
88. Ni S, Wang D, Qiu X, Pang L, Song Z, Guo K. Bone marrow mesenchymal stem cells protect against bleomycin-induced pulmonary fibrosis in rat by activating Nrf2 signaling. *Int J Clin Exp Pathol.* (2015) **8**:7752–61.
89. Lan YW, Choo KB, Chen CM, Hung TH, Chen YB, Hsieh CH, et al. Hypoxia-preconditioned mesenchymal stem cells attenuate bleomycin-induced pulmonary fibrosis. *Stem Cell Res Ther.* (2015) **6**:97. doi: 10.1186/s13287-015-0081-6
90. Hostettler KE, Gazdhar A, Khan P, Savic S, Tamo L, Lardinois D, et al. Multipotent mesenchymal stem cells in lung fibrosis. *PLoS ONE* (2017) **12**:e0181946. doi: 10.1371/journal.pone.0181946
91. Tashiro J, Rubio GA, Limper AH, Williams K, Elliot SJ, Ninou I, et al. Exploring animal models that resemble idiopathic pulmonary fibrosis. *Front Med.* (2017) **4**:118. doi: 10.3389/fmed.2017.00118
92. Ortiz LA, Dutreil M, Fattman C, Pandey AC, Torres G, Go K, et al. Interleukin 1 receptor antagonist mediates the antiinflammatory and antifibrotic effect of mesenchymal stem cells during lung injury. *Proc Natl Acad Sci USA.* (2007) **104**:11002–7. doi: 10.1073/pnas.0704421104
93. Foskett AM, Bazhanov N, Ti X, Tiblow A, Bartosh TJ, Prockop DJ. Phase-directed therapy: TSG-6 targeted to early inflammation improves bleomycin-injured lungs. *Am J Physiol Lung Cell Mol Physiol.* (2014) **306**:L120–31. doi: 10.1152/ajplung.00240.2013
94. Hecker L, Logsdon NJ, Kurundkar D, Kurundkar A, Bernard K, Hock T, et al. Reversal of persistent fibrosis in aging by targeting Nox4-Nrf2 redox imbalance. *Sci Transl Med.* (2014) **6**:231ra247. doi: 10.1126/scitranslmed.3008182
95. Lan YW, Theng SM, Huang TT, Choo KB, Chen CM, Kuo HP, et al. Oncostatin M-preconditioned mesenchymal stem cells alleviate bleomycin-induced pulmonary fibrosis through paracrine effects of the hepatocyte growth factor. *Stem Cells Transl Med.* (2017) **6**:1006–17. doi: 10.5966/sctm.2016-0054
96. Germano D, Blyszczuk P, Valaperti A, Kania G, Dirnhofer S, Landmesser U, et al. Prominin-1/CD133+ lung epithelial progenitors protect from bleomycin-induced pulmonary fibrosis. *Am J Respir Crit Care Med.* (2009) **179**:939–49. doi: 10.1164/rccm.200809-1390OC
97. Ahmad T, Mukherjee S, Pattnaik B, Kumar M, Singh S, Kumar M, et al. Miro1 regulates intercellular mitochondrial transport & enhances mesenchymal stem cell rescue efficacy. *EMBO J.* (2014) **33**:994–1010. doi: 10.1002/embj.201386030
98. Morrison TJ, Jackson MV, Cunningham EK, Kissenpfennig A, McAuley DF, O'Kane CM, et al. Mesenchymal stromal cells modulate macrophages in clinically relevant lung injury models by extracellular vesicle mitochondrial transfer. *Am J Respir Crit Care Med.* (2017) **196**:1275–86. doi: 10.1164/rccm.201701-0170OC
99. Ntolios P, Janes SM. Mesenchymal stem cell therapy for lung diseases: oasis or mirage? *Respiration* (2013) **85**:279–280. doi: 10.1159/000346642
100. Tzouvelekis A, Bouros D. Steep barriers to overcome for successful application of stem cell treatment in patients with idiopathic pulmonary fibrosis. *Am J Respir Crit Care Med.* (2013) **188**:251–2. doi: 10.1164/rccm.201301-0072LE
101. Alvarez D, Levine M, Rojas M. Regenerative medicine in the treatment of idiopathic pulmonary fibrosis: current position. *Stem Cells Cloning* (2015) **8**:61–65. doi: 10.2147/SCCAA.S49801
102. Barczyk M, Schmidt M, Mattoli S. Stem cell-based therapy in idiopathic pulmonary fibrosis. *Stem Cell Rev.* (2015) **11**:598–620. doi: 10.1007/s12015-015-9587-7
103. Tzouvelekis A, Paspaliaris V, Koliakos G, Ntolios P, Bouros E, Oikonomou A, et al. A prospective, non-randomized, no placebo-controlled, phase Ib clinical trial to study the safety of the adipose derived stromal cells-stromal vascular fraction in idiopathic pulmonary fibrosis. *J Transl Med.* (2013) **11**:171. doi: 10.1186/1479-5876-11-171
104. Tzouvelekis A, Ntolios P, Bouros D. Stem cell treatment for chronic lung diseases. *Respiration* (2013) **85**:179–192. doi: 10.1159/000346525
105. Glassberg MK, Minkiewicz J, Toonkel RL, Simonet ES, Rubio GA, DiFede D, et al. Allogeneic human mesenchymal stem cells in patients with idiopathic pulmonary fibrosis via intravenous delivery (AETHER): a phase I safety clinical trial. *Chest* (2017) **151**:971–81. doi: 10.1016/j.chest.2016.10.061
106. Glassberg MK, Toonkel RL. Moving stem cell therapy to patients with idiopathic pulmonary fibrosis. *Respirology* (2014) **19**:950–51. doi: 10.1111/resp.12364
107. Limper AH. Safety of IV human mesenchymal stem cells in patients with idiopathic pulmonary fibrosis. *Chest* (2017) **151**:951–2. doi: 10.1016/j.chest.2016.12.015
108. Glassberg MK, Hare JM, Toonkel RL, Matthay MA. Reply: idiopathic pulmonary fibrosis: a degenerative disease requiring a regenerative approach. *Am J Respir Crit Care Med.* (2013) **188**:253–4. doi: 10.1164/rccm.201302-0244LE
109. Chambers DC, Enever D, Ilic N, Sparks L, Whitelaw K, Ayres J, et al. A phase 1b study of placenta-derived mesenchymal stromal cells in patients with idiopathic pulmonary fibrosis. *Respirology* (2014) **19**:1013–8. doi: 10.1111/resp.12343
110. Weiss DJ, Casaburi R, Flannery R, LeRoux-Williams M, Tashkin DP. A placebo-controlled, randomized trial of mesenchymal stem cells in COPD. *Chest* (2013) **143**:1590–8. doi: 10.1378/chest.12-2094
111. Tzouvelekis A, Laurent G, Bouros D. Stem cell therapy in chronic obstructive pulmonary disease. Seeking the Prometheus effect. *Curr Drug Targets* (2013) **14**:246–52. doi: 10.2174/1389450111314020009
112. Hare JM, Fishman JE, Gerstenblith G, DiFede Velazquez DL, Zambrano JP, Suncion VY, et al. Comparison of allogeneic vs autologous bone marrow-derived mesenchymal stem cells delivered by transendocardial injection in patients with ischemic cardiomyopathy: the POSEIDON randomized trial. *JAMA* (2012) **308**:2369–79. doi: 10.1001/jama.2012.25321
113. Ntolios P, Manoloudi E, Tzouvelekis A, Bouros E, Steiropoulos P, Anevlavis S, et al. Longitudinal outcomes of patients enrolled in a phase Ib clinical trial of the adipose-derived stromal cells-stromal vascular fraction in idiopathic pulmonary fibrosis. *Clin Respir J.* (2018). doi: 10.1111/crj.12777. [Epub ahead of print].
114. Tzouvelekis A, Koliakos G, Ntolios P, Baira I, Bouros E, Oikonomou A, et al. Stem cell therapy for idiopathic pulmonary fibrosis: a protocol proposal. *J Transl Med.* (2011) **9**:182. doi: 10.1186/1479-5876-9-182
115. Raghu G, Collard HR, Anstrom KJ, Flaherty KR, Fleming TR, King TE, et al. Idiopathic pulmonary fibrosis: clinically meaningful primary endpoints in phase 3 clinical trials. *Am J Respir Crit Care Med* (2012) **185**:1044–1048. doi: 10.1164/rccm.201201-0006PP
116. Yang T, Jia Y, Ma Y, Cao L, Chen X, Qiao B. Comparative proteomic analysis of bleomycin-induced pulmonary fibrosis based on isobaric tag for quantitation. *Am J Med Sci.* (2017) **353**:49–58. doi: 10.1016/j.amjms.2016.11.021
117. Jenkins RG, Moore BB, Chambers RC, Eickelberg O, Königshoff M, Kolb M, et al. An Official American Thoracic Society Workshop Report: use of animal models for the preclinical assessment of potential therapies for pulmonary fibrosis. *Am J Respir Cell Mol Biol.* (2017) **56**:667–79. doi: 10.1165/rcmb.2017-0096ST
118. Tashiro J, Elliot SJ, Gerth DJ, Xia X, Pereira-Simon S, Choi R, et al. Therapeutic benefits of young, but not old, adipose-derived mesenchymal stem cells in a chronic mouse model of bleomycin-induced pulmonary fibrosis. *Transl Res.* (2015) **166**:554–567. doi: 10.1016/j.trsl.2015.09.004
119. du Bois RM, Weycker D, Albera C, Bradford WZ, Costabel U, Kartashov A, et al. Ascertainment of individual risk of mortality for patients with idiopathic pulmonary fibrosis. *Am J Respir Crit Care Med.* (2011) **184**:459–66. doi: 10.1164/rccm.201011-1790OC
120. Flaherty KR, Mumford JA, Murray S, Kazerooni EA, Gross BH, Colby TV, et al. Prognostic implications of physiologic and radiographic changes

in idiopathic interstitial pneumonia. *Am J Respir Crit Care Med.* (2003) **168**:543–8. doi: 10.1164/rccm.200209-1112OC

121. Zappala CJ, Latsi PI, Nicholson AG, Colby TV, Cramer D, Renzoni EA, et al. Marginal decline in forced vital capacity is associated with a poor outcome in idiopathic pulmonary fibrosis. *Eur Respir J.* (2010) **35**:830–6. doi: 10.1183/09031936.00155108
122. Collard HR, King TE, Bartelson BB, Vourlekis JS, Schwarz MI, Brown KK. Changes in clinical and physiologic variables predict survival in idiopathic pulmonary fibrosis. *Am J Respir Crit Care Med.* (2003) **168**:538–42. doi: 10.1164/rccm.200211-1311OC
123. du Bois RM, Nathan SD, Richeldi L, Schwarz MI, Noble PW. Idiopathic pulmonary fibrosis: lung function is a clinically meaningful endpoint for phase III trials. *Am J Respir Crit Care Med.* (2012) **186**:712–5. doi: 10.1164/rccm.201206-1010PP
124. Nathan SD, du Bois RM, Albera C, Bradford WZ, Costabel U, Kartashov A, et al. Validation of test performance characteristics and minimal clinically important difference of the 6-minute walk test in patients with idiopathic pulmonary fibrosis. *Respir Med.* (2015) **109**:914–22. doi: 10.1016/j.rmed.2015.04.008
125. du Bois RM, Weycker D, Albera C, Bradford WZ, Costabel U, Kartashov A, et al. Six-minute-walk test in idiopathic pulmonary fibrosis: test validation and minimal clinically important difference. *Am J Respir Crit Care Med.* (2011) **183**:1231–7. doi: 10.1164/rccm.201007-1179OC
126. Heresi GA, Dweik RA. Strengths and limitations of the six-minute-walk test: a model biomarker study in idiopathic pulmonary fibrosis. *Am J Respir Crit Care Med.* (2011) **183**:1122–4. doi: 10.1164/rccm.201012-2079ED
127. Richeldi L, Ryerson CJ, Lee JS, Wolters PJ, Koth LL, Ley B, et al. Relative versus absolute change in forced vital capacity in idiopathic pulmonary fibrosis. *Thorax* (2012) **67**:407–11. doi: 10.1136/thoraxjnl-2011-201184
128. du Bois RM, Weycker D, Albera C, Bradford WZ, Costabel U, Kartashov A, et al. Forced vital capacity in patients with idiopathic pulmonary fibrosis: test properties and minimal clinically important difference. *Am J Respir Crit Care Med.* (2011) **184**:1382–9. doi: 10.1164/rccm.201105-0840OC
129. Ley B, Bradford WZ, Weycker D, Vittinghoff E, du Bois RM, Collard HR. Unified baseline and longitudinal mortality prediction in idiopathic pulmonary fibrosis. *Eur Respir J.* (2015) **45**:1374–81. doi: 10.1183/09031936.00146314
130. Ikonomou L, Panoskaltsis-Mortari A, Wagner DE, Freishtat RJ, Weiss DJ Unproven stem cell treatments for lung disease-an emerging public health problem. *Am J Respir Crit Care Med.* (2017) **195**:P13–4. doi: 10.1164/rccm.201607-1461ED
131. Turner L, Knoepfler P. Selling Stem Cells in the USA: Assessing the Direct-to-Consumer Industry. *Cell Stem Cell* (2016) **19**:154–7. doi: 10.1016/j.stem.2016.06.007
132. Charo RA, Sipp D. Rejuvenating Regenerative Medicine Regulation. *N Engl J Med.* (2018) **378**:504–5. doi: 10.1056/NEJMp1715736

3

Extracorporeal Membrane Oxygenation Supported Transbronchial Cryobiopsy in the Diagnosis of Severe Organizing Pneumonia

Xiaoyan Zhang[2†], Yuqiong Wang[1,2†], Yingying Feng[2], Ling Zhao[3], Yunxia Zhang[2], Hanbo Yang[4], Bin Xing[2], Wenlin Guo[5], Ting Sun[2], Qingyuan Zhan[2] and Ye Tian[2]*

[1] Peking University China-Japan Friendship School of Clinical Medicine, Beijing, China, [2] Department of Pulmonary and Critical Care Medicine, Center of Respiratory Medicine, National Center for Respiratory Medicine, China-Japan Friendship Hospital, Beijing China, [3] Department of Pathology, China-Japan Friendship Hospital, Beijing, China, [4] Department of Rheumatology, China-Japan Friendship Hospital, Beijing, China, [5] China-Japan Union Hospital of Jilin University, Changchun, China

***Correspondence:**
Ye Tian
tychety@foxmail.com

† These authors have contributed equally to this work and share first authorship

This case report describes a 58-year-old, never-smoking housewife with chief complaints of progressively worsening cough, dyspnea, and intermittent fever, who was initially misdiagnosed with community-acquired pneumonia (CAP). However, her pulse oximetry oxygen saturation continued to decline, and eventually, she underwent an endotracheal intubation. Fortunately, transbronchial cryobiopsy (TBCB) assisted by extracorporeal membrane oxygenation (ECMO) was performed in the most critical situation, and it revealed an organizing pneumonia (OP) pattern. OP describes a histological pattern of acute or subacute pulmonary damage, which may be idiopathic or associated with a known or unknown underlying disease. A definitive diagnosis of OP usually obtained from pathology, and surgical lung biopsy with large lung tissue is recommended. However, since the surgical lung biopsy was not convenient for this patient after mechanical ventilation, bedside TBCB supported by ECMO was selected. To our knowledge, we are the first to report the pathological diagnosis of ECMO assisted TBCB in acute respiratory failure. When oxygenation cannot be maintained after endotracheal intubation and surgical lung biopsy is not feasible, ECMO-supported TBCB may be a good choice to obtain lung tissue for histopathological diagnosis in patients with acute lung injury of unknown etiology.

Keywords: organizing pneumonia, extracorporeal membrane oxygenation, mechanical ventilation, transbronchial cryobiopsy, case report

INTRODUCTION

Organizing pneumonia (OP) describes a histological pattern of acute or subacute pulmonary damage. The first description of OP can be traced back to Lange in 1901 (1). It is a clinical entity (1–3) associated with non-specific clinical manifestations, and is associated with a known or unknown underlying disease, leading to delay in diagnosis, or even misdiagnosis. A definitive diagnosis is usually obtained from lung biopsy because of the unavailability of other specific detection methodologies (4). Corticosteroid treatment represents the standard therapy in OP (5).

In this report, we present the case of a patient who was initially misdiagnosed with community-acquired pneumonia (CAP), and her respiratory failure progressed rapidly. Fortunately, transbronchial cryobiopsy (TBCB), assisted by extracorporeal membrane oxygenation (ECMO), was performed in the most critical situation, and it revealed an OP pattern. TBCB supported by ECMO has improved the pathological diagnosis rate of unexplained acute respiratory failure to a certain extent, which is significant in guiding precise treatment and disease prognosis. This study aims to suggest an alternative approach to the diagnosis of OP in the scenario of an acute respiratory failure.

CASE PRESENTATION

A 58-year-old, never-smoking housewife presented to the Department of Pulmonary and Critical Care Medicine of China-Japan Friendship Hospital with the chief complaints of cough, dyspnea, and intermittent fever. She had a history of leukopenia of unknown origin that was untreated. Chest computed tomography (CT) revealed scattered solid nodules in both lungs, with a fibrous striped shadow in the medial segment of the middle lobe of the right lung and slight enlargement in the left hilum (**Figure 1A**). Though broad-spectrum antibiotics were administered, the patient's clinical status worsened, developing a severe pneumonia with type I respiratory failure and her pulse oximetry oxygen saturation (SpO_2) decreased to 70% while on oxygen delivered at the rate of 5 L/min through a nasal cannulae. The patient was transferred to the intensive care unit (ICU) for close monitoring.

A general physical examination was performed. The patient, who was conscious, displayed the following vital signs: temperature, 38.6°C; pulse rate, 105 bpm; respiratory rate, 35 breaths/min; blood pressure, 118/77 mmHg; oxygen saturation, 93% while on oxygen delivered through a nasal cannulae at a rate of 5 L/min. Chest auscultation revealed raw breathing sounds and wet rales in both lungs. Pitting edema in both lower extremities was found as well. Results of laboratory tests were: white blood cell count 8.54*10^9/L with neutrophil predominance (89.7%); reactive protein > 200mg/L (reference value <10 mg/L); serum procalcitonin 1.67 ng/mL, alanine transaminase 48 U/L, aspartate transaminase 68 U/L. Autoimmune tests including anti-neutrophil antibody (ANA), anti-neutrophil cytoplasmic antibody (ANCA), and rheumatoid factor (RF) were negative. Results of blood culture, 1-3-β-D-glucan (BDG) assay, galactomannan (GM) tests, T-spot, cryptococcal antigen nucleic acid, blood EB virus DNA, cytomegalovirus DNA were negative. Fiberoptic bronchoscopy with bronchoalveolar lavage (BALF) revealed extensive hyperemia and edema in the bronchial mucosa, and no other abnormalities were observed. Fungal cultures were positive for *Candida albicans*. Cultures for bacteria and mycobacteria were negative. All virus, *Mycoplasma pneumoniae*, and Chlamydia nucleic acid amplification tests were negative. No pneumocystis infection was identified and tumor cytology was negative. Contrast-enhanced chest CT revealed patchy areas of ground-glass opacities (GGO) and consolidation in both lungs scattered all over and with slightly enlarged mediastinal lymph nodes (**Figure 1B**).

On ICU day 2, her respiratory status continued to decline, and bedside chest radiographs (**Figure 2A**) showed progression of bilateral infiltrates. Mechanical ventilation (PC mode, FiO_2 100%, F 35/min, PC 18 cmH_2O, PEEP 10 cmH_2O), and venovenous extracorporeal membrane oxygenation (V-V ECMO) were performed to maintain adequate oxyhemoglobin saturation. We delivered an almost constant flow of 6 L/min/m^2 *via* ECMO. A bedside TBCB was performed on the same day to obtain a definitive diagnosis. Three specimens were obtained from the outer and posterior basal segments of the lower lobe of the left lung, and histological examination revealed fibroblasts intermixed with loose connective tissue and collagen in the alveoli and the distal bronchioles (**Figures 3A,B**). These findings were typical of OP (5). Thus, an OP diagnosis was established.

The following day, the patient's treatment was changed to intravenous methylprednisolone in continuous infusion, 240 mg for 3 days, followed by 80 mg for 5 days, and then 40 mg as the maintenance dose. The fever subsided the day after the steroid was given, and her general condition improved significantly. The patient was extubated 4 days after endotracheal intubation and tracheotomized for 24 days. She remained on VV-ECMO for 15 days. Systemic heparinization is required during ECMO treatment. On the one hand, thrombus formation can be seen in front of the ECMO membrane and behind the membrane, and thrombosis can be seen around the PICC tube. On the other hand, the patient developed hemoptysis several times, hematuria, hematoma of abdominal muscle successively. For hemoptysis, we did a bronchoscopy to stop the bleeding. And we adjusted the heparin pump rate according to the APTT target value to prevent massive bleeding. After the patient was withdrawn from ECMO, heparin was stopped, and the hemoptysis was gradually relieved. There was no recurrence of hematuria and no increase in abdominal hematoma. No thrombosis was found in the deep veins of the extremities.

Bedside chest radiographs showed consolidation of both lungs decreased significantly on ICU day 10 (**Figure 2B**). On day 21 after steroid use, her chest radiograph (**Figure 1C**) showed that the consolidation was less than the previous. On day 41 after steroid use, her symptoms and chest radiograph (**Figure 1D**) were indicative of a significant improvement, with complete resolution of pulmonary symptoms.

DISCUSSION

To our knowledge, ECMO-assisted TBCB has never been reported in the pathological diagnosis of acute respiratory failure.

Clinically, patients with OP may have acute or subacute disease progression that may include constitutional symptoms with flu-like illness, including cough, fever, malaise, weight loss, and dyspnea (1, 6). OP may be idiopathic or associated with a known or unknown underlying disease, leading to

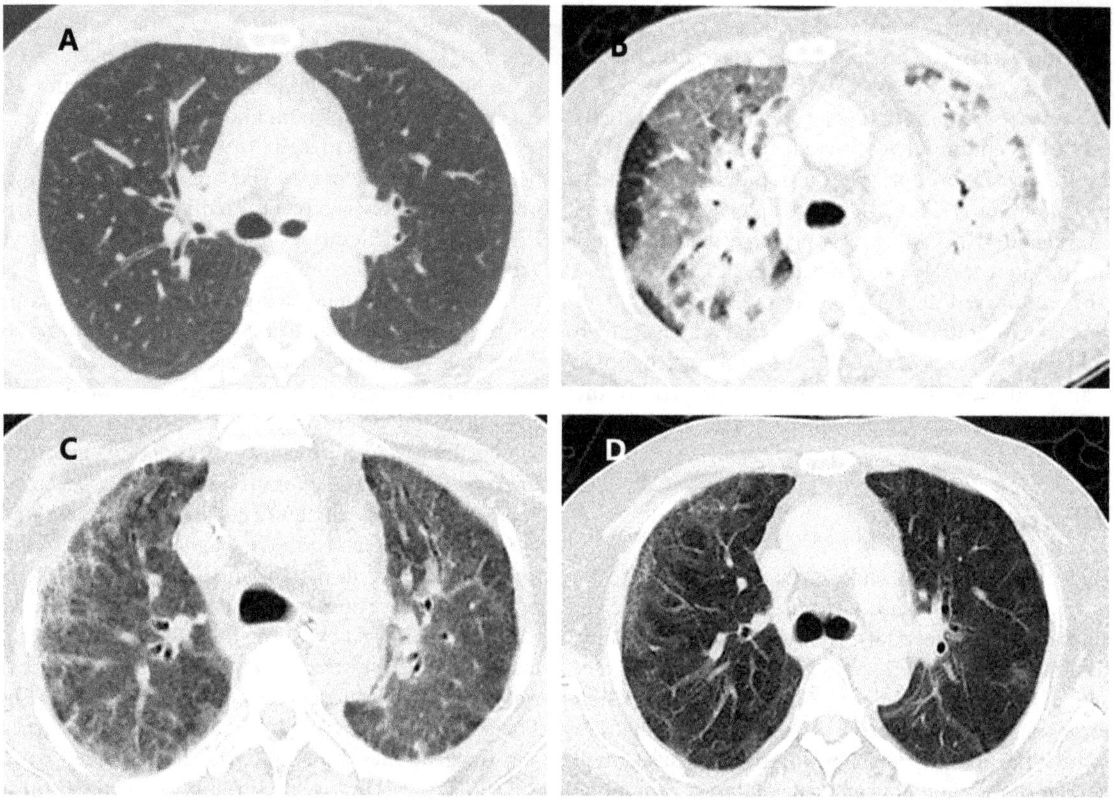

FIGURE 1 | Evolution of the computed tomography (CT) findings of the patient. **(A)** Scattered solid nodules in both lungs, with fibrous stripe shadow in the medial middle lobe of the right lung and slight enlargement in the left hilum; **(B)** patchy areas of ground glass opacities (GGO), consolidation in the double lungs scattered all over both lungs and slightly enlarged mediastinal lymph nodes; **(C)** consolidation and GGO in both lungs decreased compared with the previous one; **(D)** only a small amount of GGO and fibrous stripe shadow.

delay in diagnosis or even misdiagnosis. Similarly, our patient was diagnosed with infectious pneumonia initially and was treated with antibiotics, which may have delayed her early steroid use and led to the eventual progression of her illness. Fortunately, the patient in our case recovered, which may be because ECMO-supported TBCB was decisively performed on this patient, enabling us to develop a pathological diagnosis and use glucocorticoids at the right time.

Obtaining lung tissue for histopathological diagnosis in patients with acute lung injury of unknown etiology is helpful for precision therapy. This is because of the atypical symptoms, non-specific laboratory findings, and variable CT findings associated with OP (7). The patient had undergone ultrasound-guided percutaneous transthoracic needle biopsy in the general ward, but no valuable results were obtained. The failure of the aforementioned procedure was mainly due to the respiratory distress, which made impossible for the patient to hold her breath, resulting in unsatisfactory lung tissue sampling. A study (8) pointed out that it is difficult to diagnose OP based on bronchoscopic biopsy specimens because of its patchy distribution. Methods of obtaining large specimens, such as surgical lung biopsy, are better options for the disease. However, in our case, oxygenation could not be maintained after endotracheal intubation, making surgical lung biopsy even more challenging to perform. In our case, ECMO rendered possible a safe bedside TBCB in an otherwise extremely unstable patient.

Currently, VV-ECMO has been described for managing different lung diseases in the ICU for severe cardiorespiratory failure. However, ECMO-assisted TBCB is rarely reported in the pathological diagnosis of acute respiratory failure. Our patient's deteriorating clinical condition was a major limitation of lung biopsy. Thus, she underwent TBCB with VV-ECMO support as a bridge to diagnosis and treatment. This may show that ECMO-assisted TBCB is feasible for the histopathological diagnosis of acute respiratory failure of unknown cause. ECMO enables biopsy in critically ill patients to find the exact pathological evidence in acute lung injury management.

OP is a unique model of intraalveolar fibrotic inflammation that is fully reversible with treatment (5). However, the disease continued to progress in this case despite receiving 40 mg/day of methylprednisolone outside our hospital for 9 days, perhaps due to the inadequate treatment of steroids. The day after the patient was diagnosed, we administered pulse corticosteroid treatment of methylprednisolone 240 mg/day in continuous infusion for 3 consecutive days and then reduced it to 80 mg/day. We believe that the patient's improvement is largely dependent on appropriate steroid therapy. The standard treatment for

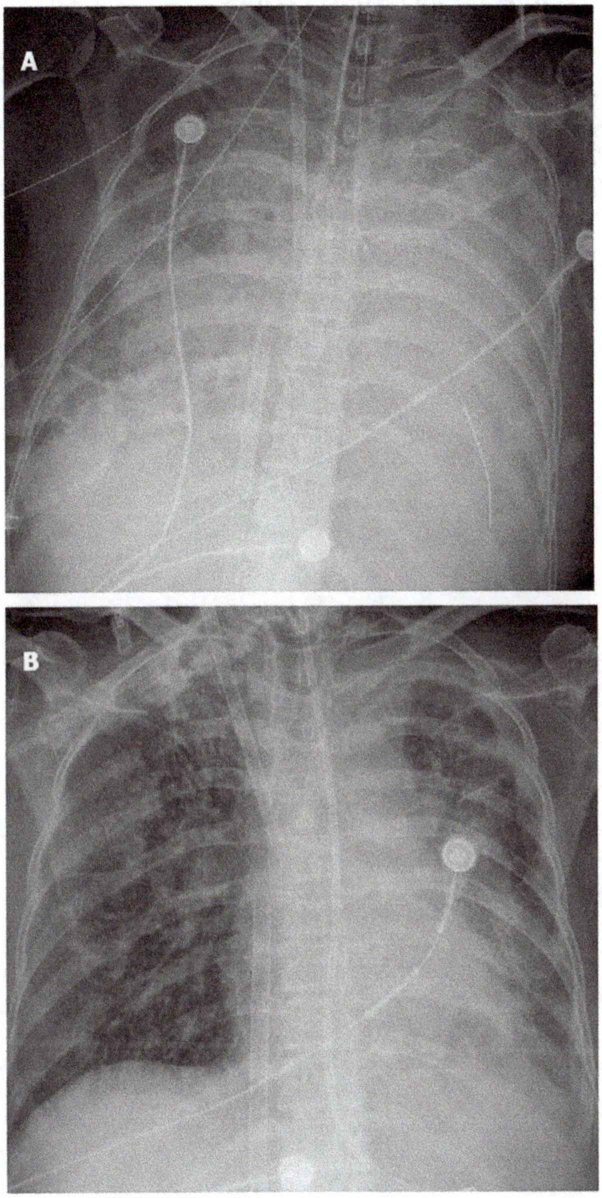

FIGURE 2 | Evolution of the chest X-ray of the patient. **(A)** Extensive consolidation of both lungs; **(B)** consolidation of both lungs decreased significantly.

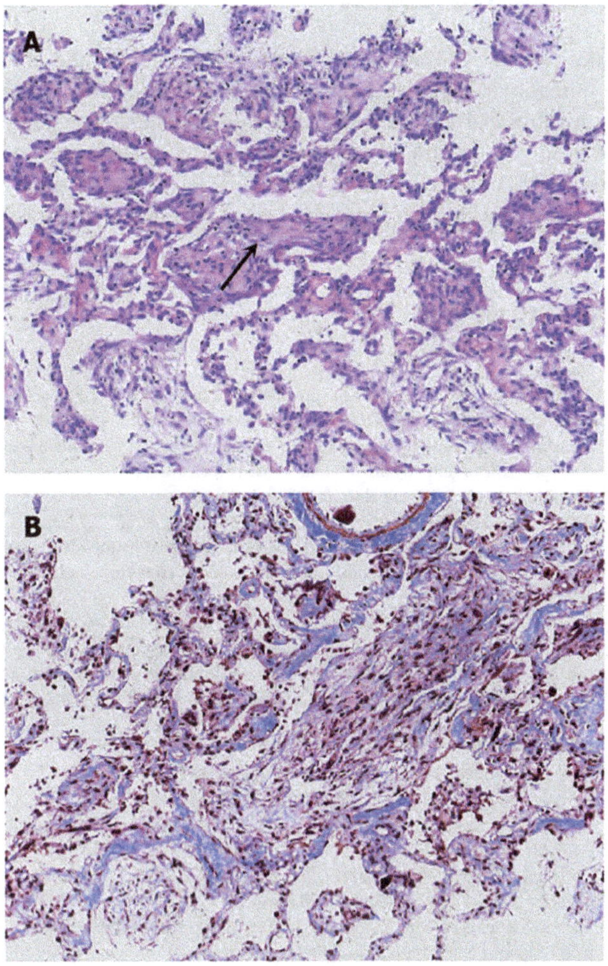

FIGURE 3 | Histological patterns of the patient's lung tissue. **(A)** Hematoxylin-eosin stain revealed the presence of fibroblasts intermixed with loose connective tissue and collagen in the alveoli and the distal bronchioles. **(B)** Masson stain showed a mass of blue collagen fibers stained with aniline blue.

OP has not yet been determined (9–11). For patients with cryptogenic OP, the recommended initial prednisone dose is 0.75 mg/kg/day for 2–4 weeks (12). However, physicians still need to adjust the dose of prednisone based on disease severity and response to therapy. In severe OP, intravenous prednisolone can be administered for 3 consecutive days (13–15) and immunosuppressive therapy with cyclophosphamide, azathioprine, or cyclosporin A can be used (16, 17), especially for acutely ill patients.

In addition, it is important to find the right opportunity to use ECMO and avoid the associated complications. Bleeding and thrombosis are serious complications of ECMO. Dealing with possible complications requires continuous management from relevant experts. One reason for the successful treatment of this patient is that we used ECMO at the right time and cleverly managed its complications.

CONCLUSION

OP is an unusual cause of acute lung injury. Diagnosis is mostly biopsy-proven. When oxygenation cannot be maintained after endotracheal intubation and surgical lung biopsy is not feasible, ECMO-supported TBCB may be a good choice to obtain lung tissue for histopathological diagnosis in patients with acute lung injury of unknown etiology, because ECMO can provide a relatively safe bedside TBCB for extremely unstable patients to avoid delayed diagnosis or even misdiagnosis. However, care should be taken to avoid ECMO-related complications.

ETHICS STATEMENT

Ethical review and approval were not required for the study on human participants in accordance with the local legislation and institutional requirements. The patient provided her written informed consent to participate in this study. Written informed consent was obtained from the individual for the publication of any potentially identifiable images or data included in this article.

AUTHOR CONTRIBUTIONS

YW, XZ, YF, and LZ produced the first draft of the manuscript. YZ, HY, BX, WG, and TS were major contributors in analyzed and interpreted the patient's data. YT, XZ, and QZ were major contributors in writing the manuscript. All authors read, approved the final manuscript, reviewed, edited, and approved the final versions of the submitted manuscript.

REFERENCES

1. Narasimhaiah DH, Chakravorty I, Swamy R, Prakash D. Organising pneumonia presenting as acute life threatening pulmonary haemorrhage. *BMJ Case Rep.* (2011) 2011:bcr0320091689. doi: 10.1136/bcr.03.2009.1689
2. Ding QL, Lv D, Wang BJ, Zhang QL, Yu YM, Sun SF, et al. Macrolide therapy in cryptogenic organizing pneumonia: a case report and literature review. *Exp Ther Med.* (2015) 9:829–34. doi: 10.3892/etm.2015.2183
3. Zhao F, Yan SX, Wang GF, Wang J, Lu PX, Chen B, et al. CT features of focal organizing pneumonia: an analysis of consecutive histopathologically confirmed 45 cases. *Eur J Radiol.* (2014) 83:73–8. doi: 10.1016/j.ejrad.2013.04.017
4. Bradley B, Branley HM, Egan JJ, Greaves MS, Hansell DM, Harrison NK, et al. Interstitial lung disease guideline: the British thoracic society in collaboration with the thoracic society of Australia and New Zealand and the Irish thoracic society. *Thorax.* (2008) 63:v1–58. doi: 10.1136/thx.2008.101691
5. Cottin V, Cordier JF. Cryptogenic organizing pneumonia. *Semin Respir Crit Care Med.* (2012) 33:462–75. doi: 10.1055/s-0032-1325157
6. Saito Z, Kaneko Y, Hasegawa T, Yoshida M, Odashima K, Horikiri T, et al. Predictive factors for relapse of cryptogenic organizing pneumonia. *BMC Pulm Med.* (2019) 19:10. doi: 10.1186/s12890-018-0764-8
7. Cordier JF. Cryptogenic organising pneumonia. *Eur Respir J.* (2006) 28:422–46. doi: 10.1183/09031936.06.00013505
8. Yao HM, Zuo W, Wang XL, Zhang W. Findings on cryptogenic organizing pneumonia: a case report and literature review. *J Int Med Res.* (2020) 48:300060520920068. doi: 10.1177/0300060520920068
9. Epler GR, Colby TV, McLoud TC, Carrington CB, Gaensler EA. Bronchiolitis obliterans organizing pneumonia. *New Engl J Med.* (1985) 312:152–8. doi: 10.1056/NEJM198501173120304
10. King TE Jr., Mortenson RL. Cryptogenic organizing pneumonitis. The North American experience. *Chest* (1992) 102:8S–13S.
11. Wells AU. Cryptogenic organizing pneumonia. *Semin Respir Crit Care Med.* (2001) 22:449–60. doi: 10.1055/s-2001-17387
12. Lazor R, Vandevenne A, Pelletier A, Leclerc P, Court-Fortune I, Cordier JF. Cryptogenic organizing pneumonia. Characteristics of relapses in a series of 48 patients. The groupe d'etudes et de recherche sur les maladles "Orphelines" pulmonaires (GERM "O"P). *Am J Respir Crit Care Med.* (2000) 162:571–7. doi: 10.1164/ajrccm.162.2.9909015
13. Nizami IY, Kissner DG, Visscher DW, Dubaybo BA. Idiopathic bronchiolitis obliterans with organizing pneumonia. An acute and life-threatening syndrome. *Chest.* (1995) 108:271–7. doi: 10.1378/chest.108.1.271
14. Perez de Llano LA, Soilan JL, Garcia Pais MJ, Mata I, Moreda M, Laserna B. Idiopathic bronchiolitis obliterans with organizing pneumonia presenting with adult respiratory distress syndrome. *Respir Med.* (1998) 92:884–6. doi: 10.1016/s0954-6111(98)90396-1
15. Schwarz MI. Diffuse pulmonary infiltrates and respiratory failure following 2 weeks of dyspnea in a 45-year-old woman. *Chest.* (1993) 104:927–9. doi: 10.1378/chest.104.3.927
16. Koinuma D, Miki M, Ebina M, Tahara M, Hagiwara K, Kondo T, et al. Successful treatment of a case with rapidly progressive bronchiolitis obliterans organizing pneumonia (BOOP) using cyclosporin a and corticosteroid. *Intern Med.* (2002) 41:26–9. doi: 10.2169/internalmedicine.41.26
17. Yousem SA, Lohr RH, Colby TV. Idiopathic bronchiolitis obliterans organizing pneumonia/cryptogenic organizing pneumonia with unfavorable outcome: pathologic predictors. *Mod Pathol.* (1997) 10:864–71.

4

Interpreting Immunoregulation in Lung Fibrosis: A New Branch of the Immune Model

*François Huaux**

Louvain Centre for Toxicology and Applied Pharmacology (LTAP), Institut de Recherche Experimentale et Clinique (IREC), Université Catholique de Louvain, Brussels, Belgium

Correspondence:
François Huaux
francois.huaux@uclouvain.be

Immunostimulation is recognized as an important contribution in lung fibrosis in some animal models and patient subsets. With this review, we illustrate an additional scenario covering the possible implication of immunoregulation during fibrogenesis. Available animal and human data indicate that pulmonary fibrosis also includes diverse and discrete immunoregulating populations comprising regulatory lymphocytes (T and B regs) and myeloid cells (immunosuppressive macrophages and myeloid-derived suppressive cells; MDSC). They are initially recruited to limit the establishment of deleterious inflammation but participate in the development of lung fibrosis by producing immunoregulatory mediators (mainly TGF-β1 and IL-10) that directly or indirectly stimulate fibroblasts and matrix protein deposition. The existence of this silent immunoregulatory environment sustains an alternative mechanism of fibrosis that explains why in some conditions neither pro-inflammatory cytokine deficiency nor steroid and immunosuppressive therapies limit lung fibrosis. Therefore, the persistent presence of immunoregulation is an important parameter to consider for refining therapeutical strategies in lung fibrotic disorders under non-immunostimulatory conditions.

Keywords: immunosuppression, inflammation, regulatory lymphocytes and myeloid cells, carbon nanotubes, silica and asbestos

DIVERSE LUNG FIBROTIC DISEASES WITH DIVERSE MECHANISMS

Repair of damaged tissue is a fundamental biological process that allows the ordered replacement of dead or injured cells. However, although initially beneficial, the healing process becomes pathogenic when it is not controlled appropriately, leading to considerable tissue remodeling and the formation of permanent scar tissue and fibrosis (1). The major site of histopathological lung fibrosis is the interstitium, which consists of alveolar epithelium, pulmonary capillary endothelium, basement membrane, and perivascular and perilymphatic tissues. There are now almost 300 distinct injurious or inflammatory causes of interstitial lung disease that can result in progressive lung scarring. Many others are referred as idiopathic (i.e. idiopathic pulmonary fibrosis, or IPF) when it arises for no obvious reason (2). Silicosis is one the oldest recorded interstitial lung disease characterized by alveolitis and progressive nodular fibrosis (3). This fibroproliferative disorder can be traced back to ancient Egypt, where it was caused by inhalation of crystalline silica. It is also well known that long-term asbestos fiber inhalation causes asbestosis also comprising persistent nodular fibrosis (4). Although the incidence of silicosis and asbestosis has diminished, it continues to be a major cause of occupational lung disease in exposed workers, particularly in developing nations (5). More recently, carbon nanotubes (CNT), which present some of the physical characteristics of asbestos (long and rigid), also induce granulomatous lung disorder characterized by persistent immune responses, culminating in the development of lung fibrosis (6). Additionally, lung fibrogenic reaction may arise from other exogenous environmental stimuli such as organic dusts (bacterial, fungal and avian antigens) (7).

Suppression of chronic inflammation by immunosuppressive therapy turn off pulmonary fibrogenesis in some sub-groups of patients (e.g. non-specific interstitial pneumonia). These findings argue that inflammation represents a major pathological pathway in lung fibrosis (8, 9). A pathogenesis paradigm that did not require inflammation and immunostimulation was, however, proposed since there is little evidence of inflammation in the histopathological samples obtained from susceptible ageing individuals developing IPF undergoing surgical lung biopsy. Treatment with anti-inflammatory agents, such as steroids or anti-cytokines, seemed to have no effect on disease progression and outcome (10, 11). These last clinical observations strongly suggested that inflammation represents an important but dispensable event and that other mechanisms than immunostimulation exist or co-exist in pulmonary fibrosis (12, 13).

THE RELEVANCE OF RELIABLE ANIMAL MODELS OF LUNG FIBROSIS

It is unanimously recognized that animal models currently available are particularly useful to discover new pro-fibrotic mediators and pathological avenues related or unrelated to the inflammatory concept. The development of experimental models producing long-lasting lesions akin to those seen in human fibrosis and defined by progressive and irreversible matrix deposition has already been the subject of many studies (14). Presently, chemical insults such as those caused by bleomycin are widely used to induce fibrotic disease. Many research studies have focused on changes in inflammatory phenomena after a single instillation of bleomycin and have yielded similar findings: the lung injuries caused by bleomycin induce acute recruitment and activation of inflammatory leukocytes which produce mediators (cytokines, chemokines, growth factors, and prostaglandins) activating fibroblast and driving fibrotic disease. While bleomycin represents the preferred molecule in this context, the lung fibrosis obtained by an unique dose of this drug is not systematically progressive and resolves itself over time after bleomycin metabolization (15).

This discrepancy led researchers to explore other models and discover new pathological avenues not apparent in the acute bleomycin-induced fibrosis model, which mainly (if not exclusively) supports that inflammation drives fibrosis. Multiple instillation of bleomycin has previously been shown to recapitulate the epithelial remodeling and fibrosis progression in the lungs of patients with IPF (16). Indeed, a repetitive alveolar epithelial injury caused by repetitive intratracheal injections of bleomycin is now proposed as the initial and major event that triggers a series of repair pathways that are in some way aberrant, leading to inappropriate fibrosis. Repeated injuries prevent epithelial cell regeneration, re-epithelialization and epithelial structure restauration and lead to a sustained disruption of alveolar epithelial morphology and fibrogenesis in injured alveoli. This experimental approach thus represents an ultimate model to address mechanistic questions on epithelial remodeling (17).

Murine models of univocal chronic lung responses and progressive fibrotic lesions using inorganic particles (crystalline silica, asbestos and CNT) are well known to cover severe fibrotic respiratory disorders in exposed human. Instillation of mineral particles into mouse and rat lungs results in the development of fibrotic nodules that resemble lesions which develop in humans. Rodents exposed to silica particles present alveolar fibrotic nodules, increased pulmonary lymphoid tissue and enhanced numbers of macrophages in the broncho-alveolar lavage fluid. Interestingly, silica, asbestos and CNT are retained in the lung and the response is characterized by a persistent and progressive fibrosis (18). Based on findings on particle-induced pulmonary fibrosis in mice, it has been recently proposed a new hypothesis that the fibrotic response may result from an exaggerated and persistent immunoregulating responses instead of or along with inflammation. This new concept have been confirmed in human silicosis but also in other animal models and patients. These results, summarized hereafter, may explain how lung fibrosis can develop in absence of immunostimulation.

HISTORY OF IMMUNOREGULATING SURVEILLANCE

The quality, magnitude, and persistence of immune reactions results from the balance between immunostimulating and immunoregulating responses. The basic mechanism of immunoregulation comprises an interconnecting system involving diverse anti-inflammatory and immunosuppressive cytokines, lymphocytes and myeloid cells. There is now evidence that this sophisticated immunoregulatory systems is crucial in maintaining immune homeostasis and resolving persistent inflammation. Immunoregulatory alterations are often implicated in the pathogenesis of several inflammatory diseases such as infection, allergy, and autoimmune disorders. Conversely, uncontrolled and exacerbated immunoregulation is strategically exploited by cancer cells to survive, proliferate and escape detection by anti-tumor effector T lymphocytes (19). A well-knowledge of immunoregulation now serves for future strategies of diagnosis and treatment. The following sections are devoted to describe (i) historical aspects of immunoregulatory mechanisms (**Figure 1**) and (ii) matching evidence supporting a deranged immunoregulation in pulmonary fibrogenesis (**Figure 2**).

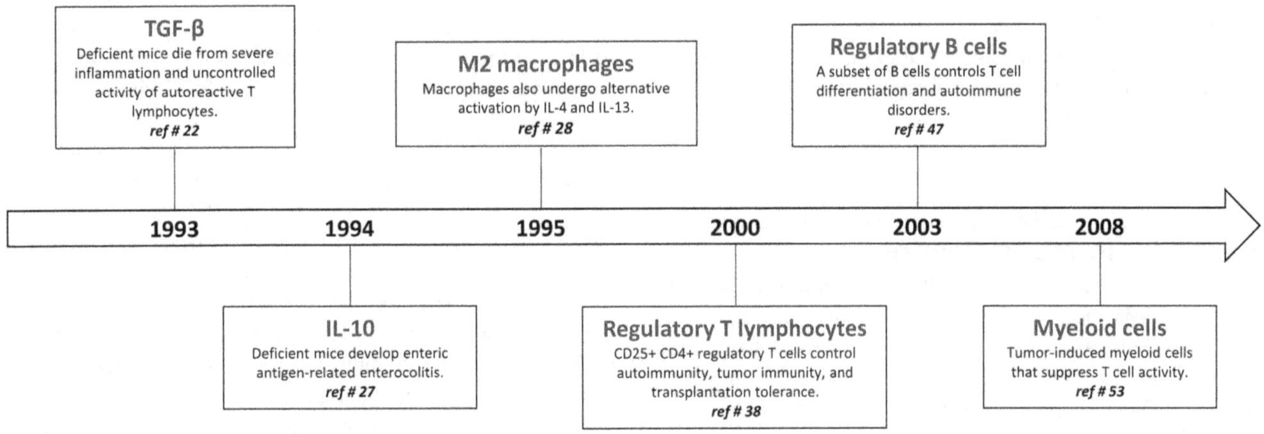

FIGURE 1 | Timeline: historical progression of immunoregulation in the literature.

TGF-β1 and IL-10 as Master Immunoregulating Cytokines

The most striking and non-redundant function of TGF-β1 is to regulate the immunostimulatory and inflammatory responses by orchestrating immunoregulation (20, 21). Indeed, in 1993, Kulkarni and Karlsson demonstrated that mice deficient for the gene encoding TGF-β1 die rapidly from a multi-systemic inflammatory syndrome related to deleterious T cell autoreactivity (22) (**Figure 1**). To become active, mature TGF-β1 must be released from the LAP (latency-associated peptide), a process referred to as TGF-β1 activation (23). The best-characterized mechanism of TGF-β1 activation imply conformational changes in the latent TGF-β1 molecule involving interaction of latent TGF-β1 with integrin αVβ8 and GARP (glycoprotein A repeats predominant protein or LRRC32) (21). The binding of the active TGF-β1 peptide to its receptors leads to a series of signaling events that are mainly mediated by SMAD2/3/4 complex that binds SMAD response elements located in the promoter regions of many genes involved in the immunoregulatory responses (21).

The cytokine interleukin-10 (IL-10) was originally described as a 'cytokine synthesis inhibitory factor' (CSIF), which was produced by mouse T helper 2 (Th2) clones and inhibited cytokine production by activated Th1 clones (24). IL-10 reportedly inhibits nuclear factor-κB (NF-κB) activation and expression of the most inducible cytokines and chemokines that are involved in inflammation. The anti-inflammatory activities of IL-10 also include induction of IL-1 receptor antagonist (IL-1ra) (24) and soluble p55 and p75 TNF receptor production, indicating that IL-10 induces a shift from production of pro-inflammatory to anti-inflammatory mediators (25). IL-10 strongly inhibits cytokine production and proliferation of CD4+ effector T cells *via* its down-regulatory effects on APC function. IL-10 also induce the differentiation of naive Th cells in a subset of regulatory T cells which are defined by their

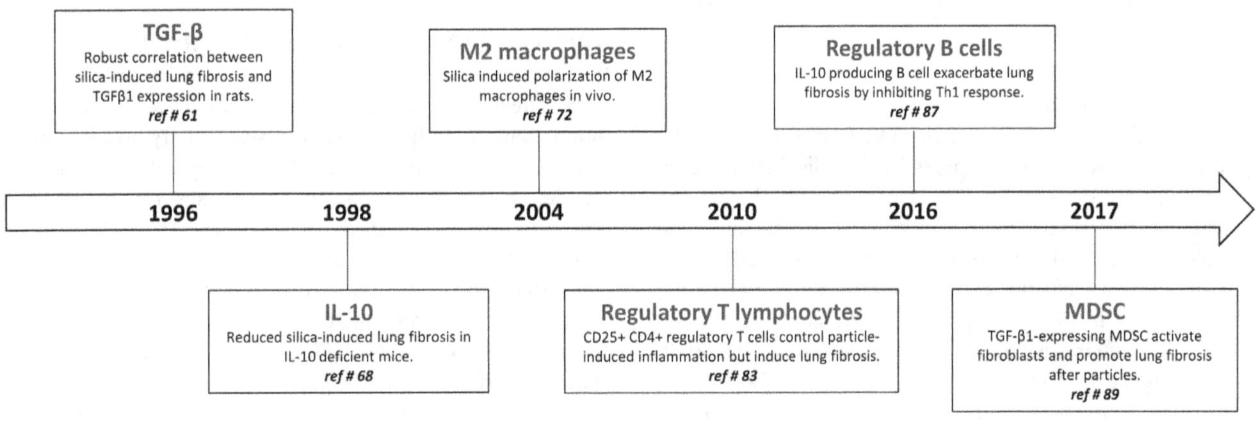

FIGURE 2 | Timeline: historical progression of immunoregulation in particle-induced lung fibrosis.

ability to produce high levels of IL-10 and TGF-β1 (26). The IL-10-related potent immunosuppressive functions and its proximity to TGF-β1 are perfectly illustrated by the work of Kuhn and colleagues demonstrating that IL-10 deficient mice suffer from chronic enterocolitis characterized by extensive inflammatory reactions and aberrant expression of major histocompatibility complex class II molecules (27) (**Figure 1**).

M2/Immunoregulatory Macrophages and Type 2 Like Immune Response

During the 1990s, Gordon and colleagues demonstrated that IL-4 and IL-13 induced an "alternative" form of activation in macrophages beside the "classically" polarized macrophages (28, 29) (**Figure 1**). In 2000, Mills and colleagues identified the fundamental M1/M2 polarization axis of macrophages and proposed that M1/inflammatory macrophages are necessary to eliminate infectious organisms and tumor cells while M2/immunoregulatory macrophages are implicated in repair process and wounds. Importantly, the uncontrolled M1 and M2 activation is associated with tissue injury and cancer progression, respectively (30, 31).

The so-called M2 phenotype express anti-inflammatory and immunosuppressive mediators such as IL-10 and TGF-β1, specific chemokines (CCL17 and CCL22, C-C motif), the subclass B scavenger receptor (CD 163), and the mannose C receptor type 1 (CD206 or MRC1) (32). The TGF-β1- and IL-10 producing M2 macrophages are thus intimately involved in the regulation of immune responses. Transcription factors such as IRF4 and STAT6 are required for M2 macrophage activation and differentiation. These different stimuli are likely to initiate during Th2-like responses (33). Th2 responses and cytokines (mainly IL-4 and IL-13) induce the differentiation of M2 macrophages.

The model categorizing macrophages (or T helper cells) in only two divergent groups M1 vs M2 (or Th1 and Th2) does not cover the intrinsic heterogeneity of macrophages (and T lymphocytes) now identified and described in diseases. A consensus now refers to M1-like or M2 like-subpopulations for avoiding oversimplified categories and highlighting the diversity and versatility of macrophages (34). M2-like macrophages possessing various functions, characteristics and deleterious activities are well known to be crucial in asthma, interstitial lung diseases and cancer (35, 36).

Regulatory T Cells

Regulatory T cells were initially described by Gershon et al. in the early 1970s and were called suppressive T cells because they practiced immune suppression (37). Unfortunately, despite the importance of these studies there was extensive skepticism in the immunological field about the existence of these cells, and suppressive T cells left the centre stage of immunology for decades. However, in 1996, Sakaguchi and colleagues rehabilitated the concept of "suppressive T cells", now renamed "regulatory T cells" (38) (**Figure 1**). CD4+ Foxp3+ regulatory T cells (T regs) constitute a thymus-derived sub-population of CD4+ T lymphocytes that constitutively express the transcription factor Foxp3 (forkhead box P3), required for their development and their anti-inflammatory and immunosuppressive function (39, 40). T regs are developed in the thymus (naturally occurring T regs; nT regs) or are differentiated from naive T cells in the presence of TGF-β1 following T-cell receptor stimulation (induced T regs; iT regs) (41). These lymphocytes are crucial to maintain tolerance by downregulating undesired immune responses to self and non-self-antigens (42, 43). Absence or defective function of regulatory T cells is correlated with the development of immuno-pathologies such as auto-immune diseases (e.g. psoriasis and rheumatoid arthritis) and asthma. In contrast, their accumulation is associated with tolerance and implicated, for instance, in the development of cancer (44). Several mechanisms have been proposed to explain immunosuppressive functions of T regs. These include secretion by T regs of immunosuppressive cytokines, cell-contact-dependent suppression and functional modulation. Most *in vivo* studies indicate that T regs mediate immunosuppression by producing IL-10 and TGF-β1 (45). The strong immunosuppressive activity T regs is also related to their capacity to regulate the polarization and function of effector T lymphocytes (T eff, i.e. Th1, Th2, and Th17).

B Regs

The historical description of the new B-cell subtype named regulatory B-cells (B regs) dates back to 1974. In a mouse model of eczema, adoptive transfer of total splenocytes had a suppressive effect, whereas adoptive transfer of splenocytes from which B-lymphocytes were removed had no effect (46). In 2003, the regulatory role of B cells was shown in a mouse model of experimental autoimmune disease and this regulatory role was attributed to the ability of B cells to produce IL-10 (47) (**Figure 1**). B cells have been shown to restore homeostasis, possess important immunosuppressive functions and play a key role in disease control and immune tolerance (48, 49). IL-10-producing B cells produce anti-inflammatory IgG4 and activate Treg cells. By promoting M2-like macrophage polarization, B regs cells also reduce auto-reactive Th1 and Th17 cell responses and limit damaging inflammatory responses. In contrast, B regs impair cytotoxic T-cell and NK cell responses to tumor cells and thereby promote progression of cancer (50). Beside IL-10, the exact mechanism by which B regs act *in vivo* remains unclear. A close contact between B-lymphocytes and the T lymphocytes, notably through the CD40-CD40L pathway are required (51, 52).

Myeloid Derived Suppressive Cells

MDSC were first identified by Van Ginderachter and his team in 2008. They detected a discrete myeloid-derived suppressor cell subpopulations with T cell-suppressive activity invading tumors. Thus, it was suggested that this MDSC population is responsible for down-regulating immune responses related to tumor progression and metastasis (53) (**Figure 1**). MDSC are now defined as heterogeneous and immature myeloid cells generated from the bone marrow and active in cancer development and inflammation regulation (54). Under normal physiological conditions, MDSC are rapidly differentiated into mature granulocytes, macrophages and dendritic cells. However, the differentiation of these cells into mature myeloid cells is blocked in chronic pathologies such as cancer (54). Two categories of these cells can be observed, one with granulocyte morphology and the other with monocyte morphology (55). MDSC suppress CD8, CD4 T cell activities and NK cell activity by inducing a suppressive environment (56). Several different mechanisms of action have been identified to explain the strong immunosuppressive activity of MDSC involving direct cell contacts and/or the production of several released mediators (54). MDSCs have the ability to induce differentiation and expansion of regulatory T cells by producing cytokines such as IL-10 and TGF-β1 or *via* CD40 (57). These cells can also deprive T cells of amino acids essential for their activity such as arginine, which is necessary for lymphocyte activation. Arginase, highly expressed by MDSCs, metabolizes arginine to urea and ornithine. Indoleamine-2.3-dioxygenase (IDO), an enzyme that catalyzes tryptophan, an essential amino acid for T cells, might also be involved in the immunosuppressive mechanisms of MDSC (54).

THE DISCOVERY OF IMMUNOREGULATION IN PARTICLE-INDUCED LUNG FIBROSIS

Inorganic particle-induced lung fibrosis consists of an uncontrolled inflammation of the respiratory system tissues characterized by a chronic macrophage and neutrophil infiltration that ultimately causes fibrosis (58). Based on the widespread study of Piguet and colleagues published in 1990 in Nature, it is accepted that silica particles activate intracellular signaling pathways that culminate in the production of the pro-inflammatory mediator TNF-α, which is crucial in driving alveolitis and lung fibrosis (59). Additionally, a recent and pivotal study demonstrated that silica activate caspase-1 in a NALP3 inflammasome-dependent manner leading to the processing and secretion of the pro-inflammatory cytokine IL-1β. Evidence demonstrate that IL-1β initiates a cascade of reactions leading to inflammation and uncontrolled fibrosis (60). These observations support the concept that inflammation and sustained expression of inflammatory cell-secreted pro-fibrotic cytokines participate in the etiology of fibroproliferative diseases associated to inorganic particles.

The interconnection between inflammation and fibrosis was, however, questioned when active TGF-β1 was pointed as a key pro-fibrotic factor in response to particles. In silicosis and asbestosis, TGF-β1 expression has been found to be increased in lung tissues from patients with accelerated fibrotic disease progression (7) (**Figure 2**). The crucial activity of TGF-β1 during fibrogenesis has been unanimously recognized in the experimental studies using silica-, asbestos- and CNT-treated mice (6, 61–63). TGF-β1 is a major profibrogenic cytokine by delaying epithelial wound healing and expanding mesenchymal compartment (64). While the activity of TGF-β1 on fibroblasts is undisputed and not anymore debated, these observations intrigued immunologists because the presence of this powerful immunosuppressive cytokine (see above) was not in line with the IL-1/TNF-related immunostimulation axis.

Additional data challenged the inflammatory concept. IL-10, another potent immunoregulatory cytokine, has also fibrogenic activities in responses to fibrogenic particles. To examine the immune responses over the whole course of the pathological process induced by fibers and particles, validated experimental models in mice and rats with contrasting sensitivities were developed (65). By comparing these models and using deficient mice, it was newly discovered that IL-10 produced by particle-activated macrophages limit neutrophilic inflammation but is a key mediator implicated in the fibrotic lung response to silica by controlling the balance between pro- and anti-fibrotic mediator production (respectively TGF-β1 and prostaglandin E2) (65–68) (**Figure 2**). IL-10 is also a prevailing inducer of type-2 immune responses in particular M2-like and Th2-like pro-fibrotic cells (69, 70). The fibrogenic activity of macrophage-derived IL-10 and M2-like macrophages is not limited to silicosis (71, 72). Indeed, these macrophages are also implicated in the fibrotic lung response induced by asbestos and CNT (6, 73, 74) (**Figure 2**).

The little evidence of inflammation in the histopathological samples obtained from silicotic patients undergoing surgical lung biopsy (75) consolidate the pathogenesis paradigm that did not require inflammation. In contrast, high levels of IL-10 in BAL or serum were detected in patients with silicosis and asbestosis in the absence of clear inflammatory reaction (73, 76). Treatment with anti-inflammatory agents, such as corticosteroids, seemed to have no effect on outcome of these fibrotic diseases (75, 77, 78). These human observation are in accordance with several animal data indicating that steroid and numerous anti-inflammatory strategies reduce particle-induced lung inflammation but not IL-10-TGF-β1 expression and lung fibrosis in sensitive animals (79, 80). At this time, it was thus suggested that these two immunoregulatory cytokines are the major event that triggers a series of repair pathways that are aberrant and lead to inappropriate fibrosis under non-inflammatory conditions.

According to the concept that inflammation is responsible for fibrogenesis and given their ability to dampen inflammatory responses, CD4+ regulatory T lymphocytes (T regs) were first supposed to slow the progression of fibrosis (81). Indeed, it is well recognized that T regs, by restraining effector T cell responses and inducing tolerance through the production of TGF-β1 and/or IL-10, control lung inflammatory disorders (82). However, CD4+ Foxp3+ regulatory T cells are persistently recruited during long-term responses to particles (69, 83) (**Figure 2**). T regs purified from the lung of silica-treated mice highly express fibrogenic mediators, stimulate fibroblast proliferation *in vitro* and increase lung collagen deposition upon transfer into naive mice. Interestingly, the effects of T regs on fibroblast proliferation recapitulate the main function of PDGF as a primary mitogen for fibroblasts during lung fibrosis. The stimulatory effect of T regs on fibroblasts *in vitro* and *in vivo* was completely abolished by a PDGF receptor inhibitor (imatinib mesylate). It is thus likely that the role of T regs is to increase tissue fibroblast numbers, and consequently, amplify the subsequent fibroblast activation and collagen deposition (83). The pro-fibrogenic functions of T regs also comprise a stimulatory activity on Th2-like pro-fibrotic cells

(69). In contrast to what it is thought, T regs thus participate in the fibrogenesis and are able to aggravate lung fibrosis induced by fibrogenic particles (i.e. silica and asbestos) in absence of inflammation (74). Finally, Xin and colleagues also observed a clear balance between inflammatory Th effector cells (Th1 and Th17) and T regs in mice treated with silica (84, 85). Neutralization of T regs-immunosuppressive activity resulted in enhanced lung inflammation and Th17 accumulation further demonstrating that T regs are initially recruited to control inflammatory responses (85, 86).

Based on the immunosuppressive profile of silica-treated mice, other immunosuppressive populations among lymphocytes have been investigated. Regulatory B lymphocytes (B regs), another immunosuppressive cell population (see above), also accumulate and participate in granuloma formation and fibrosis development by producing lung IL-10 in mice treated with silica. A heightened accumulation of inflammatory T effector cells (Th1 and Th17) but limited pulmonary fibrosis were observed in B reg-depleted mice treated with silica (87) (**Figure 2**). IL-10-producing B regs were also noted in silicotic patients in absence of inflammatory reaction (76). B regs exacerbate fibrogenesis by stimulating T regs functions and polarization *via* the release of IL-10 (88). These findings indicated that the accumulation and polarization of immunoregulatory lymphocytes is a central event during particle-induced pulmonary fibrosis with limited immunostimulation.

Finally, M-MDSC are also progressively and specifically accumulated during the development of pulmonary fibrosis. Indeed, a close relationship between the accumulation of MDSC, pulmonary immunosuppression and lung fibrosis was clearly found in mice treated with silica or CNT (89, 90) (**Figure 2**). Beside M2-like macrophages and T regs, immunosuppressive MDSC also expressed TGF-β1 conferring to these myeloid cells the capacity to down regulate T effector cell activity (91). In order to define their role in fibrosis, lung MDSC were purified from silica-treated mice and co-cultured with naive lung fibroblasts. MDSC stimulates lung fibroblasts to release tissue inhibitor of metalloproteinase and collagenolytic activity by expressing TGF-β1. They contribute to lung fibrogenesis by inducing a non-degrading collagen microenvironment (89).

The persistent accumulation of immunoregulatory macrophages, lymphocytes and myeloid cells in the lung during the progressive establishment of experimental silicosis is consistent with studies on tuberculosis (92) and lung cancer (93) that often affect the silicotic patients. Indeed, these cells control neutrophilic inflammation and anti-tumor T effector lymphocytes dedicated to microorganism and tumoral cell elimination. However, authors found that human silicosis is accompanied by a reduced number of blood regulatory T cells and speculated that the absence of these regulatory cells may explain the occurrence of autoimmune diseases (e.g. systemic scleroderma, rheumatoid arthritis and systemic lupus erythematosus) (94, 95). These conflicting results highlight the possible limitations of the mouse models. Injection of silica in mice does not fulfill all conditions encountered in patients with silicosis (infection, cancer and autoimmune diseases). Moreover, experimental models used to study the effects of silica are relatively short compared to human silicosis. These contradictory results also suggest that the fibrogenic activity of immunoregulation is only effective in a non-inflammatory environment.

INCLUSIVE IMPLICATION OF IMMUNOREGULATORY MEDIATORS AND CELLS IN LUNG FIBROTIC DISEASES

Immunoregulation is operative in different fibrotic context and not specifically concomitant to particle-induced fibrogenesis. Indeed, recent investigations using complementary mouse models of lung fibrosis also reported that inflammation is not an absolute prerequisite for fibrogenesis and that the fibrotic pathological process can develop through immunoregulation.

IL-10 induce lung collagen deposition and fibrosis when overexpressed in transgenic mice (96, 97). These observations correspond to those noted when TGF-β1 is overexpressed in murine lungs (98). Intratracheal transfer of adenoviral recombinant IL-10 or TGF-β1 to murine lung has been shown to dramatically increase fibroblast accumulation and expression of type I and type III collagen around airways as well as in the pulmonary interstitium (70, 99, 100). The pro-fibrotic function of IL-10 is associated to infiltration of fibrocytes and M2-like macrophages (97). In addition; IL-10 and TGF-β1 contribute to lung injury and fibrosis by sensitizing epithelial cells to apoptosis (98, 101). TIM-3+ M2-like macrophages that possess strong immunoregulatory functions is now considered as an important pro-fibrotic population by being a key source of TGF-β1 and IL-10. Adoptive transfer of this immunoregulatory population promoted bleomycin-induced lung fibrosis by highly secreting TGF-β1 and IL-10 (102). Recent data at single cell level suggest that pro-fibrotic macrophages did not demonstrate a shaped and clear M2-like polarization but resemble to alveolar macrophages deriving from monocytes (103). Altogether, these studies indicated that the long-term overexpression of M2 like-related immunoregulating cytokines that suppress inflammation such as TGF-β1 and IL-10 are also profibrotic factors in the lung.

In vivo expansion of lung CD4+CD25+Foxp3+ T regs cells during bleomycin-induced lung fibrosis unexpectedly led to an increase of fibrogenesis. More important, this pro-fibrotic effect was a lymphocyte-dependent process. A marked down-regulation of type 1 and an increase of type 2 immune responses in the lungs were proposed to explain T reg fibrogenic activity (104, 105). These observations were corroborated by Chakraborthy and colleagues. Depletion of T regs ameliorate bleomycin-induced acute lung fibrosis by modulating Th effector cell balance. In addition, adoptive transfer of Sema 7a1 T regs induces fibrosis in the TGF-β1–exposed murine lung by altering the production of T-cell mediators (106).

Accumulation of MDSC with functional immunosuppressive activity was also noted in bleomycin-induced experimental pulmonary fibrosis and their potential role in fibroblast activation investigated (107, 108). Purified MDSC differentiate into lung fibroblasts as manifested by significantly elevated α-smooth muscle actin and TGF-β1 expression. Differentiation of MDSC into fibrocytes could also be possible during tissue repair processes. Indeed, there is some evidence that peripheral monocytes and MDSCs differentiate into fibrocytes (109, 110). These cells have the ability to promote fibroblast proliferation, migration, and collagen production but also differentiate into myofibroblasts (111, 112). Altogether, these previous experimental studies are well in accordance with the immunoregulation concept elaborated from findings reported after particle exposure and supporting that persitent immunoregulatory environment is profibrotic in absence of immunostimulation (**Figure 3**).

The disconnection between fibrosis and inflammation is not limited to patients developing silicosis or asbestosis. Clinical measurements of inflammation in IPF patients developing fibrosis fail to correlate scar formation with inflammation and immunostimulation. Corticosteroids have never conclusively been shown to significantly alter the course of pulmonary fibrosis in patients and have, at best, limited efficacy in the treatment of scarring disease (113).

Interestingly, the expression TGF-β1 and IL-10 mainly by macrophages was increased in lung biopsies from patients with IPF compared with controls, suggesting the presence of M2-like macrophages (114, 115). Single-cell multi-omics approaches characterizing macrophage populations in health and lung fibrotic disease at high resolution tempered a clear accumulation of M2-like polarized macrophages in fibrotic tissue. Fibrotic macrophages in IPF patients are now identified as proliferating SSP1-positive macrophages (116, 117). However, it has been suggested that Th2-related cytokines such IL-4 and IL-3 as well as M-CSF activate this subset of proliferating macrophages (117). Clinical reports showed increased number and function of CD4+CD25+FoxP3+ T regs in the

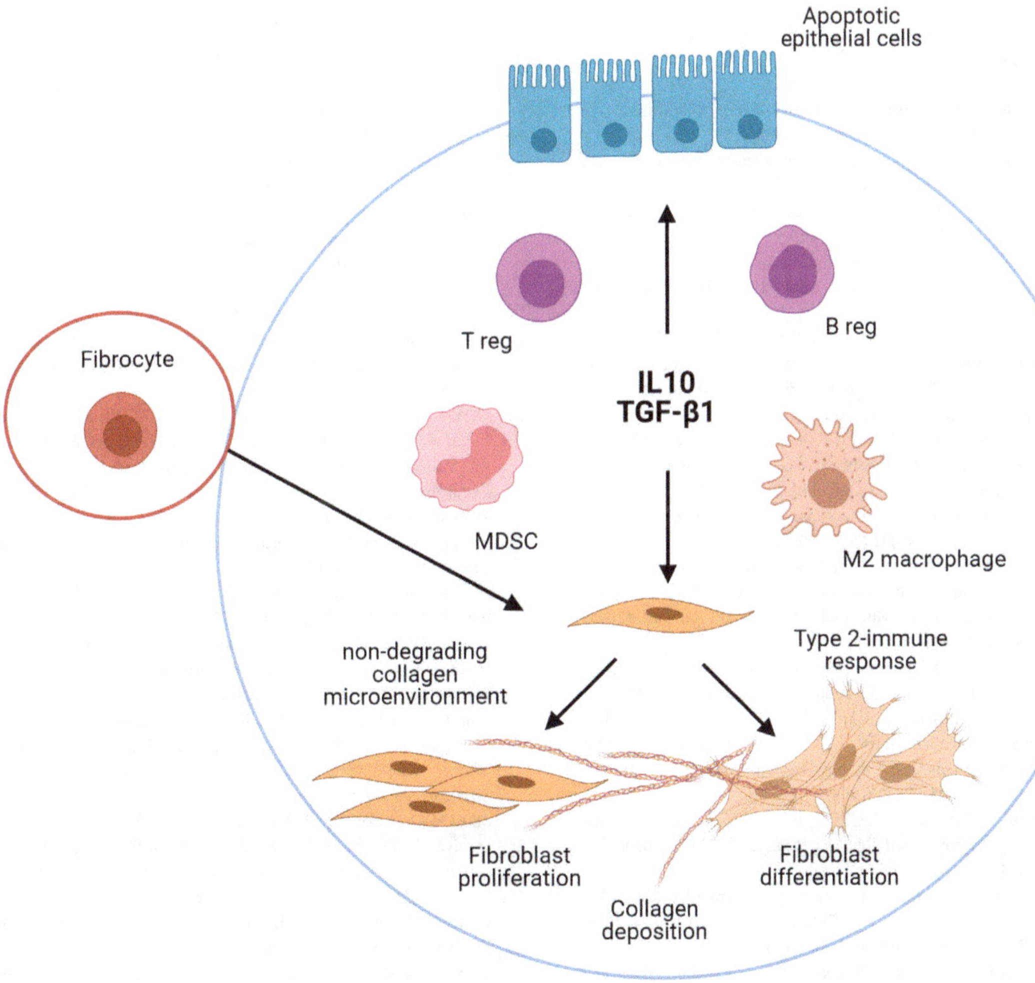

FIGURE 3 | Schematic representation of the implication of the different immunoregulatory cells and mediators in lung fibrosis. The studies on experimental lung fibrosis have highlighted a new pathological pathway, which suggests that pulmonary fibrosis is orchestrated by an immunoregulatory response characterized by a persistent accumulation of pulmonary immunoregulatory cells (regulatory T and B lymphocytes, i.e. T and B regs; regulatory myeloid cells, i.e. M2/immunosuppressive macrophages and Myeloid Derived Suppressive Cells, MDSC) and a sustained production of IL-10 and TGF-β1. The persistent accumulation of these elements to control immunostimulatory responses in the lungs contribute, however, to pulmonary fibrosis. This sustains the view that immunoregulation is important pro-fibrotic environment that could markedly explain the development of the lung fibrotic response under non-inflammatory conditions.

lungs and blood of patients with IPF associated with a more progressive clinical course (106, 116, 118–120). More recently, the importance of MDSC was also suggested by the observation of MDSC accumulation in IPF lungs (108, 121).

In conclusion, the presence of immunoregulatory microenvironment may be relevant to human pathology. Based on these recent findings, it is important to consider the possibility that regulatory lymphocytes and myeloid cells may also drive fibroproliferative wound healing. Consequently, these cells and their cytokine products could become therapeutic targets in patients developing fibrotic diseases. Particularly, these studies identified as potentially important targets the production of TGF-β1 and IL-10 by immunoregulatory cells in non-immunostimulatory conditions. The clinical separation of patients reaches from immunoregulatory or immunostimulatory scar formation could offer novel markers for the pathological assessment as well as novel regulators and drug targets to treat pulmonary fibroproliferative diseases.

AUTHOR CONTRIBUTIONS

The author confirms being the sole contributor of this work and has approved it for publication.

FUNDING

This work was funded by the Actions de Recherche Concertées, Fédération Wallonie-Bruxelles (ARC 19/24-098, CYTAID), Fondation Contre le Cancer (2019-219), Fonds de la Recherche Scientifique (FNRS, PDR T.0119.13), ANSES (Agence nationale française de sécurité sanitaire de l'alimentation, de l'environnement et du travail, MacFibOsis) and European Commission under H2020 project (Contract no. 874707, Eximious). FH is a Senior Research Associate with the FNRS, Belgium.

REFERENCES

1. Henderson NC, Rieder F, Wynn TA. Fibrosis: From Mechanisms to Medicines. *Nature* (2020) 587:555–66. doi: 10.1038/s41586-020-2938-9
2. du Bois RM. Strategies for Treating Idiopathic Pulmonary Fibrosis. *Nat Rev Drug Discov* (2010) 9:129–40. doi: 10.1038/nrd2958
3. Hoy RF, Chambers DC. Silica-Related Diseases in the Modern World. *Allergy* (2020) 75:2805–17. doi: 10.1111/all.14202
4. Gulati M, Redlich CA. Asbestosis and Environmental Causes of Usual Interstitial Pneumonia. *Curr Opin Pulm Med* (2015) 21:193–200. doi: 10.1097/MCP.0000000000000144
5. Weston A. Work-Related Lung Diseases. *IARC Sci Publ* (2011) 163:387–405.
6. Dong J, Ma Q. Type 2 Immune Mechanisms in Carbon Nanotube-Induced Lung Fibrosis. *Front Immunol* (2018) 9:1120. doi: 10.3389/fimmu.2018.01120
7. Araya J, Nishimura SL. Fibrogenic Reactions in Lung Disease. *Annu Rev Pathol* (2010) 5:77–98. doi: 10.1146/annurev.pathol.4.110807.092217
8. Kondoh Y, Taniguchi H, Yokoi T, Nishiyama O, Ohishi T, Kato T, et al. Cyclophosphamide and Low-Dose Prednisolone in Idiopathic Pulmonary Fibrosis and Fibrosing Nonspecific Interstitial Pneumonia. *Eur Respir J* (2005) 25:528–33. doi: 10.1183/09031936.05.00071004
9. Lee SH, Park MS, Kim SY, Kim DS, Kim YW, Chung MP, et al. Factors Affecting Treatment Outcome in Patients With Idiopathic Nonspecific Interstitial Pneumonia: A Nationwide Cohort Study. *Respir Res* (2017) 18:204. doi: 10.1186/s12931-017-0686-7
10. Raghu G. Idiopathic Pulmonary Fibrosis: Lessons From Clinical Trials Over the Past 25 Years. *Eur Respir J* (2017) 50:1701209. doi: 10.1183/13993003.01209-2017
11. Parker JM, Glaspole IN, Lancaster LH, Haddad TJ, She D, Roseti SL, et al. A Phase 2 Randomized Controlled Study of Tralokinumab in Subjects With Idiopathic Pulmonary Fibrosis. *Am J Respir Crit Care Med* (2018) 197:94–103. doi: 10.1164/rccm.201704-0784OC
12. Martinez FJ, Collard HR, Pardo A, Raghu G, Richeldi L, Selman M, et al. Idiopathic Pulmonary Fibrosis. *Nat Rev Dis Primers* (2017) 3:17074. doi: 10.1038/nrdp.2017.74
13. Mora AL, Rojas M, Pardo A, Selman M. Emerging Therapies for Idiopathic Pulmonary Fibrosis, A Progressive Age-Related Disease. *Nat Rev Drug Discov* (2017) 16:755–72. doi: 10.1038/nrd.2017.170
14. Moore BB, Hogaboam CM. Murine Models of Pulmonary Fibrosis. *Am J Physiol Lung Cell Mol Physiol* (2008) 294:L152–60. doi: 10.1152/ajplung.00313.2007
15. O'Dwyer DN, Moore BB. Animal Models of Pulmonary Fibrosis. *Methods Mol Biol* (2018) 1809:363–78. doi: 10.1007/978-1-4939-8570-8_24
16. Cao Z, Lis R, Ginsberg M, Chavez D, Shido K, Rabbany SY, et al. Targeting of the Pulmonary Capillary Vascular Niche Promotes Lung Alveolar Repair and Ameliorates Fibrosis. *Nat Med* (2016) 22:154–62. doi: 10.1038/nm.4035
17. Redente EF, Black BP, Backos DS, Bahadur AN, Humphries SM, Lynch DA, et al. Persistent, Progressive Pulmonary Fibrosis and Epithelial Remodeling in Mice. *Am J Respir Cell Mol Biol* (2021) 64:669–76. doi: 10.1165/rcmb.2020-0542MA
18. Dong J, Ma Q. Integration of Inflammation, Fibrosis, and Cancer Induced by Carbon Nanotubes. *Nanotoxicology* (2019) 13:1244–74. doi: 10.1080/17435390.2019.1651920
19. Chen W, Ten Dijke P. Immunoregulation by Members of the TGFbeta Superfamily. *Nat Rev Immunol* (2016) 16:723–40. doi: 10.1038/nri.2016.112
20. Theron AJ, Anderson R, Rossouw TM, Steel HC. The Role of Transforming Growth Factor Beta-1 in the Progression of HIV/AIDS and Development of Non-AIDS-Defining Fibrotic Disorders. *Front Immunol* (2017) 8:1461. doi: 10.3389/fimmu.2017.01461
21. Dedobbeleer O, Stockis J, van der Woning B, Coulie PG, Lucas S. Cutting Edge: Active TGF-Beta1 Released From GARP/TGF-Beta1 Complexes on the Surface of Stimulated Human B Lymphocytes Increases Class-Switch Recombination and Production of IgA. *J Immunol* (2017) 199:391–6. doi: 10.4049/jimmunol.1601882
22. Kulkarni AB, Huh CG, Becker D, Geiser A, Lyght M, Flanders KC, et al. Transforming Growth Factor Beta 1 Null Mutation in Mice Causes Excessive Inflammatory Response and Early Death. *Proc Natl Acad Sci USA* (1993) 90:770–4. doi: 10.1073/pnas.90.2.770
23. Taylor AW. Review of the Activation of TGF-Beta in Immunity. *J Leukoc Biol* (2009) 85:29–33. doi: 10.1189/jlb.0708415
24. Fiorentino DF, Bond MW, Mosmann TR. Two Types of Mouse T Helper Cell. IV. Th2 Clones Secrete a Factor That Inhibits Cytokine Production by Th1 Clones. *J Exp Med* (1989) 170:2081–95. doi: 10.1084/jem.170.6.2081
25. Walter MR. The Molecular Basis of IL-10 Function: From Receptor Structure to the Onset of Signaling. *Curr Top Microbiol Immunol* (2014) 380:191–212. doi: 10.1007/978-3-662-43492-5_9
26. Saraiva M, O'Garra A. The Regulation of IL-10 Production by Immune Cells. *Nat Rev Immunol* (2010) 10:170–81. doi: 10.1038/nri2711
27. Kuhn R, Lohler J, Rennick D, Rajewsky K, Muller W. Interleukin-10-Deficient Mice Develop Chronic Enterocolitis. *Cell* (1993) 75:263–74. doi: 10.1016/0092-8674(93)80068-P
28. Stein M, Keshav S, Harris N, Gordon S. Interleukin 4 Potently Enhances Murine Macrophage Mannose Receptor Activity: A Marker of Alternative Immunologic Macrophage Activation. *J Exp Med* (1992) 176:287–92. doi: 10.1084/jem.176.1.287
29. Doyle AG, Herbein G, Montaner LJ, Minty AJ, Caput D, Ferrara P, et al. Interleukin-13 Alters the Activation State of Murine Macrophages *In Vitro*: Comparison With Interleukin-4 and Interferon-Gamma. *Eur J Immunol* (1994) 24:1441–5. doi: 10.1002/eji.1830240630

30. Mills CD, Kincaid K, Alt JM, Heilman MJ, Hill AM. M-1/M-2 Macrophages and the Th1/Th2 Paradigm. *J Immunol* (2000) 164:6166–73. doi: 10.4049/jimmunol.164.12.6166
31. Gordon S, Martinez FO. Alternative Activation of Macrophages: Mechanism and Functions. *Immunity* (2010) 32:593–604. doi: 10.1016/j.immuni.2010.05.007
32. Murray PJ. Macrophage Polarization. *Annu Rev Physiol* (2017) 79:541–66. doi: 10.1146/annurev-physiol-022516-034339
33. Murray PJ, Wynn TA. Protective and Pathogenic Functions of Macrophage Subsets. *Nat Rev Immunol* (2011) 11:723–37. doi: 10.1038/nri3073
34. Mantovani A, Marchesi F, Jaillon S, Garlanda C, Allavena P. Tumor-Associated Myeloid Cells: Diversity and Therapeutic Targeting. *Cell Mol Immunol* (2021) 18:566–78. doi: 10.1038/s41423-020-00613-4
35. Ogger PP, Byrne AJ. Macrophage Metabolic Reprogramming During Chronic Lung Disease. *Mucosal Immunol* (2021) 14:282–95. doi: 10.1038/s41385-020-00356-5
36. Pan Y, Yu Y, Wang X, Zhang T. Tumor-Associated Macrophages in Tumor Immunity. *Front Immunol* (2020) 11:583084. doi: 10.3389/fimmu.2020.583084
37. Gershon RK, Kondo K. Infectious Immunological Tolerance. *Immunology* (1971) 21:903–14.
38. Sakaguchi S, Toda M, Asano M, Itoh M, Morse SS, Sakaguchi N. T Cell-Mediated Maintenance of Natural Self-Tolerance: Its Breakdown as a Possible Cause of Various Autoimmune Diseases. *J Autoimmun* (1996) 9:211–20. doi: 10.1006/jaut.1996.0026
39. Sakaguchi S. Regulatory T Cells: Key Controllers of Immunologic Self-Tolerance. *Cell* (2000) 101:455–8. doi: 10.1016/S0092-8674(00)80856-9
40. Ohkura N, Sakaguchi S. A Novel Modifier of Regulatory T Cells. *Nat Immunol* (2009) 10:685–6. doi: 10.1038/ni0709-685
41. Wan YY. Regulatory T Cells: Immune Suppression and Beyond. *Cell Mol Immunol* (2010) 7:204–10. doi: 10.1038/cmi.2010.20
42. Fehervari Z, Sakaguchi S. CD4+ Tregs and Immune Control. *J Clin Invest* (2004) 114:1209–17. doi: 10.1172/JCI200423395
43. Wing JB, Tanaka A, Sakaguchi S. Human FOXP3(+) Regulatory T Cell Heterogeneity and Function in Autoimmunity and Cancer. *Immunity* (2019) 50:302–16. doi: 10.1016/j.immuni.2019.01.020
44. Munoz-Rojas AR, Mathis D. Tissue Regulatory T Cells: Regulatory Chameleons. *Nat Rev Immunol* (2021) Online ahead of print. doi: 10.1038/s41577-021-00519-w
45. Rocamora-Reverte L, Melzer FL, Wurzner R, Weinberger B. The Complex Role of Regulatory T Cells in Immunity and Aging. *Front Immunol* (2020) 11:616949. doi: 10.3389/fimmu.2020.616949
46. Mauri C, Ehrenstein MR. The 'Short' History of Regulatory B Cells. *Trends Immunol* (2008) 29:34–40. doi: 10.1016/j.it.2007.10.004
47. Mauri C, Gray D, Mushtaq N, Londei M. Prevention of Arthritis by Interleukin 10-Producing B Cells. *J Exp Med* (2003) 197:489–501. doi: 10.1084/jem.20021293
48. Rosser EC, Mauri C. Regulatory B Cells: Origin, Phenotype, and Function. *Immunity* (2015) 42:607–12. doi: 10.1016/j.immuni.2015.04.005
49. Menon M, Hussell T, Ali Shuwa H. Regulatory B Cells in Respiratory Health and Diseases. *Immunol Rev* (2021) 299:61–73. doi: 10.1111/imr.12941
50. Jansen K, Cevhertas L, Ma S, Satitsuksanoa P, Akdis M, van de Veen W. Regulatory B Cells, A to Z. *Allergy* (2021) Online ahead of print. doi: 10.1111/all.14763
51. Mauri C, Bosma A. Immune Regulatory Function of B Cells. *Annu Rev Immunol* (2012) 30:221–41. doi: 10.1146/annurev-immunol-020711-074934
52. Mauri C. Regulation of Immunity and Autoimmunity by B Cells. *Curr Opin Immunol* (2010) 22:761–7. doi: 10.1016/j.coi.2010.10.009
53. Movahedi K, Guilliams M, Van den Bossche J, Van den Bergh R, Gysemans C, Beschin A, et al. Identification of Discrete Tumor-Induced Myeloid-Derived Suppressor Cell Subpopulations With Distinct T Cell-Suppressive Activity. *Blood* (2008) 111:4233–44. doi: 10.1182/blood-2007-07-099226
54. Veglia F, Sanseviero E, Gabrilovich DI. Myeloid-Derived Suppressor Cells in the Era of Increasing Myeloid Cell Diversity. *Nat Rev Immunol* (2021) 21:485–498. doi: 10.1038/s41577-020-00490-y
55. Bronte V, Brandau S, Chen SH, Colombo MP, Frey AB, Greten TF, et al. Recommendations for Myeloid-Derived Suppressor Cell Nomenclature and Characterization Standards. *Nat Commun* (2016) 7:12150. doi: 10.1038/ncomms12150
56. Talmadge JE, Gabrilovich DI. History of Myeloid-Derived Suppressor Cells. *Nat Rev Cancer* (2013) 13:739–52. doi: 10.1038/nrc3581
57. Pan PY, Ma G, Weber KJ, Ozao-Choy J, Wang G, Yin B, et al. Immune Stimulatory Receptor CD40 Is Required for T-Cell Suppression and T Regulatory Cell Activation Mediated by Myeloid-Derived Suppressor Cells in Cancer. *Cancer Res* (2010) 70:99–108. doi: 10.1158/0008-5472.CAN-09-1882
58. Sayan M, Mossman BT. The NLRP3 Inflammasome in Pathogenic Particle and Fibre-Associated Lung Inflammation and Diseases. *Part Fibre Toxicol* (2016) 13:51. doi: 10.1186/s12989-016-0162-4
59. Piguet PF, Collart MA, Grau GE, Sappino AP, Vassalli P. Requirement of Tumour Necrosis Factor for Development of Silica-Induced Pulmonary Fibrosis. *Nature* (1990) 344:245–7. doi: 10.1038/344245a0
60. Hornung V, Bauernfeind F, Halle A, Samstad EO, Kono H, Rock KL, et al. Silica Crystals and Aluminum Salts Activate the NALP3 Inflammasome Through Phagosomal Destabilization. *Nat Immunol* (2008) 9:847–56. doi: 10.1038/ni.1631
61. Mariani TJ, Roby JD, Mecham RP, Parks WC, Crouch E, Pierce RA. Localization of Type I Procollagen Gene Expression in Silica-Induced Granulomatous Lung Disease and Implication of Transforming Growth Factor-Beta as a Mediator of Fibrosis. *Am J Pathol* (1996) 148:151–64.
62. Ma Q. Polarization of Immune Cells in the Pathologic Response to Inhaled Particulates. *Front Immunol* (2020) 11:1060. doi: 10.3389/fimmu.2020.01060
63. Huaux F. Emerging Role of Immunosuppression in Diseases Induced by Micro- and Nano-Particles: Time to Revisit the Exclusive Inflammatory Scenario. *Front Immunol* (2018) 9:2364. doi: 10.3389/fimmu.2018.02364
64. Gharaee-Kermani M, Hu B, Phan SH, Gyetko MR. Recent Advances in Molecular Targets and Treatment of Idiopathic Pulmonary Fibrosis: Focus on TGFbeta Signaling and the Myofibroblast. *Curr Med Chem* (2009) 16:1400–17. doi: 10.2174/092986709787846497
65. Barbarin V, Nihoul A, Misson P, Arras M, Delos M, Leclercq I, et al. The Role of Pro- and Anti-Inflammatory Responses in Silica-Induced Lung Fibrosis. *Respir Res* (2005) 6:112. doi: 10.1186/1465-9921-6-112
66. Barbarin V, Arras M, Misson P, Delos M, McGarry B, Phan SH, et al. Characterization of the Effect of Interleukin-10 on Silica-Induced Lung Fibrosis in Mice. *Am J Respir Cell Mol Biol* (2004) 31:78–85. doi: 10.1165/rcmb.2003-0299OC
67. Huaux F, Arras M, Vink A, Renauld JC, Lison D. Soluble Tumor Necrosis Factor (TNF) Receptors P55 and P75 and Interleukin-10 Downregulate TNF-Alpha Activity During the Lung Response to Silica Particles in NMRI Mice. *Am J Respir Cell Mol Biol* (1999) 21:137–45. doi: 10.1165/ajrcmb.21.1.3570
68. Huaux F, Louahed J, Hudspith B, Meredith C, Delos M, Renauld JC, et al. Role of Interleukin-10 in the Lung Response to Silica in Mice. *Am J Respir Cell Mol Biol* (1998) 18:51–9. doi: 10.1165/ajrcmb.18.1.2911
69. Liu F, Liu J, Weng D, Chen Y, Song L, He Q, et al. CD4+CD25+Foxp3+ Regulatory T Cells Depletion May Attenuate the Development of Silica-Induced Lung Fibrosis in Mice. *PloS One* (2010) 5:e15404. doi: 10.1371/journal.pone.0015404
70. Barbarin V, Xing Z, Delos M, Lison D, Huaux F. Pulmonary Overexpression of IL-10 Augments Lung Fibrosis and Th2 Responses Induced by Silica Particles. *Am J Physiol Lung Cell Mol Physiol* (2005) 288:L841–8. doi: 10.1152/ajplung.00329.2004
71. Zhao Y, Hao C, Bao L, Wang D, Li Y, Qu Y, et al. Silica Particles Disorganize the Polarization of Pulmonary Macrophages in Mice. *Ecotoxicol Environ Saf* (2020) 193:110364. doi: 10.1016/j.ecoenv.2020.110364
72. Misson P, van den Brule S, Barbarin V, Lison D, Huaux F. Markers of Macrophage Differentiation in Experimental Silicosis. *J Leukoc Biol* (2004) 76:926–32. doi: 10.1189/jlb.0104019
73. Murthy S, Larson-Casey JL, Ryan AJ, He C, Kobzik L, Carter AB. Alternative Activation of Macrophages and Pulmonary Fibrosis Are Modulated by Scavenger Receptor, Macrophage Receptor With Collagenous Structure. *FASEB J* (2015) 29:3527–36. doi: 10.1096/fj.15-271304
74. Kumagai-Takei N, Lee S, Srinivas B, Shimizu Y, Sada N, Yoshitome K, et al. The Effects of Asbestos Fibers on Human T Cells. *Int J Mol Sci* (2020) 21:6987. doi: 10.3390/ijms21196987
75. Greenberg MI, Waksman J, Curtis J. Silicosis: A Review. *Dis Mon* (2007) 53:394–416. doi: 10.1016/j.disamonth.2007.09.020

76. Chen Y, Li C, Lu Y, Zhuang H, Gu W, Liu B, et al. IL-10-Producing CD1d (hi)CD5(+) Regulatory B Cells May Play a Critical Role in Modulating Immune Homeostasis in Silicosis Patients. *Front Immunol* (2017) 8:110. doi: 10.3389/fimmu.2017.00110
77. Pardo A, Selman M. Idiopathic Pulmonary Fibrosis: New Insights in Its Pathogenesis. *Int J Biochem Cell Biol* (2002) 34:1534–8. doi: 10.1016/S1357-2725(02)00091-2
78. Selman M, Rojas M, Mora AL, Pardo A. Aging and Interstitial Lung Diseases: Unraveling an Old Forgotten Player in the Pathogenesis of Lung Fibrosis. *Semin Respir Crit Care Med* (2010) 31:607–17. doi: 10.1055/s-0030-1265901
79. Rabolli V, Lo Re S, Uwambayinema F, Yakoub Y, Lison D, Huaux F. Lung Fibrosis Induced by Crystalline Silica Particles Is Uncoupled From Lung Inflammation in NMRI Mice. *Toxicol Lett* (2011) 203:127–34. doi: 10.1016/j.toxlet.2011.03.009
80. Re SL, Giordano G, Yakoub Y, Devosse R, Uwambayinema F, Couillin I, et al. Uncoupling Between Inflammatory and Fibrotic Responses to Silica: Evidence From MyD88 Knockout Mice. *PloS One* (2014) 9:e99383. doi: 10.1371/journal.pone.0099383
81. Wilson MS, Wynn TA. Pulmonary Fibrosis: Pathogenesis, Etiology and Regulation. *Mucosal Immunol* (2009) 2:103–21. doi: 10.1038/mi.2008.85
82. Scott-Browne JP, Shafiani S, Tucker-Heard G, Ishida-Tsubota K, Fontenot JD, Rudensky AY, et al. Expansion and Function of Foxp3-Expressing T Regulatory Cells During Tuberculosis. *J Exp Med* (2007) 204:2159–69. doi: 10.1084/jem.20062105
83. Lo Re S, Lecocq M, Uwambayinema F, Yakoub Y, Delos M, Demoulin JB, et al. Platelet-Derived Growth Factor-Producing CD4+ Foxp3+ Regulatory T Lymphocytes Promote Lung Fibrosis. *Am J Respir Crit Care Med* (2011) 184:1270–81. doi: 10.1164/rccm.201103-0516OC
84. Tang W, Liu F, Chen Y, Song L, Dai W, Li C, et al. Reduction of IL-17A Might Suppress the Th1 Response and Promote the Th2 Response by Boosting the Function of Treg Cells During Silica-Induced Inflammatory Response *In Vitro*. *Mediators Inflamm* (2014) 2014:570894. doi: 10.1155/2014/570894
85. Dai W, Liu F, Li C, Lu Y, Lu X, Du S, et al. Blockade of Wnt/beta-Catenin Pathway Aggravated Silica-Induced Lung Inflammation Through Tregs Regulation on Th Immune Responses. *Mediators Inflamm* (2016) 2016:6235614. doi: 10.1155/2016/6235614
86. Thakur C, Wolfarth M, Sun J, Zhang Y, Lu Y, Battelli L, et al. Oncoprotein Mdig Contributes to Silica-Induced Pulmonary Fibrosis by Altering Balance Between Th17 and Treg T Cells. *Oncotarget* (2015) 6:3722–36. doi: 10.18632/oncotarget.2914
87. Liu F, Dai W, Li C, Lu X, Chen Y, Weng D, et al. Role of IL-10-Producing Regulatory B Cells in Modulating T-Helper Cell Immune Responses During Silica-Induced Lung Inflammation and Fibrosis. *Sci Rep* (2016) 6:28911. doi: 10.1038/srep28911
88. Lu Y, Liu F, Li C, Chen Y, Weng D, Chen J. IL-10-Producing B Cells Suppress Effector T Cells Activation and Promote Regulatory T Cells in Crystalline Silica-Induced Inflammatory Response *In Vitro*. *Mediators Inflamm* (2017) 2017:8415094. doi: 10.1155/2017/8415094
89. Lebrun A, Lo Re S, Chantry M, Izquierdo Carerra X, Uwambayinema F, Ricci D, et al. CCR2(+) Monocytic Myeloid-Derived Suppressor Cells (M-MDSCs) Inhibit Collagen Degradation and Promote Lung Fibrosis by Producing Transforming Growth Factor-Beta1. *J Pathol* (2017) 243:320–30. doi: 10.1002/path.4956
90. Shvedova AA, Tkach AV, Kisin ER, Khaliullin T, Stanley S, Gutkin DW, et al. Carbon Nanotubes Enhance Metastatic Growth of Lung Carcinoma *Via* Up-Regulation of Myeloid-Derived Suppressor Cells. *Small* (2013) 9:1691–5. doi: 10.1002/smll.201201470
91. Shvedova AA, Kisin ER, Yanamala N, Tkach AV, Gutkin DW, Star A, et al. MDSC and TGFbeta Are Required for Facilitation of Tumor Growth in the Lungs of Mice Exposed to Carbon Nanotubes. *Cancer Res* (2015) 75:1615–23. doi: 10.1158/0008-5472.CAN-14-2376
92. Konecny P, Ehrlich R, Gulumian M, Jacobs M. Immunity to the Dual Threat of Silica Exposure and Mycobacterium Tuberculosis. *Front Immunol* (2018) 9:3069. doi: 10.3389/fimmu.2018.03069
93. Sato T, Shimosato T, Klinman DM. Silicosis and Lung Cancer: Current Perspectives. *Lung Cancer (Auckl)* (2018) 9:91–101. doi: 10.2147/LCTT.S156376
94. Otsuki T, Maeda M, Murakami S, Hayashi H, Miura Y, Kusaka M, et al. Immunological Effects of Silica and Asbestos. *Cell Mol Immunol* (2007) 4:261–8.
95. Brilland B, Beauvillain C, Mazurkiewicz G, Rucay P, Roquelaure Y, Tabiasco J, et al. T Cell Dysregulation in Non-Silicotic Silica Exposed Workers: A Step Toward Immune Tolerance Breakdown. *Front Immunol* (2019) 10:2743. doi: 10.3389/fimmu.2019.02743
96. Lee CG, Homer RJ, Cohn L, Link H, Jung S, Craft JE, et al. Transgenic Overexpression of Interleukin (IL)-10 in the Lung Causes Mucus Metaplasia, Tissue Inflammation, and Airway Remodeling *Via* IL-13-Dependent and -Independent Pathways. *J Biol Chem* (2002) 277:35466–74. doi: 10.1074/jbc.M206395200
97. Sun L, Louie MC, Vannella KM, Wilke CA, LeVine AM, Moore BB, et al. New Concepts of IL-10-Induced Lung Fibrosis: Fibrocyte Recruitment and M2 Activation in a CCL2/CCR2 Axis. *Am J Physiol Lung Cell Mol Physiol* (2011) 300:L341–53. doi: 10.1152/ajplung.00122.2010
98. Lee CG, Kang HR, Homer RJ, Chupp G, Elias JA. Transgenic Modeling of Transforming Growth Factor-Beta(1): Role of Apoptosis in Fibrosis and Alveolar Remodeling. *Proc Am Thorac Soc* (2006) 3:418–23. doi: 10.1513/pats.200602-017AW
99. Ask K, Bonniaud P, Maass K, Eickelberg O, Margetts PJ, Warburton D, et al. Progressive Pulmonary Fibrosis Is Mediated by TGF-Beta Isoform 1 But Not TGF-Beta3. *Int J Biochem Cell Biol* (2008) 40:484–95. doi: 10.1016/j.biocel.2007.08.016
100. Decologne N, Kolb M, Margetts PJ, Menetrier F, Artur Y, Garrido C, et al. TGF-Beta1 Induces Progressive Pleural Scarring and Subpleural Fibrosis. *J Immunol* (2007) 179:6043–51. doi: 10.4049/jimmunol.179.9.6043
101. Sun L, Hult EM, Cornell TT, Kim KK, Shanley TP, Wilke CA, et al. Loss of Myeloid-Specific Protein Phosphatase 2A Enhances Lung Injury and Fibrosis and Results in IL-10-Dependent Sensitization of Epithelial Cell Apoptosis. *Am J Physiol Lung Cell Mol Physiol* (2019) 316:L1035–48. doi: 10.1152/ajplung.00299.2018
102. Wang Y, Kuai Q, Gao F, Wang Y, He M, Zhou H, et al. Overexpression of TIM-3 in Macrophages Aggravates Pathogenesis of Pulmonary Fibrosis in Mice. *Am J Respir Cell Mol Biol* (2019) 61:727–36. doi: 10.1165/rcmb.2019-0070OC
103. Misharin AV, Morales-Nebreda L, Reyfman PA, Cuda CM, Walter JM, McQuattie-Pimentel AC, et al. Monocyte-Derived Alveolar Macrophages Drive Lung Fibrosis and Persist in the Lung Over the Life Span. *J Exp Med* (2017) 214:2387–404. doi: 10.1084/jem.20162152
104. Birjandi SZ, Palchevskiy V, Xue YY, Nunez S, Kern R, Weigt SS, et al. CD4 (+)CD25(hi)Foxp3(+) Cells Exacerbate Bleomycin-Induced Pulmonary Fibrosis. *Am J Pathol* (2016) 186:2008–20. doi: 10.1016/j.ajpath.2016.03.020
105. Moore MW, Herzog EL. Regulatory T Cells in Idiopathic Pulmonary Fibrosis: Too Much of a Good Thing? *Am J Pathol* (2016) 186:1978–81. doi: 10.1016/j.ajpath.2016.06.002
106. Reilkoff RA, Peng H, Murray LA, Peng X, Russell T, Montgomery R, et al. Semaphorin 7a+ Regulatory T Cells Are Associated With Progressive Idiopathic Pulmonary Fibrosis and Are Implicated in Transforming Growth Factor-Beta1-Induced Pulmonary Fibrosis. *Am J Respir Crit Care Med* (2013) 187:180–8. doi: 10.1164/rccm.201206-1109OC
107. Bryant AJ, Shenoy V, Fu C, Marek G, Lorentsen KJ, Herzog EL, et al. Myeloid-Derived Suppressor Cells Are Necessary for Development of Pulmonary Hypertension. *Am J Respir Cell Mol Biol* (2018) 58:170–80. doi: 10.1165/rcmb.2017-0214OC
108. Oliveira AC, Fu C, Lu Y, Williams MA, Pi L, Brantly ML, et al. Chemokine Signaling Axis Between Endothelial and Myeloid Cells Regulates Development of Pulmonary Hypertension Associated With Pulmonary Fibrosis and Hypoxia. *Am J Physiol Lung Cell Mol Physiol* (2019) 317: L434–44. doi: 10.1152/ajplung.00156.2019
109. Zhang H, Maric I, DiPrima MJ, Khan J, Orentas RJ, Kaplan RN, et al. Fibrocytes Represent a Novel MDSC Subset Circulating in Patients With Metastatic Cancer. *Blood* (2013) 122:1105–13. doi: 10.1182/blood-2012-08-449413
110. Wright AK, Newby C, Hartley RA, Mistry V, Gupta S, Berair R, et al. Myeloid-Derived Suppressor Cell-Like Fibrocytes Are Increased and Associated With Preserved Lung Function in Chronic Obstructive Pulmonary Disease. *Allergy* (2017) 72:645–55. doi: 10.1111/all.13061

111. Pilling D, Zheng Z, Vakil V, Gomer RH. Fibroblasts Secrete Slit2 to Inhibit Fibrocyte Differentiation and Fibrosis. *Proc Natl Acad Sci USA* (2014) 111:18291–6. doi: 10.1073/pnas.1417426112
112. Verstovsek S, Manshouri T, Pilling D, Bueso-Ramos CE, Newberry KJ, Prijic S, et al. Role of Neoplastic Monocyte-Derived Fibrocytes in Primary Myelofibrosis. *J Exp Med* (2016) 213:1723–40. doi: 10.1084/jem.20160283
113. Selman M, Pardo A. Idiopathic Pulmonary Fibrosis: An Epithelial/Fibroblastic Cross-Talk Disorder. *Respir Res* (2002) 3:3. doi: 10.1186/rr198
114. Bergeron A, Soler P, Kambouchner M, Loiseau P, Milleron B, Valeyre D, et al. Cytokine Profiles in Idiopathic Pulmonary Fibrosis Suggest an Important Role for TGF-Beta and IL-10. *Eur Respir J* (2003) 22:69–76. doi: 10.1183/09031936.03.00014703
115. Freeburn RW, Armstrong L, Millar AB. Cultured Alveolar Macrophages From Patients With Idiopathic Pulmonary Fibrosis (IPF) Show Dysregulation of Lipopolysaccharide-Induced Tumor Necrosis Factor-Alpha (TNF-Alpha) and Interleukin-10 (IL-10) Inductions. *Eur Cytokine Netw* (2005) 16:5–16.
116. Adams TS, Schupp JC, Poli S, Ayaub EA, Neumark N, Ahangari F, et al. Single-Cell RNA-Seq Reveals Ectopic and Aberrant Lung-Resident Cell Populations in Idiopathic Pulmonary Fibrosis. *Sci Adv* (2020) 6:eaba1983. doi: 10.1126/sciadv.aba1983
117. Morse C, Tabib T, Sembrat J, Buschur KL, Bittar HT, Valenzi E, et al. Proliferating SPP1/MERTK-Expressing Macrophages in Idiopathic Pulmonary Fibrosis. *Eur Respir J* (2019) 54:1802441. doi: 10.1183/13993003.02441-2018
118. Galati D, De Martino M, Trotta A, Rea G, Bruzzese D, Cicchitto G, et al. Peripheral Depletion of NK Cells and Imbalance of the Treg/Th17 Axis in Idiopathic Pulmonary Fibrosis Patients. *Cytokine* (2014) 66:119–26. doi: 10.1016/j.cyto.2013.12.003
119. Hou Z, Ye Q, Qiu M, Hao Y, Han J, Zeng H. Increased Activated Regulatory T Cells Proportion Correlate With the Severity of Idiopathic Pulmonary Fibrosis. *Respir Res* (2017) 18:170. doi: 10.1186/s12931-017-0653-3
120. Wang F, Xia H, Yao S. Regulatory T Cells Are a Double-Edged Sword in Pulmonary Fibrosis. *Int Immunopharmacol* (2020) 84:106443. doi: 10.1016/j.intimp.2020.106443
121. Fernandez IE, Greiffo FR, Frankenberger M, Bandres J, Heinzelmann K, Neurohr C, et al. Peripheral Blood Myeloid-Derived Suppressor Cells Reflect Disease Status in Idiopathic Pulmonary Fibrosis. *Eur Respir J* (2016) 48:1171–83. doi: 10.1183/13993003.01826-2015

5

Bleomycin Revisited: A Direct Comparison of the Intratracheal Micro-Spraying and the Oropharyngeal Aspiration Routes of Bleomycin Administration in Mice

*Ilianna Barbayianni†, Ioanna Ninou†, Argyrios Tzouvelekis and Vassilis Aidinis**

Division of Immunology, Biomedical Sciences Research Center Alexander Fleming, Athens, Greece

***Correspondence:**
Vassilis Aidinis
aidinis@fleming.gr

†These authors have contributed equally to this work

Idiopathic Pulmonary Fibrosis (IPF) is a fatal disease characterized by exuberant deposition of extracellular matrix components, deterioration of lung architecture and impairment of lung functions. Its etiopathogenesis remains incompletely understood, as reflected in the lack of an appropriate therapy. Modeling the human disease in mice via the administration of bleomycin (BLM), despite the inherent limitations, has provided valuable insights into the underlying pathogenetic mechanisms, and has been instrumental for the development and validation of new pharmacologic interventions. Here we have directly compared the, most widely used, intratracheal (IT) route of administration with oropharyngeal aspiration (OA). Our results suggest that the OA route of BLM-administration can be used as a safe and effective alternative, minimizing peri-operative and experimental mortality, while preserving a solid fibrotic profile, as assessed with a plethora of standardized readout assays.

Keywords: pulmonary fibrosis, animal model, bleomycin (BLM), intratracheal (IT), oropharyngeal (OA)

INTRODUCTION

Modelinghuman diseases in mice, despite the inherent limitations, has provided valuable insights into the underlying pathogenetic mechanisms, and has been instrumental for the development and validation of new pharmacologic interventions. In the context of Idiopathic Pulmonary Fibrosis (IPF), a fatal disease characterized by exuberant deposition of extracellular matrix components, deterioration of lung architecture and impairment of lung functions (1), the most widely used experimental model is induced by the administration of bleomycin in C57Bl6/J mice (2–4).

Bleomycin (BLM), a mixture of glycopeptides isolated from *Streptomyces verticillus*, is an anti-neoplastic/antibiotic drug for the treatment of some forms of cancer (5). It acts through DNA fragmentation, an activity modulated by many factors in different cell types including chromatin structure and DNA repair machinery, as well as antioxidant and metabolic enzymes (5).The lack of BLM hydrolase in pulmonary epithelial cells is thought to be the main reason for the observed toxicity of BLM in the lung, resulting in the development of pulmonary fibrosis as a side effect in treated cancer patients. The observed toxicity in human patients was soon translated to an animal model (6), serving the scientific community ever since. The model is characterized by alveolar epithelial cell death and the secretion of pro-inflammatory and pro-fibrotic factors, leading to fibroblast activation and collagen deposition, reproducing some, but not all, of the key features of the human disease (3, 4). The ensuing inflammation, the lack of alveolar epithelial hyperplasia and the quick resolution, the main differences with the human disease and the major drawbacks of the BLM model, can be circumvented, in part, though the repetitive administration of BLM (7).

In order to mimic the human exposure, BLM was initially administered systemically, via intravenous or intraperitoneal injections, resulting, as in humans, to the subpleural development of fibrotic lesions (4). However, intratracheal (IT) administration of a single BLM dose, resulting in bronchiolocentric fibrotic patches, has become the method of choice (3). Furthermore, the IT delivery of BLM through a microspray aerosolizer (8) has been shown to yield more reproducible results and more homogenous distribution of fibrotic lesions than IT instillation/injection (9). Following the example of other drugs and agents (10–13), an alternative way of administering BLM in the trachea, namely oropharyngeal aspiration (OA), has been recently introduced (14, 15). However, the IT and OA routes of BLM administration have not been directly compared (3). As shown here, OA of 0.8 U/Kg BLM results in similar fibrotic responses as with 3.2 U/Kg when administered IT. OA administration reduced both the peri-operative mortality, due to the ease and speed of procedures, while the lower BLM dose employed also reduced experimental mortality.

MATERIALS AND METHODS

Mice

Mice were bred under SPF conditions at the local animal facility at "20–22°C, 55 ± 5% humidity, and a 12-h light-dark cycle; water and food were given *ad libitum*" (17). All experimentation in mice was in line with the ARRIVE guidelines and has been approved by the Veterinary service and Fishery Department of the local governmental prefecture, following the approval by the Institutional Animal Ethical Committee (IAEC; #985) of BSRC Alexander Fleming.

Pulmonary fibrosis was induced through the administration of BLM (Nippon Kayaku) to anesthetized (IP ketamine/xylazine/atropine, 100/10/0.05 mg/kg, respectively) mice. The intratracheal (IT) route was applied essentially as previously published (17), and as described in the online **Supplementary Materials and Methods.** Briefly, a MicroSprayer aerosolizer attached to a high-pressure syringe was inserted from the mouth to the carina (trachea's bifurcation) and BLM (0.08 U/mouse), or saline, was sprayed directly into the lungs of mice). The oropharyngeal (OA) route was applied as follows: the tongue of the mice was carefully pulled out using blunt forceps while the mouse's neck and thorax were stabilized on a plastic wall through a rubber band in order for the neck to be minimally stretched. The latter permitted the visualization of the trachea through a laryngoscope and a fiber- optic device. BLM (in a final volume of 50 μl) was then delivered as liquid in the oropharyngeal cavity, with a blunt ended conventional pipette tip. At the same time, the nares were blocked by a tong to prevent obligate nasal breathing and force BLM inhalation. Once BLM was administered (IT or OA), mice were placed on an electrical heating blanket to ensure speedy recovery from anesthesia and to avoid hypothermia.

Bronchoalveolar Lavage Fluid (BALF) collection and analysis, lung histopathological analysis and Quantitative RT-PCR analysis were performed with standardized protocols, as previously published (16) and as described in the on-line **Supplementary Materials and Methods.**

Respiratory mechanics were analyzed with the FlexiVent ventilator system (SCIREQ) following manufacturer instructions, as previously published (17) and as described in the on-line **Supplementary Materials and Methods.**

Statistical Analysis

Statistical significance was assessed with unpaired Student's t-test in comparison with control values (GraphPad Prism 6). Data are presented as means (±SEM); $p < 0.05$ (*) was considered significant.

RESULTS AND DISCUSSION

Beyond the route of administration, the severity of BLM effects highly depends on the precise genetic background of mice (i.e., C57Bl6 J vs. N, further differing between vendors), the local genetic drift of the colony and the health status of the corresponding animal house. As a result, a wide range of BLM concentrations have been employed to induce pulmonary fibrosis in mice (2, 4). As there are only a few published protocols on the OA route of BLM administration, we first tested four different BLM doses administered by OA. The starting concentration was 3.2 U/Kg, the concentration used locally for the IT route, which has been chosen after extensive testing over the years to establish a reproducible phenotype with minimal lethality. Administering 3.2 U/Kg BLM via OA, as well as to a lesser extend 1.6 U/Kg, resulted in significant mortality rates (**Figure S1A**), so these concentrations were discontinued. On the contrary, doses of 0.4 and 0.8 U/Kg were well tolerable, while the dose of 0.8 U/Kg produced statistically significant increases in all established diseases indices (**Figures S1B–H**) with minimal mortality and was thus selected for the direct comparison of IT and OA routes.

Pulmonary fibrosis was induced by IT or OA administration of BLM (at 3.2 and 0.8 U/Kg, respectively) in both male and female, 8–12 weeks old, C57Bl6/J mice. No sex effect was observed in any readout assays, so all following experimental results concern cumulative data, of randomly assigned, sex and age matched groups of littermate mice. No statistically significant difference on overall mouse survival was found between IT and OA BLM administrations (**Figures 1A,B**); however, at these doses, no mice died upon OA administration, most likely due to the lower BLM dose employed. Similarly, both routes of BLM administration, as compared to saline-treated animals, resulted in significant weight loss (**Figure 1C**), one of the traditional indicators of BLM-induced injury. However, IT administration (of BLM or saline) always resulted in peri-operative mortality (data not shown), a feature not usually reported (or even recorded), as it concerns almost exclusively handling, skill and chance. Nevertheless, OA administration is deemed

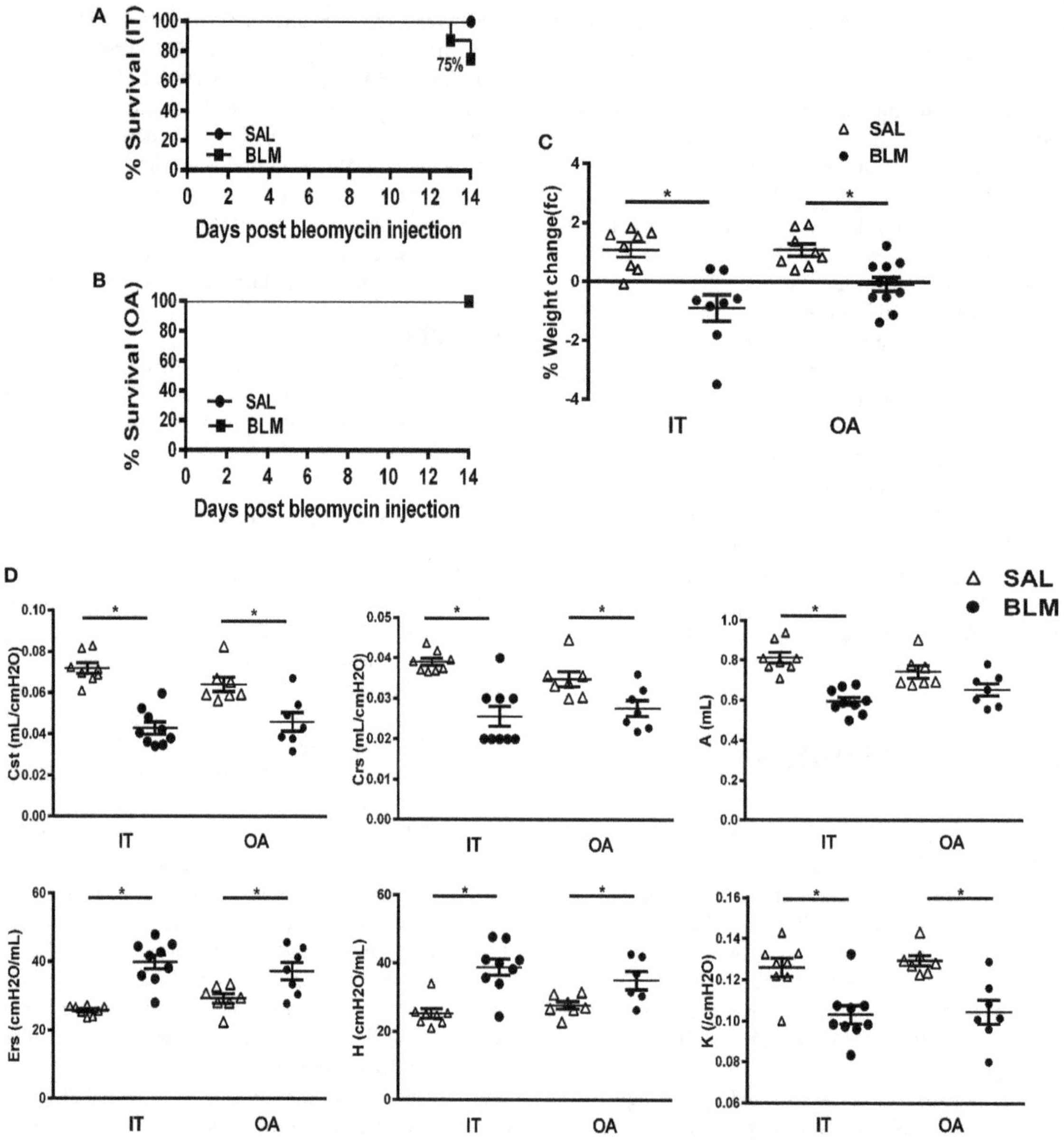

FIGURE 1 | Effects of the intratracheal microspraying (IT) or oropharyngeal aspiration (OA) routes of bleomycin (BLM) administration on mortality, weight loss and functional respiratory mechanics. 8–12 weeks-old C57BL6/J mice were challenged with BLM delivered via the IT or OA routes (at doses of 3.2 and 0.8 U/kg, respectively) and were sacrificed 14 days later. Data from two independent experiments are presented as scatter plots with horizontal bars representing mean levels (±SEM). Statistical significance was assessed with unpaired Student's *t*-test in comparison with the relative control values; *$p < 0.05$ was considered statistically significant. **(A,B)** Kaplan-Meier plot using 14-days survival data from mice treated with BLM delivered either through IT or OA route, respectively. **(C)** Both OT and IA-treated mice demonstrated marked weight loss compared to saline-treated animals 14 days following BLM-challenge. **(D)** *In-vivo* respiratory mechanics following challenge with BLM. OA administration exerted similar to IT administration significant functional impairment on respiratory mechanics compared to saline-treated controls, as assessed by: mean static lung compliance (*Cst*), mean respirator system compliance (*Crs*), mean total lung capacity (*A*), mean respiratory system elastance (*Ers*), mean tissue elastance (*H*) and the curvature of the upper portion of the deflation limp of the pressure volume (PV) curve (*K*).

advantageous on overall experimental mice survival, with both practical and ethical benefits. Moreover, the experimental OA procedure is much easier and faster, as described in detail in **Supplementary Materials and Methods**, maximizing productivity and reproducibility, while it requires much less training.

Fourteen days post BLM (or saline) administration mice were sedated, tracheotomized and connected to a mechanical ventilator to evaluate forced-oscillation lung mechanics (**Figure 1D**). OA administration exerted similar to IT administration functional impairment on respiratory mechanics compared to saline-treated controls, as assessed by significant

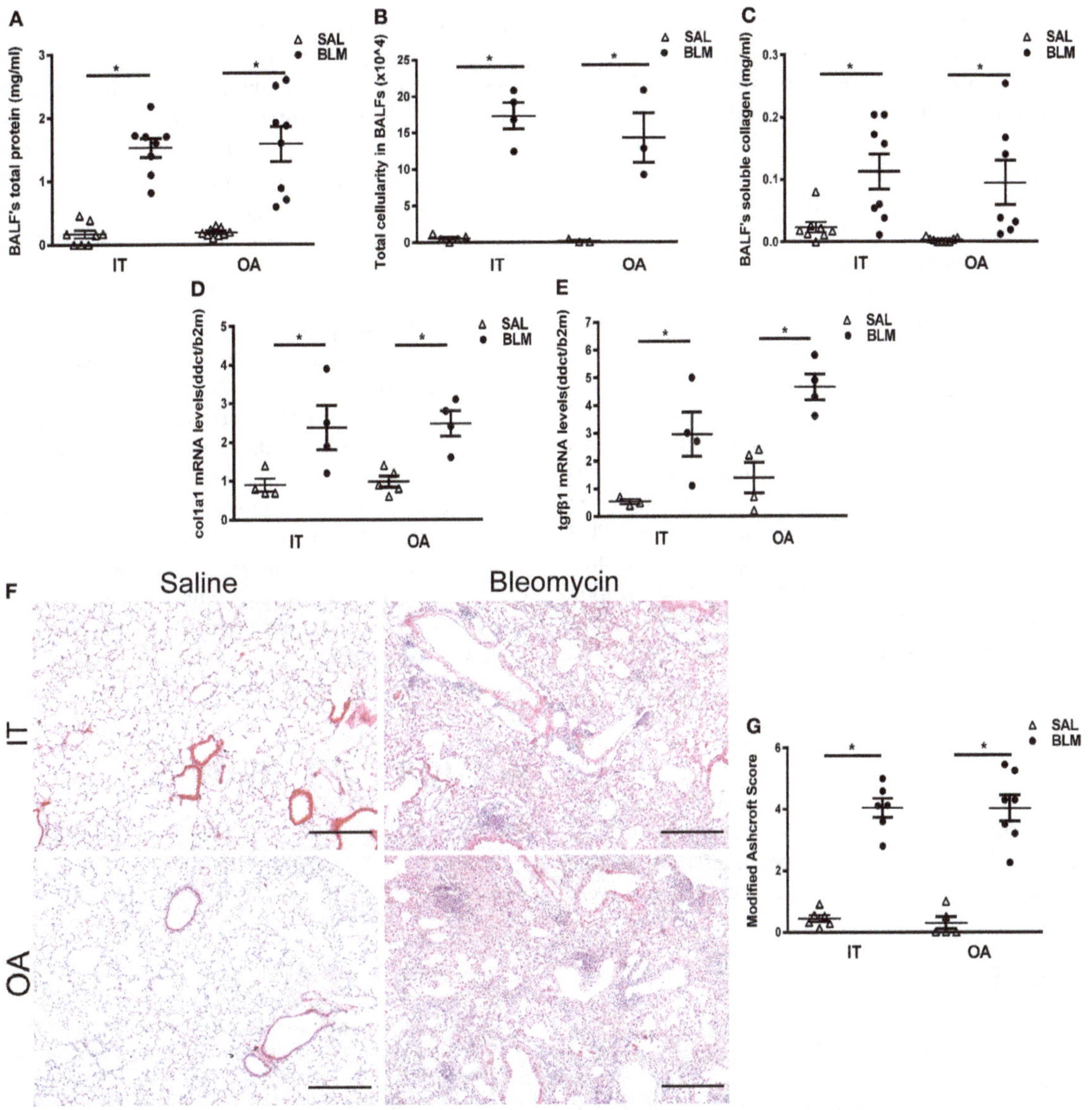

FIGURE 2 | Biochemical and histological analysis of injured lungs following intratracheal microspraying (IT) or oropharyngeal aspiration (OA) bleomycin (BLM) administration. 8–12 weeks-old C57BL6/J mice were challenged with BLM delivered via the IT or OA routes (at doses of 3.2 and 0.8 U/kg, respectively) and were sacrificed 14 days later. Data from two independent experiments are presented as scatter plots with horizontal bars representing mean levels (±SEM). Statistical significance was assessed with unpaired Student's *t*-test in comparison with the relative control values; $^{*}p < 0.05$ was considered statistically significant. **(A)** Increased total protein levels in BALF were observed with both routes of BLM delivery compared to saline-treated controls. **(B)** Both routes of delivery (IT and OA) produced significantly increases in bronchoalveolar lavage fluid (BALF) total cellularity compared to saline-treated animals. **(C)** Lung collagen was assessed by measuring BALF soluble collagen content with sirius red. Both routes of BLM administration were associated with substantial increases in BALF soluble collagen content compared to saline-treated animals. **(D,E)** Quantitative RT-PCR analysis of the *Col1a1* and *Tgfb* mRNA levels in whole mouse lungs challenged with BLM either through IT or OA route of delivery and saline-treated animals. Values were normalized to the expression values of *b2m*. **(F)** Representative H&E-stained lung sections. Scale bars 100 μm. **(G)** Quantitative analysis of histological changes and extent of fibrosis was performed by the modified Ashcroft score. Data represent mean scores obtained from two independent blind reviewers.

reductions in: (1) static lung compliance (*Cst*), (2) respiratory system compliance (*Crs*), and (3) total lung capacity (*A*), as well as increases in: (4) respiratory system elastance (*Ers*), (5) tissue elastance (*H*), (6) curvature of the upper portion of the deflation limb of the PV curve (*K*), (**Figure 1D**). Both static and dynamic lung compliance as well as elastance and total (inspiratory) lung capacity were found to be reliable indices of fibrotic lung injury, as recently suggested (18), well correlating with the Ashcroft score (**Table S1**). Therefore, and as the method is the most relevant to clinical measurements in human patients, not requiring additional mouse numbers, it is thus proposed as a valuable surrogate analysis of BLM-induced pulmonary fibrosis.

The route of BLM administration did not have an effect in BLM-induced vascular leak, as indicated by the total protein levels in the corresponding bronchoalveolar fluids (BALFs)

(**Figure 2A**). Similarly, no differences were detected in the total number of inflammatory cells in BALFs, upon measuring trypan blue stained cells in a hematocytometer (**Figure 2B**). Moreover, no qualitative differences in inflammation was detected either at this final endpoint with FACS analysis (data not shown). BALFs were also analyzed for soluble collagen content with sirius red, as an indirect indicator of tissue fibrosis. Again, no difference was noted upon the differential administration route of BLM (**Figure 2C**). It should be noted that measuring the hydroxyproline content of lung tissue is the most accurate method of determining lung collagen content and, as such, has been recommended as the optimal primary endpoint for fibrosis assessment (3). However, this technique requires at least half the lung, thus limiting the number of parallel analyses that can be performed (either in the mRNA or protein or enzymatic activity level accordingly) or requiring additional mouse numbers, that would still not allow for direct comparisons or correlations of collagen content with other disease indices. The estimation of collagen levels was complemented with Real Time RT-PCR assessment of Collagen 1a1 mRNA levels, again not revealing any differences between the two routes of BLM administration (**Figure 2D**). Similarly, no differences in TGF mRNA levels, the major profibrotic factor driving collagen expression and disease development in both mice and human, were noted (**Figure 2E**).

In line with the BALF assays, and as shown in representative images of H&E stained lung sections, BLM-challenge promoted extensive fibrotic changes and architectural distortion compared to saline-treated animals, irrespectively of the delivery method (**Figure 2F**); no major differences in the distribution and homogeneity of fibrotic lesions were observed. Moreover, collagen visualization with Sirius red and Mason trichrome staining of lung sections did not reveal any gross differences between the two methods either (**Figures S2A,B**); a recently reported automated histological image analysis of fibrotic lungs will further allow objective quantification of lung tissue density as a result of the deposited collagen (18). As expected, quantification of fibrosis by two blind reviewers using the Ashcroft score did not reveal any differences upon differential BLM delivery (**Figure 2G**).

Overall, as prompted by the recent American Thoracic Society workshop report on the use of animal models (3), we have directly compared for the first time the IT and OA routes of BLM-delivery in mice, using a plethora of readout assays including *in vivo* lung function measurements which are highly clinically relevant. Our results suggest that the OA route can be used as a safe and effective alternative route of BLM administration, allowing researchers to easily produce reproducible and robust kinetics of fibrotic lung injury combined with a beneficial safety profile sparing invasive surgical procedures of the IT administration, as well as the systemic effects of higher BLM doses. Moreover, the low BLM concentrations employed will allow drug testing in animals of a much better shape, without compromising a solid fibrotic profile.

AUTHOR CONTRIBUTIONS

VA designed the study; IB and IN performed all reported experiments; AT co-analyzed the data and wrote the paper, which was edited by VA and was critically commented by all authors.

REFERENCES

1. Martinez FJ, Collard HR, Pardo A, Raghu G, Richeldi L, Selman M, et al. Idiopathic pulmonary fibrosis. *Nat Rev Dis Primers* (2017) 3:17074. doi: 10.1038/nrdp.2017.74
2. Tashiro J, Rubio GA, Limper AH, Williams K, Elliot SJ, Ninou I, et al. Exploring animal models that resemble idiopathic pulmonary fibrosis. *Front Med.* (2017) 4:118. doi: 10.3389/fmed.2017.00118
3. Jenkins RG, Moore BB, Chambers RC, Eickelberg O, Konigshoff M, Kolb M, et al. An official american thoracic society workshop report: use of animal models for the preclinical assessment of potential therapies for pulmonary fibrosis. *Am J Respir Cell Mol Biol.* (2017) 56:667–79. doi: 10.1165/rcmb.2017-0096ST
4. Mouratis MA, Aidinis V. Modeling pulmonary fibrosis with bleomycin. *Curr Opin Pulm Med.* (2011) 17:355–61. doi: 10.1097/MCP.0b013e3283 49ac2b
5. Bolzan AD, Bianchi MS. DNA and chromosome damage induced by bleomycin in mammalian cells: an update. *Mutat Res.* (2018) 775:51–62. doi: 10.1016/j.mrrev.2018.02.003
6. Adamson IY, Bowden DH. The pathogenesis of bloemycin-induced pulmonary fibrosis in mice. *Am J Pathol.* (1974) 77:185–97.
7. Degryse AL, Lawson WE. Progress toward improving animal models for idiopathic pulmonary fibrosis. *Am J Med Sci.* (2011) 341:444–9. doi: 10.1097/MAJ.0b013e31821aa000
8. Bivas-Benita M, Zwier R, Junginger HE, Borchard G. Non-invasive pulmonary aerosol delivery in mice by the endotracheal route. *Eur J Pharm Biopharm.* (2005) 61:214–8. doi: 10.1016/j.ejpb.2005.04.009
9. Robbe A, Tassin A, Carpentier J, Declèves A-E, Ngono M, Nonclercq D, et al. Intratracheal bleomycin aerosolization: the best route of administration for a scalable and homogeneous pulmonary fibrosis rat model? *BioMed Res Int.* (2015) 2015:10. doi: 10.1155/2015/198418
10. De Vooght V, Vanoirbeek JA, Haenen S, Verbeken E, Nemery B, Hoet PH. Oropharyngeal aspiration: an alternative route for challenging in a mouse model of chemical-induced asthma. *Toxicology* (2009) 259:84–9. doi: 10.1016/j.tox.2009.02.007
11. Rao GV, Tinkle S, Weissman DN, Antonini JM, Kashon ML, Salmen R, et al. Efficacy of a technique for exposing the mouse lung to particles aspirated from the pharynx. *J Toxicol Environ Health A* (2003) 66:1441–52. doi: 10.1080/15287390306417
12. Foster WM, Walters DM, Longphre M, Macri K, Miller LM. Methodology for the measurement of mucociliary function in the mouse by scintigraphy. *J Appl Physiol.* (1985). (2001) 90:1111–7.
13. Lakatos HF, Burgess HA, Thatcher TH, Redonnet MR, Hernady E, Williams JP, et al. Oropharyngeal aspiration of a silica suspension produces a superior model of silicosis in the mouse when compared to intratracheal instillation. *Exp Lung Res.* (2006) 32:181–99. doi: 10.1080/01902140600 817465
14. Bale S, Sunkoju M, Reddy SS, Swamy V, Godugu C. Oropharyngeal aspiration of bleomycin: an alternative experimental model of pulmonary fibrosis developed in Swiss mice. *Indian J Pharmacol.* (2016) 48:643–8. doi: 10.4103/0253-7613.194859
15. Egger C, Cannet C, Gerard C, Jarman E, Jarai G, Feige A, et al. Administration of bleomycin via the oropharyngeal aspiration route leads to sustained lung fibrosis in mice and rats as quantified by UTE-MRI and histology. *PLoS ONE* (2013) 8:e63432. doi: 10.1371/journal.pone.00 63432
16. Oikonomou N, Mouratis MA, Tzouvelekis A, Kaffe E, Valavanis C, Vilaras G, et al. Pulmonary autotaxin expression contributes to the pathogenesis of pulmonary fibrosis. *Am J*

Respir Cell Mol Biol. (2012) 47:566–74. doi: 10.1165/rcmb.2012-0004OC

17. Yu G, Tzouvelekis A, Wang R, Herazo-Maya JD, Ibarra GH, Srivastava A, et al. Thyroid hormone inhibits lung fibrosis in mice by improving epithelial mitochondrial function. *Nat Med.* (2018) 24:39–49. doi: 10.1038/nm.4447
18. Gilhodes J-C, Julé Y, Kreuz S, Stierstorfer B, Stiller D, Wollin L. Quantification of pulmonary fibrosis in a bleomycin mouse model using automated histological image analysis. *PLoS ONE* (2017) 12:e0170561. doi: 10.1371/journal.pone.0170561

6

Vincristine Promotes Transdifferentiation of Fibroblasts into Myofibroblasts *via* P38 and ERK Signal Pathways

Hui Xu[1†], Jingwen Yang[2†], Mengyun Tu[3], Jie Weng[1], Mengying Xie[1], Zhiliang Zhou[1], Peisen Zhou[4], Liang Wang[5], Chan Chen[2,6] and Zhiyi Wang[1,7]**

[1]*Department of General Practice, The Second Affiliated Hospital of Wenzhou Medical University, Wenzhou, China,* [2]*Department of Geriatric Medicine, The First Affiliated Hospital of Wenzhou Medical University, Wenzhou, China,* [3]*Department of Clinical Laboratory, Hangzhou TCM Hospital Affiliated to Zhejiang Chinese Medical University, Hangzhou, China,* [4]*Department of Emergency Medicine, The Second Affiliated Hospital of Wenzhou Medical University, Wenzhou, China,* [5]*Department of Public Health, Robbins College of Health and Human Sciences, Baylor University, Waco, TX, United States,* [6]*Institute of Bioscaffold Transplantation and Immunology, School of Basic Medical Sciences, Wenzhou Medical University, Wenzhou, China,* [7]*Institute of Hypoxia Medicine, School of Basic Medical Sciences, Wenzhou Medical University, Wenzhou, China*

***Correspondence:**
Zhiyi Wang
wzy1063@126.com
Chan Chen
chenchan99@126.com

†These authors have contributed equally to this work and share first authorship

Background: Vincristine (VCR) is used in the clinic as an anti-tumor drug. VCR can cause pulmonary fibrosis (PF), leading to respiratory failure. The transformation of fibroblasts into myofibroblasts may play a key role in PF. The present study attempted to reveal the molecular mechanism of VCR-induced PF and the possible involvement of the mitogen-activated protein kinase (MAPK) signaling pathway.

Methods: Human embryonic lung fibroblasts (HELFs) were treated with different concentrations of VCR. Inhibitors of extracellular signal-regulated kinase 1/2 (ERK1/2) and p38 MAPK were added to HELFs. Cell proliferation state was assessed using cell counting kit-8 and by directly counting the number of cells. The expressions of vimentin and α-smooth muscle actin (α-SMA) were investigated using western blot and immunofluorescence analyses. Activation of ERK and P38 was estimated by the expression of phosphorylated p38 MAPK (p-p38), p38 MAPK, phosphorylated ERK1/2 (p-ERK1/2) and ERK1/2 using western blot analysis. Enzyme-linked immunosorbent assay was used to estimate the level of collagen I in cell culture supernatants.

Results: Results showed that VCR promoted cellular proliferation, secretion of collagen I and the expression of vimentin and α-SMA. High expression of p-p38 and p-ERK1/2 was associated with the activation of the MAPK signaling pathway. MAPK inhibitors SB203580 and PD98059 suppressed the expression of the above proteins.

Abbreviations: α-SMA, A-smooth muscle actin; CCK-8, Cell counting kit -8; DAPI, 4,6-diamidino-2-phenylindole; ECM, Extracellular matrix; ELISA, Enzyme-Linked Immunosorbent Assay; ERK1/2, Extracellular signal-regulated kinase 1/2; FB, Fibroblasts; FCS, Fetal calf serum; helfs, Human Embryonic Lung Fibroblasts; MAPK, Mitogen-activated protein kinase; MB, Myofibroblast; PBS, Phosphate-buffered saline; p-ERK1/2, Phosphorylated ERK1/2; PF, Pulmonary fibrosis; p-p38, Phosphorylated p38 MAPK; RIPA, Radioimmunoprecipitation assay; VCR, Vincristine.

Conclusion: Our study revealed that VCR could promote the differentiation of fibroblasts into myofibroblasts by regulating the MAPK signal pathway, which may be a promising way to treat VCR-induced PF.

Keywords: vincristine, pulmonary fibrosis, fibroblast, myofibroblast, MAPK

INTRODUCTION

Pulmonary fibrosis (PF) is a life-threatening pulmonary disease with multiple causes, including environmental factors (such as inhalation of particulates) (Biondini et al., 2020; Türkkan et al., 2021), various kinds of diseases ((such as the COVID-19 pandemic, Antisynthetase syndrome) (Baratella et al., 2021; Orlandi et al., 2021) and adverse effects of specific drugs (Wang et al., 2015; Wan et al., 2020; Weng et al., 2020). Some specific drugs, especially for carcinoma, can lead to PF, which is one of the major causes of death worldwide (Xu et al., 2021). Vincristine (VCR) is an alkaloid extracted from *Catharanthus roseus* of the Apocynaceae family. It is effective in treating acute lymphoblastic leukemia, Hodgkin's disease, lymphosarcoma and breast cancer (Okamoto et al., 2016; Yao et al., 2019). However, one of the most important adverse effects is PF. Although several studies have shown that VCR-induced PF may be associated with oxidative stress, inflammation or pulmonary epithelial cells, the underlying mechanism remains elusive (K. Zhang & Xu, 2020). Therefore, exploring the exact mechanism of VCR-induced PF will be of significant clinical importance.

Fibroblasts (FB) play a very essential role in the process of PF (H. Zhao et al., 2020). In pathological conditions, FBs are involved in the process of PF mainly through their abnormal proliferation and transformation and secretion of large amounts of extracellular matrix (ECM) (Chanda et al., 2019; Y.; Zhang et al., 2019). Moreover, several factors, especially the stimulation of a large number of cytokines, can cause FBs proliferation and transformation into myofibroblast (MB) during PF, leading to the secretion of a large amount of ECM. The MBs express α-smooth muscle actin (α-SMA), which is considered to be a crucial marker for MB (Xie et al., 2015; L.; Zhang et al., 2020).

Accumulating evidence has proved that MB differentiation is related to the pathogenesis of PF (Wei et al., 2019; Li N et al., 2020). MBs proliferate continuously, the survival time of single cells is greatly prolonged and a large number of collagen fibers are produced, which indicate MBs are important promoters of PF. Some studies showed that the mRNA expression of type I collagen increased in a-SMA positive cells, which proved that MBs were the key source of collagen gene expression. These pieces of evidence suggest that MBs are the primary cell types causing abnormal deposition of ECM. MBs can also accelerate the course of fibrosis by aggravating the epithelial injury and inflammatory reaction (Wei et al., 2019; Andugulapati et al., 2020).

Thus, inhibiting the transformation of lung FBs into MBs may be a promising strategy to treat VCR-induced PF. The signaling pathway of p38 and extracellular signal-regulated kinase (ERK) are considered to play an important role in cell proliferation and differentiation (Sun et al., 2015; Lavoie et al., 2020). Previous studies showed that p38 and ERK participated in the process of PF (Weng et al., 2019; Yu et al., 2019). Here, we attempted to reveal the molecular mechanism of VCR-induced PF and the potential effect of mitogen-activated protein kinase (MAPK) signaling pathway.

MATERIALS AND METHODS

Antibodies and Reagents

VCR injection was provided by Selleck Corporation (Beijing, China). Human embryonic lung fibroblasts (HELFs) were obtained from the Shanghai Cell Bank of the Chinese Academy of Sciences (Shanghai, China). Antibodies against vimentin, α-SMA, p-ERK, ERK, p-p38MAPK and p38MAPK were purchased from Cell Signaling Technologies (Boston, MASS, United States). Collagen I concentration was determined by the enzyme-linked immunosorbent assay (ELISA) kit (Abcam, Cambridge, UK). Cell counting kit -8 (CCK-8) was acquired from Abcam (Cambridge, UK). Antibodies to GAPDH were purchased from Proteintech (Wuhan, China).

Cell Culture and Treatment

HELFs were cultured in Eagles minimum essential medium (Corning Inc., Corning, NY, United States) supplemented with 10% fetal calf serum (FCS), streptomycin and penicillin (both 100 U/ml) under a 5% CO2-containing humidified atmosphere at 37°C. Cells were subcultured in T-flasks about every 5 days (Corning, United States). After washing twice with 10 ml of phosphate-buffered saline (PBS) and treating with trypsin (0.25%) and EDTA (0.02%) PBS, cells were removed from flasks after reaching 80–90% confluence. Cells were resuspended in a culture medium after incubating for 5 min at 37°C and seeded on a dish at a density of 4 × 106 cells/100-mm. HELFs were treated with different concentrations of VCR (0, 0.35, 0.7 and 1.4 μg/ml) for 24 h after overnight serum starvation.

Cell Proliferation Assay

HELFs (1 × 104 cells/well) were maintained in a complete culture medium in 96-well plates until they reached 60–70% confluence. Cells were incubated with CCK8 solution (10 μL) at 37°C for 3 h in the presence or absence of SB203580 or PD98059 (MedChemExpress, United States) after stimulation with VCR. The cell proliferation rate was then determined by measuring the absorbance at a wavelength of 450 nm using a microplate reader.

ELISA

As an indicator of PF, the amount of collagen I in cell culture supernatants was measured using commercial ELISA kits.

Supernatants were collected after centrifugation (2500 × g) at 4°C for 10 min. All of the samples were measured in triplicate, according to the manufacturer's instructions.

Western Blotting Analysis

Total cell protein was extracted by radioimmunoprecipitation assay (RIPA) buffer, and the protein concentration was detected using the Bicinchoninic Protein Assay kit (BCA, Beyotime Biotechnology, China). The cells were washed thrice in PBS and then re-suspended in cold RIPA buffer. The cell lysates were centrifuged at 12,000 × g at 4°C for 15 min, and supernatants were collected. Total proteins (5–10 μg) were exposed to 10% sodium dodecyl sulfate-polyacrylamide gel electrophoresis (SDS-PAGE, Beyotime Biotechnology, China) and then transferred to nitrocellulose membranes (Pall Corporation, United States). Next, the membranes were sealed for 2 h with 5% fat-free milk at room temperature, and then co-incubated overnight at 4°C with primary antibodies: anti-p-ERK1/2, anti-ERK1/2, anti-p-p38, anti-p38, anti-vimentin and anti-α-SMA. The membranes were washed and then incubated with secondary antibody goat anti-rabbit IgG at room temperature for 1 h. An anti-GAPDH antibody was used as the internal reference. Signals were detected using an enhanced chemiluminescence-detecting kit according to the manufacturer's protocol (Bio-Rad Laboratories, Hercules, CA, United States). The band intensity was analyzed using ImageJ software (National Institutes of Health, Bethesda, MD, United States).

Immunofluorescence Analysis

Cells were fixed with 4% paraformaldehyde at room temperature for 20 min. Cells were then treated with 0.3% Triton X-100 for 6 min. Non-specific staining was prevented using 5% goat serum. Cells were incubated with combinations of primary antibodies: anti-vimentin or anti-α-SMA at 4°C overnight in a humidified chamber. Cells were washed thrice and then cultured with combinations of secondary antibodies for 1 h. After washing with PBS, cell nuclei were stained with 4,6-diamidino-2-phenylindole (DAPI). The sections were cover-slipped and then examined using a fluorescence microscope (Leica Microsystems, Wetzlar, Germany).

Statistical Analysis

SPSS 19.0 statistical software (Armonk, New York: IBM Corp.) was used for data analysis. All data were presented as the mean ± SEM from at least three independent experiments. Comparisons between groups were performed by one-way analysis of variance (ANOVA) and Tukey's multiple comparison test. $p < 0.05$ was considered statistically significant.

RESULTS

VCR Induces HELF Proliferation in a Concentration-Dependent Manner

As VCR was observed to be cytotoxic *in vitro* at high concentrations (J. E. Sun et al., 2016). The proliferation of HELFs treated with different concentrations of VCR (0, 0.35, 0.7 and 1.4 μg/ml) for 24 h was assessed using CCK-8 assay. The number of cells was also counted. Results showed that compared with the control group, VCR treatment significantly increased HELF proliferation in a concentration-dependent manner ($F = 71.18$, $p < 0.05$ and $F = 62.98$, $p < 0.05$ respectively) (**Figures 1A,C**). HELF proliferation was the most significant at a concentration of 1.4 μg/ml. Therefore, 1.4 μg/ml was used in subsequent experiments.

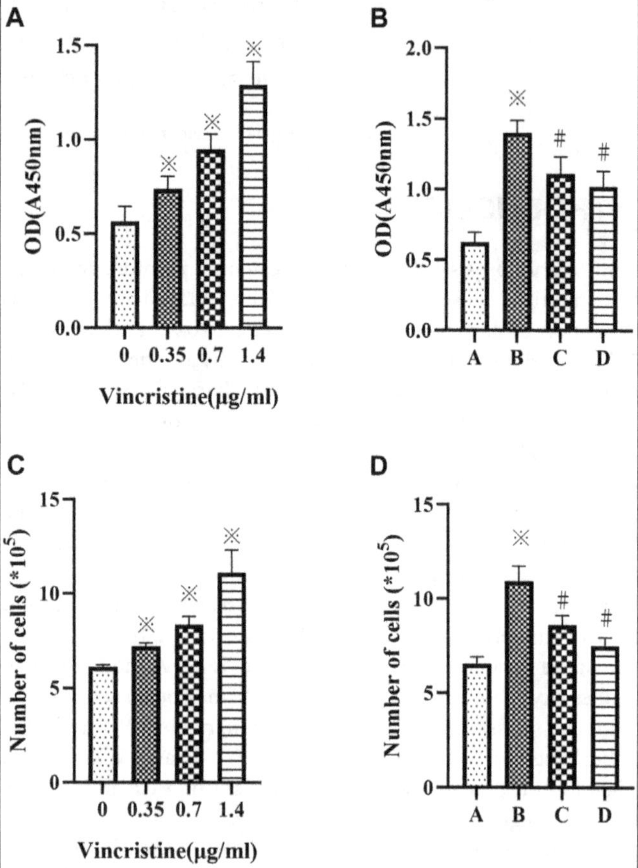

FIGURE 1 | (A,C): Vincristine (VCR) increases cell proliferation in HELFs. Cells were treated with different concentration of vincristine (0, 0.35, 0.7 and 1.4 μg/ml) for 24 h *$p < 0.05$ *vs.* the control group. **(B,D)**: VCR-induced cells proliferation was decreased by SB203580 and PD98059 in HELFs (cells were treated with 1.4 μg/ml VCR for 24 h). Cell proliferation was assessed by CCK8 assay. *$p < 0.05$ *vs.* the control group; #$p < 0.05$ *vs.* the VCR group. A: control group, B: VCR group, C: SB203580 group, D: PD98059 group.

HELFs were treated with VCR (1.4 μg/ml) for 24 h in the presence or absence of p38 MAPK inhibitor SB203580 or ERK1/2 inhibitor PD98059. It was found that HELF proliferation was markedly inhibited by SB203580 or PD98059. Similar results were obtained by counting the number of cells ($F = 62.33$, $p < 0.05$ and $F = 70.35$, $p < 0.05$, respectively) (**Figures 1B,D**).

VCR Induces Collagen I Secretion in a Concentration-Dependent Manner

Compared with the control group, treatment with VCR significantly increased the level of collagen I in a

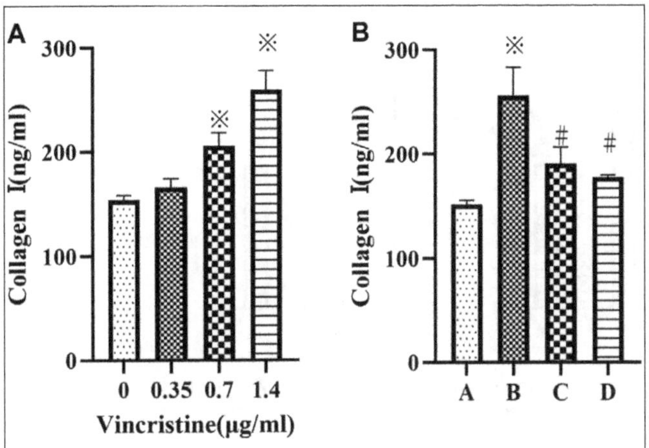

FIGURE 2 | (A): Cells were treated with different concentration of vincristine (0, 0.35, 0.7 and 1.4 μg/ml) for 24 h *$p < 0.05$ *vs*. the control group. **(B)**: VCR-induced collagen I production was decreased by SB203580 and PD98059 (cells were treated with 1.4 μg/ml VCR for 24 h). We measured the level of collagen I using ELISA assay. *$p < 0.05$ *vs*. the control group; #$p < 0.05$ *vs*. the VCR group. A: control group, B VCR group, C: SB203580 group, D: PD98059 group.

concentration-dependent manner ($F = 92.98$, $p < 0.05$) (**Figure 2A**). The most dramatic increase was detected at a concentration of 1.4 μg/ml. Furthermore, the level of collagen I decreased significantly in the presence of SB203580 or PD98059 incubation with 1.4 μg/ml VCR ($F = 47.93$, $p < 0.05$) (**Figure 2B**).

VCR Induces HELF Differentiation *via* p38 and ERK Signal Pathways

The expression of vimentin and α-SMA was detected using western blotting to confirm lung FB differentiation. The result showed that incubation of HELFs with different concentrations of VCR significantly increased the expression of vimentin and α-SMA in a dose-dependent manner. The most significant increase was detected at a concentration of 1.4 μg/ml. ($F = 87.93$, $p < 0.05$ and $F = 78.05$, $p < 0.05$, respectively) (**Figures 3A–C**).

In addition, the phosphorylation and total levels of p38 MAPK and ERK1/2 were detected using western blot analysis. The results revealed that compared with the control group, incubation with VCR significantly increased the amount of p-p38 MAPK, t-p38 MAPK, p-ERK1/2 and t-ERK1/2 in a dose-dependent manner. The most significant increase was detected at a concentration of 1.4 μg/ml. ($F = 80.03$, $p < 0.05$ and $F = 78.20$, $p < 0.05$, respectively) (**Figures 3A,D,E**). Collectively, these findings suggest that VCR induced MB differentiation *via* p38 MAPK and ERK signal pathways.

Inhibition of p38 MAPK and ERK Signaling Pathways Suppresses VCR-Induced PF

To further determine the mechanism of p38 MAPK and ERK signaling pathways in VCR-induced PF, SB203580 and PD98059 were used to inhibit p38 MAPK and ERK1/2 signaling pathways. Western blot and immunofluorescence assays were used to detect the level of α-SMA.

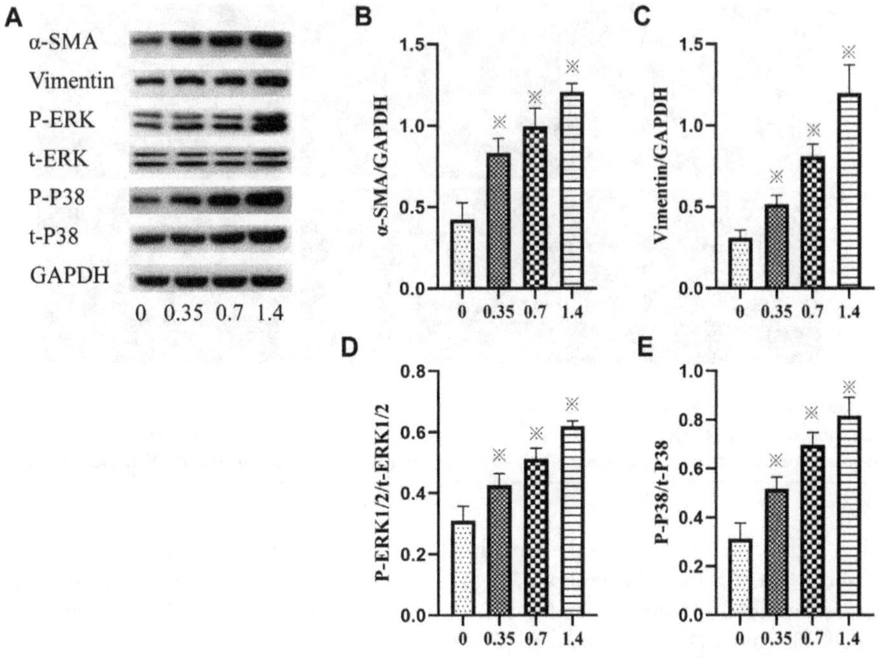

FIGURE 3 | (A–E): α-SMA, vimentin, p-ERK1/2, ERK1/2, p-p38 and p38 levels in HELFs were detected using Western blotting. Cells were incubated with different concentration of VCR (0, 0.35, 0.7 and 1.4 μg/ml) for 24 h. Data were presented as mean ± SEM from three independent experiments. *$p < 0.05$ *vs*. the control group. **(A–D)**: 0,0, 0.35,0.7 and 1.4 μg/ml VCR group.

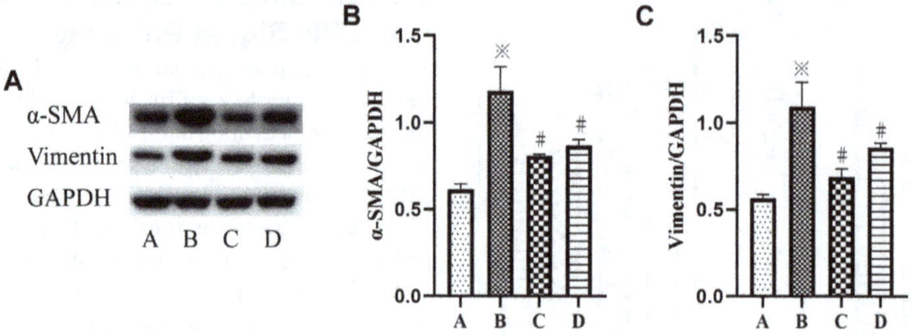

FIGURE 4 | (A–C): α-SMA and vimentin levels in HELFs were detected using Western blotting. Cells were which were stimulated with VCR (1.4 μg/ml) for 24 h in presence of SB203580 and PD98059. Data were presented as mean ± SEM from three independent experiments. $^{*}p < 0.05$ *vs*. the control group; $\#p < 0.05$ *vs*. the VCR group. A: control group, B: VCR group, C: SB203580 group, D: PD98059 group.

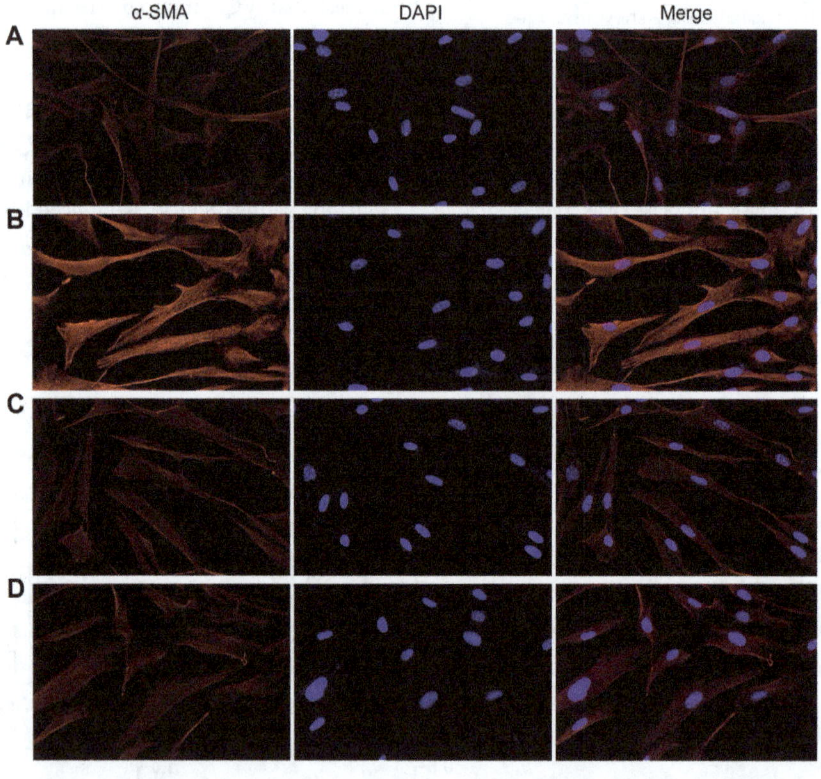

FIGURE 5 | Expression of α-SMA induced by VCR in HELFs (original magnification, ×400). HELFs were cultured with VCR (1.4 μg/ml) for 24 h. Immunocytochemical analysis showed that α-SMA expression was markedly increased in the VCR group compared with the control group, but was decreased in the two inhibitor groups. Red represents α-SMA; blue represents nuclei. **(A)**: control group, **(B)**: VCR group, **(C)**: SB203580 group, **(D)**: PD98059 group.

The results showed a significant increase in the protein expression of vimentin and α-SMA in the VCR group (1.4 μg/ml), and the protein expression level of vimentin and α-SMA were decreased after SB203580 and PD98059 treatment ($F = 55.95$, $p < 0.05$ and $F = 61.40$, $p < 0.05$) (**Figures 4A–C**).

Similarly, fluorescence analysis results showed that α-SMA expression was significantly increased in the VCR group (1.4 μg/ml) compared with the control group (**Figure 5**). α-SMA expression levels were dramatically reduced in groups pretreated with SB203580 and PD98059. Together, these results indicate that p38 MAPK and ERK are involved in the modulatory effects of VCR-induced PF.

DISCUSSION

While VCR is being widely in the clinic for the treatment of various conditions (such as breast cancer, bronchogenic carcinoma, soft tissue sarcoma and neuroblastoma) (Chao et al., 2015), it may cause several adverse effects in the long term, for instance, lung toxicity, especially PF, which is life-threatening. Moreover, relatively little research has been conducted on molecular mechanisms of VCR-induced PF. Thus, revealing the underlying mechanism of VCR-induced lung injury may help to optimize the treatment strategy and reduce its adverse effect in clinical practice. Studies have shown that the proliferation of MBs is one of the main characteristic features of PF (Huang et al., 2017; J.; Li J et al., 2020). Our study shows that VCR could lead to the transformation of FBs into MBs, revealing the important role of FB proliferation in the pathogenesis of VCR-induced PF.

Pulmonary FBs are important effector cells in the occurrence and development of PF. HELFs have been widely used to study the transdifferentiation of fibroblasts into myofibroblasts and the mechanism of PF *in vitro* (Zhang et al., 2018; Gu et al., 2021). Therefore, we also regard HELFs as fibroblasts in this study. The expression of α-SMA is considered to be one of the markers of MBs and a phenotypic marker of FB differentiation (Shinde et al., 2017). In PF, there are a large number of FBs, mainly MBs, accumulating in lung connective tissues, which are speculated to be formed by the transformation of FBs in lung stroma (Pechkovsky et al., 2012; Lin et al., 2020). Dense bundles of α-SMA in MB cytoplasm have a contractile function and reduce lung compliance, which is closely related to its fibrogenic function. Vimentin is a member of the intermediate fiber family (Yang et al., 2021). It constitutes the main intermediate fiber in interstitial cells. Its primary function is to form the cell scaffold network with microtubule and microfilaments to maintain their integrity. It plays an important role in cell adhesion, migration, metastasis, proliferation and apoptosis. Vimentin is derived from MBs and endothelial cells. It is also a typical marker of mesenchymal cells. In the present study, we analyzed the specific protein levels of MBs. The expression of α-SMA and vimentin was assayed using western blot analysis. It was found that the protein expression of α-SMA and vimentin increased significantly after 12-h treatment with VCR. Hence, it was inferred that VCR promotes the development of PF by stimulating the transformation of FBs into MBs.

The mitogen-activated protein kinase (MAPK) is the most important growth regulatory protein. It is the key connection between the cytoplasm and nucleus. It influences the response of cells to changes in the external environment. It can regulate various inflammatory mediators and the expression of cytokines. It plays an important regulatory role in the physiological processes of cell growth, differentiation, development, neural function, immune function, etc. (P. Zhao et al., 2018). It is also reported to play a key role in MB differentiation and ECM deposition.

P38 MAPK, as an important member of the MAPK family, is mainly in the cytoplasm in the resting state. It can be phosphorylated and transferred to the nucleus after stimulation by hypoxia, ultraviolet and other factors. It plays a key role in the regulation of inflammatory response and wound healing by regulating the activity of transcription factors and the synthesis of cytokines (Deng et al., 2021).

The activation of the ERK signaling pathway is associated with many pro-fibrotic cytokines and kinases, such as transforming growth factor-β (TGF-β), platelet-derived growth factor, matrix metalloproteinases, etc. The expression of activated ERK1/2 protein was up-regulated in human or animal models of PF (Liu et al., 2021). The degree of PF was significantly reduced after the administration of inhibitors of ERK signaling pathway PD98059, indicating that this signal pathway is involved in the process of PF. Another study revealed that TGF-β-induced protein expression of human basic fibroblast growth factor (bFGF) could stimulate ERK phosphorylation, which can be inhibited by nonspecific inhibitors of the ERK signaling pathway PD98059. It showed that the ERK signaling pathway plays an important role in MB proliferation, apoptosis and type I collagen proliferation. Limiting the activity of the ERK signaling pathway can inhibit FB proliferation and reduce the production of ECM (Dong et al., 2017).

The current study showed that VCR induced increased protein and gene levels of p-p38 and p-ERK, and P38 and ERK signaling pathways were activated in the cell model of MBs. Our data showed that p38 MAPK and ERK are involved in the modulatory effects of VCR-induced PF.

In summary, for the first time, our study demonstrated that VCR could promote the transformation of FBs into MBs by inducing the phosphorylation of ERK and p38 MAPK. It means that the regulation of ERK and p38 MAPK may provide a target for clinical treatment of VCR-induced PF.

AUTHOR CONTRIBUTIONS

CC and ZW were primarily responsible for making experiment plans and designed the experiments. HX and JY performed the experiments and took charge of paper writing. MT and JW analyzed the data and took charge of paper writing. MX and ZZ created figures. PZ and LW gave experimental technical support.

REFERENCES

1. Andugulapati, S. B., Gourishetti, K., Tirunavalli, S. K., Shaikh, T. B., and Sistla, R. (2020). Biochanin-A Ameliorates Pulmonary Fibrosis by Suppressing the TGF- β Mediated EMT, Myofibroblasts Differentiation and Collagen Deposition in *In Vitro* and *In Vivo* Systems. *Phytomedicine* 78, 153298. doi:10.1016/j.phymed. 2020.153298
2. Baratella, E., Marrocchio, C., Cifaldi, R., Santagiuliana, M., Bozzato, A. M., Crivelli, P., et al. (2021). Interstitial Lung Disease in Patients with Antisynthetase Syndrome: a Retrospective Case Series Study. *Jpn. J. Radiol.* 39 (1), 40–46. doi:10.1007/s11604-020-01030-3
3. Biondini, D., Balestro, E., Sverzellati, N., Cocconcelli, E., Bernardinello, N., Ryerson, C. J., et al. (2020). Acute Exacerbations of Idiopathic Pulmonary Fibrosis (AE-IPF): an Overview of Current and Future Therapeutic Strategies. *Expert Rev. Respir. Med.* 14 (4), 405–414. doi:10.1080/17476348.2020.1724096
4. Chanda, D., Otoupalova, E., Smith, S. R., Volckaert, T., De Langhe, S. P., and Thannickal, V. J. (2019). Developmental Pathways in the Pathogenesis of Lung Fibrosis. *Mol. Aspects Med.* 65, 56–69. doi:10.1016/j.mam.2018.08.004
5. Chao, M. W., Lai, M. J., Liou, J. P., Chang, Y. L., Wang, J. C., Pan, S. L., et al. (2015). The Synergic Effect of Vincristine and Vorinostat in Leukemia *In Vitro* and *In Vivo*. *J. Hematol. Oncol.* 8, 82. doi:10.1186/s13045-015-0176-7

6. Deng, J., Xiong, M., Liao, C., and Xiang, T. (2021). Effects of Propofol on Inflammatory Response and Activation of P38 MAPK Signaling Pathway in Rats with Ventilator-Induced Lung Injury. *Acta Cir Bras* 36 (10), e361004. doi:10.1590/acb361004
7. Dong, H., Luo, L., Zou, M., Huang, C., Wan, X., Hu, Y., et al. (2017). Blockade of Extracellular Heat Shock Protein 90α by 1G6-D7 Attenuates Pulmonary Fibrosis through Inhibiting ERK Signaling. *Am. J. Physiol. Lung Cel Mol Physiol* 313 (6), L1006–l1015. doi:10.1152/ajplung.00489.2016
8. Gu, P., Wang, D., Zhang, J., Wang, X., Chen, Z., Gu, L., et al. (2021). Protective Function of Interleukin-22 in Pulmonary Fibrosis. *Clin. Transl Med.* 11 (8), e509. doi:10.1002/ctm2.509
9. Huang, C., Xiao, X., Yang, Y., Mishra, A., Liang, Y., Zeng, X., et al. (2017). MicroRNA-101 Attenuates Pulmonary Fibrosis by Inhibiting Fibroblast Proliferation and Activation. *J. Biol. Chem.* 292 (40), 16420–16439. doi:10.1074/jbc.M117.805747
10. Lavoie, H., Gagnon, J., and Therrien, M. (2020). ERK Signalling: a Master Regulator of Cell Behaviour, Life and Fate. *Nat. Rev. Mol. Cel Biol* 21 (10), 607–632. doi:10.1038/s41580-020-0255-7
11. Li, J., Feng, M., Sun, R., Li, Z., Hu, L., Peng, G., et al. (2020). Andrographolide Ameliorates Bleomycin-Induced Pulmonary FIbrosis by Suppressing Cell Proliferation and Myofibroblast Differentiation of Fibroblasts *via* the TGF- B1-Mediated Smad-dependent and -independent Pathwaysfibrosis by Suppressing Cell Proliferation and Myofibroblast Differentiation of Fibroblasts *via* the TGF-B1-Mediated Smad-dependent and -independent Pathways. *Toxicol. Lett.* 321, 103–113. doi:10.1016/j.toxlet.2019.11.003
12. Li, N., Wang, Z., Gao, F., Lei, Y., and Li, Z. (2020). Melatonin Ameliorates Renal Fibroblast-Myofibroblast Transdifferentiation and Renal Fibrosis through miR- 21-5p Regulation. *J. Cel Mol Med* 24 (10), 5615–5628. doi:10.1111/jcmm.15221
13. Lin, H., Wu, C., Zhu, F., Zhang, G., Xie, Y., Cui, Y., et al. (2020). Anti-fibrotic Effect of Iguratimod on Pulm onary Fibrosis by Inhibiting the Fibroblast-To- Myofibroblast Transition. *Adv. Med. Sci.* 65 (2), 338–347. doi:10.1016/j.advms.2020.05.006
14. Liu, Y., Wang, Y., Lu, F., Wang, L., Miao, L., and Wang, X. (2021). BTB and CNC Homology 1 Inhibition Ameliorates Fibrosis and Inflammation *via* Blocking ERK Pathway in Pulmonary Fibrosis. *Exp. Lung Res.* 47 (2), 67–77. doi:10.1080/ 01902148.2020.1849448
15. Okamoto, Y., Koga, Y., Inagaki, J., Ozono, S., Ueda, K., Shimoura, M., et al. (2016). Effective VCR/DEX Pulse Maintenance Therapy in the KYCCSG ALL-02 Protocol for Pediatric Acute Lymphoblastic Leukemia. *Int. J. Hematol.* 103 (2), 202–209. doi:10.1007/s12185-015-1910-1
16. Orlandi, M., Landini, N., Sambataro, G., Nardi, C., Tofani, L., Bruni, C., et al. (2021). The Role of Chest CT in Deciphering Interstitial Lung Involvement: Systemic Sclerosis versus Covid-19. *Rheumatology (Oxford)* 61 (4), 1600–1609. doi:10.1093/rheumatology/keab615
17. Pechkovsky, D. V., Prêle, C. M., Wong, J., Hogaboam, C. M., McAnulty, R. J., Laurent, G. J., et al. (2012). STAT3-mediated Signaling Dysregulates Lung Fibroblast-Myofibroblast Activation and Differentiation in UIP/IPF. *Am. J. Pathol.* 180 (4), 1398–1412. doi:10.1016/j.ajpath.2011.12.022
18. Shinde, A. V., Humeres, C., and Frangogiannis, N. G. (2017). The Role of α-smooth Muscle Actin in Fibroblast-Mediated Matrix Contraction and Remodeling. *Biochim. Biophys. Acta Mol. Basis Dis.* 1863 (1), 298–309. doi:10.1016/j.bbadis. 2016.11.006
19. Sun, J. E., Stewart, B., Litan, A., Lee, S. J., Schneider, J. P., Langhans, S. A., et al. (2016). Sustained Release of Active Chemotherapeutics from Injectable-Solid β-hairpin Peptide Hydrogel. *Biomater. Sci.* 4 (5), 839–848. doi:10.1039/c5bm00538h
20. Sun, Y., Liu, W. Z., Liu, T., Feng, X., Yang, N., and Zhou, H. F. (2015). Signaling Pathway of MAPK/ERK in Cell Proliferation, Differentiation, Migration, Senescence and Apoptosis. *J. Recept Signal. Transduct Res.* 35 (6), 600–604. doi:10.3109/10799893.2015.1030412
21. Türkkan, G., Willems, Y., Hendriks, L. E. L., Mostard, R., Conemans, L., Gietema, H. A., et al. (2021). Idiopathic Pulmonary Fibrosis: Current Knowledge, Future Perspectives and its Importance in Radiation Oncology. *Radiother. Oncol.* 155, 269–277. doi:10.1016/j.radonc.2020.11.020
22. Wan, X. L., Zhou, Z. L., Wang, P., Zhou, X. M., Xie, M. Y., Mei, J., et al. (2020). Small Molecule Proteomics Quantifies Differences between normal and Fibrotic Pulmonary Extracellular Matrices. *Chin. Med. J. (Engl)* 133 (10), 1192–1202. doi:10.1097/cm9.0000000000000754
23. Wang, Z., Ma, J., Zhang, M., Wen, C., Huang, X., Sun, F., et al. (2015). Serum Metabolomics in Rats after Acute Paraquat Poisoning. *Biol. Pharm. Bull.* 38 (7), 1049–1053. doi:10.1248/bpb.b15-00147
24. Wei, P., Xie, Y., Abel, P. W., Huang, Y., Ma, Q., Li, L., et al. (2019). Transforming Growth Factor (TGF)-β1-induced miR-133a Inhibits Myofibroblast Differentiation and Pulmonary Fibrosis. *Cell Death Dis* 10 (9), 670. doi:10.1038/s41419-019-1873-x
25. Weng, J., Chen, H., Wu, H., Tu, M., Wang, Z., Chen, D., et al. (2020). Amiodarone Induces Epithelial-Mesenchymal Transition in A549 Cells *via* Activation of TGF-B1. *Drug Chem. Toxicol.* 43 (4), 415–422. doi:10.1080/01480545.2018. 1497055
26. Weng, J., Tu, M., Wang, P., Zhou, X., Wang, C., Wan, X., et al. (2019). Amiodarone Induces Cell Proliferation and Myofibroblast Differentiation *via* ERK1/2 and P38 MAPK Signaling in Fibroblasts. *Biomed. Pharmacother.* 115, 108889. doi:10.1016/j.biopha.2019.108889
27. Xie, N., Tan, Z., Banerjee, S., Cui, H., Ge, J., Liu, R. M., et al. (2015). Glycolytic Reprogramming in Myofibroblast Differentiation and Lung Fibrosis. *Am. J. Respir. Crit. Care Med.* 192 (12), 1462–1474. doi:10.1164/rccm.201504-0780OC
28. Xu, J., Weng, J., Yang, J., Shi, X., Hou, R., Zhou, X., et al. (2021). Development and Validation of a Nomogram to Predict the Mortality Risk in Elderly Patients with ARF. *PeerJ* 9, e11016. doi:10.7717/peerj.11016
29. Yang, F., Whelan, E. C., Guan, X., Deng, B., Wang, S., Sun, J., et al. (2021). FGF9 Promotes Mouse Spermatogonial Stem Cell Proliferation Mediated by P38 MAPK Signalling. *Cell Prolif* 54 (1), e12933. doi:10.1111/cpr.12933
30. Yao, W., Li, K., Wang, Z., Pei, J., Liu, X., Zheng, S., et al. (2019). Comparison of Corticosteroid and Vincristine in Treating Kaposiform Hemangioendothelioma and Tufted Angioma: A Systematic Review and Meta-Analysis. *Eur. J. Pediatr. Surg.* 29 (5), 401–407. doi:10.1055/s-0038-1673708
31. Yu, W., Song, X., and Liu, Y. (2019). TRB3 Regulates Pulmonary Interstitial Fibrosis through the MAPK Signaling Pathway. *Int. J. Clin. Exp. Pathol.* 12 (9), 3247–3257.
32. Zhang, K., and Xu, Y. (2020). Suppressing BRD4 Exhibits Protective Effects against Vincristine-Induced Peripheral Neuropathy by Alleviating Inflammation and Oxidative Stress. *Biochem. Biophys. Res. Commun.* 532 (2), 271–279. doi:10. 1016/j.bbrc.2020.06.142
33. Zhang, L., Chi, X., Luo, W., Yu, S., Zhang, J., Guo, Y., et al. (2020). Lung Myofi broblast Transition and Fibrosis Is Regulated by Circ0044226. *Int. J. Biochem. Cel Biol* 118, 105660. doi:10.1016/j.biocel.2019.105660
34. Zhang, X., Cai, Y., Zhang, W., and Chen, X. (2018). Quercetin Ameliorates Pulmonary Fibrosis by Inhibiting SphK1/S1 P Signaling. *Biochem. Cel Biol* 96 (6), 742–751. doi:10.1139/bcb-2017-0302
35. Zhang, Y., Jiao, H., Wu, Y., and Sun, X. (2019). P120-catenin Regulates Pulmonary Fibrosis and TGF-β Induced Lung Fibroblast Differentiation. *Life Sci.* 230, 35–44. doi:10.1016/j.lfs.2019.05.052
36. Zhao, H., Li, C., Li, L., Liu, J., Gao, Y., Mu, K., et al. (2020). Baicalin Alleviates Bleomycin-induced P-ulmonary F-ibrosis and F-ibroblast P-roliferation in R-ats *via* the PI3K/AKT S-ignaling P-athway. *Mol. Med. Rep.* 21 (6), 2321–2334. doi:10.3892/mmr.2020.11046
37. Zhao, P., Xiao, L., Peng, J., Qian, Y. Q., and Huang, C. C. (2018). Exosomes Derived from Bone Marrow Mesenchymal Stem Cells Improve Osteoporosis through Promoting Osteoblast Proliferation *via* MAPK Pathway. *Eur. Rev. Med. Pharmacol. Sci.* 22 (12), 3962–3970. doi:10.26355/eurrev_201806_15280

7

Regulatory Immune Cells in Idiopathic Pulmonary Fibrosis: Friends or Foes?

Chiel van Geffen[1], Astrid Deißler[1,2], Markus Quante[2], Harald Renz[3,4], Dominik Hartl[5,6] and Saeed Kolahian[1,3,4]*

[1] Department of Experimental and Clinical Pharmacology and Pharmacogenomics, University Hospital Tübingen, Tübingen, Germany, [2] Department of General, Visceral and Transplant Surgery, University Hospital Tübingen, Tübingen, Germany, [3] Institute of Laboratory Medicine and Pathobiochemistry, Molecular Diagnostics, Philipps University of Marburg, Marburg, Germany, [4] Universities of Giessen and Marburg Lung Center, German Center for Lung Research (DZL), Marburg, Germany, [5] Department of Pediatrics I, Eberhard Karls University of Tübingen, Tübingen, Germany, [6] Dominik Hartl, Novartis Institutes for BioMedical Research, Basel, Switzerland

***Correspondence:**
Saeed Kolahian
saeed.kolahian@med.uni-tuebingen.de

The immune system is receiving increasing attention for interstitial lung diseases, as knowledge on its role in fibrosis development and response to therapies is expanding. Uncontrolled immune responses and unbalanced injury-inflammation-repair processes drive the initiation and progression of idiopathic pulmonary fibrosis. The regulatory immune system plays important roles in controlling pathogenic immune responses, regulating inflammation and modulating the transition of inflammation to fibrosis. This review aims to summarize and critically discuss the current knowledge on the potential role of regulatory immune cells, including mesenchymal stromal/stem cells, regulatory T cells, regulatory B cells, macrophages, dendritic cells and myeloid-derived suppressor cells in idiopathic pulmonary fibrosis. Furthermore, we review the emerging role of regulatory immune cells in anti-fibrotic therapy and lung transplantation. A comprehensive understanding of immune regulation could pave the way towards new therapeutic or preventive approaches in idiopathic pulmonary fibrosis.

Keywords: idiopathic pulmonary fibrosis, mesenchymal stem/stromal cells, regulatory T cells, regulatory B cells, macrophages, myeloid-derived suppressor cells, pharmacotherapy, transplantation

INTRODUCTION

Pulmonary fibrosis (PF) is a chronic lung disease characterized by progressive fibrotic tissue remodeling and scarring of lung tissue (1). Various factors, such as smoking, chronic aspiration due to gastroesophageal reflux, infections, toxins, radiation, autoimmune reactions (e.g. rheumatoid arthritis, scleroderma, polymyositis, dermatomyositis, Sjögren's syndrome or systemic lupus erythematosus) and exposure to environmental pollutants can trigger chronic lung tissue damage resulting in fibrotic remodeling (2–6). However, PF can also occur without an identifiable underlying cause, known as idiopathic pulmonary fibrosis (IPF). IPF is an age-related interstitial lung disease, affecting mainly patients of 50 years and older with an incidence of 2.8–18 per 100,000 people and a prevalence of 1.25–27.9 per 100,000 people in Europe and North America (3). Unfortunately, IPF patients have a poor prognosis with a median survival of 2-4 years after diagnosis (3). A gain-of-function mutation in the *MUC5B* gene represents the highest genetic risk factor for the development of IPF (3). IPF is difficult to treat with pharmacological therapies and to date, the only effective curative therapy for IPF patients is lung transplantation (3).

Chronic alveolar-micro injuries presumably lead to a maintained and dysregulated wound healing process, which drives IPF (3). Fibrogenesis is marked by a massive accumulation of extracellular matrix (ECM) produced by myofibroblasts such as collagen, elastin, laminin, fibronectin, hyaluronan and glycoproteins, resulting in irreversible thickening of alveolar walls, compromising the exchange of oxygen and carbon dioxide between blood and alveolar air (7, 8). At the cellular level, repeating lung injuries mostly affect type I alveolar epithelial cells (AECs), which mainly form the alveolar surface. In response to this cell loss, type II AECs proliferate in a hyperplastic manner to mask the exposed basement membrane (2). Under healthy conditions, the cells would differentiate into type I AECs and hyperplastic type II AECs would undergo apoptosis (2). However, under the influence of transforming growth factor (TGF)-β, hyperplastic type II AECs remain at the alveolar surface resulting in alveolar collapse (2). Fibroblasts are the most frequent cell type in fibrotic tissues that produce ECM-producing cells which are recruited into the lung compartment (2). Fibroblasts differentiate into contractile myofibroblasts with massive ECM productive capacity (2). Cytokines and growth factors activating fibroblasts and myofibroblasts and inducing further fibrotic tissue remodeling include TGF-β, interleukin (IL)-1, IL-6, IL-13, IL-33, platelet-derived growth factor (PDGF), fibroblast growth factor (FGF), tumor necrosis factor (TNF)-α and leukotrienes (7). Activated fibroblasts produce TGF-β, IL-1β, IL-33, reactive oxygen species, C-X-C motif chemokines (CXC), C-C motif chemokines (CC) maintaining fibrogenesis and attracting immune cells to promote chronic inflammation, resulting in a positive feedback loop supporting fibrogenesis through differentiation of fibroblasts into myofibroblasts (7). TGF-β itself contributes to fibrosis progression *via* TGF-β/SMAD signaling by stimulation of ECM production, inhibition of ECM breakdown through matrix metalloproteinases (MMPs), and epithelial-mesenchymal transition (EMT) induction (9).

Cells of both the innate and adaptive immune system such as mesenchymal stem/stromal cells (MSCs), regulatory T cells (Tregs), regulatory B cells (Bregs), macrophages, dendritic cells (DCs) and myeloid-derived suppressor cells (MDSCs) have been linked to the pathogenesis of IPF, often with contradicting findings (**Figure 1**) (10–14). Immunomodulation by regulatory immune cells is crucial in dampening pathogenic immune responses and inhibiting the transition from inflammation to fibrosis. Identifying the role of regulatory immune cells in IPF is therefore key in understanding the imbalanced immune responses underlying IPF. In this review, we summarize and critically discuss the role of regulatory immune cells in IPF, and assess their interaction with current pharmacological therapies and lung transplantation in IPF.

REGULATORY IMMUNE CELLS IN IPF

Mesenchymal Stem/Stromal Cells

MSCs are multipotent stem cells that can differentiate into various cell types, including osteoblasts, chondrocytes, adipocytes, myocytes, fibroblasts and endothelial cells (15). Furthermore, MSCs play an important role in modulating immunity (16). MSC phenotype and function are dependent on environmental cues (17). Lung-resident (LR)-MSCs have been proposed to play a role in lung regeneration. The expression of high levels of telomerase by LR-MSCs provides self-renewal, survival and replication capacity which may promote lung regeneration by repopulating structural lung cells (17). LR-MSCs have also been suggested to play an important role in IPF. Several profibrotic factors, as mentioned above, have been found to induce myofibroblastic transition (MFT) of MSCs, which in turn promotes collagen production and ECM accumulation driving PF (17–21). Bleomycin-induced pulmonary fibrosis (BPF) in mice resulted in the loss of LR-MSCs, likely due to MFT induced by the upregulation of previously mentioned profibrotic factors (22). Inhibition of the underlying signals mediating MFT, such as Hedgehog, Wnt/β-catenin, Shh/Gli – Wnt or nuclear factor (NF) - κB signaling, were shown to reduce myofibroblast differentiation of LR-MSCs and attenuated BPF in mice (18, 23–25). Dysregulations in these pathways have been found to modulate TGF-β, MMPs, ECM production and EMT (9, 26). Manipulating the MFT of LR-MSCs by regulating microRNA-497 expression understated their detrimental effect in BPF (27). The expression and activity of collagen prolyl hydroxylase, an enzyme crucial for collagen synthesis, by fibrotic lung mesenchymal cells was observed to be one of the mechanisms underlying the TGF-β-mediated profibrotic effects (28). Suppression of collagen prolyl hydroxylase by pyridine-2,5-dicarboxylate attenuated TGF-β-mediated collagen production in both cultured fibroblasts as well as in BPF (28). Promotion of REVERBα, a transcriptional repressor that is upregulated in IPF, has been shown to inhibit both myofibroblast differentiation and collagen secretion in organotypic cultures from IPF patients (29).

In contrast, there is an increasing scientific interest in MSCs due to their immunomodulatory and anti-inflammatory effects (15) as well as an increasing amount of evidence showing anti-fibrotic effects of MSCs in rodents. MSC therapy in BPF models in rodents showed reductions in lung collagen deposition (22, 30–43), lung fibrosis (22, 32, 34, 35, 37, 38), TGF-β levels (22, 30–36, 38–41) and total and/or neutrophil cell count in the bronchoalveolar lavage fluid (BALF) (34, 36, 37, 39) and improved 14-day survival (22, 34, 36) after bleomycin administration. A large body of research is focused on MSC therapies in a variety of human diseases, including graft versus host disease (GVHD), autoimmune disorders, acute respiratory distress syndrome (ARDS), chronic obstructive pulmonary disease (COPD) and asthma (44) as well as in novel diseases like COVID-19 (45, 46). Autologous or allogeneic MSCs are harvested from the peripheral blood, adipose tissue, bone marrow, umbilical cord, placenta, dental pulp, synovial fluid, endometrium, skin or muscle. Due to low numbers, harvested

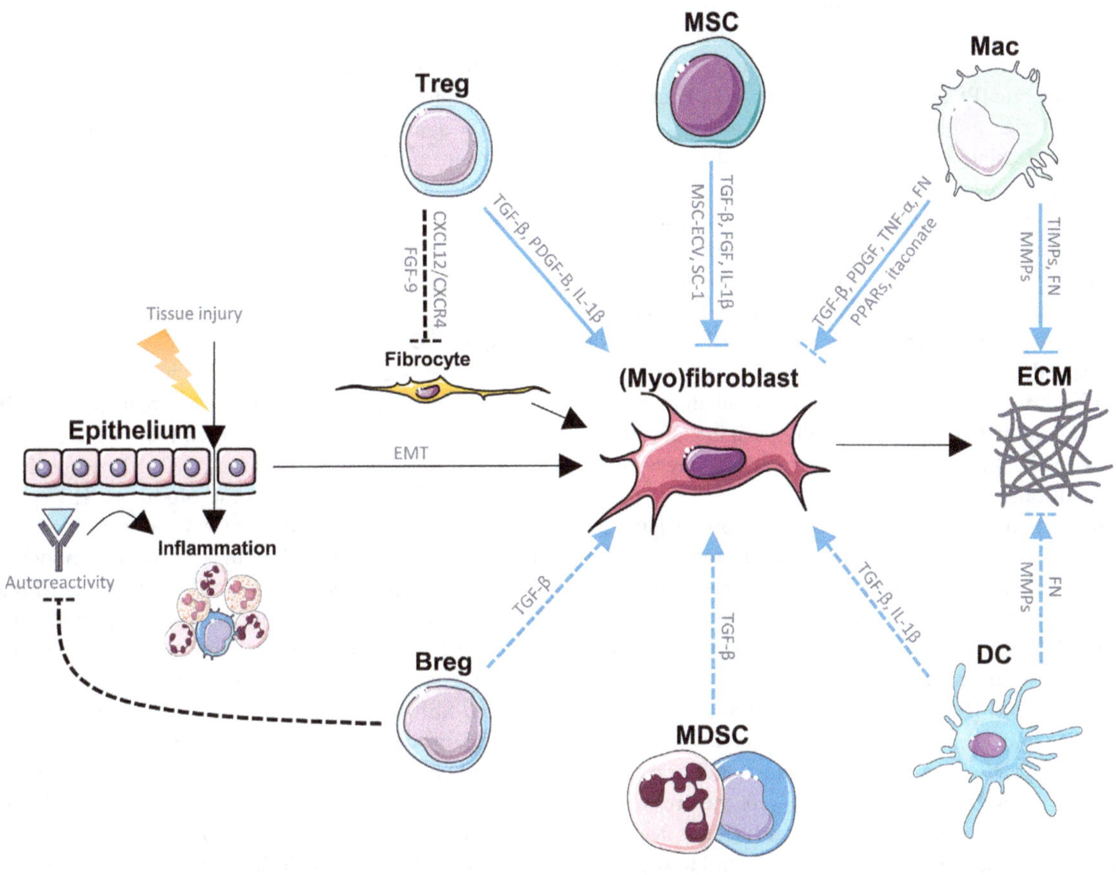

FIGURE 1 | Direct effects of regulatory immune cells on (myo)fibroblasts and extracellular matrix (ECM) in idiopathic pulmonary fibrosis (IPF). Repeated tissue injury triggering chronic tissue damage resulting in inflammation, epithelial mesenchymal transition (EMT) and ultimately in excessive production and buildup of ECM by fibrocytes and (myo)fibroblasts (fibrosis) in the lungs, represents the main paradigm involved in the pathology of IPF. Immune cells with regulatory functions modulate (myo)fibroblast generation, (myo)fibroblast function and ECM homeostasis through various signaling pathways, and known direct pathways are listed here. Mesenchymal stem/stromal cells (MSCs) promote (myo)fibroblasts through fibroblast growth factor (FGF), transforming growth factor (TGF)-β and interleukin (IL)-1β, while MSC-derived extracellular vesicles (MSC-ECV) and stanniocalcin (SC)-1 have opposite effects. MSCs are also prone to myofibroblastic transition. Tregs promote fibrogenesis through TGF-β, platelet-derived growth factor (PDGF)-B and IL-1β, while inhibiting the recruitment of fibrocytes by inhibition of the CXCL12/CXCR4 axis as well as FGF-9. Macrophages enhance fibrosis through TGF-β, PDGF, tumor necrosis factor (TNF)-α, fibronectin (FN) and inhibit fibroblasts *via* itaconate and peroxisome proliferator-activated receptor (PPAR) ligands. Myeloid-derived suppressor cells (MDSCs) and regulatory B cells (Bregs) have been suggested to activate lung fibroblasts, possibly through TGF-β. Bregs inhibit autoreactive immunoglobulins, which may deposit in lung tissue and promote inflammation and IPF. Dendritic cells (DCs) have been shown to produce pro-fibrotic TGF-β and IL-1β. Macrophages (Macs) as well as DCs break down the ECM *via* matrix metalloproteinases (MMPs), a process that is inhibited by tissue inhibitors of metalloproteinases (TIMPs) produced by other macrophage subtypes. Both Macs and DCs have been found to produce fibronectin (FN), another ECM component. Blue lines represent the direct effects of regulatory immune cells on (myo)fibroblasts and ECM in IPF. Dashed lines represent interactions that are not firmly established in IPF. This figure was created using Servier Medical Art templates, which are licensed under a Creative Commons Attribution 3.0 Unported License; https://smart.servier.com.

MSCs are usually expanded *in vitro* in culture medium supplemented with fetal bovine serum, before being transferred to patients (44). The use of MSC-derived products, such as MSC-derived vesicles and exosomes were also reported (47).

At the time of writing, there are five clinical trials using MSC therapy to treat IPF, as registered on the National Institute of Health (NIH) clinical trial database (48)[1]. A phase Ib clinical trial, completed in 2015, studied the intravenous administration of 1 to $2*10^6$ MSC/kg allogeneic placenta-derived MSCs in patients with moderately severe IPF (NCT01385644) (49). The phase I AETHER trial, completed in 2016, studied the administration of a single intravenous infusion of 20, 100, or $200*10^6$ allogeneic bone marrow-derived MSCs in patients with mild-to-moderate IPF (NCT02013700) (50). Another phase I clinical trial, completed in 2018, studied the safety and feasibility of endobronchial administrated autologous bone marrow-derived MSCs in patients with mild-to-moderate IPF (NCT01919827). An uncompleted phase I/II clinical trial that planned to study adipose-derived MSCs in IPF has not recently been updated on its status (NCT02135380). Finally, a phase I/II clinical trial, completed in 2018, studied the intravenous administration of two doses of $2*10^8$ allogeneic bone marrow-derived MSCs every

[1] https://www.clinicaltrials.gov/

3 months for a total of $1.6*10^9$ MSCs in patients with moderate-to-severe IPF (NCT02594839) (51). Another phase Ib clinical trial studied the safety of $1.5*10^6$ autologous adipose-derived MSCs-stromal vascular fraction/kg infused into the lungs of patients with mild-to-moderate IPF at monthly intervals (52). Four of the completed clinical trials published their results showing that MSC therapy is a safe, feasible and promising method to treat IPF patients (49–52). However, more clinical trials are necessary to prove the efficacy of MSC therapy in IPF patients. Due to the urgency and severity of many diseases, including IPF, there are many reports of unapproved stem cell therapies being used, often due to a lack of regulation (53, 54). There remain key challenges in MSC therapy, such as identifying the most valuable source of MSCs, the ideal donors and recipients and the most effective handling and administration routes. Other challenges are in identifying during which stages of IPF patients are most susceptible to MSC therapy as well as possible interactions with pharmaceuticals.

Beneficial effects of MSC therapy in IPF have been suggested to be modulated by MSCs promoting alveolar repair by the secretion of growth factors (55), suppressing inflammation by the production of nitric oxide (NO) and indoleamine 2,3-dioxygenase (IDO) (56), promotion of Treg expansion (57), decreasing pro-inflammatory cytokines such as TNF-α, interferon (IFN)-γ and IL-2 by secreting IL-10 and soluble IL-1β receptor (56) and by protecting lung injury by restituting alveolar bioenergetics through mediating mitochondrial transfer (58). Other observed anti-fibrotic pathways were the production of stanniocalcin-1 which is shown to dampen BPF in mice (41), MSC-derived extracellular vesicles which were found to suppress TGF-β1-induced MFT (47, 59, 60), and MSCs ability to differentiate into type II lung cells expressing surfactant (60). MSCs are also immunoprivileged, lacking human leukocyte antigen (HLA) class II combined with low HLA class I expression, allowing the administration to immunocompetent patients without the need for further immunosuppression (61). However, transferred MSCs have been shown to secrete pro-fibrotic TGF-β1 and underwent MFT in BPF in mice (57). In contrast, MSCs secreting higher levels of TGF-β1 have been suggested to have optimal anti-fibrotic efficacy in BPF in mice (57).

Recent evidence suggests an increase in senescent bone marrow-derived (BM-) MSCs (expressing the senescence markers p21, $p16^{INK4A}$, p53 and senescence-associated β-galactosidase) in IPF patients contribute to disease progression (62, 63). Accumulation of DNA damage in senescent IPF BM-MSCs resulted in decreased mitochondrial and cellular function (62). These findings are in line with the observed decrease in migration capacity and reduced anti-fibrotic effects of BM-MSCs derived from IPF patients, which were adoptively transferred in BPF mice (62). Administrated MSCs derived from older mice were found to be less successful in ameliorating BPF compared to those derived from younger rodents, supporting the contribution of MSC senescence (64). DNA protein kinase catalytic subunits, involved in DNA repair mechanisms, were found to be reduced in IPF lung tissue, which was suggested to result in the expansion of stage-specific embryonic antigen-4^+ mesenchymal progenitors, and the senescence of mesenchymal progeny (63). The possible involvement of senescent MSCs in IPF disease progression may be correlated with age being the most important risk factor (62).

Taken together, literature suggests that an increase in MFT of LR-MSCs as well as an increase in MSC senescence are detrimental to IPF progression. However, the immune regulatory role of MSC has been linked with beneficial effects in IPF, and, as evidenced by the positive findings of studies investigating MSC therapy, seem to provide promising treatment strategies.

Regulatory T cells

Tregs have been found crucial in modulating immunity and maintaining immune tolerance, but their role in IPF remains contradicting and unclearly defined (65, 66). Activated $CD4^+$ T cells (67–69) as well as Tregs (70–73) were found to be upregulated in the peripheral blood of IPF patients and positively correlated with disease severity (67, 68, 70, 71, 73). Tregs were recruited to the lungs of murine models of PF (74, 75). In contrast, several studies observed reduced Treg numbers with reduced suppressive functions in the peripheral blood and BALF of IPF patients correlating to disease severity (76, 77).

Tregs have been suggested to be able to protect from TGF-β1-induced fibrosis *via* the release of IL-10, as Th1 cells exposed to TGF-β1 produce IL-10 (78). TGF-1β was shown to ameliorate BPF in wild-type mice, but not in IL-10-deficient mice (78). IL-10 also has been found to down-regulate type I collagen synthesis in human scar tissue-derived fibroblasts (79) and protect against BPF (80). However, TGF-β1 may also mediate the potential negative role that Tregs play in IPF (81). Tregs have been shown to increase collagen deposition through TGF-β1 in fibroblasts (82) and in lymphatic tissue (83) as well as in the lungs (74) of mice. TGF-β1 autocrine signaling in Tregs was also shown to induce secretion of pro-fibrotic PDGF-B in non-inflammatory conditions (74). Early depletion of Tregs indeed reduced TGF-β levels and lung fibrosis in BPF in mice (81). Semaphorin 7A is an immunomodulating protein involved in many processes such as monocyte chemotaxis (84) and DC migration (85). Adoptive transfer of semaphorin 7A-positive Tregs was found to exaggerate TGF-β1-induced lung fibrosis in TGF-β1-transgenic mice (70). However, the regulation of TGF-β1 levels is not limited to Tregs, confirmed by the finding that reduced Tregs and Foxp3 expression in mice lacking phosphatase and tensin homolog (an antagonist of phosphatidylinositol 3-kinases, which mediate myeloid effector function) was combined with a massive upregulation of TGF-β1 in the lungs (86).

The importance of the CXCL12/CXCR4 axis in IPF has previously been described, and is thought to contribute to fibrosis through recruitment and modulation of fibrocytes (77, 87, 88). Fibrocytes are cells expressing CD45, collagen-1 and CXCR4, exhibit pro-inflammatory and ECM-remodeling properties and share key features with fibroblasts (89, 90). Indeed, the recruitment of $CXCR4^+$ fibrocytes to the lungs of IPF patients was confirmed and blockage of CXCR4 ameliorated BPF in mice (87, 88). Tregs were found to decrease CXCL12 expression and may therefore play a key role in reducing fibrocyte recruitment (91). Similarly, Tregs have been found to inhibit fibrocyte recruitment *via* suppression of FGF-9 (92).

Another pathway by which Tregs may influence IPF progression is by mediating the balance between T helper (Th) 1, Th2, and Th17 responses. Th1 cells were shown to exhibit anti-fibrotic effects through the production of IFN-γ and IL-12 (93), and IFN-γ production by T cells was found to be suppressed by Tregs (94). Th2 immune responses were shown to stimulate myofibroblasts and the progression of the disease through the production of IL-4, IL-5, IL-13 and IL-17A (95, 96). In radiation-induced lung disease in mice, an increase in Th17 was linked to enhanced lung fibrosis, while an increase in Th1 was found to have the opposite effect (97). The downregulation and depletion of Tregs as well as the neutralization of Treg-immunosuppressive activity has been shown to switch Th2-driven responses to Th1-driven responses (74, 98, 99) and attenuated PF progression in a silica-induced (99) as well as in an irradiation-induced murine model (100). Tregs were suggested to promote Th17 through TGF-β and IL-1β (100, 101). However, Th17 cells were found to be decreased in the peripheral blood (while Tregs were found upregulated) resulting in increased TGF-β/IL-17 ratio in IPF patients (72). Adoptive transfer of Tregs into recombination activating gene (Rag) 2 protein-deficient mice (lacking lymphocytes) was found to promote BPF progression and a loss of Foxp3 expression after transfer (10, 102). These findings suggest Tregs might lose their suppressor ability and adopt a Th2 phenotype through which they may promote disease progression (10, 102). In contrast, pro-inflammatory $CD4^{+}CD28^{null}$ helper T cells were found to be upregulated in IPF and were found to be unresponsive to Treg immunomodulation (103).

Treg expansion using IL-2 therapies was shown successful in treating diseases like vasculitis and GVHD (104, 105). Soluble IL-2 complexed to an IL-2 receptor neutralizing antibody allows for hyperstimulation of CD25 (IL-2 receptor alpha chain) by depleting the IL-2 receptor, which in turn promotes Treg expansion. Administration of IL-2 complex in a mouse model of BPF was found to exacerbate PF by increasing collagen deposition as well as inducing lung remodeling (102). The immune response was found to be switched from a Th1 to a Th2 response, while TGF-β production remained unaltered (102).

The adoptive transfer of Tregs did show positive effects in mice models of acute lung injury (91, 106). Adoptive transfer of Tregs was observed to reduce delayed lung recovery in $Rag1^{-/-}$ mice (lacking mature T and B cells) (106) as well as fibroproliferation (91) in lipopolysaccharide-induced acute lung injury. Interestingly, while early depletion of Tregs was found to reduce lung fibrosis and TGF-β1 expression in BPF in mice, late depletion of Tregs showed opposite effects (81). Late stage (after 21 days) increase of Tregs in BPF in CC receptor (CCR) 7 (receptor involved in B and T cell activation, T cell homing and DC maturation) deficient mice showed a positive suppressive effect of Tregs in IPF as well (107). These results suggest several translational limitations relating to animal models of PF that likely resulted in several contradicting results regarding the role of Tregs in IPF (10). Commonly used animal models, such as BPF, are not specific to IPF and rather poorly replicate the core characteristics of the disease, such as the slow development and its irreversible nature. Combined with the already existing gap between animals and humans, as well as the complexity of Tregs, it further complicates translation to the clinical setting.

Literature on the role of Tregs in IPF is often contradictory and the explanation to this phenomenon may be hiding in several factors (10). First of all, the phase of IPF progression appears to be of vital importance when assessing the role of Tregs. Second, there seems to be a high likelihood of discrepancies in the number of Tregs found in the periphery (i.e. the blood) versus the number of Tregs observed in the lungs. Third, there are translational limitations relating to animal models of IPF. Combined with the diverse role of Tregs, it is reasonable to assume these factors contributed to the contradicting observations regarding their role in IPF. All in all, Tregs appear to be both friend and foe in relation to IPF, which suggests that Treg modulation requires careful assessment of the phase of IPF disease state.

Regulatory B Cells

B cells mediate the humoral immunity of the adaptive immune system by secreting antibodies (as plasma cells), and mediate immunity by functioning as antigen-presenting cells (APCs) and by producing cytokines (108). The amount of circulating B cells in the peripheral blood (109, 110) and B cells in the lungs (110–114) of IPF patients were found to be increased together with CXCL 13 (a critical chemokine for the homing of B cells) (115, 116), correlating with disease progression. Similarly, there was an increase in IL-6, IL-13 and B-cell-activating factor (BAFF) (all factors that promote B cells) found in IPF patients (110). $Rag1^{-/-}$ mice as well as gp130(757F);$uMT^{-/-}$ compound mutant mice (deprived of mature B cells) were protected from BPF, suggesting a negative role of B cells in IPF progression (117).

Bregs, however, have been shown to dampen T-cell driven immune responses, to support immunological tolerance, and have been shown to produce anti-inflammatory IL-10 and TGF-β (118). A loss of Bregs in both allergic and autoimmune diseases was found to exacerbate disease progression (119). Decreased numbers of Bregs were found in IPF patients, as well as an increase in the proliferation and activation of T follicular helper (Tfh) cells (12). Tfh cells are a specialized Th cell subset that assist B cells by the secretion of IL-4, IL-10 and IL-21 and CD40 ligand expression, which promotes the growth, differentiation and initiates class switching of B cells as well as induce antigen-specific antibody responses (120). Bregs were shown to suppress Tfh-cell maturation and inhibit Tfh cell-mediated antibody secretion (121). Increases of circulating antigen differentiated B cells (110), plasmablasts (110), autoreactive immunoglobulin (Ig) A in the lungs (109), Ig in BALF (122) and immune complexes were observed in the BALF and lungs of IPF patients (123–126). These findings are in line with the observed reduction of Bregs and observed increase of both Tfh and non-regulatory B cells in IPF. Autoreactive immune complexes are able to deposit in the lung and promote inflammation, while antibodies mediate antibody-dependent cellular cytotoxicity (mediated *via* complement activation or natural killer cells), processes that may drive IPF progression (127).

Antibodies, such as Rituximab, target the CD20 marker that is expressed on the surface of all B cells starting at the pre-B cell stage (128). These antibodies therefore inhibit $CD20^+$ B cells, which as described above were found to be positively correlated to IPF progression (109–117). Rituximab indeed may be a viable treatment option of IPF (129, 130), and is included in 6 NIH registered clinical trials treating IPF at the time of writing (48)[2]. Unfortunately, CD20 antibodies also target CD20 expressing Bregs, showing a downside to unspecific downregulation of B cells. However, levels of CD20 expression differs among different B cells populations, with Bregs generally expressing lower levels of CD20 (131). Depletion of most $CD20^+$ B cells by rituximab was found to enrich $CD20^{low}$ Bregs in mice and human cancer (131). The specific targeting of Bregs or non-regulatory B cells is limited by the lack of specific surface markers (132). However, Bregs might be targeted and upregulated *via* other pathways such as immunomodulation by MDSC (133). A study by Wu et al. found that PGE2 in the exosomes derived from polymorphonuclear (PMN)- MDSCs promote $IL\text{-}10^+$ B cells and ameliorates collagen-induced arthritis in mice (133).

Collectively, Bregs seem to be able to play a vital role in the suppression of IPF. Progress in the specific depletion of non-regulatory B cells or in the expansion of Bregs may provide promising clues for future treatment strategies.

Macrophages

Macrophages play an important role in mediating tissue homeostasis and inflammation as well as phagocytosing viral, bacterial and parasitic pathogens and inducing the adaptive immune response by functioning as an APC (134). The disturbed balance in wound healing processes underlying IPF is thought to be primarily mediated by macrophages (11). Furthermore, the interplay of MMPs and tissue inhibitors of metalloproteinase (TIMPs), secreted by macrophages, among other secreted factors, such as collagen, shape the ECM. Macrophages thereby contribute to IPF in either a pro- or anti-fibrotic manner (135).

Increased number of macrophages was observed in the lungs of IPF patients (136), yet their functional role remains a matter of active discussion. Lung macrophages have been shown to play a crucial role during the fibrotic phase of BPF in mice (136). Low numbers of macrophages during the resolution phase were found to reduce ECM degradation and exacerbate PF (137). Depletion of macrophages in an early phase of fibrosis was, however, shown protective in a murine model of liver fibrosis (137). Previously, the M1/M2 macrophage polarization nomenclature, inspired by the Th1/Th2 paradigm, was commonly used to classify macrophages (86, 96, 138–149). M1-like macrophages have been found to promote fibrosis by secreting pro-inflammatory IL-6 and TNF-α as well as promoting the Th17 and neutrophilic immune response (86, 139–141). M2-like macrophages have been linked to fibrotic processes through the promotion of CC ligand (CCL) 2 and 17, TIMPs, fibronectin, Th2 response through IL-4 production, fibroblasts and the MFT of LR-MSCs (96, 142–149). On the other hand, the production of arginase-1 and MMPs, as well as anti-inflammatory IL-10, TGF-β1 and heme oxygenase 1 by M2-like macrophages suggest a protective role in IPF (96, 142, 143, 149). Peroxisome proliferator-activated receptor (PPAR-) α and PPAR-γ activation has been found to inhibit inflammation by inducing M2-like macrophages, which in turn may inhibit pro-inflammatory cytokine production (150, 151). These findings suggest PPAR ligands may be interesting therapeutic targets in IPF, especially considering they have also been found to directly inhibit fibroblast activation induced by TGF-β1 (152). However, as the M1/M2 paradigm is based on findings from *ex vivo* cultured cells, it is unable to accurately recapitulate the complexity of macrophage phenotypes *in vivo*, and, especially those observed in the IPF lung (153).

Recent studies have begun profiling individual cells, including macrophages, in IPF in great detail through single-cell RNA sequencing (scRNA-seq) (154). Several research groups made their scRNA-seq findings on thousands of cells derived from the lungs of IPF and healthy control available (154). Analysis of such data sets enables the identification of many novel macrophage subsets and their specific ontogeny relating to different stages of IPF. Highly proliferative osteopontin-expressing macrophages were identified through scRNA-seq and were found to mediate myofibroblast activation in the lungs of IPF patients (155). Similarly, another expanded population of pro-fibrotic $CD36^+CD84^+$ macrophages in IPF were identified, which also showed increased expression of genes involved in ECM remodeling (156, PREPRINT).

On the other hand, itaconate has recently been described to mediate anti-fibrotic effects of macrophages in the lungs (157). Decreased levels of pulmonary itaconate as well as reduced itaconate-synthesizing cis-aconitate decarboxylase (*ACOD1*) expression (which mediates itaconate production) in lung macrophages were observed in IPF patients (157). *Acod1* deficient mice developed more severe BPF, while adoptive transfer of lung-derived monocytic macrophages from healthy donor mice alleviated the developed persistent fibrosis (157). Furthermore, itaconate was shown to decrease fibroblast proliferation and wound healing capacity of cultured fibroblasts (157).

The pentraxin-2 analogue, PRM-151, which inhibits the differentiation of monocytes into pro-inflammatory and pro-fibrotic macrophages (and fibrocytes), is therefore a promising therapy and is currently undergoing clinical trial for the treatment of IPF (158). However, several studies suggest possible anti-fibrotic and immunomodulating roles of macrophages, which may be suppressed in IPF, and therefore might provide interesting therapeutic targets. Furthermore, the recent unraveling of specialized macrophage subsets through tools such as scRNA-seq is rapidly increasing the understanding of the complex role they play in IPF and is expected to accelerate future research development substantially.

Dendritic Cells

DCs bridge the innate and adaptive immunity through their role as APCs (159). Besides their primary role as immune activators, DCs have also been described to play tolerogenic and regulatory roles (13). These tolerogenic DCs are crucial in the maintenance

[2] https://www.clinicaltrials.gov/

of central and peripheral tolerance by inducing clonal T cell deletion, T cell anergy, inhibition of memory and effector T cell responses and promoting Tregs (160).

DCs accumulate in the fibrotic lungs of BPF in mice (161, 162) as well as in the BALF and lungs of IPF patients (163–165), while circulating DCs were decreased (166). Fms-like tyrosine kinase-3 ligand (Flt3L), a cytokine that promotes differentiation and proliferation of DCs, was found to be upregulated in the peripheral blood and lungs together with an increase in DCs in the lungs of TGF-β1-induced murine model of PF as well as in IPF patients (167). The unspecific deprivation of DCs in mice lacking Flt3L resulted in more severe PF, while unspecific upregulation of DCs, by supplementing Flt3L, resulted in reduced PF progression in a TGF-β1-induced PF mouse model (167). Specific depletion of DCs by diphtheria toxin (DT) in a mouse strain expressing zinc-finger and BTB domain containing 46 (*Zbtb46*; transcription factor keeping DCs in a quiescent state)-DT receptors was found to result in severe PF in a TGF-β1-induced mouse model of PF (167). In contrast, depletion of DCs by the administration of DT to CD11c-DT receptor-transgenic mice attenuated BPF (168). However, in the latter study it is important to note that CD11c-expressing macrophages were depleted as well, which may explain the discrepancy between the two studies (168). Inactivating DCs using VAG539, a pro-drug of VAF347, which activates the transcription factor aryl hydrocarbon, attenuated BPF lung injury in mice (162). However, VAG539 modulates the cell physiology by binding the transcription factor aryl hydrocarbon receptor expressed in many other cell types besides DCs (169), and has been shown to promote the development of IL-22-secreting Th cells (170), making it questionable whether the attenuation can be attributed solely to DC inactivation. $CD11b^+$ DCs have been found to upregulate the expression of several MMPs, promoting collagen and ECM degradation (171). CXCL4 has recently been identified to be crucial in altering DC development into a pro-inflammatory and pro-fibrotic phenotype that induces ECM accumulation and MFT (172).

Taken together, these findings suggests that besides their tolerogenic role, DCs may also play a detrimental role in IPF disease progression. However, due to a lack of convincing evidence on immune regulation by DCs in IPF, their role remains unclear and needs to be studied in more detail.

Myeloid-Derived Suppressor Cells

MDSCs are immature myeloid-derived cells that potently suppress the immune response, and are mainly subdivided into PMN- and monocytic (M)- MDSCs (173). Due to MDSCs plasticity they have also been found to differentiate into M2-like macrophages and tolerogenic-like DCs (174). The role of MDSCs in cancer is well established, however, their role in many other diseases, such as IPF, remains incompletely defined (14). Increased numbers of PMN-MDSCs were found in the lungs of BPF (and clodronate-treated) mice, likely through increased CXCR 2 expression (40). PMN-MDSCs were also increased in the peripheral blood of patients with interstitial pulmonary disease, while M-MDSC numbers remained unaltered (175). Increased numbers of $CD33^+CD11b^+$ cells (suggestive of MDSCs, particularly M-MDSCs) were found in the peripheral blood in the lungs of IPF patients (69). Increased MDSC numbers were suggested to correlate to poor lung function and increased number of Tregs in IPF patients (69). Depletion of MDSCs was found to enhance fibrosis markers in both kidney and liver models of fibrosis in mice (176), while adoptively transferred MDSCs ameliorated renal fibrosis modeled in mice (177), suggesting a protective role. Increased number of PMN-MDSCs were suggested to be correlated to a decrease in parenchymal fibrosis and attenuation of BPF in mice (175). Another study reported a population of circulating MDSC-like fibrocytes in cancer (178). Furthermore, cells generated from $CD11b^+CD115^+Gr1^+$ MDSCs were shown to contribute to renal deposition of collagen type I in a murine model of renal fibrosis (179). As mentioned above, PMN-MDSCs have been found to promote Bregs, which was suggested to promote the potential protective role MDSCs play in IPF (133). Bone marrow-derived MSCs have been suggested to drive the differentiation of $Gr1^{high}CD11b^+$ cells (mainly PMN-MDSCs) towards a $Gr1^{low}CD11b^+$ phenotype (indicative of M-MDSCs), which was found to inhibit BPF progression in mice (180).

In summary, literature suggests that the immune regulatory functions of anti-inflammatory MDSCs may promote anti-fibrotic effects, making them potentially interesting cells to target in the treatment of IPF. However, there remains a lot of uncertainty on their role, partly attributed to MDSCs plasticity, and more research is needed to further clarify their significance in IPF.

INTERACTION OF PHARMACOLOGICAL THERAPY AND IMMUNE RESPONSES IN IPF

Previously, immune suppressive medications including glucocorticoids and azathioprine or cyclophosphamide were used in the treatment of IPF (181). In 2015, a new guideline for treatment of IPF formulated strong recommendations against the use of immunosuppressive drugs in IPF (182). This suggestion was primarily based on a single multicenter study, PANTHER-IPF, which was terminated prematurely due to the major safety concerns in patients receiving combination therapy of prednisone, azathioprine, and N-acetylcysteine compared with placebo (183). However, the question remained whether immunosuppressants should be tested once more in combination with anti-fibrotics like nintedanib and pirfenidone in the context of IPF. Further long-term studies are needed to determine the safety and efficacy of the combination of immunosuppressive and anti-fibrotic therapy in IPF.

Pirfenidone

Pirfenidone is an anti-fibrotic, anti-inflammatory, and antioxidant drug that has been found to interfere with fibroblast proliferation and MFT and the synthesis of ECM (184, 185). Three double blind randomized placebo-controlled

Phase III trials (CAPACITY 1 and 2 and ASCEND) approved the efficacy and safety of pirfenidone in PF (186, 187). These studies showed that pirfenidone reduced the rate of decline in forced vital capacity (FVC) over a period of 1 year, by approximately 50%, in IPF patients with mild, moderate and severe impairment in lung function (187, 188). Pirfenidone improved life expectancy in IPF patients, however, its use is unfortunately not associated with significant improvement in clinical symptoms like cough or shortness of breath (187). Pirfenidone has been shown to inhibit pro-inflammatory and pro-fibrotic cytokine production such as TGF-β, IL-4, IL-13, and TNF-α and promotes the production of anti-inflammatory IL-10 (189–194). The beneficial effect of pirfenidone in IPF may indeed be the result of the modulation of immune responses through modulating cytokines. However, the direct modulatory effects of pirfenidone on immune responses were not described for a long time. The direct immune modulatory properties of pirfenidone were first studied by Visner GA., et al., 2009, in a murine model of cardiac allograft transplantation (195). This study demonstrated the direct inhibitory role of pirfenidone on $CD4^+$ and $CD8^+$ cell proliferation index *in vivo*, whereas pirfenidone showed no effect on the immunosuppressive properties of Tregs (195). The same group of researchers studied the immunomodulatory role of pirfenidone in a murine model of lung allograft transplantation in 2012 (196). Here they showed that pirfenidone suppressed the activation of lung DCs *in vivo* (196). In this respect, *in vitro* treatment of DCs with pirfenidone reduced the expression of major histocompatibility complex (MHC) class II and costimulatory molecules and impaired DC's capacity to stimulate T cell activation (196). Considering the prolonged allograft survival and robust inhibitory effects of pirfenidone observed in *in vivo* models, as compared to *in vitro* conditions, it may be postulated that other regulatory immune mechanisms are involved in the immunosuppressive effect of pirfenidone besides its direct T cell inhibitory effects. Du et al. showed that pirfenidone reduced splenic germinal center B-cell and Tfh frequencies and reduced infiltration of M2-like macrophages into the lung as well as TGF-β production in a murine model of chronic GVHD (197). Recent studies attempted to investigate the efficacy of pirfenidone co-administered with standard chemotherapy, in cancer. A recent *in vitro* study suggested the inhibitory effect of pirfenidone on metastasis and immune suppressive capacity of cancer-associated fibroblasts (CAFs) in the tumor microenvironment (TME) through inhibition of expression of programmed death-ligand (PD-L) 1 on CAFs and cancer-promoting cytokines and chemokines secretion like TNF-β and CCL17 (198). The immunomodulatory role of pirfenidone needs to be studied in more detail in the TME of cancer models. Although the Food and Drug Administration (FDA) approved pirfenidone for the treatment of IPF since 2014, there remains a lack of robust evidence on the interaction of pirfenidone and the immune system in IPF. Considering the important role of immune responses in IPF, the interaction between pirfenidone and the immune system needs to be studied in more detail, especially in IPF patients receiving long-term pirfenidone treatment.

Nintedanib

Nintedanib is a triple tyrosine kinase inhibitor targeting PDGF, vascular endothelial growth factor and FGF receptors as well as the non-receptor members of the Src family (199, 200). Nintedanib is an anti-fibrotic and anti-inflammatory drug, and was found to reduce fibroblast proliferation, recruitment, and myofibroblast differentiation, and hinders the secretion of ECM in the lung (199). Two replicate Phase II randomized control studies (INPULSIS-1 and 2) confirmed the safety and tolerability profile of Nintedanib in PF (201). Nintedanib reduced the decline of lung function, improved life expectancy, and reduced the risk of acute exacerbations and mortality (201). Recently, the high affinity of nintedanib to FGF receptors and its favorable toxicity profile resulted in the successful application of nintedanib in combination with conventional chemotherapy in cancer patients, such as second-line therapy for rapidly progressing advanced non-small-cell lung cancer (NSCLC) (202–207). However, the direct impact of nintedanib on the host immune response in the clinical cancer setting as well as in IPF is not completely understood. A recent study showed that nintedanib in combination with paclitaxel, a widely used chemotherapy medication, reduced the number of leukocytes and MDSCs in peripheral blood, and reduced the number of $CD8^+$ and B cells in the tumors of Lewis lung carcinoma tumor bearing mice (208). However, nintedanib alone only reduced the mobilization of MDSCs into peripheral blood (208). Overed-Sayer et al., 2020, found that the number of lung mast cells is increased in IPF and was found to be negatively correlated with baseline lung function in humans (209). Additionally, they found that nintedanib, but not pirfenidone, inhibited human fibroblast mediated mast cell survival through stem cell factor receptors and reduced the recruitment of mast cells into the lungs of BPF in rats (209). Although there is a growing body of evidence supporting a dynamic interaction between nintedanib and immune cells, there remains limited understanding on its details, thus warranting further studies.

Novel Therapies for the Treatment of IPF

Future therapies in IPF would ideally target the phenotype and molecular endotype of IPF patients to further personalize treatments based on guided molecular testing. Completed or still ongoing clinical trials of other pharmacological therapies in IPF are listed (**Table 1**). Although some of the listed medications provided encouraging results on the safety and efficacy in IPF patients (227), several other medications failed to demonstrate benefits in treating patients with IPF in recent clinical trials (213–216). However, many of these new medications may potentially interact with the immune system and be beneficial in some endotype of the IPF patient population but both the exact effects of these medications on immune responses and the beneficial effects remain unclear. In recent years, novel revolutionary anti-cancer agents were also suggested to be used in IPF patients. A recent review article analyzed the available literature on the use of immune checkpoint inhibitors in IPF and suggested only a slight beneficial effect for PD-1/PD-L1 inhibitors (228). Cross talk between PD-1, expressed on $CD4^+$ T cells, and PD-L1,

TABLE 1 | Last completed and/or ongoing clinical trials in idiopathic pulmonary fibrosis.

Drug	Mechanism	Phase	NCT identifier (48)[3]	Ref.
Sirolimus (Rapamycin)	Phosphoinositide 3-kinase (PI3K)/mammalian target of rapamycin (mTOR) inhibitor	N/A	NCT01462006	–
Omipalisib (GSK2126458)	PI3K/mTOR inhibitor	I	NCT01725139*	(210)
HEC68498	PI3K/mTOR inhibitor	I	NCT03502902	–
Fresolimumab (GC1008)	Anti-TGF-ß monoclonal antibody	I	NCT00125385*	–
TD139	Galectin-3 inhibitor	II	NCT02257177*/NCT03832946	(211)
Tipelukast (MN-001)	Leukotriene antagonist	II	NCT02503657	–
Belumosudil (KD025)	Rho-associated coiled-coil kinase 2 (ROCK2) inhibitor	II	NCT02688647	(212)
CC-90001	Jun N-terminal kinase inhibitor	II	NCT03142191	–
Dactrekumab (QAX576)	Anti-IL-13 monoclonal antibody	II	NCT00532233*/NCT01266135#	–
Lebrikizumab	Anti-IL-13 monoclonal antibody	II	NCT01872689*	(213)
Tralokinumab (CAT354)	Anti-IL-13 monoclonal antibody	II	NCT02036580*/NCT01629667#	(214)
Romilkimab (SAR156597)	Anti-IgG4 monoclonal antibody that neutralizes IL-4 and IL-13	II	NCT02345070*	(215, 216)
BG00011 (STX-100)§	Anti-integrin (αvβ6) monoclonal antibody	II	NCT01371305*/NCT03573505#	–
Simtuzumab (GS-6624)§	Anti-lysyl oxidase like-2 (LOXL2) monoclonal antibody	II	NCT01769196#	(217)
Ianalumab (VAY-736)	Anti-B-cell activation factor (BAFF) receptor monoclonal antibody	II	NCT03287414	–
Rituximab	Anti-CD20 monoclonal antibody	II	NCT01969409/NCT03286556	–
Carlumab (CNTO 888)§	Anti-CCL2 monoclonal antibody	II	NCT00786201*	(218)
Fezagepras (PBI-4050)	Ligand of probable G-protein coupled receptor (GPR) 40 and 84	II	NCT02538536*	(219)
BMS-986020	Autotaxin-Lysophosphatidic acid pathway (ATX-LPA) inhibitor	II	NCT01766817*	(220)
GLPG1690	ATX-LPA inhibitor	III	NCT03711162/NCT03733444	(221)
PRM-151	Pentraxin-2 analogue	III	NCT04552899/NCT04594707	(158, 222)
ART-123	Recombinant thrombomodulin	III	NCT02739165*	(223)
Treprostinil	Prostacyclin	III	NCT04708782	–
Cotrimoxazole	Antimicrobial	III	NCT01777737#/NCT02759120#	(224)
Doxycycline	Antimicrobial	III	NCT02759120#	(224)
Sildenafil	Phosphodiesterase type 5 (PDE5) inhibitor	III	NCT00517933*/NCT02802345*	(225, 226)
Pamrevlumab (FG-3019)	Anti-connective tissue growth factor (CTGF) monoclonal antibody	III	NCT03955146/NCT04419558	(227)

**Completed clinical trial.*
#Clinical trial withdrawn or terminated.
§Development in IPF discontinued.

expressed on fibroblasts, was proposed to lead to IL17A and TGF-β production by $CD4^+$ T cells, which in turn promoted fibrogenesis (228). Recent research also highlighted promising novel drug targets, such as IL-11 in PF, that warrant further studies (229).

However, our incomplete understanding of IPF pathogenesis, particularly of the role of both structural cells and immune cells in the initiation and progression of IPF, and interaction of current as well as novel therapies with the immune system represent important challenges on the way to success for future precision medicine. To this end, considering the high inter-individual variation in IPF patients, responses to any medication will presumably result in similar variation, thus underscoring the importance of the identification of biomarkers predicting treatment response.

IMMUNOREGULATORY CELLS AND LUNG TRANSPLANTATION IN IPF

Progressive fibrosis in IPF can ultimately result in respiratory failure and death. Here, lung transplantation represents the only therapeutic option that has been linked with a survival benefit in patients suffering from IPF (230). In 2018, a total of 2562 lung transplants were performed in the US, with >60% for underlying disease of IPF (231). However, persisting donor organ scarcity is still limiting the availability of this life-saving therapeutic option. As a result, single-lung transplants (SLT) might represent an effective strategy to serve the increasing demand on donor organs. However, recent analysis of >9.000 patients undergoing lung transplantation for IPF within the United Network of Organ Sharing (UNOS) area demonstrated that double-lung transplantations (DLTs) have improved survival compared to SLTs in patients suffering from IPF (232). Still, five-year survival rates after lung transplantation for IPF are worse compared to other indications (233) with chronic lung allograft dysfunction (CLAD) affecting more than 50% of transplanted lungs after 5 years. Of note, fibrotic processes in the engrafted lung exhibit striking similarities to those in IPF (234).

Since the first report that Tregs are involved in preventing allograft rejection two decades ago (235), immunoregulatory cells have also been widely reported to play a significant role in the context of transplantation and graft tolerance. In more detail, graft acceptance could be linked to complex immunological cross-talk between many more cells, including Bregs, regulatory DCs and especially MDSCs. For example, MDSCs were shown to inhibit GVHD after cell transplantation *via* an

[3]https://www.clinicaltrials.gov/

arginase-1–dependent mechanism in an experimental model (236). In the clinical context, 50 patients with biopsy-proven acute T cell-mediated rejection (ATCMR) showed increased frequencies of MDSCs in peripheral blood mononuclear cells (PBMC) after renal transplantation, which were linked to improved allograft function compared with the MDSCs low group (237). In addition, MDSCs isolated from 29 adult kidney transplant recipients were demonstrated to expand Tregs *in vitro*, while their accumulation overtime after transplantation linearly correlated with an increase of Tregs *in vivo*, thus providing further evidence for an interactive cross-talk between regulatory cell types (238).

Immunoregulatory cells have also entered the stage in the context of both experimental and clinical lung transplantation. Experimental data demonstrated that long-term lung acceptance is associated with the induction of bronchus-associated lymphoid tissue (BALT), where Tregs accumulate and recipient T cells interact with CD11c$^+$ DCs, ultimately resulting in an immune quiescent state (239). Mechanistically, the depletion of Tregs from the BALT of tolerant lungs was shown to result in antibody-mediated rejection, which was characterized by the generation of donor-specific antibodies, complement deposition, and the destruction of airway epithelium. In contrast, the undepleted control group showed no evidence of rejection (240). Of note, a recent prospective human observational study could demonstrate that increased Treg frequencies after lung transplantations were reciprocal associated with chronic lung allograft dysfunction (241). Of particular interest, monocyte-derived DCs, isolated from the peripheral blood of lung transplant patients without bronchiolitis obliterans syndrome, were found to have higher IDO expression, implicating the involvement of MDSCs (242). A recent clinical study focused on MDSCs, assessing their phenotype and frequency in peripheral blood from 20 lung transplant recipients and its relationship to post-transplant complications and immunosuppression (243). In detail, MDSCs were isolated from PBMCs and their functionality was assessed *in vitro* by their capability to block CD4$^+$ and CD8$^+$ T cell proliferation. As a result, MDSCs were increased in stable lung transplant recipients (n=6) vs. non-transplant controls (n=4). Furthermore, patients with infection (n=5) or CLAD (n=9) had lower MDSCs compared to stable recipients. Of note, MDSCs tended to correlate with blood levels of immunosuppressive medication (i.e. cyclosporine A and tacrolimus).

In addition, Bregs have also been shown to interact during the immunological cross-talk subsequent to allotransplantation by mainly promoting the development of Tregs while at the same time suppressing effector CD4$^+$ and CD8$^+$ T cells, as demonstrated in experimental models (244). The first clinical study in 117 lung transplant recipients recently revealed that CD19+CD24^{high}CD38^{high} Breg cells were associated with chronic rejection while no significant correlation with Tregs was found (245).

Interestingly, a recent publication could demonstrate that the application of MSC-based therapy during *ex vivo* lung perfusion (EVLP) before lung transplantation ameliorated ischemic injury in an experimental pig model. In detail, the MSC group showed significantly lower IL-18 and IFN-γ levels and a significantly higher IL-4 level in lung tissue at 12 hours of EVLP compared to the control group thus reflecting a shift of the inflammatory network towards protective conditions. Of critical relevance, the pathological acute lung injury score after transplantation was significantly lower in the MSC-treated group compared to the control group (246). These experimental data are intriguing and might already point towards future directions where immunoregulatory cells might represent promising candidates for cell therapies.

Thus, there is robust and growing evidence that immunoregulatory cells play a pivotal role in allograft acceptance from both experimental and clinical science (247). Coming back to MDSCs, current data attribute the immunoregulatory properties of these cells mainly to two mechanisms of action upstream of T cells to shift the immune response towards peripheral tolerance: First, to their capacity to inhibit the proliferation of allogeneic T cells (243); Second, to their capacity of Treg induction (248, 249). Interestingly, the impact of concomitant immunosuppressive therapy, to prevent allograft rejection, while at the same time acting on the immune cells in general, and MDSCs in particular, has also become a field of increasing research activities. Here, cyclosporine A, a widely used immunosuppressive drug from the group of calcineurin inhibitors, could be mechanistically linked to increased expression of IDO resulting in increased suppressive activities of MDSCs in a mouse skin transplant model (250).

Tacrolimus, another calcineurin inhibitor used to maintain immunosuppression, has recently been shown to increase the immunosuppressive capacity of MDSCs derived from human kidney allograft recipients *in vitro* (251). In the context of experimental trachea transplantation, the impact of Rapamycin combined with immature DCs (Rapa-imDC), isolated from bone marrow, was investigated in trachea recipient rats receiving Rapa-imDCs for 10 consecutive days after transplantation. Here, Rapa-imDC treatment induced T cell hyporesponsiveness by attenuating T cell differentiation into IFN-γ-producing Th1 cells while at the same time increasing Tregs. In addition, Rapa-imDC administration ameliorated airway obliteration symptoms and CD4$^+$ and CD8$^+$ T cell infiltration (252).

Taken together, immunoregulatory cells have been shown to play a central role in mediating the alloimmune response towards graft tolerance, thus becoming a promising target for new pharmacologic strategies in the clinical context of transplantation. However, our current understanding of how immunoregulatory cells are interacting in the clinical context of lung transplantation and IPF is still at its infancy, as particular data are missing thus far. Furthermore, we still have to foster our current understanding of how these cells are shaping the alloimmune response while interacting with current immunosuppressive drugs. Here, the clinical background of IPF patients undergoing lung transplantation with poor prognosis is calling for intensive research activities while the concept of tailored cell therapy is already arising from experimental science.

CONCLUSION

IPF is the most devastating interstitial lung disease, yet remains poorly characterized and understood. Lack of mechanistic understanding of the complex disease causality and the devastating chronic nature complicate research and development. There remains a lack of efficacy of pharmaceutical therapies and lung transplantation is currently still the only truly effective treatment IPF. Despite recent advances in our understanding of IPF, particularly the role of regulatory immune cells remains contradictory and poorly understood. Indeed most, if not all, of the regulatory immune cells involved exhibit both detrimental as well as beneficial effects in IPF. Substantial evidence underlines the negative role of macrophages in IPF, through the involvement in the dysregulated wound healing process and ECM build-up. On the other hand, the suppressed anti-fibrotic effects observed in lung macrophages hint to potential beneficial effects, resulting in a complex and controversially-discussed role for macrophages in IPF. There are several lines of evidence on the pro-fibrotic role of MSCs in IPF, mainly related to myofibroblast differentiation and cellular senescence. However, recent research on MSCs points to a beneficial role in IPF, mainly related to their anti-inflammatory characteristics. Tregs were also found to act beneficial or detrimental in IPF models, likely influenced by the state of the disease or the disease model used. The role of more recently discovered regulatory immune cells, namely Bregs, tolerogenic DCs, MDSCs and novel macrophage phenotypes in IPF remains unclear as well and needs to be studied in more detail. An increased understanding of the potential role of regulatory immune cells in IPF mouse models and, particularly, in human IPF will be of vital importance to design novel effective pharmaceutical treatments as well as improving the success of lung transplantation and to prevent related GVHD. This is especially true with regards to precision medicine that might define future healthcare frameworks. Therefore, further preclinical and human studies are crucial to better understand and define the role of immune regulatory cells in IPF pathogenesis.

AUTHOR CONTRIBUTIONS

SK conceptualized the review. CG, AD, MQ, and SK contributed to the original draft. CG, AD, MQ, HR, DH, and SK contributed to revising and final approval of the manuscript. All authors contributed to the article and approved the submitted version.

REFERENCES

1. Martinez FJ, Collard HR, Pardo A, Raghu G, Richeldi L, Selman M, et al. Idiopathic pulmonary fibrosis. *Nat Rev Dis Primers* (2017) 3:17074. doi: 10.1038/nrdp.2017.74
2. Loomis-King H, Flaherty KR, Moore BB. Pathogenesis, current treatments and future directions for idiopathic pulmonary fibrosis. *Curr Opin Pharmacol* (2013) 13(3):377–85. doi: 10.1016/j.coph.2013.03.015
3. Richeldi L, Collard HR, Jones MG. Idiopathic pulmonary fibrosis. *Lancet* (2017) 389(10082):1941–52. doi: 10.1016/S0140-6736(17)30866-8
4. Molyneaux PL, Maher TM. The role of infection in the pathogenesis of idiopathic pulmonary fibrosis. *Eur Respir Rev* (2013) 22(129):376–81. doi: 10.1183/09059180.00000713
5. Wynn TA. Cellular and molecular mechanisms of fibrosis. *J Pathol* (2008) 214(2):199–210. doi: 10.1002/path.2277
6. Olson AL, Gifford AH, Inase N, Fernandez Perez ER, Suda T. The epidemiology of idiopathic pulmonary fibrosis and interstitial lung diseases at risk of a progressive-fibrosing phenotype. *Eur Respir Rev* (2018) 27(150):180077. doi: 10.1183/16000617.0077-2018
7. Kendall RT, Feghali-Bostwick CA. Fibroblasts in fibrosis: novel roles and mediators. *Front Pharmacol* (2014) 5:123. doi: 10.3389/fphar.2014.00123
8. Fernandez IE, Eickelberg O. New cellular and molecular mechanisms of lung injury and fibrosis in idiopathic pulmonary fibrosis. *Lancet* (2012) 380 (9842):680–8. doi: 10.1016/S0140-6736(12)61144-1
9. Chanda D, Otoupalova E, Smith SR, Volckaert T, De Langhe SP, Thannickal VJ. Developmental pathways in the pathogenesis of lung fibrosis. *Mol Aspects Med* (2019) 65:56–69. doi: 10.1016/j.mam.2018.08.004
10. Moore MW, Herzog EL. Regulatory T Cells in Idiopathic Pulmonary Fibrosis: Too Much of a Good Thing? *Am J Pathol* (2016) 186(8):1978–81. doi: 10.1016/j.ajpath.2016.06.002
11. Zhang L, Wang Y, Wu G, Xiong W, Gu W, Wang CY. Macrophages: friend or foe in idiopathic pulmonary fibrosis? *Respir Res* (2018) 19(1):170. doi: 10.1186/s12931-018-0864-2
12. Asai Y, Chiba H, Nishikiori H, Kamekura R, Yabe H, Kondo S, et al. Aberrant populations of circulating T follicular helper cells and regulatory B cells underlying idiopathic pulmonary fibrosis. *Respir Res* (2019) 20(1):244. doi: 10.1186/s12931-019-1216-6
13. Schmidt SV, Nino-Castro AC, Schultze JL. Regulatory dendritic cells: there is more than just immune activation. *Front Immunol* (2012) 3:274. doi: 10.3389/fimmu.2012.00274
14. Kolahian S, Oz HH, Zhou B, Griessinger CM, Rieber N, Hartl D. The emerging role of myeloid-derived suppressor cells in lung diseases. *Eur Respir J* (2016) 47(3):967–77. doi: 10.1183/13993003.01572-2015
15. Pittenger MF, Discher DE, Peault BM, Phinney DG, Hare JM, Caplan AI. Mesenchymal stem cell perspective: cell biology to clinical progress. *NPJ Regener Med* (2019) 4:22. doi: 10.1038/s41536-019-0083-6
16. Weiss ARR, Dahlke MH. Immunomodulation by Mesenchymal Stem Cells (MSCs): Mechanisms of Action of Living, Apoptotic, and Dead MSCs. *Front Immunol* (2019) 10:1191. doi: 10.3389/fimmu.2019.01191
17. Foronjy RF, Majka SM. The potential for resident lung mesenchymal stem cells to promote functional tissue regeneration: understanding microenvironmental cues. *Cells* (2012) 1(4):874. doi: 10.3390/cells1040874
18. Hou J, Ma T, Cao H, Chen Y, Wang C, Chen X, et al. TNF-alpha-induced NF-kappaB activation promotes myofibroblast differentiation of LR-MSCs and exacerbates bleomycin-induced pulmonary fibrosis. *J Cell Physiol* (2018) 233(3):2409–19. doi: 10.1002/jcp.26112
19. Xia H, Bodempudi V, Benyumov A, Hergert P, Tank D, Herrera J, et al. Identification of a cell-of-origin for fibroblasts comprising the fibrotic reticulum in idiopathic pulmonary fibrosis. *Am J Pathol* (2014) 184 (5):1369–83. doi: 10.1016/j.ajpath.2014.01.012
20. Yang L, Herrera J, Gilbertsen A, Xia H, Smith K, Benyumov A, et al. IL-8 mediates idiopathic pulmonary fibrosis mesenchymal progenitor cell fibrogenicity. *Am J Physiol Lung Cell Mol Physiol* (2018) 314(1):L127–L36. doi: 10.1152/ajplung.00200.2017
21. Chanda D, Kurundkar A, Rangarajan S, Locy M, Bernard K, Sharma NS, et al. Developmental Reprogramming in Mesenchymal Stromal Cells of

Human Subjects with Idiopathic Pulmonary Fibrosis. *Sci Rep* (2016) 6:37445. doi: 10.1038/srep37445

22. Jun D, Garat C, West J, Thorn N, Chow K, Cleaver T, et al. The pathology of bleomycin-induced fibrosis is associated with loss of resident lung mesenchymal stem cells that regulate effector T-cell proliferation. *Stem Cells* (2011) 29(4):725–35. doi: 10.1002/stem.604
23. Chen X, Shi C, Cao H, Chen L, Hou J, Xiang Z, et al. The hedgehog and Wnt/beta-catenin system machinery mediate myofibroblast differentiation of LR-MSCs in pulmonary fibrogenesis. *Cell Death Dis* (2018) 9(6):639. doi: 10.1038/s41419-018-0692-9
24. Cao H, Chen X, Hou J, Wang C, Xiang Z, Shen Y, et al. The Shh/Gli signaling cascade regulates myofibroblastic activation of lung-resident mesenchymal stem cells via the modulation of Wnt10a expression during pulmonary fibrogenesis. *Lab Invest* (2020) 100(3):363–77. doi: 10.1038/s41374-019-0316-8
25. Wang C, Zhu H, Sun Z, Xiang Z, Ge Y, Ni C, et al. Inhibition of Wnt/beta-catenin signaling promotes epithelial differentiation of mesenchymal stem cells and repairs bleomycin-induced lung injury. *Am J Physiol Cell Physiol* (2014) 307(3):C234–44. doi: 10.1152/ajpcell.00366.2013
26. Shi J, Li F, Luo M, Wei J, Liu X. Distinct Roles of Wnt/beta-Catenin Signaling in the Pathogenesis of Chronic Obstructive Pulmonary Disease and Idiopathic Pulmonary Fibrosis. *Mediators Inflamm* (2017) 2017:3520581. doi: 10.1155/2017/3520581
27. Chen X, Shi C, Wang C, Liu W, Chu Y, Xiang Z, et al. The role of miR-497-5p in myofibroblast differentiation of LR-MSCs and pulmonary fibrogenesis. *Sci Rep* (2017) 7:40958. doi: 10.1038/srep40958
28. Luo Y, Xu W, Chen H, Warburton D, Dong R, Qian B, et al. A novel profibrotic mechanism mediated by TGFbeta-stimulated collagen prolyl hydroxylase expression in fibrotic lung mesenchymal cells. *J Pathol* (2015) 236(3):384–94. doi: 10.1002/path.4530
29. Cunningham PS, Meijer P, Nazgiewicz A, Anderson SG, Borthwick LA, Bagnall J, et al. The circadian clock protein REVERBalpha inhibits pulmonary fibrosis development. *Proc Natl Acad Sci USA* (2020) 117 (2):1139–47. doi: 10.1073/pnas.1912109117
30. Ortiz LA, Gambelli F, McBride C, Gaupp D, Baddoo M, Kaminski N, et al. Mesenchymal stem cell engraftment in lung is enhanced in response to bleomycin exposure and ameliorates its fibrotic effects. *Proc Natl Acad Sci USA* (2003) 100(14):8407–11. doi: 10.1073/pnas.1432929100
31. Zhao F, Zhang YF, Liu YG, Zhou JJ, Li ZK, Wu CG, et al. Therapeutic effects of bone marrow-derived mesenchymal stem cells engraftment on bleomycin-induced lung injury in rats. *Transplant Proc* (2008) 40 (5):1700–5. doi: 10.1016/j.transproceed.2008.01.080
32. Aguilar S, Scotton CJ, McNulty K, Nye E, Stamp G, Laurent G, et al. Bone marrow stem cells expressing keratinocyte growth factor via an inducible lentivirus protects against bleomycin-induced pulmonary fibrosis. *PloS One* (2009) 4(11):e8013. doi: 10.1371/journal.pone.0008013
33. Cargnoni A, Gibelli L, Tosini A, Signoroni PB, Nassuato C, Arienti D, et al. Transplantation of allogeneic and xenogeneic placenta-derived cells reduces bleomycin-induced lung fibrosis. *Cell Transplant* (2009) 18(4):405–22. doi: 10.3727/096368909788809857
34. Kumamoto M, Nishiwaki T, Matsuo N, Kimura H, Matsushima K. Minimally cultured bone marrow mesenchymal stem cells ameliorate fibrotic lung injury. *Eur Respir J* (2009) 34(3):740–8. doi: 10.1183/09031936.00128508
35. Moodley Y, Atienza D, Manuelpillai U, Samuel CS, Tchongue J, Ilancheran S, et al. Human umbilical cord mesenchymal stem cells reduce fibrosis of bleomycin-induced lung injury. *Am J Pathol* (2009) 175(1):303–13. doi: 10.2353/ajpath.2009.080629
36. Lee SH, Jang AS, Kim YE, Cha JY, Kim TH, Jung S, et al. Modulation of cytokine and nitric oxide by mesenchymal stem cell transfer in lung injury/fibrosis. *Respir Res* (2010) 11:16. doi: 10.1186/1465-9921-11-16
37. Garcia O, Carraro G, Turcatel G, Hall M, Sedrakyan S, Roche T, et al. Amniotic fluid stem cells inhibit the progression of bleomycin-induced pulmonary fibrosis via CCL2 modulation in bronchoalveolar lavage. *PloS One* (2013) 8(8):e71679. doi: 10.1371/journal.pone.0071679
38. Gazdhar A, Susuri N, Hostettler K, Gugger M, Knudsen L, Roth M, et al. HGF Expressing Stem Cells in Usual Interstitial Pneumonia Originate from the Bone Marrow and Are Antifibrotic. *PloS One* (2013) 8(6):e65453. doi: 10.1371/journal.pone.0065453
39. Lee SH, Lee EJ, Lee SY, Kim JH, Shim JJ, Shin C, et al. The effect of adipose stem cell therapy on pulmonary fibrosis induced by repetitive intratracheal bleomycin in mice. *Exp Lung Res* (2014) 40(3):117–25. doi: 10.3109/01902148.2014.881930
40. Huang K, Kang X, Wang X, Wu S, Xiao J, Li Z, et al. Conversion of bone marrow mesenchymal stem cells into type II alveolar epithelial cells reduces pulmonary fibrosis by decreasing oxidative stress in rats. *Mol Med Rep* (2015) 11(3):1685–92. doi: 10.3892/mmr.2014.2981
41. Ono M, Ohkouchi S, Kanehira M, Tode N, Kobayashi M, Ebina M, et al. Mesenchymal stem cells correct inappropriate epithelial-mesenchyme relation in pulmonary fibrosis using stanniocalcin-1. *Mol Ther* (2015) 23 (3):549–60. doi: 10.1038/mt.2014.217
42. Reddy M, Fonseca L, Gowda S, Chougule B, Hari A, Totey S. Human Adipose-derived Mesenchymal Stem Cells Attenuate Early Stage of Bleomycin Induced Pulmonary Fibrosis: Comparison with Pirfenidone. *Int J Stem Cells* (2016) 9(2):192–206. doi: 10.15283/ijsc16041
43. Perez JR, Lee S, Ybarra N, Maria O, Serban M, Jeyaseelan K, et al. A comparative analysis of longitudinal computed tomography and histopathology for evaluating the potential of mesenchymal stem cells in mitigating radiation-induced pulmonary fibrosis. *Sci Rep* (2017) 7(1):9056. doi: 10.1038/s41598-017-09021-7
44. Tzouvelekis A, Toonkel R, Karampitsakos T, Medapalli K, Ninou I, Aidinis V, et al. Mesenchymal Stem Cells for the Treatment of Idiopathic Pulmonary Fibrosis. *Front Med (Lausanne)* (2018) 5:142. doi: 10.3389/fmed.2018.00142
45. Liu S, Peng D, Qiu H, Yang K, Fu Z, Zou L. Mesenchymal stem cells as a potential therapy for COVID-19. *Stem Cell Res Ther* (2020) 11(1):169. doi: 10.1186/s13287-020-01678-8
46. Yen BL, Yen ML, Wang LT, Liu KJ, Sytwu HK. Current status of mesenchymal stem cell therapy for immune/inflammatory lung disorders: Gleaning insights for possible use in COVID-19. *Stem Cells Transl Med* (2020) 9(10):1163–73. doi: 10.1002/sctm.20-0186
47. Harrell CR, Jovicic N, Djonov V, Arsenijevic N, Volarevic V. Mesenchymal Stem Cell-Derived Exosomes and Other Extracellular Vesicles as New Remedies in the Therapy of Inflammatory Diseases. *Cells* (2019) 8 (12):1605. doi: 10.3390/cells8121605
48. U.S. National Library of Medicine. *Registered clinical trials* . Available at: https://www.clinicaltrials.gov/ (Accessed January, 2021).
49. Chambers DC, Enever D, Ilic N, Sparks L, Whitelaw K, Ayres J, et al. A phase 1b study of placenta-derived mesenchymal stromal cells in patients with idiopathic pulmonary fibrosis. *Respirology* (2014) 19(7):1013–8. doi: 10.1111/resp.12343
50. Glassberg MK, Minkiewicz J, Toonkel RL, Simonet ES, Rubio GA, DiFede D, et al. Allogeneic Human Mesenchymal Stem Cells in Patients With Idiopathic Pulmonary Fibrosis via Intravenous Delivery (AETHER): A Phase I Safety Clinical Trial. *Chest* (2017) 151(5):971–81. doi: 10.1016/j.chest.2016.10.061
51. Averyanov A, Koroleva I, Konoplyannikov M, Revkova V, Lesnyak V, Kalsin V, et al. First-in-human high-cumulative-dose stem cell therapy in idiopathic pulmonary fibrosis with rapid lung function decline. *Stem Cells Transl Med* (2020) 9(1):6–16. doi: 10.1002/sctm.19-0037
52. Tzouvelekis A, Paspaliaris V, Koliakos G, Ntolios P, Bouros E, Oikonomou A, et al. A prospective, non-randomized, no placebo-controlled, phase Ib clinical trial to study the safety of the adipose derived stromal cells-stromal vascular fraction in idiopathic pulmonary fibrosis. *J Transl Med* (2013) 11:171. doi: 10.1186/1479-5876-11-171
53. Charo RA, Sipp D. Rejuvenating Regenerative Medicine Regulation. *N Engl J Med* (2018) 378(6):504–5. doi: 10.1056/NEJMp1715736
54. Marks PW, Witten CM, Califf RM. Clarifying Stem-Cell Therapy's Benefits and Risks. *N Engl J Med* (2017) 376(11):1007–9. doi: 10.1056/NEJMp1613723
55. Leeman KT, Pessina P, Lee JH, Kim CF. Mesenchymal Stem Cells Increase Alveolar Differentiation in Lung Progenitor Organoid Cultures. *Sci Rep* (2019) 9(1):6479. doi: 10.1038/s41598-019-42819-1
56. Li X, Yue S, Luo Z. Mesenchymal stem cells in idiopathic pulmonary fibrosis. *Oncotarget* (2017) 8(60):102600–16. doi: 10.18632/oncotarget.18126
57. Liu M, Zeng X, Wang J, Fu Z, Wang J, Liu M, et al. Immunomodulation by mesenchymal stem cells in treating human autoimmune disease-associated

lung fibrosis. *Stem Cell Res Ther* (2016) 7(1):63. doi: 10.1186/s13287-016-0319-y
58. Islam MN, Das SR, Emin MT, Wei M, Sun L, Westphalen K, et al. Mitochondrial transfer from bone-marrow-derived stromal cells to pulmonary alveoli protects against acute lung injury. *Nat Med* (2012) 18 (5):759–65. doi: 10.1038/nm.2736
59. Shentu TP, Huang TS, Cernelc-Kohan M, Chan J, Wong SS, Espinoza CR, et al. Thy-1 dependent uptake of mesenchymal stem cell-derived extracellular vesicles blocks myofibroblastic differentiation. *Sci Rep* (2017) 7(1):18052. doi: 10.1038/s41598-017-18288-9
60. Choi M, Ban T, Rhim T. Therapeutic use of stem cell transplantation for cell replacement or cytoprotective effect of microvesicle released from mesenchymal stem cell. *Mol Cells* (2014) 37(2):133–9. doi: 10.14348/molcells.2014.2317
61. Sinclair K, Yerkovich ST, Chambers DC. Mesenchymal stem cells and the lung. *Respirology* (2013) 18(3):397–411. doi: 10.1111/resp.12050
62. Cardenes N, Alvarez D, Sellares J, Peng Y, Corey C, Wecht S, et al. Senescence of bone marrow-derived mesenchymal stem cells from patients with idiopathic pulmonary fibrosis. *Stem Cell Res Ther* (2018) 9(1):257. doi: 10.1186/s13287-018-0970-6
63. Habiel DM, Hohmann MS, Espindola MS, Coelho AL, Jones I, Jones H, et al. DNA-PKcs modulates progenitor cell proliferation and fibroblast senescence in idiopathic pulmonary fibrosis. *BMC Pulm Med* (2019) 19(1):165. doi: 10.1186/s12890-019-0922-7
64. Tashiro J, Elliot SJ, Gerth DJ, Xia X, Pereira-Simon S, Choi R, et al. Therapeutic benefits of young, but not old, adipose-derived mesenchymal stem cells in a chronic mouse model of bleomycin-induced pulmonary fibrosis. *Transl Res* (2015) 166(6):554–67. doi: 10.1016/j.trsl.2015.09.004
65. Kolahian S, Fernandez IE, Eickelberg O, Hartl D. Immune Mechanisms in Pulmonary Fibrosis. *Am J Respir Cell Mol Biol* (2016) 55(3):309–22. doi: 10.1165/rcmb.2016-0121TR
66. Desai O, Winkler J, Minasyan M, Herzog EL. The Role of Immune and Inflammatory Cells in Idiopathic Pulmonary Fibrosis. *Front Med (Lausanne)* (2018) 5:43. doi: 10.3389/fmed.2018.00043
67. Gilani SR, Vuga LJ, Lindell KO, Gibson KF, Xue J, Kaminski N, et al. CD28 down-regulation on circulating CD4 T-cells is associated with poor prognoses of patients with idiopathic pulmonary fibrosis. *PloS One* (2010) 5(1):e8959. doi: 10.1371/journal.pone.0008959
68. Herazo-Maya JD, Noth I, Duncan SR, Kim S, Ma SF, Tseng GC, et al. Peripheral blood mononuclear cell gene expression profiles predict poor outcome in idiopathic pulmonary fibrosis. *Sci Transl Med* (2013) 5 (205):205ra136. doi: 10.1126/scitranslmed.3005964
69. Fernandez IE, Greiffo FR, Frankenberger M, Bandres J, Heinzelmann K, Neurohr C, et al. Peripheral blood myeloid-derived suppressor cells reflect disease status in idiopathic pulmonary fibrosis. *Eur Respir J* (2016) 48 (4):1171–83. doi: 10.1183/13993003.01826-2015
70. Reilkoff RA, Peng H, Murray LA, Peng X, Russell T, Montgomery R, et al. Semaphorin 7a+ regulatory T cells are associated with progressive idiopathic pulmonary fibrosis and are implicated in transforming growth factor-beta1-induced pulmonary fibrosis. *Am J Respir Crit Care Med* (2013) 187(2):180–8. doi: 10.1164/rccm.201206-1109OC
71. Moore BB, Fry C, Zhou Y, Murray S, Han MK, Martinez FJ, et al. Inflammatory leukocyte phenotypes correlate with disease progression in idiopathic pulmonary fibrosis. *Front Med* (2014) 1(56):56. doi: 10.3389/fmed.2014.00056
72. Galati D, De Martino M, Trotta A, Rea G, Bruzzese D, Cicchitto G, et al. Peripheral depletion of NK cells and imbalance of the Treg/Th17 axis in idiopathic pulmonary fibrosis patients. *Cytokine* (2014) 66(2):119–26. doi: 10.1016/j.cyto.2013.12.003
73. Hou Z, Ye Q, Qiu M, Hao Y, Han J, Zeng H. Increased activated regulatory T cells proportion correlate with the severity of idiopathic pulmonary fibrosis. *Respir Res* (2017) 18(1):170. doi: 10.1186/s12931-017-0653-3
74. Lo Re S, Lecocq M, Uwambayinema F, Yakoub Y, Delos M, Demoulin JB, et al. Platelet-derived growth factor-producing CD4+ Foxp3+ regulatory T lymphocytes promote lung fibrosis. *Am J Respir Crit Care Med* (2011) 184 (11):1270–81. doi: 10.1164/rccm.201103-0516OC
75. D'Alessandro-Gabazza CN, Kobayashi T, Yasuma T, Toda M, Kim H, Fujimoto H, et al. A Staphylococcus pro-apoptotic peptide induces acute exacerbation of pulmonary fibrosis. *Nat Commun* (2020) 11(1):1539. doi: 10.1038/s41467-020-15344-3
76. Kotsianidis I, Nakou E, Bouchliou I, Tzouvelekis A, Spanoudakis E, Steiropoulos P, et al. Global impairment of CD4+CD25+FOXP3+ regulatory T cells in idiopathic pulmonary fibrosis. *Am J Respir Crit Care Med* (2009) 179(12):1121–30. doi: 10.1164/rccm.200812-1936OC
77. Shimizu Y, Dobashi K, Endou K, Ono A, Yanagitani N, Utsugi M, et al. Decreased interstitial FOXP3(+) lymphocytes in usual interstitial pneumonia with discrepancy of CXCL12/CXCR4 axis. *Int J Immunopathol Pharmacol* (2010) 23(2):449–61. doi: 10.1177/039463201002300207
78. Kitani A, Fuss I, Nakamura K, Kumaki F, Usui T, Strober W. Transforming growth factor (TGF)-beta1-producing regulatory T cells induce Smad-mediated interleukin 10 secretion that facilitates coordinated immunoregulatory activity and amelioration of TGF-beta1-mediated fibrosis. *J Exp Med* (2003) 198(8):1179–88. doi: 10.1084/jem.20030917
79. Wangoo A, Laban C, Cook HT, Glenville B, Shaw RJ. Interleukin-10- and corticosteroid-induced reduction in type I procollagen in a human ex vivo scar culture. *Int J Exp Pathol* (1997) 78(1):33–41. doi: 10.1046/j.1365-2613.1997.d01-241.x
80. Arai T, Abe K, Matsuoka H, Yoshida M, Mori M, Goya S, et al. Introduction of the interleukin-10 gene into mice inhibited bleomycin-induced lung injury in vivo. *Am J Physiol Lung Cell Mol Physiol* (2000) 278(5):L914–22. doi: 10.1152/ajplung.2000.278.5.L914
81. Boveda-Ruiz D, D'Alessandro-Gabazza CN, Toda M, Takagi T, Naito M, Matsushima Y, et al. Differential role of regulatory T cells in early and late stages of pulmonary fibrosis. *Immunobiology* (2013) 218(2):245–54. doi: 10.1016/j.imbio.2012.05.020
82. Zeng M, Smith AJ, Wietgrefe SW, Southern PJ, Schacker TW, Reilly CS, et al. Cumulative mechanisms of lymphoid tissue fibrosis and T cell depletion in HIV-1 and SIV infections. *J Clin Invest* (2011) 121(3):998–1008. doi: 10.1172/JCI45157
83. Estes JD, Wietgrefe S, Schacker T, Southern P, Beilman G, Reilly C, et al. Simian immunodeficiency virus-induced lymphatic tissue fibrosis is mediated by transforming growth factor beta 1-positive regulatory T cells and begins in early infection. *J Infect Dis* (2007) 195(4):551–61. doi: 10.1086/510852
84. Holmes S, Downs AM, Fosberry A, Hayes PD, Michalovich D, Murdoch P, et al. Sema7A is a potent monocyte stimulator. *Scand J Immunol* (2002) 56 (3):270–5. doi: 10.1046/j.1365-3083.2002.01129.x
85. van Rijn A, Paulis L, te Riet J, Vasaturo A, Reinieren-Beeren I, van der Schaaf A, et al. Semaphorin 7A Promotes Chemokine-Driven Dendritic Cell Migration. *J Immunol* (2016) 196(1):459–68. doi: 10.4049/jimmunol.1403096
86. Kral JB, Kuttke M, Schrottmaier WC, Birnecker B, Warszawska J, Wernig C, et al. Sustained PI3K Activation exacerbates BLM-induced Lung Fibrosis via activation of pro-inflammatory and pro-fibrotic pathways. *Sci Rep* (2016) 6:23034. doi: 10.1038/srep23034
87. Griffiths K, Habiel DM, Jaffar J, Binder U, Darby WG, Hosking CG, et al. Anti-fibrotic Effects of CXCR4-Targeting i-body AD-114 in Preclinical Models of Pulmonary Fibrosis. *Sci Rep* (2018) 8(1):3212. doi: 10.1038/s41598-018-20811-5
88. Jaffar J, Griffiths K, Oveissi S, Duan M, Foley M, Glaspole I, et al. CXCR4(+) cells are increased in lung tissue of patients with idiopathic pulmonary fibrosis. *Respir Res* (2020) 21(1):221. doi: 10.1186/s12931-020-01467-0
89. Phillips RJ, Burdick MD, Hong K, Lutz MA, Murray LA, Xue YY, et al. Circulating fibrocytes traffic to the lungs in response to CXCL12 and mediate fibrosis. *J Clin Invest* (2004) 114(3):438–46. doi: 10.1172/JCI20997
90. Reilkoff RA, Bucala R, Herzog EL. Fibrocytes: emerging effector cells in chronic inflammation. *Nat Rev Immunol* (2011) 11(6):427–35. doi: 10.1038/nri2990
91. Garibaldi BT, D'Alessio FR, Mock JR, Files DC, Chau E, Eto Y, et al. Regulatory T cells reduce acute lung injury fibroproliferation by decreasing fibrocyte recruitment. *Am J Respir Cell Mol Biol* (2013) 48(1):35–43. doi: 10.1165/rcmb.2012-0198OC
92. Peng X, Moore MW, Peng H, Sun H, Gan Y, Homer RJ, et al. CD4+CD25+FoxP3+ Regulatory Tregs inhibit fibrocyte recruitment and fibrosis via suppression of FGF-9 production in the TGF-beta1 exposed murine lung. *Front Pharmacol* (2014) 5:80. doi: 10.3389/fphar.2014.00080

93. Oldroyd SD, Thomas GL, Gabbiani G, El Nahas AM. Interferon-gamma inhibits experimental renal fibrosis. *Kidney Int* (1999) 56(6):2116–27. doi: 10.1046/j.1523-1755.1999.00775.x
94. Park Y, Oh SJ, Chung DH. CD4(+)CD25(+) regulatory T cells attenuate Hypersensitivity Pneumonitis by suppressing IFN-gamma production by CD4(+) and CD8(+) T cells. *J Leukoc Biol* (2009) 86(6):1427–37. doi: 10.1189/jlb.0908542
95. Wilson MS, Madala SK, Ramalingam TR, Gochuico BR, Rosas IO, Cheever AW, et al. Bleomycin and IL-1beta-mediated pulmonary fibrosis is IL-17A dependent. *J Exp Med* (2010) 207(3):535–52. doi: 10.1084/jem.20092121
96. Barron L, Wynn TA. Fibrosis is regulated by Th2 and Th17 responses and by dynamic interactions between fibroblasts and macrophages. *Am J Physiol Gastrointest Liver Physiol* (2011) 300(5):G723–8. doi: 10.1152/ajpgi.00414.2010
97. Paun A, Bergeron ME, Haston CK. The Thl/Th17 balance dictates the fibrosis response in murine radiation-induced lung disease. *Sci Rep* (2017) 7 (1):11586. doi: 10.1038/s41598-017-11656-5
98. Cao Q, Wang L, Du F, Sheng H, Zhang Y, Wu J, et al. Downregulation of CD4+CD25+ regulatory T cells may underlie enhanced Thl immunity caused by immunization with activated autologous T cells. *Cell Res* (2007) 17(7):627–37. doi: 10.1038/cr.2007.46
99. Liu F, Liu J, Weng D, Chen Y, Song L, He Q, et al. CD4+CD25+Foxp3+ regulatory T cells depletion may attenuate the development of silica-induced lung fibrosis in mice. *PloS One* (2010) 5(11):e15404. doi: 10.1371/journal.pone.0015404
100. Xiong S, Guo R, Yang Z, Xu L, Du L, Li R, et al. Treg depletion attenuates irradiation-induced pulmonary fibrosis by reducing fibrocyte accumulation, inducing Th17 response, and shifting IFN-gamma, IL-12/IL-4, IL-5 balance. *Immunobiology* (2015) 220(11):1284–91. doi: 10.1016/j.imbio.2015.07.001
101. Song L, Weng D, Liu F, Chen Y, Li C, Dong L, et al. Tregs promote the differentiation of Th17 cells in silica-induced lung fibrosis in mice. *PloS One* (2012) 7(5):e37286. doi: 10.1371/journal.pone.0037286
102. Birjandi SZ, Palchevskiy V, Xue YY, Nunez S, Kern R, Weigt SS, et al. CD4 (+)CD25(hi)Foxp3(+) Cells Exacerbate Bleomycin-Induced Pulmonary Fibrosis. *Am J Pathol* (2016) 186(8):2008–20. doi: 10.1016/j.ajpath.2016.03.020
103. Habiel DM, Espindola MS, Kitson C, Azzara AV, Coelho AL, Stripp B, et al. Characterization of CD28(null) T cells in idiopathic pulmonary fibrosis. *Mucosal Immunol* (2019) 12(1):212–22. doi: 10.1038/s41385-018-0082-8
104. Koreth J, Matsuoka K, Kim HT, McDonough SM, Bindra B, Alyea EP,3, et al. Interleukin-2 and regulatory T cells in graft-versus-host disease. *N Engl J Med* (2011) 365(22):2055–66. doi: 10.1056/NEJMoa1108188
105. Saadoun D, Rosenzwajg M, Joly F, Six A, Carrat F, Thibault V, et al. Regulatory T-cell responses to low-dose interleukin-2 in HCV-induced vasculitis. *N Engl J Med* (2011) 365(22):2067–77. doi: 10.1056/NEJMoa1105143
106. D'Alessio FR, Tsushima K, Aggarwal NR, West EE, Willett MH, Britos MF, et al. CD4+CD25+Foxp3+ Tregs resolve experimental lung injury in mice and are present in humans with acute lung injury. *J Clin Invest* (2009) 119 (10):2898–913. doi: 10.1172/JCI36498
107. Trujillo G, Hartigan AJ, Hogaboam CM. T regulatory cells and attenuated bleomycin-induced fibrosis in lungs of CCR7-/- mice. *Fibrogenesis Tissue Repair* (2010) 3:18. doi: 10.1186/1755-1536-3-18
108. LeBien TW, Tedder TF. B lymphocytes: how they develop and function. *Blood* (2008) 112(5):1570–80. doi: 10.1182/blood-2008-02-078071
109. Heukels P, van Hulst JAC, van Nimwegen M, Boorsma CE, Melgert BN, von der Thusen JH, et al. Enhanced Bruton's tyrosine kinase in B-cells and autoreactive IgA in patients with idiopathic pulmonary fibrosis. *Respir Res* (2019) 20(1):232. doi: 10.1186/s12931-019-1195-7
110. Xue J, Kass DJ, Bon J, Vuga L, Tan J, Csizmadia E, et al. Plasma B lymphocyte stimulator and B cell differentiation in idiopathic pulmonary fibrosis patients. *J Immunol* (2013) 191(5):2089–95. doi: 10.4049/jimmunol.1203476
111. Todd NW, Scheraga RG, Galvin JR, Iacono AT, Britt EJ, Luzina IG, et al. Lymphocyte aggregates persist and accumulate in the lungs of patients with idiopathic pulmonary fibrosis. *J Inflammation Res* (2013) 6:63–70. doi: 10.2147/JIR.S40673
112. Nuovo GJ, Hagood JS, Magro CM, Chin N, Kapil R, Davis L, et al. The distribution of immunomodulatory cells in the lungs of patients with idiopathic pulmonary fibrosis. *Mod Pathol* (2012) 25(3):416–33. doi: 10.1038/modpathol.2011.166
113. Campbell DA, Poulter LW, Janossy G, du Bois RM. Immunohistological analysis of lung tissue from patients with cryptogenic fibrosing alveolitis suggesting local expression of immune hypersensitivity. *Thorax* (1985) 40 (6):405–11. doi: 10.1136/thx.40.6.405
114. Tzouvelekis A, Zacharis G, Oikonomou A, Mikroulis D, Margaritopoulos G, Koutsopoulos A, et al. Increased incidence of autoimmune markers in patients with combined pulmonary fibrosis and emphysema. *BMC Pulm Med* (2013) 13:31. doi: 10.1186/1471-2466-13-31
115. Vuga LJ, Tedrow JR, Pandit KV, Tan J, Kass DJ, Xue J, et al. C-X-C motif chemokine 13 (CXCL13) is a prognostic biomarker of idiopathic pulmonary fibrosis. *Am J Respir Crit Care Med* (2014) 189(8):966–74. doi: 10.1164/rccm.201309-1592OC
116. DePianto DJ, Chandriani S, Abbas AR, Jia G, N'Diaye EN, Caplazi P, et al. Heterogeneous gene expression signatures correspond to distinct lung pathologies and biomarkers of disease severity in idiopathic pulmonary fibrosis. *Thorax* (2015) 70(1):48–56. doi: 10.1136/thoraxjnl-2013-204596
117. O'Donoghue RJ, Knight DA, Richards CD, Prele CM, Lau HL, Jarnicki AG, et al. Genetic partitioning of interleukin-6 signalling in mice dissociates Stat3 from Smad3-mediated lung fibrosis. *EMBO Mol Med* (2012) 4(9):939–51. doi: 10.1002/emmm.201100604
118. Rosser EC, Mauri C. Regulatory B cells: origin, phenotype, and function. *Immunity* (2015) 42(4):607–12. doi: 10.1016/j.immuni.2015.04.005
119. Palomares O, Martin-Fontecha M, Lauener R, Traidl-Hoffmann C, Cavkaytar O, Akdis M, et al. Regulatory T cells and immune regulation of allergic diseases: roles of IL-10 and TGF-beta. *Genes Immun* (2014) 15 (8):511–20. doi: 10.1038/gene.2014.45
120. Crotty S. T follicular helper cell differentiation, function, and roles in disease. *Immunity* (2014) 41(4):529–42. doi: 10.1016/j.immuni.2014.10.004
121. Achour A, Simon Q, Mohr A, Seite JF, Youinou P, Bendaoud B, et al. Human regulatory B cells control the TFH cell response. *J Allergy Clin Immunol* (2017) 140(1):215–22. doi: 10.1016/j.jaci.2016.09.042
122. Groot Kormelink T, Pardo A, Knipping K, Buendia-Roldan I, Garcia-de-Alba C, Blokhuis BR, et al. Immunoglobulin free light chains are increased in hypersensitivity pneumonitis and idiopathic pulmonary fibrosis. *PloS One* (2011) 6(9):e25392. doi: 10.1371/journal.pone.0025392
123. Wallace WA, Roberts SN, Caldwell H, Thornton E, Greening AP, Lamb D, et al. Circulating antibodies to lung protein(s) in patients with cryptogenic fibrosing alveolitis. *Thorax* (1994) 49(3):218–24. doi: 10.1136/thx.49.3.218
124. Dall'Aglio PP, Pesci A, Bertorelli G, Brianti E, Scarpa S. Study of immune complexes in bronchoalveolar lavage fluids. *Respiration* (1988) 54 Suppl 1:36–41. doi: 10.1159/000195495
125. Dobashi N, Fujita J, Murota M, Ohtsuki Y, Yamadori I, Yoshinouchi T, et al. Elevation of anti-cytokeratin 18 antibody and circulating cytokeratin 18: anti-cytokeratin 18 antibody immune complexes in sera of patients with idiopathic pulmonary fibrosis. *Lung* (2000) 178(3):171–9. doi: 10.1007/s004080000020
126. Kahloon RA, Xue J, Bhargava A, Csizmadia E, Otterbein L, Kass DJ, et al. Patients with idiopathic pulmonary fibrosis with antibodies to heat shock protein 70 have poor prognoses. *Am J Respir Crit Care Med* (2013) 187 (7):768–75. doi: 10.1164/rccm.201203-0506OC
127. Hoyne GF, Elliott H, Mutsaers SE, Prele CM. Idiopathic pulmonary fibrosis and a role for autoimmunity. *Immunol Cell Biol* (2017) 95(7):577–83. doi: 10.1038/icb.2017.22
128. Ernst JA, Li H, Kim HS, Nakamura GR, Yansura DG, Vandlen RL. Isolation and characterization of the B-cell marker CD20. *Biochemistry* (2005) 44 (46):15150–8. doi: 10.1021/bi0511078
129. Donahoe M, Valentine VG, Chien N, Gibson KF, Raval JS, Saul M, et al. Autoantibody-Targeted Treatments for Acute Exacerbations of Idiopathic Pulmonary Fibrosis. *PloS One* (2015) 10(6):e0127771. doi: 10.1371/journal.pone.0127771
130. Brito Y, Glassberg MK, Ascherman DP. Rheumatoid Arthritis-Associated Interstitial Lung Disease: Current Concepts. *Curr Rheumatol Rep* (2017) 19 (12):79. doi: 10.1007/s11926-017-0701-5
131. Bodogai M, Lee Chang C, Wejksza K, Lai J, Merino M, Wersto RP, et al. Anti-CD20 antibody promotes cancer escape via enrichment of tumor-evoked regulatory B cells expressing low levels of CD20 and CD137L. *Cancer Res* (2013) 73(7):2127–38. doi: 10.1158/0008-5472.CAN-12-4184

132. Mauri C, Menon M. Human regulatory B cells in health and disease: therapeutic potential. *J Clin Invest* (2017) 127(3):772–9. doi: 10.1172/JCI85113
133. Wu X, Zhu D, Tian J, Tang X, Guo H, Ma J, et al. Granulocytic Myeloid-Derived Suppressor Cell Exosomal Prostaglandin E2 Ameliorates Collagen-Induced Arthritis by Enhancing IL-10(+) B Cells. *Front Immunol* (2020) 11:588500. doi: 10.3389/fimmu.2020.588500
134. Geissmann F, Manz MG, Jung S, Sieweke MH, Merad M, Ley K. Development of monocytes, macrophages, and dendritic cells. *Science* (2010) 327(5966):656–61. doi: 10.1126/science.1178331
135. Craig VJ, Zhang L, Hagood JS, Owen CA. Matrix metalloproteinases as therapeutic targets for idiopathic pulmonary fibrosis. *Am J Respir Cell Mol Biol* (2015) 53(5):585–600. doi: 10.1165/rcmb.2015-0020TR
136. Gibbons MA, MacKinnon AC, Ramachandran P, Dhaliwal K, Duffin R, Phythian-Adams AT, et al. Ly6Chi monocytes direct alternatively activated profibrotic macrophage regulation of lung fibrosis. *Am J Respir Crit Care Med* (2011) 184(5):569–81. doi: 10.1164/rccm.201010-1719OC
137. Duffield JS, Forbes SJ, Constandinou CM, Clay S, Partolina M, Vuthoori S, et al. Selective depletion of macrophages reveals distinct, opposing roles during liver injury and repair. *J Clin Invest* (2005) 115(1):56–65. doi: 10.1172/JCI22675
138. Mills CD, Kincaid K, Alt JM, Heilman MJ, Hill AM. M-1/M-2 macrophages and the Th1/Th2 paradigm. *J Immunol* (2000) 164(12):6166–73. doi: 10.4049/jimmunol.164.12.6166
139. Raghu G, Brown KK, Costabel U, Cottin V, du Bois RM, Lasky JA, et al. Treatment of idiopathic pulmonary fibrosis with etanercept: an exploratory, placebo-controlled trial. *Am J Respir Crit Care Med* (2008) 178(9):948–55. doi: 10.1164/rccm.200709-1446OC
140. Siwik DA, Chang DL, Colucci WS. Interleukin-1beta and tumor necrosis factor-alpha decrease collagen synthesis and increase matrix metalloproteinase activity in cardiac fibroblasts in vitro. *Circ Res* (2000) 86 (12):1259–65. doi: 10.1161/01.res.86.12.1259
141. Jiang D, Liang J, Fan J, Yu S, Chen S, Luo Y, et al. Regulation of lung injury and repair by Toll-like receptors and hyaluronan. *Nat Med* (2005) 11 (11):1173–9. doi: 10.1038/nm1315
142. Song E, Ouyang N, Horbelt M, Antus B, Wang M, Exton MS. Influence of alternatively and classically activated macrophages on fibrogenic activities of human fibroblasts. *Cell Immunol* (2000) 204(1):19–28. doi: 10.1006/cimm.2000.1687
143. Sun L, Louie MC, Vannella KM, Wilke CA, LeVine AM, Moore BB, et al. New concepts of IL-10-induced lung fibrosis: fibrocyte recruitment and M2 activation in a CCL2/CCR2 axis. *Am J Physiol Lung Cell Mol Physiol* (2011) 300(3):L341–53. doi: 10.1152/ajplung.00122.2010
144. Murthy S, Larson-Casey JL, Ryan AJ, He C, Kobzik L, Carter AB. Alternative activation of macrophages and pulmonary fibrosis are modulated by scavenger receptor, macrophage receptor with collagenous structure. *FASEB J* (2015) 29(8):3527–36. doi: 10.1096/fj.15-271304
145. Pechkovsky DV, Prasse A, Kollert F, Engel KM, Dentler J, Luttmann W, et al. Alternatively activated alveolar macrophages in pulmonary fibrosis-mediator production and intracellular signal transduction. *Clin Immunol* (2010) 137 (1):89–101. doi: 10.1016/j.clim.2010.06.017
146. Gratchev A, Guillot P, Hakiy N, Politz O, Orfanos CE, Schledzewski K, et al. lternatively activated macrophages differentially express fibronectin and its splice variants and the extracellular matrix protein betaIG-H3. A*Scand J Immunol* (2001) 53(4):386–92. doi: 10.1046/j.1365-3083.2001.00885.x
147. Selman M, Ruiz V, Cabrera S, Segura L, Ramirez R, Barrios R, et al. TIMP-1, -2, -3, and -4 in idiopathic pulmonary fibrosis. A prevailing nondegradative lung microenvironment? *Am J Physiol Lung Cell Mol Physiol* (2000) 279(3): L562–74. doi: 10.1152/ajplung.2000.279.3.L562
148. Hou J, Shi J, Chen L, Lv Z, Chen X, Cao H, et al. M2 macrophages promote myofibroblast differentiation of LR-MSCs and are associated with pulmonary fibrogenesis. *Cell Commun Signal* (2018) 16(1):89. doi: 10.1186/s12964-018-0300-8
149. Murray PJ, Wynn TA. Protective and pathogenic functions of macrophage subsets. *Nat Rev Immunol* (2011) 11(11):723–37. doi: 10.1038/nri3073
150. Ricote M, Li AC, Willson TM, Kelly CJ, Glass CK. The peroxisome proliferator-activated receptor-gamma is a negative regulator of macrophage activation. *Nature* (1998) 391(6662):79–82. doi: 10.1038/34178
151. Odegaard JI, Ricardo-Gonzalez RR, Goforth MH, Morel CR, Subramanian V, Mukundan L, et al. Macrophage-specific PPARgamma controls alternative activation and improves insulin resistance. *Nature* (2007) 447 (7148):1116–20. doi: 10.1038/nature05894
152. Kulkarni AA, Thatcher TH, Olsen KC, Maggirwar SB, Phipps RP, Sime PJ. PPAR-gamma ligands repress TGFbeta-induced myofibroblast differentiation by targeting the PI3K/Akt pathway: implications for therapy of fibrosis. *PloS One* (2011) 6(1):e15909. doi: 10.1371/journal.pone.0015909
153. Ogger PP, Byrne AJ. Macrophage metabolic reprogramming during chronic lung disease. *Mucosal Immunol* (2021) 14(2):282–95. doi: 10.1038/s41385-020-00356-5
154. Neumark N, Cosme C Jr, Rose KA, Kaminski N. The Idiopathic Pulmonary Fibrosis Cell Atlas. *Am J Physiol Lung Cell Mol Physiol* (2020) 319(6):L887–L93. doi: 10.1152/ajplung.00451.2020
155. Morse C, Tabib T, Sembrat J, Buschur KL, Bittar HT, Valenzi E, et al. Proliferating SPP1/MERTK-expressing macrophages in idiopathic pulmonary fibrosis. *Eur Respir J* (2019) 54(2):1802441. doi: 10.1183/13993003.02441-2018
156. Ayaub E, Poli S, Ng J, Adams T, Schupp J, Quesada-Arias L, et al. Single Cell RNA-seq and Mass Cytometry Reveals a Novel and a Targetable Population of Macrophages in Idiopathic Pulmonary Fibrosis. *bioRxiv* (2021), 2021.01.04.425268. doi: 10.1101/2021.01.04.425268
157. Ogger PP, Albers GJ, Hewitt RJ, O'Sullivan BJ, Powell JE, Calamita E, et al. Itaconate controls the severity of pulmonary fibrosis. *Sci Immunol* (2020) 5 (52):eabc1884. doi: 10.1126/sciimmunol.abc1884
158. Duffield JS, Lupher ML Jr. PRM-151 (recombinant human serum amyloid P/pentraxin 2) for the treatment of fibrosis. *Drug News Perspect* (2010) 23 (5):305–15. doi: 10.1358/dnp.2010.23.5.1444206
159. Steinman RM, Inaba K, Turley S, Pierre P, Mellman I. Antigen capture, processing, and presentation by dendritic cells: recent cell biological studies. *Hum Immunol* (1999) 60(7):562–7. doi: 10.1016/s0198-8859(99)00030-0
160. Domogalla MP, Rostan PV, Raker VK, Steinbrink K. Tolerance through Education: How Tolerogenic Dendritic Cells Shape Immunity. *Front Immunol* (2017) 8:1764. doi: 10.3389/fimmu.2017.01764
161. Chakraborty K, Chatterjee S, Bhattacharyya A. Modulation of CD11c+ lung dendritic cells in respect to TGF-beta in experimental pulmonary fibrosis. *Cell Biol Int* (2017) 41(9):991–1000. doi: 10.1002/cbin.10800
162. Bantsimba-Malanda C, Marchal-Somme J, Goven D, Freynet O, Michel L, Crestani B, et al. A role for dendritic cells in bleomycin-induced pulmonary fibrosis in mice? *Am J Respir Crit Care Med* (2010) 182(3):385–95. doi: 10.1164/rccm.200907-1164OC
163. Greer AM, Matthay MA, Kukreja J, Bhakta NR, Nguyen CP, Wolters PJ, et al. Accumulation of BDCA1(+) dendritic cells in interstitial fibrotic lung diseases and Th2-high asthma. *PloS One* (2014) 9(6):e99084. doi: 10.1371/journal.pone.0099084
164. Tsoumakidou M, Karagiannis KP, Bouloukaki I, Zakynthinos S, Tzanakis N, Siafakas NM. Increased bronchoalveolar lavage fluid CD1c expressing dendritic cells in idiopathic pulmonary fibrosis. *Respiration* (2009) 78 (4):446–52. doi: 10.1159/000226244
165. Marchal-Somme J, Uzunhan Y, Marchand-Adam S, Kambouchner M, Valeyre D, Crestani B, et al. Dendritic cells accumulate in human fibrotic interstitial lung disease. *Am J Respir Crit Care Med* (2007) 176(10):1007–14. doi: 10.1164/rccm.200609-1347OC
166. Galati D, Zanotta S, Polistina GE, Coppola A, Capitelli L, Bocchino M. Circulating dendritic cells are severely decreased in idiopathic pulmonary fibrosis with a potential value for prognosis prediction. *Clin Immunol* (2020) 215:108454. doi: 10.1016/j.clim.2020.108454
167. Tort Tarres M, Aschenbrenner F, Maus R, Stolper J, Schuette L, Knudsen L, et al. The FMS-like tyrosine kinase-3 ligand/lung dendritic cell axis contributes to regulation of pulmonary fibrosis. *Thorax* (2019) 74(10):947–57. doi: 10.1136/thoraxjnl-2018-212603
168. Ding L, Liu T, Wu Z, Hu B, Nakashima T, Ullenbruch M, et al. Bone Marrow CD11c+ Cell-Derived Amphiregulin Promotes Pulmonary Fibrosis. *J Immunol* (2016) 197(1):303–12. doi: 10.4049/jimmunol.1502479
169. Hauben E, Gregori S, Draghici E, Migliavacca B, Olivieri S, Woisetschlager M, et al. Activation of the aryl hydrocarbon receptor promotes allograft-specific tolerance through direct and dendritic cell-mediated effects on regulatory T cells. *Blood* (2008) 112(4):1214–22. doi: 10.1182/blood-2007-08-109843

170. Baba N, Rubio M, Kenins L, Regairaz C, Woisetschlager M, Carballido JM, et al. The aryl hydrocarbon receptor (AhR) ligand VAF347 selectively acts on monocytes and naive CD4(+) Th cells to promote the development of IL-22-secreting Th cells. *Hum Immunol* (2012) 73(8):795–800. doi: 10.1016/j.humimm.2012.05.002
171. Yen JH, Khayrullina T, Ganea D. PGE2-induced metalloproteinase-9 is essential for dendritic cell migration. *Blood* (2008) 111(1):260–70. doi: 10.1182/blood-2007-05-090613
172. Silva-Cardoso SC, Tao W, Angiolilli C, Lopes AP, Bekker CPJ, Devaprasad A, et al. CXCL4 Links Inflammation and Fibrosis by Reprogramming Monocyte-Derived Dendritic Cells in vitro. *Front Immunol* (2020) 11:2149. doi: 10.3389/fimmu.2020.02149
173. Bronte V, Brandau S, Chen SH, Colombo MP, Frey AB, Greten TF, et al. Recommendations for myeloid-derived suppressor cell nomenclature and characterization standards. *Nat Commun* (2016) 7:12150. doi: 10.1038/ncomms12150
174. Narita Y, Wakita D, Ohkur T, Chamoto K, Nishimura T. Potential differentiation of tumor bearing mouse CD11b+Gr-1+ immature myeloid cells into both suppressor macrophages and immunostimulatory dendritic cells. *BioMed Res* (2009) 30(1):7–15. doi: 10.2220/biomedres.30.7
175. Bryant AJ, Shenoy V, Fu C, Marek G, Lorentsen KJ, Herzog EL, et al. Myeloid-derived Suppressor Cells Are Necessary for Development of Pulmonary Hypertension. *Am J Respir Cell Mol Biol* (2018) 58(2):170–80. doi: 10.1165/rcmb.2017-0214OC
176. Hochst B, Mikulec J, Baccega T, Metzger C, Welz M, Peusquens J, et al. Differential induction of Ly6G and Ly6C positive myeloid derived suppressor cells in chronic kidney and liver inflammation and fibrosis. *PloS One* (2015) 10(3):e0119662. doi: 10.1371/journal.pone.0119662
177. Hsieh CC, Lin CL, He JT, Chiang M, Wang Y, Tsai YC, et al. Administration of cytokine-induced myeloid-derived suppressor cells ameliorates renal fibrosis in diabetic mice. *Stem Cell Res Ther* (2018) 9(1):183. doi: 10.1186/s13287-018-0915-0
178. Zhang H, Maric I, DiPrima MJ, Khan J, Orentas RJ, Kaplan RN, et al. Fibrocytes represent a novel MDSC subset circulating in patients with metastatic cancer. *Blood* (2013) 122(7):1105–13. doi: 10.1182/blood-2012-08-449413
179. Niedermeier M, Reich B, Rodriguez Gomez M, Denzel A, Schmidbauer K, Gobel N, et al. CD4+ T cells control the differentiation of Gr1+ monocytes into fibrocytes. *Proc Natl Acad Sci USA* (2009) 106(42):17892–7. doi: 10.1073/pnas.0906070106
180. Su X, Yang L, Yin Y, Huang J, Qiao F, Fang Y, et al. Bone marrow mesenchymal stem cells tune the differentiation of myeloid-derived suppressor cells in bleomycin-induced lung injury. *Stem Cell Res Ther* (2018) 9(1):253. doi: 10.1186/s13287-018-0983-1
181. American Thoracic Society. Idiopathic pulmonary fibrosis: diagnosis and treatment. International consensus statement. American Thoracic Society (ATS), and the European Respiratory Society (ERS). *Am J Respir Crit Care Med* (2000) 161(2 Pt 1):646–64. doi: 10.1164/ajrccm.161.2.ats3-00
182. Raghu G, Rochwerg B, Zhang Y, Garcia CA, Azuma A, Behr J, et al. An Official ATS/ERS/JRS/ALAT Clinical Practice Guideline: Treatment of Idiopathic Pulmonary Fibrosis. An Update of the 2011 Clinical Practice Guideline. *Am J Respir Crit Care Med* (2015) 192(2):e3–19. doi: 10.1164/rccm.201506-1063ST
183. Idiopathic Pulmonary Fibrosis Clinical Research N, Raghu G, Anstrom KJ, King TE Jr, Lasky JA, Martinez FJ. Prednisone, azathioprine, and N-acetylcysteine for pulmonary fibrosis. *N Engl J Med* (2012) 366(21):1968–77. doi: 10.1056/NEJMoa1113354
184. Lehtonen ST, Veijola A, Karvonen H, Lappi-Blanco E, Sormunen R, Korpela S, et al. Pirfenidone and nintedanib modulate properties of fibroblasts and myofibroblasts in idiopathic pulmonary fibrosis. *Respir Res* (2016) 17:14. doi: 10.1186/s12931-016-0328-5
185. Ahluwalia N, Shea BS, Tager AM. New therapeutic targets in idiopathic pulmonary fibrosis. Aiming to rein in runaway wound-healing responses. *Am J Respir Crit Care Med* (2014) 190(8):867–78. doi: 10.1164/rccm.201403-0509PP
186. King TE Jr, Bradford WZ, Castro-Bernardini S, Fagan EA, Glaspole I, Glassberg MK, et al. A phase 3 trial of pirfenidone in patients with idiopathic pulmonary fibrosis. *N Engl J Med* (2014) 370(22):2083–92. doi: 10.1056/NEJMoa1402582
187. Noble PW, Albera C, Bradford WZ, Costabel U, Glassberg MK, Kardatzke D, et al. Pirfenidone in patients with idiopathic pulmonary fibrosis (CAPACITY): two randomised trials. *Lancet* (2011) 377(9779):1760–9. doi: 10.1016/S0140-6736(11)60405-4
188. Costabel U, Albera C, Glassberg MK, Lancaster LH, Wuyts WA, Petzinger U, et al. Effect of pirfenidone in patients with more advanced idiopathic pulmonary fibrosis. *Respir Res* (2019) 20(1):55. doi: 10.1186/s12931-019-1021-2
189. Liu H, Drew P, Gaugler AC, Cheng Y, Visner GA. Pirfenidone inhibits lung allograft fibrosis through L-arginine-arginase pathway. *Am J Transpl* (2005) 5(6):1256–63. doi: 10.1111/j.1600-6143.2005.00876.x
190. Hirano A, Kanehiro A, Ono K, Ito W, Yoshida A, Okada C, et al. Pirfenidone modulates airway responsiveness, inflammation, and remodeling after repeated challenge. *Am J Respir Cell Mol Biol* (2006) 35(3):366–77. doi: 10.1165/rcmb.2005-0452OC
191. Shihab FS, Bennett WM, Yi H, Andoh TF. Pirfenidone treatment decreases transforming growth factor-beta1 and matrix proteins and ameliorates fibrosis in chronic cyclosporine nephrotoxicity. *Am J Transpl* (2002) 2 (2):111–9. doi: 10.1034/j.1600-6143.2002.020201.x
192. Cain WC, Stuart RW, Lefkowitz DL, Starnes JD, Margolin S, Lefkowitz SS. Inhibition of tumor necrosis factor and subsequent endotoxin shock by pirfenidone. *Int J Immunopharmacol* (1998) 20(12):685–95. doi: 10.1016/s0192-0561(98)00042-3
193. Nakazato H, Oku H, Yamane S, Tsuruta Y, Suzuki R. A novel anti-fibrotic agent pirfenidone suppresses tumor necrosis factor-alpha at the translational level. *Eur J Pharmacol* (2002) 446(1-3):177–85. doi: 10.1016/s0014-2999(02)01758-2
194. Oku H, Nakazato H, Horikawa T, Tsuruta Y, Suzuki R. Pirfenidone suppresses tumor necrosis factor-alpha, enhances interleukin-10 and protects mice from endotoxic shock. *Eur J Pharmacol* (2002) 446(1-3):167–76. doi: 10.1016/s0014-2999(02)01757-0
195. Visner GA, Liu F, Bizargity P, Liu H, Liu K, Yang J, et al. Pirfenidone inhibits T-cell activation, proliferation, cytokine and chemokine production, and host alloresponses. *Transplantation* (2009) 88(3):330–8. doi: 10.1097/TP.0b013e3181ae3392
196. Bizargity P, Liu K, Wang L, Hancock WW, Visner GA. Inhibitory effects of pirfenidone on dendritic cells and lung allograft rejection. *Transplantation* (2012) 94(2):114–22. doi: 10.1097/TP.0b013e3182584879
197. Du J, Paz K, Flynn R, Vulic A, Robinson TM, Lineburg KE, et al. Pirfenidone ameliorates murine chronic GVHD through inhibition of macrophage infiltration and TGF-beta production. *Blood* (2017) 129(18):2570–80. doi: 10.1182/blood-2017-01-758854
198. Aboulkheyr Es H, Zhand S, Thiery JP, Warkiani ME. Pirfenidone reduces immune-suppressive capacity of cancer-associated fibroblasts through targeting CCL17 and TNF-beta. *Integr Biol (Camb)* (2020) 12(7):188–97. doi: 10.1093/intbio/zyaa014
199. Wollin L, Wex E, Pautsch A, Schnapp G, Hostettler KE, Stowasser S, et al. Mode of action of nintedanib in the treatment of idiopathic pulmonary fibrosis. *Eur Respir J* (2015) 45(5):1434–45. doi: 10.1183/09031936.00174914
200. Hilberg F, Tontsch-Grunt U, Baum A, Le AT, Doebele RC, Lieb S, et al. Triple Angiokinase Inhibitor Nintedanib Directly Inhibits Tumor Cell Growth and Induces Tumor Shrinkage via Blocking Oncogenic Receptor Tyrosine Kinases. *J Pharmacol Exp Ther* (2018) 364(3):494–503. doi: 10.1124/jpet.117.244129
201. Richeldi L, du Bois RM, Raghu G, Azuma A, Brown KK, Costabel U, et al. Efficacy and safety of nintedanib in idiopathic pulmonary fibrosis. *N Engl J Med* (2014) 370(22):2071–82. doi: 10.1056/NEJMoa1402584
202. Reck M, Kaiser R, Mellemgaard A, Douillard JY, Orlov S, Krzakowski M, et al. Docetaxel plus nintedanib versus docetaxel plus placebo in patients with previously treated non-small-cell lung cancer (LUME-Lung 1): a phase 3, double-blind, randomised controlled trial. *Lancet Oncol* (2014) 15(2):143–55. doi: 10.1016/S1470-2045(13)70586-2
203. Awasthi N, Schwarz RE. Profile of nintedanib in the treatment of solid tumors: the evidence to date. *Onco Targets Ther* (2015) 8:3691–701. doi: 10.2147/OTT.S78805
204. Reck M, Mellemgaard A, von Pawel J, Gottfried M, Bondarenko I, Cheng Y, et al. Anti-angiogenic-specific adverse events in patients with non-small cell lung cancer treated with nintedanib and docetaxel. *Lung Cancer* (2015) 90 (2):267–73. doi: 10.1016/j.lungcan.2015.08.003

205. du Bois A, Huober J, Stopfer P, Pfisterer J, Wimberger P, Loibl S, et al. A phase I open-label dose-escalation study of oral BIBF 1120 combined with standard paclitaxel and carboplatin in patients with advanced gynecological malignancies. *Ann Oncol* (2010) 21(2):370–5. doi: 10.1093/annonc/mdp506
206. Doebele RC, Conkling P, Traynor AM, Otterson GA, Zhao Y, Wind S, et al. A phase I, open-label dose-escalation study of continuous treatment with BIBF 1120 in combination with paclitaxel and carboplatin as first-line treatment in patients with advanced non-small-cell lung cancer. *Ann Oncol* (2012) 23(8):2094–102. doi: 10.1093/annonc/mdr596
207. Quintela-Fandino M, Urruticoechea A, Guerra J, Gil M, Gonzalez-Martin A, Marquez R, et al. Phase I clinical trial of nintedanib plus paclitaxel in early HER-2-negative breast cancer (CNIO-BR-01-2010/GEICAM-2010-10 study). *Br J Cancer* (2014) 111(6):1060–4. doi: 10.1038/bjc.2014.397
208. Reguera-Nunez E, Man S, Xu P, Hilberg F, Kerbel RS. Variable impact of three different antiangiogenic drugs alone or in combination with chemotherapy on multiple bone marrow-derived cell populations involved in angiogenesis and immunity. *Angiogenesis* (2019) 22(4):535–46. doi: 10.1007/s10456-019-09677-x
209. Overed-Sayer C, Miranda E, Dunmore R, Liarte Marin E, Beloki L, Rassl D, et al. Inhibition of mast cells: a novel mechanism by which nintedanib may elicit anti-fibrotic effects. *Thorax* (2020) 75(9):754–63. doi: 10.1136/thoraxjnl-2019-214000
210. Lukey PT, Harrison SA, Yang S, Man Y, Holman BF, Rashidnasab A, et al. A randomised, placebo-controlled study of omipalisib (PI3K/mTOR) in idiopathic pulmonary fibrosis. *Eur Respir J* (2019) 53(3):1801992. doi: 10.1183/13993003.01992-2018
211. Hirani N, MacKinnon AC, Nicol L, Ford P, Schambye H, Pedersen A, et al. Target-inhibition of Galectin-3 by Inhaled TD139 in Patients with Idiopathic Pulmonary Fibrosis. *Eur Respir J* (2020). doi: 10.1183/13993003.02559-2020
212. Knipe RS, Tager AM, Liao JK. The Rho kinases: critical mediators of multiple profibrotic processes and rational targets for new therapies for pulmonary fibrosis. *Pharmacol Rev* (2015) 67(1):103–17. doi: 10.1124/pr.114.009381
213. Maher TM, Costabel U, Glassberg MK, Kondoh Y, Ogura T, Scholand MB, et al. Phase 2 trial to assess lebrikizumab in patients with idiopathic pulmonary fibrosis. *Eur Respir J* (2020) 57:1902442. doi: 10.1183/13993003.02442-2019
214. Parker JM, Glaspole IN, Lancaster LH, Haddad TJ, She D, Roseti SL, et al. A Phase 2 Randomized Controlled Study of Tralokinumab in Subjects with Idiopathic Pulmonary Fibrosis. *Am J Respir Crit Care Med* (2018) 197(1):94–103. doi: 10.1164/rccm.201704-0784OC
215. Wijsenbeek MS, Kool M, Cottin V. Targeting interleukin-13 in idiopathic pulmonary fibrosis: from promising path to dead end. *Eur Respir J* (2018) 52 (6):1802111. doi: 10.1183/13993003.02111-2018
216. Raghu G, Richeldi L, Crestani B, Wung P, Bejuit R, Esperet C, et al. SAR156597 in idiopathic pulmonary fibrosis: a phase 2 placebo-controlled study (DRI11772). *Eur Respir J* (2018) 52(6):1801130. doi: 10.1183/13993003.01130-2018
217. Raghu G, Brown KK, Collard HR, Cottin V, Gibson KF, Kaner RJ, et al. Efficacy of simtuzumab versus placebo in patients with idiopathic pulmonary fibrosis: a randomised, double-blind, controlled, phase 2 trial. *Lancet Respir Med* (2017) 5(1):22–32. doi: 10.1016/S2213-2600(16)30421-0
218. Raghu G, Martinez FJ, Brown KK, Costabel U, Cottin V, Wells AU, et al. CC-chemokine ligand 2 inhibition in idiopathic pulmonary fibrosis: a phase 2 trial of carlumab. *Eur Respir J* (2015) 46(6):1740–50. doi: 10.1183/13993003.01558-2014
219. Khalil N, Manganas H, Ryerson CJ, Shapera S, Cantin AM, Hernandez P, et al. Phase 2 clinical trial of PBI-4050 in patients with idiopathic pulmonary fibrosis. *Eur Respir J* (2019) 53(3):1800663. doi: 10.1183/13993003.00663-2018
220. Palmer SM, Snyder L, Todd JL, Soule B, Christian R, Anstrom K, et al. Randomized, Double-Blind, Placebo-Controlled, Phase 2 Trial of BMS-986020, a Lysophosphatidic Acid Receptor Antagonist for the Treatment of Idiopathic Pulmonary Fibrosis. *Chest* (2018) 154(5):1061–9. doi: 10.1016/j.chest.2018.08.1058
221. Maher TM, Kreuter M, Lederer DJ, Brown KK, Wuyts W, Verbruggen N, et al. Rationale, design and objectives of two phase III, randomised, placebo-controlled studies of GLPG1690, a novel autotaxin inhibitor, in idiopathic pulmonary fibrosis (ISABELA 1 and 2). *BMJ Open Respir Res* (2019) 6(1): e000422. doi: 10.1136/bmjresp-2019-000422
222. Dillingh MR, van den Blink B, Moerland M, van Dongen MG, Levi M, Kleinjan A, et al. Recombinant human serum amyloid P in healthy volunteers and patients with pulmonary fibrosis. *Pulm Pharmacol Ther* (2013) 26(6):672–6. doi: 10.1016/j.pupt.2013.01.008
223. Kondoh Y, Azuma A, Inoue Y, Ogura T, Sakamoto S, Tsushima K, et al. Thrombomodulin Alfa for Acute Exacerbation of Idiopathic Pulmonary Fibrosis. A Randomized, Double-Blind Placebo-controlled Trial. *Am J Respir Crit Care Med* (2020) 201(9):1110–9. doi: 10.1164/rccm.201909-1818OC
224. Anstrom KJ, Noth I, Flaherty KR, Edwards RH, Albright J, Baucom A, et al. Design and rationale of a multi-center, pragmatic, open-label randomized trial of antimicrobial therapy - the study of clinical efficacy of antimicrobial therapy strategy using pragmatic design in Idiopathic Pulmonary Fibrosis (CleanUP-IPF) clinical trial. *Respir Res* (2020) 21(1):68. doi: 10.1186/s12931-020-1326-1
225. Durheim MT, Collard HR, Roberts RS, Brown KK, Flaherty KR, King TE Jr, et al. Association of hospital admission and forced vital capacity endpoints with survival in patients with idiopathic pulmonary fibrosis: analysis of a pooled cohort from three clinical trials. *Lancet Respir Med* (2015) 3(5):388–96. doi: 10.1016/S2213-2600(15)00093-4
226. Behr J, Kolb M, Song JW, Luppi F, Schinzel B, Stowasser S, et al. Nintedanib and Sildenafil in Patients with Idiopathic Pulmonary Fibrosis and Right Heart Dysfunction. A Prespecified Subgroup Analysis of a Double-Blind Randomized Clinical Trial (INSTAGE). *Am J Respir Crit Care Med* (2019) 200(12):1505–12. doi: 10.1164/rccm.201903-0488OC
227. Sgalla G, Franciosa C, Simonetti J, Richeldi L. Pamrevlumab for the treatment of idiopathic pulmonary fibrosis. *Expert Opin Investig Drugs* (2020) 29(8):771–7. doi: 10.1080/13543784.2020.1773790
228. Duitman J, van den Ende T, Spek CA. Immune Checkpoints as Promising Targets for the Treatment of Idiopathic Pulmonary Fibrosis? *J Clin Med* (2019) 8(10):1547. doi: 10.3390/jcm8101547
229. Ng B, Dong J, D'Agostino G, Viswanathan S, Widjaja AA, Lim WW, et al. Interleukin-11 is a therapeutic target in idiopathic pulmonary fibrosis. *Sci Transl Med* (2019) 11(511):eaaw1237. doi: 10.1126/scitranslmed.aaw1237
230. Kumar A, Kapnadak SG, Girgis RE, Raghu G. Lung transplantation in idiopathic pulmonary fibrosis. *Expert Rev Respir Med* (2018) 12(5):375–85. doi: 10.1080/17476348.2018.1462704
231. Valapour M, Lehr CJ, Skeans MA, Smith JM, Carrico R, Uccellini K, et al. OPTN/SRTR 2016 Annual Data Report: Lung. *Am J Transplant* (2018) 18 Suppl 1:363–433. doi: 10.1111/ajt.14562
232. Villavicencio MA, Axtell AL, Osho A, Astor T, Roy N, Melnitchouk S, et al. Single- Versus Double-Lung Transplantation in Pulmonary Fibrosis: Impact of Age and Pulmonary Hypertension. *Ann Thorac Surg* (2018) 106(3):856–63. doi: 10.1016/j.athoracsur.2018.04.060
233. Tuyls S, Verleden SE, Wuyts WA, Yserbyt J, Vos R, Verleden GM. Determinants of survival in lung transplantation patients with idiopathic pulmonary fibrosis: a retrospective cohort study. *Transpl Int* (2019) 32 (4):399–409. doi: 10.1111/tri.13382
234. Fernandez IE, Heinzelmann K, Verleden S, Eickelberg O. Characteristic patterns in the fibrotic lung. Comparing idiopathic pulmonary fibrosis with chronic lung allograft dysfunction. *Ann Am Thorac Soc* (2015) 12 Suppl 1: S34–41. doi: 10.1513/AnnalsATS.201410-476MG
235. Kingsley CI, Karim M, Bushell AR, Wood KJ. CD25+CD4+ regulatory T cells prevent graft rejection: CTLA-4- and IL-10-dependent immunoregulation of alloresponses. *J Immunol* (2002) 168(3):1080–6. doi: 10.4049/jimmunol.168.3.1080
236. Highfill SL, Rodriguez PC, Zhou Q, Goetz CA, Koehn BH, Veenstra R, et al. Bone marrow myeloid-derived suppressor cells (MDSCs) inhibit graft-versus-host disease (GVHD) via an arginase-1-dependent mechanism that is up-regulated by interleukin-13. *Blood* (2010) 116(25):5738–47. doi: 10.1182/blood-2010-06-287839
237. Meng F, Chen S, Guo X, Chen Z, Huang X, Lai Y, et al. Clinical significance of myeloid-derived suppressor cells in human renal transplantation with acute T cell-mediated rejection. *Inflammation* (2014) 37(5):1799–805. doi: 10.1007/s10753-014-9910-5
238. Luan Y, Mosheir E, Menon MC, Wilson D, Woytovich C, Ochando J, et al. Monocytic myeloid-derived suppressor cells accumulate in renal transplant patients and mediate CD4(+) Foxp3(+) Treg expansion. *Am J Transplant* (2013) 13(12):3123–31. doi: 10.1111/ajt.12461

239. Li W, Bribriesco AC, Nava RG, Brescia AA, Ibricevic A, Spahn JH, et al. Lung transplant acceptance is facilitated by early events in the graft and is associated with lymphoid neogenesis. *Mucosal Immunol* (2012) 5(5):544–54. doi: 10.1038/mi.2012.30
240. Li W, Gauthier JM, Higashikubo R, Hsiao HM, Tanaka S, Vuong L, et al. Bronchus-associated lymphoid tissue-resident Foxp3+ T lymphocytes prevent antibody-mediated lung rejection. *J Clin Invest* (2019) 129(2):556–68. doi: 10.1172/JCI122083
241. Salman J, Ius F, Knoefel AK, Sommer W, Siemeni T, Kuehn C, et al. Association of Higher CD4(+) CD25(high) CD127(low) , FoxP3(+) , and IL-2(+) T Cell Frequencies Early After Lung Transplantation With Less Chronic Lung Allograft Dysfunction at Two Years. *Am J Transplant* (2017) 17 (6):1637–48. doi: 10.1111/ajt.14148
242. Botturi K, Lacoeuille Y, Thomas P, Boniface S, Reynaud-Gaubert M, Magnan A. CTLA-4-mediated regulatory phenotype of T-cells in tolerant lung recipients. *Eur Respir J* (2008) 31(6):1167–76. doi: 10.1183/09031936.00093207
243. Heigl T, Singh A, Saez-Gimenez B, Kaes J, Van Herck A, Sacreas A, et al. Myeloid-Derived Suppressor Cells in Lung Transplantation. *Front Immunol* (2019) 10:900. doi: 10.3389/fimmu.2019.00900
244. Wortel CM, Heidt S. Regulatory B cells: Phenotype, function and role in transplantation. *Transpl Immunol* (2017) 41:1–9. doi: 10.1016/j.trim.2017.02.004
245. Piloni D, Morosini M, Magni S, Balderacchi A, Inghilleri S, Cova E, et al. Peripheral CD19+CD24(high)CD38(high) B-regulatory cells in lung transplant recipients. *Transpl Immunol* (2019) 57:101245. doi: 10.1016/j.trim.2019.101245
246. Nakajima D, Watanabe Y, Ohsumi A, Pipkin M, Chen M, Mordant P, et al. Mesenchymal stromal cell therapy during ex vivo lung perfusion ameliorates ischemia-reperfusion injury in lung transplantation. *J Heart Lung Transplant* (2019) 38(11):1214–23. doi: 10.1016/j.healun.2019.07.006
247. D'Aveni M, Notarantonio AB, Bertrand A, Boulange L, Pochon C, Rubio MT. Myeloid-Derived Suppressor Cells in the Context of Allogeneic Hematopoietic Stem Cell Transplantation. *Front Immunol* (2020) 11:989. doi: 10.3389/fimmu.2020.00989
248. MacDonald KP, Rowe V, Clouston AD, Welply JK, Kuns RD, Ferrara JL, et al. Cytokine expanded myeloid precursors function as regulatory antigen-presenting cells and promote tolerance through IL-10-producing regulatory T cells. *J Immunol* (2005) 174(4):1841–50. doi: 10.4049/jimmunol.174.4.1841
249. Perobelli SM, Mercadante AC, Galvani RG, Goncalves-Silva T, Alves AP, Pereira-Neves A, et al. G-CSF-Induced Suppressor IL-10+ Neutrophils Promote Regulatory T Cells That Inhibit Graft-Versus-Host Disease in a Long-Lasting and Specific Way. *J Immunol* (2016) 197(9):3725–34. doi: 10.4049/jimmunol.1502023
250. Wang X, Bi Y, Xue L, Liao J, Chen X, Lu Y, et al. The calcineurin-NFAT axis controls allograft immunity in myeloid-derived suppressor cells through reprogramming T cell differentiation. *Mol Cell Biol* (2015) 35(3):598–609. doi: 10.1128/MCB.01251-14
251. Iglesias-Escudero M, Sansegundo-Arribas D, Riquelme P, Merino-Fernandez D, Guiral-Foz S, Perez C, et al. Myeloid-Derived Suppressor Cells in Kidney Transplant Recipients and the Effect of Maintenance Immunotherapy. *Front Immunol* (2020) 11:643. doi: 10.3389/fimmu.2020.00643
252. Dong M, Wang X, Liu J, Zhao YX, Chen XL, Li KQ, et al. Rapamycin Combined with Immature Dendritic Cells Attenuates Obliterative Bronchiolitis in Trachea Allograft Rats by Regulating the Balance of Regulatory and Effector T Cells. *Int Arch Allergy Immunol* (2015) 167 (3):177–85. doi: 10.1159/000437207

8

The Management of Patients with Idiopathic Pulmonary Fibrosis

Paolo Spagnolo [1*]***, Argyris Tzouvelekis*** [2] ***and Francesco Bonella*** [3]

[1] *Respiratory Disease Unit, Department of Cardiac, Thoracic and Vascular Sciences, University of Padova, Padova, Italy,* [2] *Division of Immunology, Biomedical Sciences Research Center "Alexander Fleming", Athens, Greece,* [3] *Interstitial and Rare Lung Disease Unit, Ruhrlandklinik, University of Duisburg-Essen, Essen, Germany*

***Correspondence:**
Paolo Spagnolo
paolo.spagnolo@unipd.it

Idiopathic pulmonary fibrosis (IPF), the most common form of fibrosing idiopathic interstitial pneumonia, is an inexorably progressive disease with a 5-year survival of ~20%. In the last decade, our understanding of disease pathobiology has increased significantly and this has inevitably impacted on the approach to treatment. Indeed, the paradigm shift from a chronic inflammatory disorder to a primarily fibrotic one coupled with a more precise disease definition and redefined diagnostic criteria have resulted in a massive increase in the number of clinical trials evaluating novel candidate drugs. Most of these trials, however, have been negative, probably because of the multitude and redundancy of cell types, growth factors and profibrotic pathways involved in disease pathogenesis. As a consequence, until recently IPF has lacked effective therapies. Finally, in 2014, two large phase 3 clinical trials have provided robust evidence that pirfenidone, a compound with anti-fibrotic, anti-oxidant and anti-inflammatory properties, and nintedanib, a tyrosine kinase inhibitor with selectivity for vascular endothelial growth factor, platelet-derived growth factor and fibroblast growth factor receptors are able to slow down functional decline and disease progression with an acceptable safety profile. While this is a major achievement, neither pirfenidone nor nintedanib cures IPF and most patients continue to experience disease progression and/or exacerbation despite treatment. Therefore, in recent years increasingly more attention has been paid to preservation of quality of life and, in the advanced phase of the disease, palliation of symptoms. Lung transplantation, the only curative treatment, remains a viable option for only a minority of highly selected patients. The unmet medical need in IPF remains high, and more efficacious and better tolerated drugs are urgently needed. However, a truly effective therapeutic approach should also address quality of life and highly prevalent concomitant conditions and complications of IPF.

Keywords: idiopathic pulmonary fibrosis, pharmacologic treatment, pirfenidone, nintedanib, non-pharmacological treatment, therapy

INTRODUCTION

The approach to treatment of idiopathic pulmonary fibrosis (IPF) has changed dramatically in the last decade. A number of factors have contributed to this, including improved, though still incomplete, knowledge of disease pathobiology, refined disease definition and diagnostic criteria, and advances in clinical trial design and conductance (1–3). Historically, corticosteroids and immunosuppressive agents have represented the standard of care for patients with IPF based on the prevailing hypothesis that chronic inflammation may precede and progresses to pulmonary fibrosis. However, the IPFnet-sponsored PANTHER-IPF (Evaluating the Effectiveness of Prednisone, Azathioprine, and N-acetylcysteine in Patients With IPF) trial was terminated prematurely following an interim safety analysis revealing that combination (triple) therapy of prednisone, azathioprine and N-acetylcysteine was associated with increased rates of all-cause mortality, hospitalization and serious adverse events compared to placebo (4). Accordingly, this therapy no longer represents a therapeutic option in patients with IPF (5).

Current paradigm of disease pathogenesis involves recurrent alveolar epithelial cell injury followed by an aberrant wound healing response characterized by uncontrolled migration and proliferation of lung fibroblasts and differentiation of fibroblasts to myofibroblasts resulting in excessive collagen deposition, scarring of the lung parenchyma and irreversible loss of function (6, 7). Accordingly, recent clinical trials have evaluated the efficacy of compounds targeting the wound healing cascade and fibrogenesis, but, overall, with disappointing results, probably because of the multitude of mediators, growth factors and signaling pathways involved in the fibrotic process (8). More recently, two compounds pleiotropic in their mechanisms of action—pirfenidone and nintedanib—have been approved for the treatment of IPF based on their ability to slow down the pace of functional decline and disease progression in phase 3 clinical trials (9, 10). Management of physical debility and palliation of symptoms are similarly important, while lung transplantation represents a realistic therapeutic option only in a small fraction of highly selected patients.

In this article, we summarize and discuss the most recent literature on pharmacological and non-pharmacological treatment of this dreadful disease.

THE ATS/ERS/JRS/ALAT GUIDELINE DOCUMENT ON TREATMENT OF IPF

Originally published in 2011 (11), these evidence-based guidelines have been updated in 2015 to incorporate the most relevant data reported since publication of the previous document (5). For each treatment regimen, a multidisciplinary expert committee graded the certainty (e.g., the *confidence*) in effect estimate as *high*, *moderate*, *low*, or *very low* according to the GRADE (Grading of Recommendations Assessment, Development and Evaluation) methodology (12) and made a recommendation either "strong" or "conditional" *for* or *against* a given intervention. The recommendations were based, among others, on the strength of evidence, outcomes studies, and associated importance to patients, desirable and undesirable consequences of treatment, costs, feasibility of treatment, and acceptability of treatment to stakeholders. Current recommendations for treatment of IPF are summarized in **Table 1**.

Three therapeutic interventions received a *conditional* (e.g., weak) recommendation for use (e.g., pirfenidone, nintedanib, and antacid medication), and they are discussed below.

TABLE 1 | Key recommendations on pharmacological treatment of IPF according to current guideline.

	2015 Guideline	2011 Guideline
THERAPEUTIC AGENT		
Pirfenidone	Conditional recommendation for use*	Weak recommendation against use
Nintedanib	Conditional recommendation for use	Not addressed
Antiacid therapy	Conditional recommendation for use	Weak recommendation for use
Phosphodiesterase-5 inhibitor (sildenafil)	Conditional recommendation against use	Not addressed
Dual endothelin receptor antagonists (bosentan, macitentan)	Conditional recommendation against use	Strong recommendation against use
N-acetylcysteine (NAC)	Conditional recommendation against use	Weak recommendation against use
Azathioprine + corticosteroids + NAC	Strong recommendation against use	Weak recommendation against use
Warfarin	Strong recommendation against use	Weak recommendation against use
Imatinib	Strong recommendation against use	Not addressed
Selective endothelin receptor antagonist (ambrisentan)	Strong recommendation against use	Not addressed

**Conditional recommendations are synonymous with weak recommendations*

PIRFENIDONE

Pirfenidone (5-methyl-1-phenyl-2-(1H)-pyridone) is an orally available, synthetic compound that exerts anti-fibrotic, anti-inflammatory, and anti-oxidant activities (13). While its exact mechanism of action remains to be elucidated, pirfenidone's biological effects are believed to occur mainly through suppression of tumor necrosis factor (TNF)-α, an early mediator of inflammation (14), and mediators in the transforming growth factor (TGF)-β pathway, such as the cytoplasmic Smad proteins (15), resulting in inhibition of fibroblast proliferation and differentiation to myofibroblasts, and decreased collagen production (16).

Four phase 3 randomized controlled trials have assessed the efficacy of pirfenidone in patients with IPF. In a Japanese study led by Taniguchi [Shionogi Phase 3 (SP3)], 275 patients were randomized in a 2:1:2 ratio to high-dose pirfenidone (1,800 mg/day), low-dose pirfenidone (1,200 mg/day), or placebo (17). As compared to placebo, both high-dose and low-dose pirfenidone reduced significantly the rate of decline in vital capacity (VC) (−0.16 vs. −0.09 L and −0.08 L; $p = 0.042$ and $p = 0.039$, respectively). Additional significant differences in favor of pirfenidone were observed in progression-free survival (PFS) (defined as decline in VC of >10% from baseline or death) and change in total lung capacity (TLC). Limitations of the study, however, included the change of the primary endpoint before unblinding and the handling of missing data (e.g., last observation carried forward, which may inflate the type 1 error rate). At the time of this trial, pirfenidone had already been approved for treatment of IPF in Japan based on a secondary endpoint analysis of a previous study [Shionogi Phase 2 (SP2)] showing a significantly reduced rate of acute exacerbations (AE) of IPF (AE-IPF) in patients randomized to pirfenidone (18).

The CAPACITY (Clinical Studies Assessing Pirfenidone in IPF: Research on Efficacy and Safety Outcomes) program consisted of two nearly identical trials (PIPF-004 and PIPF-006) that evaluated the efficacy of pirfenidone in IPF patients with mild to moderate functional impairment [predicted forced vital capacity (FVC) ≥50%, predicted carbon monoxide diffusing capacity (DL_{CO}) ≥35%, either predicted FVC or predicted DL_{CO} ≤90%, and 6-minute walk test (6MWT) distance ≥150 m] (19). Study 004 enrolled 435 patients who were randomized in a 2:1:2 dosing ratio to pirfenidone 2,403 mg/day ($n = 174$), pirfenidone 1,197 mg/day ($n = 87$), or placebo ($n = 174$), whereas study 006 had only two arms (e.g., pirfenidone 2,403 mg/day, $n = 173$ and placebo, $n = 171$). The change in percentage predicted FVC from baseline to week 72 was the primary outcome in both trials. In study PIPF-004, mean FVC change at week 72 was −8.0% in the pirfenidone 2,403 mg/day arm and −12.4% in the placebo arm ($p = 0.001$). In addition, 35/174 (20%) patients in the pirfenidone 2,403 mg/day group vs. 60/174 (35%) in the placebo group had a decline in FVC of at least 10% ($p = 0.001$). In the pirfenidone low-dose group, change in FVC was intermediate to that of the pirfenidone 2,403 mg/day and placebo groups. Conversely, in study PIPF-006, the FVC change at week 72 did not differ significantly between the two groups (−9.0% in the pirfenidone group vs. −9.6% in the placebo group; $p = 0.51$). Based on these data, pirfenidone was approved by the European Medicines Agency (EMA), whereas the U.S. Food and Drug Administration (FDA) requested an additional phase 3 study to confirm drug efficacy before pirfenidone could be approved. The ASCEND (Assessment of Pirfenidone to Confirm Efficacy and Safety in IPF) trial enrolled 555 patients with IPF who were randomly assigned to either pirfenidone 2,403 mg/day ($n = 278$) or placebo ($n = 277$) (9). The primary outcome was the change in percentage of predicted FVC or death from baseline to week 52. Notably, in order to enrol patients at higher risk for disease progression, thus maximizing the likelihood of detecting a treatment effect, patients suspected to have airflow limitation [ratio of the forced expiratory volume in one second (FEV1) to FVC <0.80] were excluded while the minimum DL_{CO} for enrolment was reduced from 35 to 30% of the predicted value. Pirfenidone treatment, as compared with placebo, was associated with a relative reduction of 47.9% in the proportion of patients who had an absolute decline of ≥10% in percentage predicted FVC or who died (46/278 [16.5%] vs. 88/277 [31.8%]; $p < 0.001$), and with a relative increase of 132.5% in the proportion of patients whose FVC remained stable (63/278 [22.7%] vs. 27/277 [9.7%]; $p < 0.001$). A series of sensitivity analyses corroborated the robustness of these findings and the magnitude of pirfenidone effect (20). Pirfenidone treatment was also associated with a reduced decline in the 6-minute walk distance (6MWD) ($p = 0.04$) and improved progression-free survival (defined as the time to a decrease of ≥10% in the percentage of the predicted FVC, a decrease of ≥50 m in the 6MWD, or death, whichever occurred first; $p < 0.001$). Conversely, pirfenidone was not superior to placebo with regard to dyspnea scores ($p = 0.16$), or all-cause (4.0 vs. 7.2%; $p = 0.10$) or IPF-related mortality (1.1 vs. 2.5%; $p = 0.23$). However, a pre-specified pooled analysis of the ASCEND and CAPACITY trials revealed that pirfenidone was associated with a significant reduction of both all-cause [3.5 vs. 6.7%; hazard ratio (HR): 0.52; $p = 0.01$] and IPF-related mortality (1.1 vs. 3.5%; HR: 0.32; $p = 0.006$) at week 52 compared with placebo (9). Pooled analyses of ASCEND and CAPACITY trials and meta-analyses, which included also data from the SP2 and SP3 Japanese trials, confirmed that pirfenidone treatment reduced significant the risk of mortality compared with placebo over 120 weeks (21). In addition, pooled analysis of the phase 3 clinical trials ASCEND and CAPACITY showed that pirfenidone beneficial effect extends to non-elective respiratory-related hospitalization, which is reduced by ~50% compared to placebo (7 vs. 12%, HR 0.52, p-value = 0.001) (22), and is consistent across a broad range of patient subsets (e.g., U.S. vs. non-U.S. patients, gender, age, race, various measures and degrees of lung function impairment, use of supplemental oxygen, smoking status, or time since diagnosis) (23, 24). Several recent publications, including "real world" experiences, have confirmed the long-term efficacy and safety profiles of pirfenidone in patients with IPF (25–27). These studies exemplified the difference between efficacy and effectiveness of pirfenidone use in patient with IPF, as pirfenidone was the first drug for IPF to show longitudinal effectiveness within the real-life clinical setting and not only within the "controlled" environment of a clinical trial (28).

Data on safety and efficacy of pirfenidone in patients with severe functional impairment (i.e., FVC% predicted <50% and/or DL_{CO} <35%) are limited. In a recent retrospective study of such patients ($n = 43$), pirfenidone was associated with a trend toward a reduced functional decline compared to the 6-month period preceding treatment initiation, but did not show any benefit after 1 year of treatment (29). At present, there are insufficient data to justify the use of pirfenidone in patients with severe functional impairment.

Common side effects of the drug include gastrointestinal intolerance (e.g., nausea, dyspepsia, vomiting, abdominal discomfort, diarrhea) and skin reactions (photosensitivity, rash), which in most cases are mild to moderate in severity, reversible, and without clinically significant sequelae. Gastrointestinal side effects can be prevented/mitigated by taking pirfenidone during a meal, following a gradual initial dosing titration, and taking prokinetic agents and/or proton-pump inhibitors, whereas avoiding direct sun exposure, applying a broad-spectrum sunscreen with high ultraviolet (UV) A and UVB protection, and wearing protective clothing generally reduces the risk of photosensitivity skin reactions (30). Rare cases of eosinophilic pneumonia have also been described (www.pneumotox.com). Pirfenidone has been granted approval for treatment of IPF by the FDA in October 2014.

NINTEDANIB

Nintedanib, previously known by its development code BIBF 1120, is an intracellular inhibitor of the tyrosine kinases vascular endothelial growth factor receptor (VEGFR) 1-3, fibroblast growth factor receptor (FGFR) 1-3, and platelet-derived growth factor receptor (PDGFR) a and b (31). By inhibiting VEGFR, FGFR, and PDGFR, nintedanib interferes with a number of processes that have been implicated in the pathogenesis of IPF, namely proliferation and migration of primary human lung fibroblasts, fibroblast to myofibroblast transformation, and TGF-β-stimulated secretion and deposition of collagen by primary human lung fibroblasts, resulting in an inhibitory effect on extracellular matrix secretion and deposition (32). In patients with IPF, the safety and efficacy of four different doses of BIBF 1120 (e.g., 50 mg once daily [$n = 86$], and 50 mg [$n = 86$], 100 mg [$n = 86$] and 150 mg [$n = 85$] all twice daily) compared with placebo ($n = 85$) were initially evaluated in the TOMORROW (To Improve Pulmonary Fibrosis With BIBF 1120), a phase 2, proof-of-concept study, in which the primary endpoint was the annual rate of decline in FVC (33). In the BIBF 1120 150 mg twice daily group, FVC declined by 0.06 L per year compared with 0.19 L per year in the placebo group, corresponding to a 68.4% reduction in the rate of decline. In addition, BIBF 1120 150 mg twice daily was associated with a lower incidence of AE-IPF (15.7 vs. 2.4 vs. per 100-patient-years; risk ratio: 0.16; $p = 0.02$) and improved quality of life as assessed by the St. George's Respiratory Questionnaire (SGRQ) compared with placebo. The INPULSIS program consisted of two parallel 52-week, phase 3 trials (INPULSIS-1 and INPULSIS-2) designed to confirm the efficacy and safety of nintedanib 150 mg twice daily in patients with IPF (10). One thousand sixty-six patients were randomly assigned in a 3:2 ratio to either nintedanib 150 mg twice daily ($n = 309$ in INPULSIS-1 and $n = 329$ in INPULSIS-2) or placebo ($n = 204$ in INPULSIS-1 and $n = 219$ in INPULSIS-2). Similar to the TOMORROW trial, the primary outcome was the annual rate of decline in FVC. Both studies met the primary endpoint. Specifically, the adjusted annual rate of change in FVC was −114.7 ml in the nintedanib group and −239.9 ml in the placebo group in INPULSIS-1 (between group difference: 125.3 ml; $p < 0.001$) and −113.6 and −207.3 ml in INPULSIS-2 (between group difference: 93.7 ml; $p < 0.001$), respectively. In both trials, the robustness of the results of the primary analysis and the magnitude of treatment effect were confirmed by a series of prespecified sensitivity analyses. In addition, nintedanib treatment, compared with placebo, was associated with a reduced risk of disease progression—defined as absolute decline in percent predicted FVC of ≥10% or death—by 47% in INPULSIS-1 (24.3 vs. 40.7%; HR: 0.53; $p = 0.0001$) and by 33% in INPULSIS-2 (29.8 vs. 42.0%; HR: 0.67; $p = 0.0054$) (34). Furthermore, in both trials, patients receiving nintedanib were more likely to be stable (e.g., to have a decline in the percentage of predicted FVC of ≤5%) at week 52 compared with patients randomized to placebo (52.8 vs. 38.2% in INPULSIS-1, $p = 0.001$; and 53.2 vs. 39.3% in INPULSIS-2, $p = 0.001$) (32). A pooled analysis and a meta-analysis of data from the TOMORROW and INPULSIS trials confirmed the beneficial effect of nintedanib in slowing down disease progression (35).

Time to first investigator-reported AE, one of the two key secondary end points (the other being SGRQ), was significantly delayed with nintedanib vs. placebo in INPULSIS-2 (HR: 0.38, $p = 0.005$) but not in INPULSIS-1 (HR: 1.15, $p = 0.67$). However, a pre-specified sensitivity analysis of pooled data from the INPULSIS trials showed that nintedanib compared to placebo delayed significantly the first adjudicated AE-IPF (either confirmed or suspected) (HR: 0.32, $p = 0.001$) (10). More extensive analysis of the INPULSIS data showed that nintedanib treatment reduces by ~40% mortality following AE, although this result did not reach statistical significance (36). Nintedanib treatment was associated with a significantly smaller increase in the total SGRQ score (consistent with more preserved quality of life) in INPULSIS-2 (2.80 points vs. 5.48 points in the placebo group; $p = 0.02$) but not in INPULSIS-1 (4.34 points vs. 4.39 points, respectively; $p = 0.97$). In addition, in a pre-specified analysis of pooled data from the INPULSIS trials, the adjusted mean change in the SGRQ total score from baseline to week 52 was similar in the nintedanib and placebo groups. Finally, in a pre-specified pooled analysis of the INPULSIS data, the nintedanib and placebo arms did not differ significantly in terms of death from any cause (5.5 vs. 7.8%, respectively; HR: 0.70; $p = 0.14$) or death from a respiratory cause (3.8 vs. 5.0%, respectively; HR: 0.74; $p = 0.34$).

IPF is a highly heterogeneous disease and patients with varying clinical phenotypes may respond differently to antifibrotic therapies. A number of subgroup analyses however have confirmed the broad therapeutic efficacy of nintedanib in patients with IPF. Using pooled data from the INPULSIS trials, Costabel and colleagues showed that treatment effects, examined against sex, age (<65, ≥65 years), race (White, Asian), smoking status (never, ex/current), baseline FVC % predicted (≤70%, >70%), baseline SGRQ total score (≤40, >40), corticosteroid use (yes, no) and bronchodilator use (yes, no) did not differ significantly for the primary (annual rate of decline in FVC) or key secondary (time to first AE and change from baseline in the SGRQ) end points (37). In a *post-hoc* subgroup analysis of pooled data from the INPULSIS trials ($n = 1{,}061$), Raghu and colleagues demonstrated that the rate of decline in FVC in patients with possible UIP on high-resolution CT (HRCT) [i.e., reticular abnormality and traction bronchiectasis in the absence of features inconsistent with usual interstitial pneumonia (UIP)] and no confirmatory surgical lung biopsy is similar as in patients with a diagnosis of IPF according to current guidelines (i.e., honeycombing on HRCT and/or UIP on surgical lung biopsy) (38). A further *post-hoc* subgroup analysis of pooled data from the INPULSIS trials revealed that patients with IPF and preserved lung volumes (FVC >90% predicted) experience the same rate of functional decline and receive the same benefit from nintedanib as patients with more impaired lung function (FVC <90%), thus supporting the concept of offering early treatment to patients with IPF (39).

The most frequent adverse event associated with nintedanib treatment was diarrhea (~60% within the first 3 months of treatment), which in most cases was of mild or moderate intensity and led to premature study discontinuation in 4.5% of patients (vs. none in the placebo group) in INPULSIS-1 and 4.3% of patients (vs. 0.5% in the placebo group) in INPULSIS-2 (10). However, in both trials, the same proportion of patients in the nintedanib and placebo groups experienced serious adverse events. Nintedanib has been approved by the FDA in October 2014 and in Europe in early 2015.

ANTACID THERAPY

Gastroesophageal reflux (GER), both symptomatic and asymptomatic, occurs in a high proportion of patients with IPF, and chronic microaspiration secondary to GER is believed to play a role in the pathogenesis and progression of the disease (40, 41). Accordingly, a number of studies have explored the possibility that antacid therapy (AAT) may be beneficial in terms of slowing disease progression and even improving survival in patients with IPF. In an uncontrolled retrospective study of 204 IPF patients from two major academic medical centers in the U.S., GER medications [either proton pump inhibitors (PPI) or H2 blockers] were associated with reduced radiological fibrosis and improved survival (42). Furthermore, a *post-hoc* analysis of data from patients randomized to placebo in three IPFnet-sponsored clinical trials ($n = 242$, 124 of whom [51%] were taking either PPI or H2 blockers at the time of enrolment) showed that the use of AAT was associated with a smaller decrease in FVC (estimated change over 30-weeks of −0.06 vs. −0.12 L in patients not taking AAT; $p = 0.05$) and fewer AEs (no events vs. 9 events in patients not taking AAT; $p < 0.01$) (43). The 2015 guidelines conditionally recommend the use of GER medications in patients with IPF based on the potential benefit and favorable side effect profile of these drugs (5). However, a more recent *post-hoc* analysis of patients assigned to placebo in three clinical trials of pirfenidone (CAPACITY 004, CAPACITY 006, and ASCEND) ($n =$ 624, 291 of whom [47%] received AAT) questioned the efficacy of GER medications in IPF (44). Indeed, in this study AAT did not improve progression-free survival (defined as FVC decrease ≥10%, 6MWD decrease ≥50 m, or death), FVC decline, hospitalization and all-cause and IPF-related mortality. Moreover, use of GER medications was associated with a significantly higher rate of overall infections ($p = 0.02$) and pulmonary infections ($p = 0.02$) in patients with advanced IPF (e.g., FVC <70%). The role of AAT in the treatment of patients with IPF remains highly controversial and needs to be addressed in prospective randomized trials (45). One such study, which is currently ongoing, will test the hypothesis that treatment with laparoscopic antireflux surgery in patients with IPF and abnormal GER (WRAP-IPF; NCT01982968) may slow the decline in FVC over the 48-week study duration by abolishing acid and non-acid reflux, both believed to be pathogenic in IPF (41).

MANAGEMENT OF ACUTE EXACERBATIONS

The term "acute exacerbations" (AE) refers to episodes of acute respiratory deterioration accompanied by the development of new radiologic abnormalities (i.e., ground glass opacities and/or consolidation on a background of reticulation and traction bronchiectasis with or without honeycomb changes) on chest X-ray or HRCT (46). The annual incidence of AE ranges between 4 and 20% and is significantly higher in patients with more severe disease (46). The prognosis following an AE is poor with a median survival of ~3 months (47). At present, there are no therapies of proven efficacy for AE-IPF so that the treating physician is left with supportive care (i.e., palliation of symptoms and relief of hypoxemia with supplemental oxygen) and unproven interventions. Therefore, searching for (and ruling out) known causes of clinical deterioration, including drug toxicity, is warranted.

Corticosteroids

The 2011 guidelines make a weak recommendation *for* the use of corticosteroids in patients with AE-IPF, although randomized controlled clinical trials are lacking (11). The appropriate dose and duration of therapy remain unclear, but in most series the dose has ranged between prednisone 1 mg/kg per day orally and methylprednisolone 1 g per day intravenously for 3 days followed by a gradual taper, based on clinical response. The role of high-dose corticosteroids in AE-IPF remains highly controversial (48–50).

Antibiotics

The rationale behind the use of broad-spectrum antibiotics to treat AE-IPF is that many patients present with flu-like symptoms and have elevated neutrophil count in bronchoalveolar lavage fluid (51). More recently, in a retrospective single-center study of IPF patients hospitalized for AE ($n = 85$), Kawamura and co-workers showed that early administration of azithromycin 500 mg/day for 5 days is associated with a significantly lower mortality compared with a fluoroquinolone-based regimen (26 vs. 70%; $p < 0.001$) (52). This study however has a number of limitations, including its small sample size, retrospective nature and the choice of fluoroquinolone-treated patients as control group; accordingly, these findings need to be confirmed in prospective studies. Ding and colleagues evaluated the use of procalcitonin (PCT)-guided antibiotic treatment vs. standard clinician-determined antibiotic treatment in patients with AE-IPF (53). PCT guidance reduced significantly the duration of antibiotic use, but the duration of mechanical ventilation and overall mortality were similar in both groups.

Mechanical Ventilation

The role of invasive mechanical ventilation (IMV) and non-invasive ventilation (NIV) in the management of AE-IPF has not been formally studied and remains unclear. The 2011 guideline document makes a weak recommendation *against* the use of MV to treat AE-IPF, thus suggesting this may be a reasonable intervention only in a minority of selected patients (11); however, a recent U.S. nationwide retrospective cohort analysis suggested that mortality rates of IPF patients who received IMV or NIV for acute respiratory failure (51.6 and 30.9%, respectively, in this study) may be lower than previously reported (54). Prospective studies are needed to identify IPF patients more likely to benefit from MV and NIV.

Novel Approaches

Recombinant Human Soluble Thrombomodulin (rhTM)

It is a regulator of intravascular coagulation expressed on the endothelial cell surface (55). A number of studies have consistently shown that rhTM improves 3-month survival in patients with AE-IPF (56–58). However, these results need to be confirmed in the setting of randomized controlled trials.

Hemoperfusion With Polymyxin B Immobilized Fiber

Originally developed to remove gram-negative bacterial endotoxins, polymyxin B direct hemoperfusion (PMX-DHP) may also remove cytokines involved in lung injury (59). A number of retrospective studies, mostly from Japan, have shown that PMX-DHP improves oxygenation and survival in patients with AE-IPF, although most patients received also high-dose systemic corticosteroids (60–62). PMX-DHP is a promising therapeutic approach in patients with AE-IPF, but its safety and efficacy need to be validated in larger prospective clinical trials.

Autoantibody-Targeted Treatment

Recent evidence suggests that immune dysregulation may contribute to IPF progression and that treatments that reduce autoantibodies may be beneficial in a significant minority of patients (63). Donahoe and colleagues treated 11 patients with AE-IPF with plasma exchange and rituximab ± intravenous immunoglobulin (64). Compared to historical controls treated with high-dose corticosteroids, trial subjects had significantly better 1-year survival (1/20, 5% vs. 9/11, 82%). These data suggest considering a trial of autoantibody-targeted therapies in patients with AE-IPF.

MESENCHYMAL STEM CELLS

Mesenchymal stem cells (MSCs) are multipotent stromal cells with the potential of transdifferentiation, clonality, and self-renewal. MSC properties include also immunomodulation, epithelial repair, and secretion of growth factors (65). MSCs have been shown to ameliorate inflammation and mitigate parenchymal remodeling in bleomycin-induced pulmonary fibrosis (66), but the bleomycin model recapitulates only partially the complex pathobiology of IPF (67). Therefore, the application of MSCs in patients with IPF is controversial and under study (68). In a small cohort of patients with IPF (n = 14), Tzouvelekis and colleagues have shown that endobronchial infusion of autologous adipose derived stem cells was not associated with serious adverse events (69). Yet, results should be interpreted cautiously before rigid conclusions can be drawn. Significant limitations severely hampering the widespread implementation of stem cell use in IPF relate mainly to our limited knowledge of the fate of these cells within the pro-fibrotic microenvironment given their mesenchymal origin and their potential to differentiate into myofibroblasts, thus causing disease progression. In addition, there are many unanswered questions including the time (early or advanced disease) and optimal route of administration (intravenous or endobronchial), source of mesenchymal stem cells (MSCs) (eg, adipose tissue, bone marrow, or umbilical cord), frequency of infusions as well as the choice of the appropriate primary end-points to show benefit (70). An FDA approved RCT investigating safety and efficacy of a single intravenous administration of allogeneic bone-marrow derived MSCs is currently recruiting patients (NCT02611167) and results are eagerly awaited.

NON-PHARMACOLOGICAL MANAGEMENT

Besides pharmacological treatment and lung transplantation, there is increasing evidence that supportive measures such as pulmonary rehabilitation, adequate nutrition, prevention of infections and timely initiation of palliative care can improve and maintain health status and quality of life of patients with IPF (**Figure 1**). The most recent advances in lung transplantation, rehabilitation, and palliative care are discussed below.

Lung Transplantation

In the last 5 years, IPF has become the most common indication for lung transplantation (71). In the 2011 guideline document, lung transplantation was strongly recommended in IPF, though in highly selected patients (11). According to the Organ Procurement and Transplantation Network (OPTN) report, the proportion of patients transplanted with IPF has increased constantly in recent years and reached 49.6% in 2015. At present, the worldwide frequency of the procedure is ~4,000 per year with 5-year survival rates ranging from 50 to 60%, whereas 10 years survival is around 30% (72). Recipients aged 65 years or older and those with a *lung allocation score* (LAS) of 60 or higher show the lowest survival (72). Recent analyses performed after implementation of the LAS suggest that lung transplantation in patients older than 70 years of age may

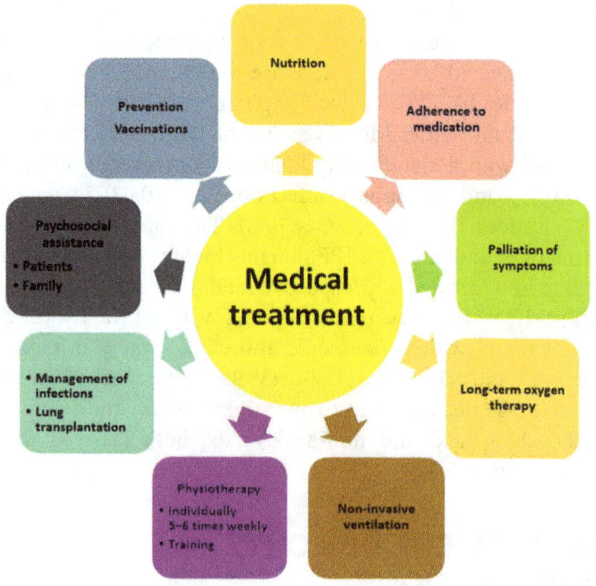

FIGURE 1 | Multidisciplinary approach to the management of patients with IPF.

have outcomes comparable to those of younger patients (73). The trend in transplanting older patients may increase in the future due to greater experience of transplant centers and the raising awareness of IPF patient advocacy groups, which in the IPF Charter on patients' rights raised the point that *age restrictions for lung transplantations exclude many healthy, viable patients* (74).

Worldwide, bilateral lung transplants are preferentially performed (about 70% of all procedures) (72), while most patients with interstitial lung disease (ILD) undergo single lung transplant (75). Bilateral lung transplants in patients with IPF appear to be associated with longer survival, although the long-term survival advantage is counterbalanced by longer time on the waiting list and higher risk of mortality (76). There are several factors that influence the selection procedure, such as age, comorbidities, anatomical features, predicted pre-transplant survival, organ availability, and center experience, but further long-term data are needed to draw firm conclusions on this highly debated topic (77). Early referral of IPF patients to transplant is highly recommended due to their poor prognosis, high mortality on the waiting list and the unpredictable disease course. After the LAS implementation and the revision of the selection criteria (78), change over time in lung function (FVC and DL_{CO}) has become the driving factor for early referral to lung transplant and has led to a reduction of the waiting list mortality of 10–20% (72).

Overall, the median survival of patients with ILD after lung transplant is 4.7 years, significantly less than that of patients with chronic obstructive pulmonary disease (COPD) and cystic fibrosis (CF) (5.5 and 8.3 years, respectively) (71, 72). Older age at the time of the transplant, prevalence of age-related comorbidities, and higher prevalence of bronchiolitis obliterans syndrome (BOS) represent the main factors that influence outcome (77). Although the incidence of pulmonary and extra-pulmonary post-transplant complications does not appear to be higher in patients with IPF than in those with other ILDs or lung diseases, there is an increasing risk for IPF patients to develop thromboembolism before and after lung transplantation (79). In addition, GER, which is highly prevalent in patients with IPF (80) and often complicates lung transplantation, is strongly associated with the development of BOS (81) and its presence should be carefully evaluated both pre- and post-transplantation (77). Fundoplication after lung transplantation and antireflux surgery pre- and post-transplantation have shown to preserve lung function and prevent reflux-associated BOS (82). On the other hand, there are no data to suggest that IPF patients are at higher risk to develop restrictive chronic lung allograft dysfunction (CLAD), a condition characterized by concomitant decrease in FVC and FEV_1, and usually accompanied by parenchymal infiltrates (77).

Pulmonary Rehabilitation

The natural history of IPF is characterized by a progressive impairment of exercise capacity and mobility, as a consequence of shortness of breath and exercise-induced hypoxemia, which induce patients to reduce and eventually avoid physical activity (83). In addition, sarcopenia, the age-related loss of muscle mass quality and strength, contributes to inactivity in these patients, which are typically 60–80 years old. In the general population and in chronic respiratory diseases, inactivity is associated with poorer health-related outcomes, including higher mortality risk (84). Exercise training in healthy subjects has been shown to positively affect the physiology of cardiovascular, respiratory, and musculoskeletal systems (85). In ILDs, pulmonary rehabilitation has been shown to alleviate respiratory and psychological symptoms, particularly dyspnea and anxiety, and improve exercise tolerance, 6MWD and quality of life scores (86–88). Possible mechanisms underlying these beneficial effects include chest expansion during deep-breathing exercises and stretching of the thoracic muscles resulting in a more efficient breathing pattern, improved respiratory muscle strength, enhanced pleural elasticity and pulmonary compliance (89).

The majority of studies on pulmonary rehabilitation in IPF combined aerobic activity (walking and/or cycling) with resistance and flexibility exercises for peripheral skeletal muscles (90). In a recent meta-analysis, 9 out of 10 of the exercise training studies examined showed a benefit in 6MWD (range 35–81 meters), peak aerobic capacity, and improvement of dyspnea and quality of life (91). Overall, supervised exercise training programs appear to provide the best results in terms of compliance and maintenance of physical activity, while home-based programs seem to be associated with a lower level of improvement (92). Pulmonary rehabilitation should be considered at any stage of IPF and in patients awaiting lung transplantation, since its timely administration correlates with a clinically significant improvement in physical activity and health-related quality of life (93). While the short-term effects of pulmonary rehabilitation on IPF outcomes are supported by several retrospective and prospective studies, its long-term effects have not been extensively studied and systematic investigation in this regard is needed.

Oxygen Treatment

Prescription of long-term oxygen treatment (LTOT) is a challenging step in the management of IPF not only for the patients but also for their relatives and treating physicians. Patients tend not to accept LTOT as the disease becomes more "visible." In addition, their training with the devices is often inadequate and problematic. Although supplemental oxygen therapy is likely to improve symptoms and overall quality of life in IPF patients, especially those with resting or nocturnal hypoxemia (11), a recent systematic review showed no effects of oxygen therapy on dyspnoea during exercise in ILD, although exercise capacity was increased (94). The *ambulatory oxygen in fibrotic lung disease* (AmbOx) trial is the first randomized control trial investigating the effects of ambulatory oxygen during daily life on health status and breathlessness in patients with ILD (95). In this study, patients with fibrotic lung disease with oxygen saturation (SaO_2) $\geq$94% at rest but $\leq$88% during a 6MWT were treated with ambulatory oxygen for a 2-week period compared to 2 weeks off. Preliminary data show that ambulatory oxygen is associated with significantly improved health status in patients with ILD (96).

TABLE 2 | Most developed drug candidates for idiopathic pulmonary fibrosis.

Compound	Mechanism of action	Study design	Primary outcome/study duration	Developmental phase/status	Clinical trial identifier
Inhaled TD139	Galectin-3 inhibitor	Phase 1: randomized, placebo-controlled, single ascending dose. Phase 2: randomized, placebo-controlled, multiple dose expansion cohort	Safety and tolerability (number of participant with adverse events over 2 weeks)	Phase I/II; completed, awaiting results	NCT02257177
PRM-151	Recombinant human Pentraxin-2 (serum amyloid P). Antifibrotic immunomodulator.	Randomized, placebo-controlled	Change in FVC % predicted from baseline through week 28	Phase II; active, not recruiting	NCT02550873
KD025	ROCK2 inhibitor	Randomized, open-label, active comparator	Change in FVC from baseline through week 24	Phase II; recruiting	NCT02688647
Tipelukast	LT receptor antagonist, PDE 3 and 4 inhibitor, 5-LO inhibitor	Randomized, placebo-controlled	Change in FVC from baseline through week 26	Phase II; recruiting	NCT02503657
PBI-4050	CTGF, α-SMA and collagen I expression inhibitor	Open-label, single-arm	Safety and tolerability (number of participant with abnormal laboratory values and/or adverse events over 9 months)	Phase II; completed, awaiting results	NCT02538536
GLPG1690	Autotaxin inhibitor	Randomized, placebo-controlled	Safety and tolerability over 12 weeks; pharmacokinetics; concentration of lysophosphatidic acid in blood/bronchoalveolar lavage	Phase II; Completed, awaiting results	NCT02738801
CC-90001	JNK inhibitor	Randomized, placebo-controlled	Change in FVC % predicted from baseline through week 24	Phase II; recruiting	NCT03142191
BMS-986020	LPA receptor inhibitor	Randomized, placebo-controlled	Rate of change in FVC at week 26	Phase II; completed, awaiting results	NCT01766817
BG00011 (formerly STX-100)	$\alpha_V\beta_6$ inhibitor	Randomized, placebo-controlled, dose escalation	Safety and tolerability (number of participant experiencing adverse events over 16 weeks)	Phase II; completed, awaiting results	NCT01371305
Pamrevlumab/FG-3019	CTGF inhibitor	Randomized, placebo-controlled	Change in FVC from baseline through week 48	Phase II; active, not recruiting	NCT01890265
Rituximab	CD20 inhibitor	Randomized, placebo-controlled	Change in titers of Autoantibodies to HEp-2 Cells over 9 months	Phase II; completed, awaiting results	NCT01969409
Lebrikizumab	IL-13 inhibitor	Randomized, placebo-controlled and active drug (i.e., pirfenidone) controlled	Rate of decline in FVC % predicted from baseline through week 52	Phase II; completed, awaiting results	NCT01872689
SAR156597	IL-4 and IL-13 inhibitor	Randomized, placebo-controlled	Absolute change in FVC from baseline through week 52	Phase II; completed, awaiting results	NCT02345070

CTGF, connective tissue growth factor; FVC, forced vital capacity; HEp-2, Human epithelial type 2; IL, interleukin; JNK, c-Jun N-Terminal Kinase; 5-LO, 5-lipoxygenase; LPA, lysophosphatidic acid; LT, leukotriene; PDE, phosphodiesterase; ROCK2, Rho associated kinase 2; α-SMA, α-smooth muscle actin; TGF-β, transforming growth factor-β.

Palliation of Symptoms

The aim of palliative care in IPF is to reduce the impact of symptoms on quality of life and minimize stress and psychological consequences, mainly depression and anxiety, which are related to the inexorably progressive nature of the disease. Dyspnea and cough appear early in the disease course, while fatigue, reduced appetite, and weight loss are typically seen in advanced stages of the disease. Dyspnea is strongly associated with reduced quality of life (97, 98) and has been shown to correlate with a worse prognosis (99). The mechanisms behind dyspnea are not fully understood but neuroimaging studies have shown how dyspnea and pain activate common areas in the brain and share a cerebral network (100). In a recent systematic review on the use of opioids for dyspnea in patients with IPF, Kohberg and colleagues observed that only systemic morphine administration improved significantly the dyspnea score on a visual analog scale without severe side effects (101). The majority of these studies used an individually titrated dose between 10 and 30 mg, which appears to be associated with a beneficial effect on dyspnea. Conversely, nebulized morphine did not show any effect on dyspnea, although this was probably due to the sub-therapeutic dosage (102). The concern of morphine-induced respiratory depression was addressed by almost all studies, but only minor side effects, such as nausea and constipation, were reported (103). However, strict dosage is necessary, and the risk of tolerance should be considered. Only randomized placebo-controlled trials will clarify whether morphine is effective and safe in the treatment of dyspnea in patients with IPF.

Chronic cough is another major issue in the management of IPF, since patients are often refractory to conventional anti-tussive therapy (104). A small non-randomized study with oral corticosteroids showed a reduction of cough reflex in IPF patients (103), somehow supporting the beneficial effect of low-dose steroids observed in clinical practice (102). Thalidomide has also been investigated as a potential treatment of cough in a single-center study, but despite the positive effect on quality of life, only 20% of the subjects completed the study due to adverse events (104). Recently, Birring and colleagues assessed the safety and efficacy of PA101, a novel formulation of sodium cromoglicate delivered via a high-efficiency eFlow nebuliser, in patients with IPF and chronic cough (105). IPF patients and patients with chronic idiopathic cough (CIC) were randomized 1:1 to receive PA101 (40 mg) or placebo three times daily for 2 weeks, followed by a 2-week washout, and then crossed over to the other arm. Compared to placebo, PA101 reduced daytime cough frequency by 31% at day 14 in patients with IPF but not in those with CIC, suggesting that the mechanism of cough in IPF may be disease specific. More recently, pirfenidone has been shown to significantly reduce objective 24-h cough counts and to improve subjective measures of cough, although the study had a short follow-up period and was not placebo-controlled (106).

Access to palliative care is one of the most relevant unmet needs in the management of IPF (74). It is, therefore, strongly recommended to treat respiratory symptoms irrespective of disease severity (11). Early referral of patients to individual counseling, patient support groups and comprehensive rehabilitation programs, which should also include psychological support, can have a positive impact on perception of dyspnea and quality of life, and prepare patients to face the final stages of the disease (107, 108).

Outlook

With improved clinical and basic understanding of IPF, an evidence-based approach to treatment is evolving. However, access to approved therapies remains suboptimal and problematic. Maher and colleagues have recently reported that ~40% of patients with confirmed IPF across Europe do not receive antifibrotic treatment (109). In particular, there appears to be a tendency to adopt a "wait and watch" approach in patients with mild functional impairment or stable disease. This observation underscores the need for increasing physician awareness of the progressive nature of IPF and the benefit associated with early treatment. In addition, compared to treated patients, a lower proportion of untreated patients had a multidisciplinary team evaluation at diagnosis, highlighting the importance of encouraging and facilitating patient referral to expert centers.

The need for safer and more efficacious treatment options has led to an exponential increase in the number of high-quality clinical trials of pharmacological interventions (**Table 2**). Yet, drug development in IPF poses major challenges, ranging from the lack of animal models that mimic all pathologic changes of IPF to the choice of the appropriate primary outcome on which to judge drug efficacy and the clinical meaningfulness of the observed effects. FVC is acknowledged as the preferred endpoint in IPF clinical trials (110), but how often the FVC should be measured remains unknown. Indeed, while the preferred time interval has been every 3 months, this may result in "missing events" in the case of patients who progress and die within this timeframe without documentation of a significant decline of their FVC (111). Recently, Russell and colleagues have shown that unsupervised daily home spirometry is a feasible and clinically informative tool for monitoring disease behavior in patients with IPF (112). From a clinical trial perspective, daily home spirometry may significantly reduce both the required sample size and duration of the trial by increasing the number of recorded measurements. Daily home spirometry may benefit particularly early phase clinical trials.

CONCLUSIONS

The management of patients with IPF is highly complex due to the progressive nature of the disease, the debilitating symptoms that severely impair quality of life and the highly prevalent comorbidities and complications. Currently, there is significant lack of knowledge regarding management of comorbid conditions including pulmonary hypertension and lung cancer as well as disease acute exacerbations that severely limit patients' survival. In the terminal phase of the disease palliative care becomes critically important. Developing a real cure for patients suffering from this terrible disease requires a close collaborative interplay between the scientific, professional, and patient community and the pharmaceutical industry. Only a comprehensive approach to disease management will eventually prove truly efficacious. Clinical trials focusing on disease biology and mechanisms by applying personalized medicine approaches seems to be the way forward (113, 114).

AUTHOR CONTRIBUTIONS

PS: conception and drafting of the article, final approval of the manuscript; AT and FB: drafting and critical revision of the article, final approval of the manuscript.

REFERENCES

1. Richeldi L, Collard HR, and Jones MG. Idiopathic pulmonary fibrosis. *Lancet* (2017) 389:1941–52. doi: 10.1016/S0140-6736(17)30866-8
2. Martinez FJ, Chisholm A, Collard HR, Flaherty KR, Myers J, Raghu G, et al. The diagnosis of idiopathic pulmonary fibrosis: current and future approaches. *Lancet Respir Med.* (2017) 5:61–71. doi: 10.1016/S2213-2600(16)30325-3
3. Collard HR, Bradford WZ, Cottin V, Flaherty KR, King TE, Koch GG, et al. A new era in idiopathic pulmonary fibrosis: considerations for future clinical trials. *Eur Respir J.* (2015) 46:243–9. doi: 10.1183/09031936.00200614
4. Idiopathic Pulmonary Fibrosis Clinical Research Network K, Raghu G, Anstrom KJ, King TE Jr, Lasky JA, and Martinez FJ. Prednisone, azathioprine, and N-acetylcysteine for pulmonary fibrosis. *N Engl J Med.* (2012) 366:1968–77. doi: 10.1056/NEJMoa1113354
5. Raghu G, Rochwerg B, Zhang Y, Garcia CA, Azuma A, Behr J, et al. An official ATS/ERS/JRS/ALAT clinical practice guideline: treatment of idiopathic pulmonary fibrosis. an update of the 2011 clinical practice guideline. *Am J Respir Crit Care Med.* (2015) 192:e3–19. doi: 10.1164/rccm.201506-1063ST
6. Spagnolo P, Rossi G, and Cavazza A. Pathogenesis of idiopathic pulmonary fibrosis and its clinical implications. *Expert Rev Clin Immunol.* (2014) 10:1005–17. doi: 10.1586/1744666X.2014.917050
7. Wolters PJ, Collard HR, and Jones KD. Pathogenesis of idiopathic pulmonary fibrosis. *Annu Rev Pathol.* (2014) 9:157–79. doi: 10.1146/annurev-pathol-012513-104706
8. Maher TM. Idiopathic pulmonary fibrosis: pathobiology and novel approaches to treatment. *Clin Chest Med.* (2012) 33:69–83. doi: 10.1016/j.ccm.2011.11.002
9. King TE, Bradford WZ, Castro-Bernardini S, Fagan EA, Glaspole I, Glassberg MK, et al. A phase 3 trial of pirfenidone in patients with idiopathic pulmonary fibrosis. *N Engl J Med.* (2014) 370:2083–92. doi: 10.1056/NEJMoa1402582
10. Richeldi L, du Bois RM, Raghu G, Azuma A, Brown KK, Costabel U, et al. Efficacy and safety of nintedanib in idiopathic pulmonary fibrosis. *N Engl J Med.* (2014) 370:2071–82. doi: 10.1056/NEJMoa1402584
11. Raghu G, Collard HR, Egan JJ, Martinez FJ, Behr J, Brown KK, et al. Idiopathic pulmonary fibrosis: evidence based guidelines for diagnosis and management. *Am J Respir Crit Care Med.* (2011) 183:788–824. doi: 10.1164/rccm.2009-040GL
12. Balshem H, Helfand M, Schünemann HJ, Oxman AD, Kunz R, Brozek J, et al. GRADE guidelines: 3 rating the quality of evidence. *J Clin Epidemiol.* (2011) 64:401–6. doi: 10.1016/j.jclinepi.2010.07.015
13. Kim ES, and Keating GM. Pirfenidone: a review of its use in idiopathic pulmonary fibrosis. *Drugs* (2015) 75:219–30. doi: 10.1007/s40265-015-0350-9
14. Oku H, Nakazato H, Horikawa T, Tsuruta Y, and Suzuki R. Pirfenidone suppresses tumor necrosis factor-alpha, enhances interleukin-10 and protects mice from endotoxic shock. *Eur J Pharmacol.* (2002) 446:167–76. doi: 10.1016/S0014-2999(02)01757-0
15. Conte E, Gili E, Fagone E, Fruciano M, Iemmolo M, and Vancheri C. Effect of pirfenidone on proliferation, TGF-β-induced myofibroblast differentiation and fibrogenic activity of primary human lung fibroblasts. *Eur J Pharm Sci.* (2014) 58:13–9. doi: 10.1016/j.ejps.2014.02.014
16. Selvaggio AS, and Noble PW. Pirfenidone initiates a new era in the treatment of idiopathic pulmonary fibrosis. *Annu Rev Med.* (2016) 67:487–95. doi: 10.1146/annurev-med-120214-013614
17. Taniguchi H, Ebina M, Kondoh Y, Ogura T, Azuma A, Suga M, et al. Pirfenidone in idiopathic pulmonary fibrosis. *Eur Respir J.* (2010) 35:821–29. doi: 10.1183/09031936.00005209
18. Azuma A, Nukiwa T, Tsuboi E, Suga M, Abe S, Nakata K, et al. Double-blind, placebo-controlled trial of pirfenidone in patients with idiopathic pulmonary fibrosis. *Am J Respir Crit Care Med.* (2005) 171:1040–47. doi: 10.1164/rccm.200404-571OC
19. Noble PW, Albera C, Bradford WZ, Costabel U, Glassberg MK, Kardatzke D, et al. Pirfenidone in patients with idiopathic pulmonary fibrosis (CAPACITY): two randomised trials. *Lancet* (2011) 77:1760–9. doi: 10.1016/S0140-6736(11)60405-4
20. Lederer DJ, Bradford WZ, Fagan EA, Glaspole I, Glassberg MK, Glasscock KF, et al. Sensitivity analyses of the change in FVC in a phase 3 trial of pirfenidone for idiopathic pulmonary fibrosis. *Chest* (2015) 148:196–201. doi: 10.1378/chest.14-2817
21. Nathan SD, Albera C, Bradford WZ, Costabel U, Glaspole I, Glassberg MK, et al. Effect of pirfenidone on mortality: pooled analyses and meta-analyses of clinical trials in idiopathic pulmonary fibrosis. *Lancet Respir Med.* (2017) 5:33–41. doi: 10.1016/S2213-2600(16)30326-5
22. Ley B, Swigris J, Day BM, Stauffer JL, Raimundo K, Chou W, et al. Pirfenidone reduces respiratory-related hospitalizations in idiopathic pulmonary fibrosis. *Am J Respir Crit Care Med.* (2017) 196:756–61. doi: 10.1164/rccm.201701-0091OC
23. Noble PW, Albera C, Bradford WZ, Costabel U, du Bois RM, Fagan EA, et al. Pirfenidone for idiopathic pulmonary fibrosis: analysis of pooled data from three multinational phase 3 trials. *Eur Respir J.* (2016) 47:243–53. doi: 10.1183/13993003.00026-2015
24. Albera C, Costabel U, Fagan EA, Glassberg MK, Gorina E, Lancaster L, et al. Efficacy of pirfenidone in patients with idiopathic pulmonary fibrosis with more preserved lung function. *Eur Respir J.* (2016) 48:843–51. doi: 10.1183/13993003.01966-2015
25. Lancaster L, Albera C, Bradford WZ, Costabel U, du Bois RM, Fagan EA, et al. Safety of pirfenidone in patients with idiopathic pulmonary fibrosis: integrated analysis of cumulative data from 5 clinical trials. *BMJ Open Respir Res.* (2016) 3:e000105. doi: 10.1136/bmjresp-2015-000105
26. Costabel U, Albera C, Lancaster LH, Lin CY, Hormel P, Hulter HN, et al. Open-label study of the long-term safety of pirfenidone in patients with idiopathic pulmonary fibrosis (RECAP). *Respiration* (2017) 94:408–15. doi: 10.1159/000479976
27. Ogura T, Azuma A, Inoue Y, Taniguchi H, Chida K, Bando M, et al. All-case post-marketing surveillance of 1371 patients treated with pirfenidone for idiopathic pulmonary fibrosis. *Respir Investig.* (2015) 53:232–41. doi: 10.1016/j.resinv.2015.06.001
28. Tzouvelekis A, Bouros E, Tzilas V, and Bouros D. Pirfenidone in idiopathic pulmonary fibrosis "RECAP-itulating Safety into the Real World". *Respiration* (2017) 94:405–7. doi: 10.1159/000480299
29. Tzouvelekis A, Ntolios P, Karampitsakos T, Tzilas V, Anevlavis S, Bouros E, et al. Safety and efficacy of pirfenidone in severe idiopathic pulmonary fibrosis: a real-world observational study. *Pulm Pharmacol Ther.* (2017) 46:48–53. doi: 10.1016/j.pupt.2017.08.011
30. Costabel U, Bendstrup E, Cottin V, Dewint P, Egan JJ, Ferguson J, et al. Pirfenidone in idiopathic pulmonary fibrosis: expert panel discussion on the management of drug-related adverse events. *Adv Ther.* (2014) 31:375–91. doi: 10.1007/s12325-014-0112-1
31. Hilberg F, Roth GJ, Krssak M, Kautschitsch S, Sommergruber W, Tontsch-Grunt U, et al. BIBF 1120: triple angiokinase inhibitor with sustained receptor blockade and good antitumor efficacy. *Cancer Res.* (2008) 2008:4774–82. doi: 10.1158/0008-5472.CAN-07-6307
32. Wollin L, Wex E, Pautsch A, Schnapp G, Hostettler KE, Stowasser S, et al. Mode of action of nintedanib in the treatment of idiopathic pulmonary fibrosis. *Eur Respir J.* (2015) 45:1434–45. doi: 10.1183/09031936.00174914
33. Richeldi L, Costabel U, Selman M, Kim DS, Hansell DM, Nicholson AG, et al. Efficacy of a tyrosine kinase inhibitor in idiopathic pulmonary fibrosis. *N Engl J Med.* (2011) 365:1079–87. doi: 10.1056/NEJMoa1103690
34. Keating GM. Nintedanib: a review of its use in patients with idiopathic pulmonary fibrosis. *Drugs* (2015) 75:1131–40. doi: 10.1007/s40265-015-0418-6
35. Richeldi L, Cottin V, du Bois RM, Selman M, Kimura T, Bailes Z, et al. Nintedanib in patients with idiopathic pulmonary fibrosis: combined evidence from the TOMORROW and INPULSIS® trials. *Respir Med.* (2016) 113:74–79. doi: 10.1016/j.rmed.2016.02.001
36. Collard HR, Richeldi L, Kim DS, Taniguchi H, Tschoepe I, Luisetti M, et al. Acute exacerbations in the INPULSIS trials of nintedanib in idiopathic pulmonary fibrosis. *Eur Respir J.* (2017) 49:1601339. doi: 10.1183/13993003.01339-2016
37. Costabel U, Inoue Y, Richeldi L, Collard HR, Tschoepe I, Stowasser S, et al. Efficacy of nintedanib in idiopathic pulmonary fibrosis across pre-specified subgroups in INPULSIS®. *Am J Respir Crit Care Med.* (2016) 193:178–85. doi: 10.1164/rccm.201503-0562OC

38. Raghu G, Wells AU, Nicholson AG, Richeldi L, Flaherty KR, Le Maulf F, et al. Effect of nintedanib in subgroups of idiopathic pulmonary fibrosis by diagnostic criteria. *Am J Respir Crit Care Med.* (2017) 195:78–85. doi: 10.1164/rccm.201602-0402OC
39. Kolb M, Richeldi L, Behr J, Maher TM, Tang W, Stowasser S, et al. Nintedanib in patients with idiopathic pulmonary fibrosis and preserved lung volume. *Thorax* (2017) 72:340–6. doi: 10.1136/thoraxjnl-2016-208710
40. Raghu G, Amatto VC, Behr J, and Stowasser S. Comorbidities in idiopathic pulmonary fibrosis patients: a systematic literature review. *Eur Respir J.* (2015) 46:1113–30. doi: 10.1183/13993003.02316-2014
41. Savarino E, Carbone R, Marabotto E, Furnari M, Sconfienza L, Ghio M, et al. Gastro-oesophageal reflux and gastric aspiration in idiopathic pulmonary fibrosis patients. *Eur Respir J.* (2013) 42:1322–31. doi: 10.1183/09031936.00101212
42. Lee JS, Ryu JH, Elicker BM, Lydell CP, Jones KD, Wolters PJ, et al. Gastroesophageal reflux therapy is associated with longer survival in patients with idiopathic pulmonary fibrosis. *Am J Respir Crit Care Med.* (2011) 184:1390–94. doi: 10.1164/rccm.201101-0138OC
43. Lee JS, Collard HR, Anstrom KJ, Martinez FJ, Noth I, Roberts RS, et al. Anti-acid treatment and disease progression in idiopathic pulmonary fibrosis: an analysis of data from three randomised controlled trials. *Lancet Resp Med.* (2013) 1:369–76. doi: 10.1016/S2213-2600(13)70105-X
44. Kreuter M, Wuyts W, Renzoni E, Koschel D, Maher TM, Kolb M, et al. Antacid therapy and disease outcomes in idiopathic pulmonary fibrosis: a pooled analysis. *Lancet Respir Med.* (2016) 4:381–9. doi: 10.1016/S2213-2600(16)00067-9
45. Johannson KA, Strâmbu I, Ravaglia C, Grutters JC, Valenzuela C, Mogulkoc N, et al. Antacid therapy in idiopathic pulmonary fibrosis: more questions than answers? *Lancet Respir Med.* (2017) 5:591–8. doi: 10.1016/S2213-2600(17)30219-9
46. Collard HR, Ryerson CJ, Corte TJ, Jenkins G, Kondoh Y, Lederer DJ, et al. Acute exacerbation of idiopathic pulmonary fibrosis. An international working group report. *Am J Respir Crit Care Med.* (2016) 194:265–75. doi: 10.1164/rccm.201604-0801CI
47. Song JW, Hong SB, Lim CM, Koh Y, and Kim DS. Acute exacerbation of idiopathic pulmonary fibrosis: incidence, risk factors and outcome. *Eur Respir J.* (2011) 37:356–63. doi: 10.1183/09031936.00159709
48. Papiris SA, Kagouridis K, Kolilekas L, Papaioannou AI, Roussou A, Triantafillidou C, et al. Survival in idiopathic pulmonary fibrosis acute exacerbations: the non-steroid approach. *BMC Pulm Med.* (2015) 15:162. doi: 10.1186/s12890-015-0146-4
49. Naccache JM, Cadranel J, and Nunes H. Acute exacerbation of idiopathic pulmonary fibrosis. *Am J Respir Crit Care Med.* (2017) 195:541–2. doi: 10.1164/rccm.201609-1802LE
50. Arai T, Tachibana K, Sugimoto C, Inoue Y, Tokura S, Okuma T, et al. High-dose prednisolone after intravenous methylprednisolone improves prognosis of acute exacerbation in idiopathic interstitial pneumonias. *Respirology* (2017) 22:1363–70. doi: 10.1111/resp.13065
51. Kim DS, Park JH, Park BK, Lee JS, Nicholson AG, and Colby T. Acute exacerbation of idiopathic pulmonary fibrosis: frequency and clinical features. *Eur Respir J.* (2006) 27:143–50. doi: 10.1183/09031936.06.00114004
52. Kawamura K, Ichikado K, Yasuda Y, Anan K, and Suga M. Azithromycin for idiopathic acute exacerbation of idiopathic pulmonary fibrosis: a retrospective single-center study. *BMC Pulm Med.* (2017) 17:94. doi: 10.1186/s12890-017-0437-z
53. Ding J, Chen Z, and Feng K. Procalcitonin-guided antibiotic use in acute exacerbations of idiopathic pulmonary fibrosis. *Int J Med Sci.* (2013) 10:903–7. doi: 10.7150/ijms.4972
54. Rush B, Wiskar K, Berger L, and Griesdale D. The use of mechanical ventilation in patients with idiopathic pulmonary fibrosis in the United States: a nationwide retrospective cohort analysis. *Respir Med.* (2016) 111:72–6. doi: 10.1016/j.rmed.2015.12.005
55. Conway EM. Thrombomodulin and its role in inflammation. *Semin Immunopathol.* (2012) 34:107–25. doi: 10.1007/s00281-011-0282-8
56. Isshiki T, Sakamoto S, Kinoshita A, Sugino K, Kurosaki A, and Homma S. Recombinant human soluble thrombomodulin treatment for acute exacerbation of idiopathic pulmonary fibrosis: a retrospective study. *Respiration* (2015) 89:201–7. doi: 10.1159/000369828
57. Kataoka K, Taniguchi H, Kondoh Y, Nishiyama O, Kimura T, Matsuda T, et al. Recombinant human thrombomodulin in acute exacerbation of idiopathic pulmonary fibrosis. *Chest* (2015) 148:436–43. doi: 10.1378/chest.14-2746
58. Abe M, Tsushima K, Matsumura T, Ishiwata T, Ichimura Y, Ikari J, et al. Efficacy of thrombomodulin for acute exacerbation of idiopathic pulmonary fibrosis and nonspecific interstitial pneumonia: a nonrandomized prospective study. *Drug Des Devel Ther.* (2015) 9:5755–62. doi: 10.2147/DDDT.S90739
59. Cruz DN, Perazella MA, Bellomo R, de Cal M, Polanco N, Corradi V, et al. Effectiveness of polymyxin B-immobilized fiber column in sepsis: a systematic review. *Crit Care* (2007) 11:R47. doi: 10.1186/cc5780
60. Oishi K, Aoe K, Mimura Y, Murata Y, Sakamoto K, Koutoku W, et al. Survival from an acute exacerbation of idiopathic pulmonary fibrosis with or without direct hemoperfusion with a polymyxin B-immobilized fiber column: a retrospective analysis. *Intern Med.* (2016) 55:3551–9. doi: 10.2169/internalmedicine.55.6056
61. Enomoto N, Mikamo M, Oyama Y, Kono M, Hashimoto D, Fujisawa T, et al. Treatment of acute exacerbation of idiopathic pulmonary fibrosis with direct hemoperfusion using a polymyxin B-immobilized fiber column improves survival. *BMC Pulm Med.* (2015) 15:15. doi: 10.1186/s12890-015-0004-4
62. Abe S, Azuma A, Mukae H, Ogura T, Taniguchi H, Bando M, et al. Polymyxin B-immobilized fiber column (PMX) treatment for idiopathic pulmonary fibrosis with acute exacerbation: a multicenter retrospective analysis. *Intern Med.* (2012) 51:1487–91. doi: 10.2169/internalmedicine.51.6965
63. Kahloon RA, Xue J, Bhargava A, Csizmadia E, Otterbein L, Kass DJ, et al. Patients with idiopathic pulmonary fibrosis with antibodies to heat shock protein 70 have poor prognoses. *Am J Respir Crit Care Med.* (2013) 187:768–75. doi: 10.1164/rccm.201203-0506OC
64. Donahoe M, Valentine VG, Chien N, Gibson KF, Raval JS, Saul M, et al. Autoantibody-targeted treatments for acute exacerbations of idiopathic pulmonary fibrosis. *PLoS ONE* (2015) 10:e0127771. doi: 10.1371/journal.pone.0127771
65. Huleihel L, Levine M, Rojas M. The potential of cell-based therapy in lung diseases. *Expert Opin Biol Ther.* (2013) 13:1429–40. doi: 10.1517/14712598.2013.833603
66. Weiss DJ, Ortiz LA. Cell therapy trials for lung diseases: progress and cautions. *Am J Respir Crit Care Med.* (2013) 188:123–5. doi: 10.1164/rccm.201302-0351ED
67. Moeller A, Ask K, Warburton D, Gauldie J, Kolb M. The bleomycin animal model: a useful tool to investigate treatment options for idiopathic pulmonary fibrosis? *Int J Biochem Cell Biol.* (2008) 40:362–82. doi: 10.1016/j.biocel.2007.08.011
68. McNulty K, Janes SM. Stem cells and pulmonary fibrosis: cause or cure? *Proc Am Thorac Soc.* (2012) 9:164–71. doi: 10.1513/pats.201201-010AW
69. Tzouvelekis A, Paspaliaris V, Koliakos G, Ntolios P, Bouros E, Oikonomou A, et al. A prospective, non-randomized, no placebo-controlled, phase Ib clinical trial to study the safety of the adipose derived stromal cells-stromal vascular fraction in idiopathic pulmonary fibrosis. *J Transl Med.* (2013) 11:171. doi: 10.1186/1479-5876-11-171
70. Tzouvelekis A, Bouros D. Steep barriers to overcome for successful application of stem cell treatment in patients with idiopathic pulmonary fibrosis. *Am J Respir Crit Care Med.* (2013) 188:251–2. doi: 10.1164/rccm.201301-0072LE
71. Yusen RD, Edwards LB, Kucheryavaya AY, Benden C, Dipchand AI, Dobbels F, et al. The registry of the international society for heart and lung transplantation: thirty-first adult lung and heart-lung transplant report—2014; focus theme: retransplantation. *J Heart Lung Transplant.* (2014) 33:1009–24. doi: 10.1016/j.healun.2014.08.004
72. Valapour M, Skeans MA, Heubner BM, Smith JM, Hertz MI, Edwards LB, et al. OPTN/SRTR 2013 annual data report: lung. *Am J Transplant.* (2015) 15:1–28. doi: 10.1111/ajt.13200

73. Kilic A, Merlo CA, Conte JV, and Shah AS. Lung transplantation in patients 70 years old or older: have outcomes changed after implementation of the lung allocation score? *J Thorac Cardiovasc Surg.* (2012) 144:1133–1138. doi: 10.1016/j.jtcvs.2012.07.080
74. Bonella F, Wijsenbeek M, Molina-Molina M, Duck A, Mele R, Geissler K, et al. European IPF patient charter: unmet needs and a call to action for healthcare policymakers. *Eur Respir J.* (2016) 47:597–606. doi: 10.1183/13993003.01204-2015
75. Thabut G, Mal H, Castier Y, Groussard O, Brugière O, Marrash-Chahla R, et al. Survival benefit of lung transplantation for patients with idiopathic pulmonary fibrosis. *J Thorac Cardiovasc Surg.* (2003) 126:469–75. doi: 10.1016/S0022-5223(03)00600-7
76. Nathan SD, Shlobin OA, Ahmad S, Burton NA, Barnett SD, Edwards E, et al. Comparison of wait times and mortality for idiopathic pulmonary fibrosis patients listed for single or bilateral lung transplantation. *J Heart Lung Transplant.* (2010) 29:1165–71. doi: 10.1016/j.healun.2010.05.014
77. Brown AW, Kaya H, and Nathan SD. Lung transplantation in IIP: a review. *Respirology* (2016) 21:1173–84. doi: 10.1111/resp.12691
78. Weill D, Benden C, Corris PA, Dark JH, Davis RD, Keshavjee S, et al. A consensus document for the selection of lung transplant candidates: 2014–an update from the pulmonary transplantation council of the international society for heart and lung transplantation. *J Heart Lung Transplant.* (2015) 34:1–15. doi: 10.1016/j.healun.2014.06.014
79. Nathan SD, Barnett SD, Urban BA, Nowalk C, Moran BR, and Burton N. Pulmonary embolism in idiopathic pulmonary fibrosis transplant recipients. *Chest* (2003) 123:1758–63. doi: 10.1378/chest.123.5.1758
80. Raghu G, Freudenberger TD, Yang S, Curtis JR, Spada C, Hayes J, et al. High prevalence of abnormal acid gastro-oesophageal reflux in idiopathic pulmonary fibrosis. *Eur Respir J.* (2006) 27:136–42. doi: 10.1183/09031936.06.00037005
81. Robertson AG, Ward C, Pearson JP, Corris PA, Dark JH, and Griffin SM. Lung transplantation, gastroesophageal reflux, and fundoplication. *Ann Thorac Surg.* (2010) 89:653–60. doi: 10.1016/j.athoracsur.2009.09.001
82. Hartwig MG, Anderson DJ, Onaitis MW, Reddy S, Snyder LD, Lin SS, et al. Fundoplication after lung transplantation prevents the allograft dysfunction associated with reflux. *Ann Thorac Surg.* (2011) 92:462–8. doi: 10.1016/j.athoracsur.2011.04.035
83. Holland AE. Exercise limitation in interstitial lung disease - mechanisms, significance and therapeutic options. *Chron Respir Dis.* (2010) 7:101–11. doi: 10.1177/1479972309354689
84. Spruit MA, Singh SJ, Garvey C, ZuWallack R, Nici L, Rochester C, et al. An official american thoracic society/european respiratory society statement: key concepts and advances in pulmonary rehabilitation. *Am J Respir Crit Care Med.* (2013) 188, e13–64. Erratum *Am J Respir Crit Care Med.* 189:1570. doi: 10.1164/rccm.201309-1634ST
85. Borjesson M, Urhausen A, Kouidi E, Dugmore D, Sharma S, Halle M, et al. Cardiovascular evaluation of middle-aged/ senior individuals engaged in leisure-time sport activities: position stand from the sections of exercise physiology and sports cardiology of the European Association of Cardiovascular Prevention and Rehabilitation. *Eur J Cardiovasc Prev Rehabil.* (2011) 18:446–58. doi: 10.1097/HJR.0b013e32833bo969
86. Swigris JJ, Fairclough DL, Morrison M, Make B, Kozora E, Brown KK, et al. Benefits of pulmonary rehabilitation in idiopathic pulmonary fibrosis. *Respir Care* (2011) 56:783–89. doi: 10.4187/respcare.00939
87. Huppmann P, Sczepanski B, Boensch M, Winterkamp S, Schönheit-Kenn U, Neurohr C, et al. Effects of inpatient pulmonary rehabilitation in patients with interstitial lung disease. *Eur Respir J.* (2013) 42:444–53. doi: 10.1183/09031936.00081512
88. Spagnolo P, Maher TM, and Richeldi L. Idiopathic pulmonary fibrosis: recent advances on pharmacological therapy. *Pharmacol Ther.* (2015) 152:18–27. doi: 10.1016/j.pharmthera.2015.04.005
89. Kenn K, Gloeckl R, and Behr J. Pulmonary rehabilitation in patients with idiopathic pulmonary fibrosis–a review. *Respiration* (2013) 86:89–99. doi: 10.1159/000354112
90. Vainshelboim B. Exercise training in idiopathic pulmonary fibrosis: is it of benefit? *Breathe* (2016) 12:130–138. doi: 10.1183/20734735.006916
91. Vainshelboim B, Fox BD, Oliveira J, and Kramer MR. Exercise training in idiopathic pulmonary fibrosis. *Expert Rev Respir Med.* (2016) 10:69–77. doi: 10.1586/17476348.2016.1121104
92. Vainshelboim B, Kramer MR, Fox BD, Izhakian S, Sagie A, and Oliveira J. Supervised exercise training improves exercise cardiovascular function in idiopathic pulmonary fibrosis. *Eur J Phys Rehabil Med.* (2017) 53:209–18. doi: 10.23736/S1973-9087.16.04319-7
93. Kenn K, Gloeckl R, Soennichsen A, Sczepanski B, Winterkamp S, Boensch M, et al. Predictors of success for pulmonary rehabilitation in patients awaiting lung transplantation. *Transplantation* (2015) 99:1072–7. doi: 10.1097/TP.0000000000000472
94. Bell EC, Cox NS, Goh N, Glaspole I, Westall GP, Watson A, et al. Oxygen therapy for interstitial lung disease: a systematic review. *Eur Respir Rev.* (2017) 26:160080. doi: 10.1183/16000617.0080-2016
95. Visca D, Tsipouri V, Mori L, Firouzi A, Fleming S, Farquhar M, et al. Ambulatory oxygen in fibrotic lung disease (AmbOx): study protocol for a randomised controlled trial. *Trials* (2017) 18:201. doi: 10.1186/s13063-017-1912-9
96. Visca D, Mori L, Tsipouri V, Canu S, Bonini M, Pavitt M, et al. Ambox: a randomised controlled, crossover trial evaluating the effects of ambulatory oxygen on health status in patients with fibrotic interstitial lung disease. *Am J Respir Crit Care Med.* (2017) 195:A7603.
97. Swigris JJ, Gould MK, and Wilson SR. Health-related quality of life among patients with idiopathic pulmonary fibrosis. *Chest* (2005) 127:284–294. doi: 10.1378/chest.127.1.284
98. Kreuter M, Swigris J, Pittrow D, Geier S, Klotsche J, Prasse A, et al. Health related quality of life in patients with idiopathic pulmonary fibrosis in clinical practice: insights-IPF registry. *Respir Res.* (2017) 18:139. doi: 10.1186/s12931-017-0621-y
99. Nishiyama O, Taniguchi H, Kondoh Y, Kimura T, Kato K, Kataoka K, et al. A simple assessment of dyspnoea as a prognostic indicator in idiopathic pulmonary fibrosis. *Eur Respir J.* (2010) 36:1067–72. doi: 10.1183/09031936.00152609
100. von Leupoldt A, Sommer T, Kegat S, Baumann HJ, Klose H, Dahme B, et al. Dyspnea and pain share emotion-related brain network. *Neuroimage* (2009) 48:200–6. doi: 10.1016/j.neuroimage.2009.06.015
101. Kohberg C, Andersen CU, and Bendstrup E. Opioids: an unexplored option for treatment of dyspnea in IPF. *Eur Clin Respir J.* (2016) 3:30629. doi: 10.3402/ecrj.v3.30629
102. van Manen MJ, Birring SS, Vancheri C, Cottin V, Renzoni EA, Russell AM, et al. Cough in idiopathic pulmonary fibrosis. *Eur Respir Rev.* (2016) 25:278–86. doi: 10.1183/16000617.0090-2015
103. Hope-Gill BD, Hilldrup S, Davies C, Newton RP, and Harrison NK. A study of the cough reflex in idiopathic pulmonary fibrosis. *Am J Respir Crit Care Med.* (2003) 168:995–1002. doi: 10.1164/rccm.200304-597OC
104. Horton MR, Santopietro V, Mathew L, Horton KM, Polito AJ, Liu MC, et al. Thalidomide for the treatment of cough in idiopathic pulmonary fibrosis: a randomized trial. *Ann Intern Med.* (2012) 157:398–406. doi: 10.7326/0003-4819-157-6-201209180-00003
105. Birring SS, Wijsenbeek MS, Agrawal S, van den Berg JWK, Stone H, Maher TM, et al. A novel formulation of inhaled sodium cromoglicate (PA101) in idiopathic pulmonary fibrosis and chronic cough: a randomised, double-blind, proof-of-concept, phase 2 trial. *Lancet Respir Med.* (2017) 5:806–15. doi: 10.1016/S2213-2600(17)30310-7
106. van Manen MJG, Birring SS, Vancheri C, Vindigni V, Renzoni E, Russell AM, et al. Effect of pirfenidone on cough in patients with idiopathic pulmonary fibrosis. *Eur Respir J.* (2017) 50:1701157. doi: 10.1183/13993003.01157-2017
107. Spagnolo P, Wells AU, and Collard HR. Pharmacological treatment of idiopathic pulmonary fibrosis: an update. *Drug Discov Today* (2015) 20:514–24. doi: 10.1016/j.drudis.2015.01.001
108. van Manen MJ, Geelhoed JJ, Tak NC, and Wijsenbeek MS. Optimizing quality of life in patients with idiopathic pulmonary fibrosis. *Ther Adv Respir Dis.* (2017) 11:157–69. doi: 10.1177/1753465816686743
109. Maher TM, Molina-Molina M, Russell AM, Bonella F, Jouneau S, Ripamonti E, et al. Unmet needs in the treatment of idiopathic pulmonary fibrosis-insights from patient chart review in five European countries. *BMC Pulm Med.* (2017) 17:124. doi: 10.1186/s12890-017-0468-5

110. Karimi-Shah BA, and Chowdhury BA. Forced vital capacity in idiopathic pulmonary fibrosis–FDA review of pirfenidone and nintedanib. *N Engl J Med.* (2015) 372:1189–91. doi: 10.1056/NEJMp 1500526
111. Martinez FJ, Safrin S, Weycker D, Starko KM, Bradford WZ, King TE Jr, et al. The clinical course of patients with idiopathic pulmonary fibrosis. *Ann Intern Med.* (2005) 142:963–7. doi: 10.7326/0003-4819-142-12_Part_1-200506210-00005
112. Russell AM, Adamali H, Molyneaux PL, Lukey PT, Marshall RP, Renzoni EA, et al. Daily home spirometry: an effective tool for detecting progression in idiopathic pulmonary fibrosis. *Am J Respir Crit Care Med.* (2016) 194:989–97. doi: 10.1164/rccm.201511-2152OC
113. Spagnolo P, Tzouvelekis A, and Maher TM. Personalized medicine in idiopathic pulmonary fibrosis: facts and promises. *Curr Opin Pulm Med.* (2015) 21:470–8. doi: 10.1097/MCP.0000000000000187
114. Tzouvelekis A, Antoniadis A, Bouros D. Stem cell therapy in pulmonary fibrosis. *Curr Opin Pulm Med.* (2011) 17:368–73. doi: 10.1097/MCP.0b013e328348744f

9

TRAF6 Suppresses the Development of Pulmonary Fibrosis by Attenuating the Activation of Fibroblasts

*Jiali Min[1], Qiao Li[1], Suosi Liu[1], Qianrong Wang[1], Min Yin[1], Yan Zhang[1], Jun Yan[2], Bing Cui[3] and Shanshan Liu[1]**

[1]National Clinical Research Center for Metabolic Diseases, Key Laboratory of Diabetes Immunology, Ministry of Education, Department of Metabolism and Endocrinology, The Second Xiangya Hospital of Central South University, Changsha, China, [2]Beijing Institute of Brain Disorders, Capital Medical University, Beijing, China, [3]State Key Laboratory of Bioactive Substance and Function of Natural Medicines, Institute of Materia Medica, Chinese Academy of Medical Sciences and Peking Union Medical College, Beijing, China

Correspondence:
Shanshan Liu
lss0625@csu.edu.cn

Pulmonary fibrosis (PF) has a high mortality rate, and its pathogenesis is unknown. TNF receptor-associated factor 6 (TRAF6), a signal transducer for inflammatory signaling, plays crucial roles in the pathogenesis of immune diseases. However, its function in PF remains unknown. Herein, we demonstrated that lungs from mice with bleomycin (BLM)-induced PF were characterized by decreased expression of TRAF6 in lung fibroblasts. Enhancing TRAF6 expression protected mice from BLM-induced PF coupled with a significant reduction in fibroblast differentiation. Furthermore, we demonstrated that overexpression of TRAF6 reversed the activation of myofibroblasts from PF mice by reducing the expression of Wnt3a and subsequently suppressing Wnt/β-catenin signaling. Additionally, the abundance of Tribbles pseudokinase 3 (TRIB3), a stress sensor, was negatively correlated with the abundance of TRAF6 in lung fibroblasts. TRIB3 overexpression decreased TRAF6 abundance by reducing TRAF6 stability in lung fibroblasts during PF. Mechanistic studies revealed that TRIB3 bound to TRAF6 and accelerated basal TRAF6 ubiquitination and degradation. Collectively, our data indicate that reduced TRAF6 expression in fibroblasts is essential for the progression of PF, and therefore, genetically increasing TRAF6 expression or disrupting the TRIB3-TRAF6 interaction could be potential therapeutic strategies for fibroproliferative lung diseases in clinical settings.

Keywords: pulmonary fibrosis, TRAF6, lung fibroblast, TRIB3, ubiquitination, protein degradation, Wnt3a

INTRODUCTION

Pulmonary fibrosis (PF) is a type of chronic, progressive, and irreversible fibrotic lung disease characterized by an excess of extracellular matrix (ECM), destruction of normal lung architecture, and ultimately, respiratory failure (Sgalla et al., 2019; George et al., 2020). To date, only two therapies, pirfenidone and nintedanib, have been approved for use in PF. However, neither treatment is known to be curative. Lung transplantation remains the final and life-saving therapeutic option for PF. The lack of a successful treatment of PF is due to a lack of understanding of the underlying cellular and molecular mechanisms. Therefore, an in-depth investigation of the molecular pathogenesis of PF is urgently needed.

Although the cause of PF remains unclear, existing evidence suggests that lung fibroblasts play a crucial role in the pathogenesis of PF (Hinz and Lagares, 2020; Liu G. et al., 2021). Upon stimulation of fibrotic factors, such as chemokine (C-C motif) ligand 1 (CCL1), transforming growth factor-β1 (TGF-β1), and platelet-derived growth factor (PDGF), fibroblasts differentiate into myofibroblasts, which secrete excessive amounts of ECM proteins, including type I collagen, and fibronectin (Lo Re et al., 2011; Frangogiannis, 2020; Liu S. S. et al., 2021). Increased accumulation of ECM obliterates functional alveolar units, thereby decreasing gas exchange and reducing lung function. It is critically important to identify the key mediators contributing to the activation of myofibroblasts during PF development.

TRAF6 (TNF receptor-associated factor 6), a member of the TRAF protein family, plays a pivotal role in immune signal transduction pathways triggered by members of the TNF receptor superfamily and the IL-1 receptor superfamily (Cao et al., 1996; Walsh et al., 2015). By acting as a ubiquitin ligase (E3) catalyzing the formation of Lys63-linked polyubiquitin on itself and its substrates, TRAF6 participates in many biological processes, such as the operation of the innate immune system, lymph node organogenesis, and osteoclast formation (Naito et al., 1999; Wu and Arron, 2003; Yang et al., 2009). TRAF6 contains a RING-finger domain in the N-terminus, which is responsible for its E3 ligase activity, followed by several zinc-finger domains and a conserved C-terminal TRAF domain that enables interaction with receptors and adaptor proteins. Recent studies have revealed the role of

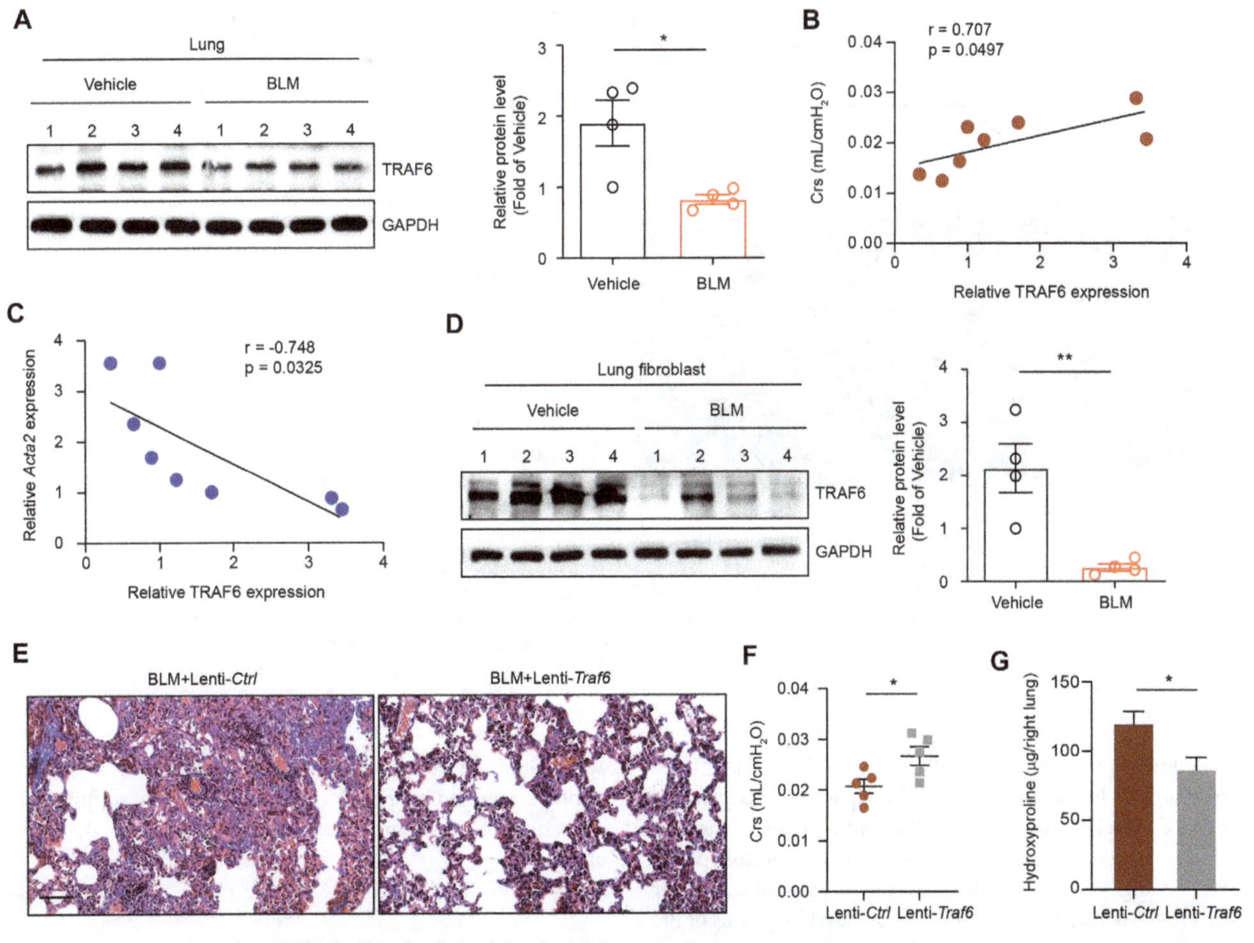

FIGURE 1 | TRAF6 expression in lung fibroblasts is negatively correlated with PF progression. **(A)** Western blot analysis of TRAF6 expression in the lungs of mice following BLM induction. **(B)** Correlation analysis between TRAF6 expression in the lungs of PF mice and respiratory system compliance (Crs) in mice. Each point represents the value of one mouse. Spearman's rank correlation test was employed to determine statistical significance. **(C)** Correlation analysis between TRAF6 expression and *Acta2* expression in the lungs of PF mice. Each point represents the value of one mouse. Spearman's rank correlation test was employed to determine statistical significance. **(D)** Western blot analysis of TRAF6 expression in lung fibroblasts isolated from the lungs of mice following BLM induction. **(E)** Masson staining was performed to evaluate fibrotic changes in the indicated mice (Group 1: BLM + Lenti-Ctrl, Group 2: BLM + Lenti-Traf6; n = 5 per group). Scale bars, 100 μm. Crs **(F)** and hydroxyproline content in the right lung **(G)** were assessed to evaluate pulmonary fibrosis and lung function (Group 1: BLM + Lenti-Ctrl, Group 2: BLM + Lenti-Traf6; $n = 5$ per group). Data are representative of 3 independent experiments. Data represent means ± SEM Statistical significance: $^{*}p < 0.05$ or $^{**}p < 0.01$.

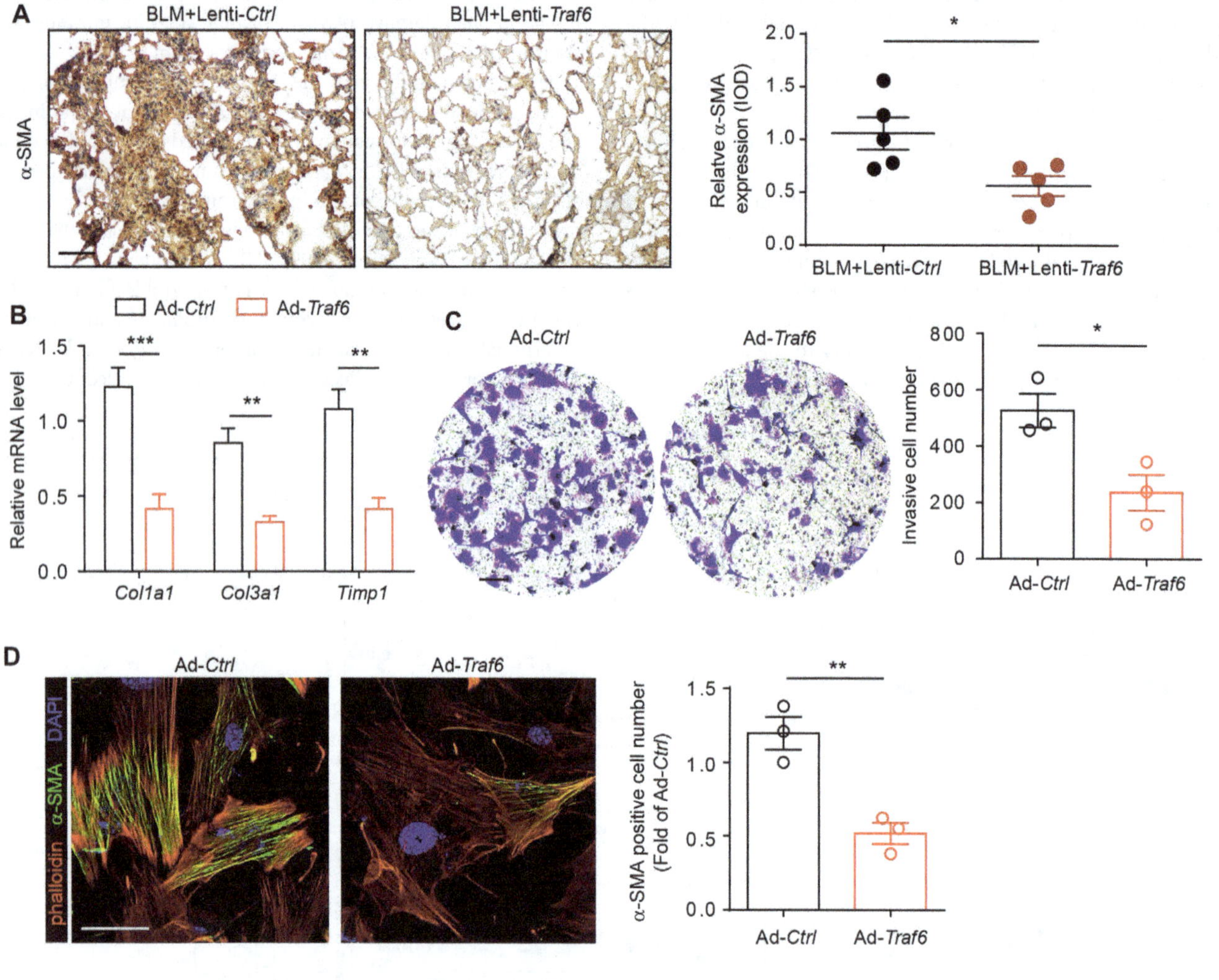

FIGURE 2 | Overexpression of TRAF6 suppresses fibroblast activation. **(A)** IHC staining showing the expression of α-SMA in lung tissues. Representative data and quantified results are shown (Group 1: BLM + Lenti-*Ctrl*, Group 2: BLM + Lenti-*Traf6*; $n = 5$ per group). Scale bar, 100 μm. **(B)** mRNA expression of fibrosis genes in mouse PF lung fibroblasts with or without TRAF6 overexpression. **(C)** Representative images and quantification of the invasion experiment results for mouse PF lung fibroblasts with or without TRAF6 overexpression. Scale bars, 100 μm. **(D)** Representative images and quantification of α-SMA immunostaining in mouse PF fibroblasts with or without TRAF6 overexpression. Scale bars, 50 μm. Data are representative of 3 independent experiments. Data represent means ± SEM Statistical significance: $^{*}p < 0.05$, $^{**}p < 0.01$ or $^{***}p < 0.001$.

TRAF6 in fibrosis (Wang et al., 2020; Zhang et al., 2021). TRAF6 overexpression in hepatocytes promotes ubiquitination-dependent activation of ASK1, contributing to the pathogenesis of hepatic fibrosis during the progression of nonalcoholic steatohepatitis (NASH) (Wang et al., 2020). However, it remains unclear whether TRAF6 plays any important roles in the pathogenesis of PF.

In the present study, we observed reduced protein levels of TRAF6 in the lungs of PF mice, supporting a role for TRAF6 in PF development. Using the classical bleomycin (BLM)-induced PF mouse model, we found that overexpression of TRAF6 reduced BLM-induced PF changes. Using gain- and loss-of-function approaches *in vitro*, we demonstrated that the downregulation of TRAF6 expression is induced by the upregulation of expression of TRIB3 in lung fibroblasts during chronic lung injury. Furthermore, the loss of TRAF6 aggravated the progression of PF by acting as a novel negative regulator of Wnt3a, thereby activating lung fibroblasts into myofibroblasts. Collectively, our findings revealed a critical role for TRAF6 in suppressing the activation of lung fibroblasts and preventing the development of PF.

MATERIALS AND METHODS

Antibodies and Reagents

Antibodies against TRAF6 and TRIB3 were purchased from Abcam (Cambridge, MA, United States); antibodies against Axin 2, c-Myc, and cyclin D1 were obtained from Cell Signaling Technology (Danvers, MA, United States); an antibody against α-SMA was purchased from BOSTER (Wuhan, China); and antibodies against DDK, Myc and HA were obtained from MBL BIOTECH (Beijing, China). CoraLite® 594-phalloidin was obtained from Proteintech

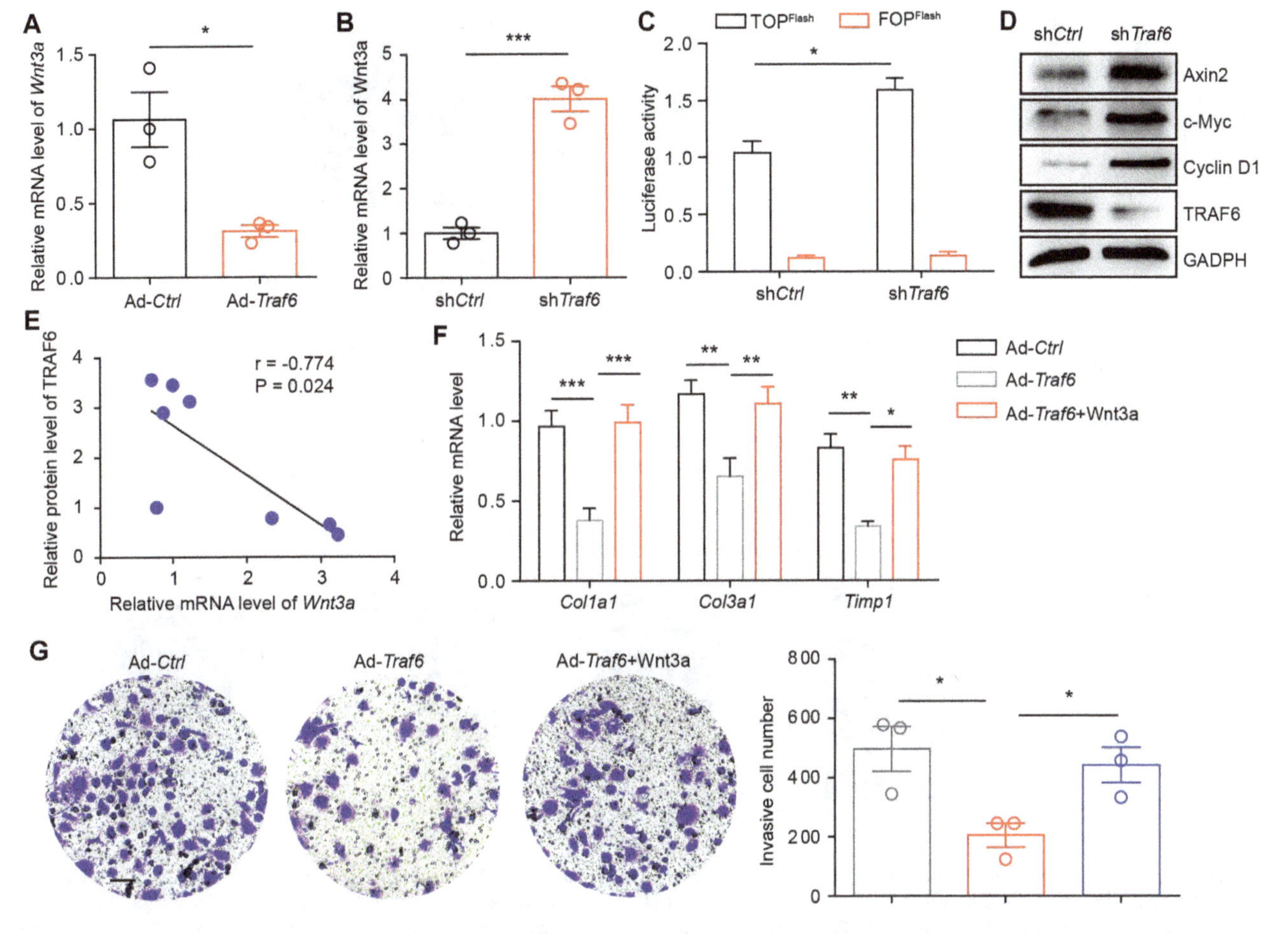

FIGURE 3 | TRAF6 suppresses fibroblast activation by reducing Wnt3a expression. **(A)** mRNA levels of *Wnt3a* as measured by qRT–PCR in TRAF6-overexpressing lung fibroblasts. **(B)** mRNA levels of *Wnt3a* as measured by qRT–PCR in TRAF6-depleted lung fibroblasts. **(C)** Wnt-reporter luciferase activity in PF lung fibroblasts with or without TRAF6 depletion. **(D)** Western blot analysis of β-catenin target gene expression in PF lung fibroblasts with or without TRAF6 depletion. **(E)** Correlation analysis of TRAF6 protein expression and *Wnt3a* mRNA levels in mouse PF lung fibroblasts. **(F)** qRT–PCR analysis of the expression of fibrosis genes in TRAF6-overexpressing mouse lung fibroblasts with or without Wnt3a stimulation. **(G)** Transwell assay for the evaluation of the invasion of TRAF6-overexpressing lung fibroblasts with or without Wnt3a stimulation. Scale bars, 100 μm. Data are representative of 3 independent experiments. Data represent means ± SEM Statistical significance: $^{*}p < 0.05$, $^{**}p < 0.01$ or $^{***}p < 0.001$.

(Wuhan, China). CHX was purchased from Sigma (St Louis, MO, United States). Bleomycin (BLM), MG132, and 3-Methyladenine (3-MA) were obtained from MCE (Shanghai, China).

Bleomycin (BLM) Induction of Pulmonary Fibrosis

C57BL/6J male mice (8 weeks old) were purchased from SJA Laboratory Animal Co., Ltd. (Hunan, China). The mouse PF model was induced as previously reported (Liu et al., 2019). In brief, mice were anesthetized with 400 mg/kg avertin (Sigma-Aldrich) via intraperitoneal injection and then treated with 1 mg/kg BLM in 50 μl PBS via intratracheal injection. This was conducted 6 times, with 14 days between each challenge. Mice were sacrificed by excessive anesthesia at Day 40 after the last BLM challenge, and then lungs were obtained for immunoblotting and RT–PCR analysis.

Lentiviral Treatment in Vivo

For lentivirus administration, lentiviruses (5×10^7 I.U.) overexpressing *Traf6* in 50 μl of PBS were administered to mice via intratracheal instillation for a total of two treatments at 2-weeks intervals beginning on Day 10 after the last BLM administration.

Isolation of Lung Fibroblasts

Lung fibroblasts were obtained from mice as reported previously (Liu S. S. et al., 2021). The chests of mice sacrificed by excessive anesthesia were cut open, and the lungs were removed, rinsed with sterile PBS and cut into 1 mm^3 pieces in culture medium. After centrifugation at 1,500 rpm for 10 min, the tissue suspension was suspended in DMEM containing 15% FBS and spread evenly in a 10-cm dish. After 5–7 days of culture, the adherent fibroblasts were harvested for passage or for assays.

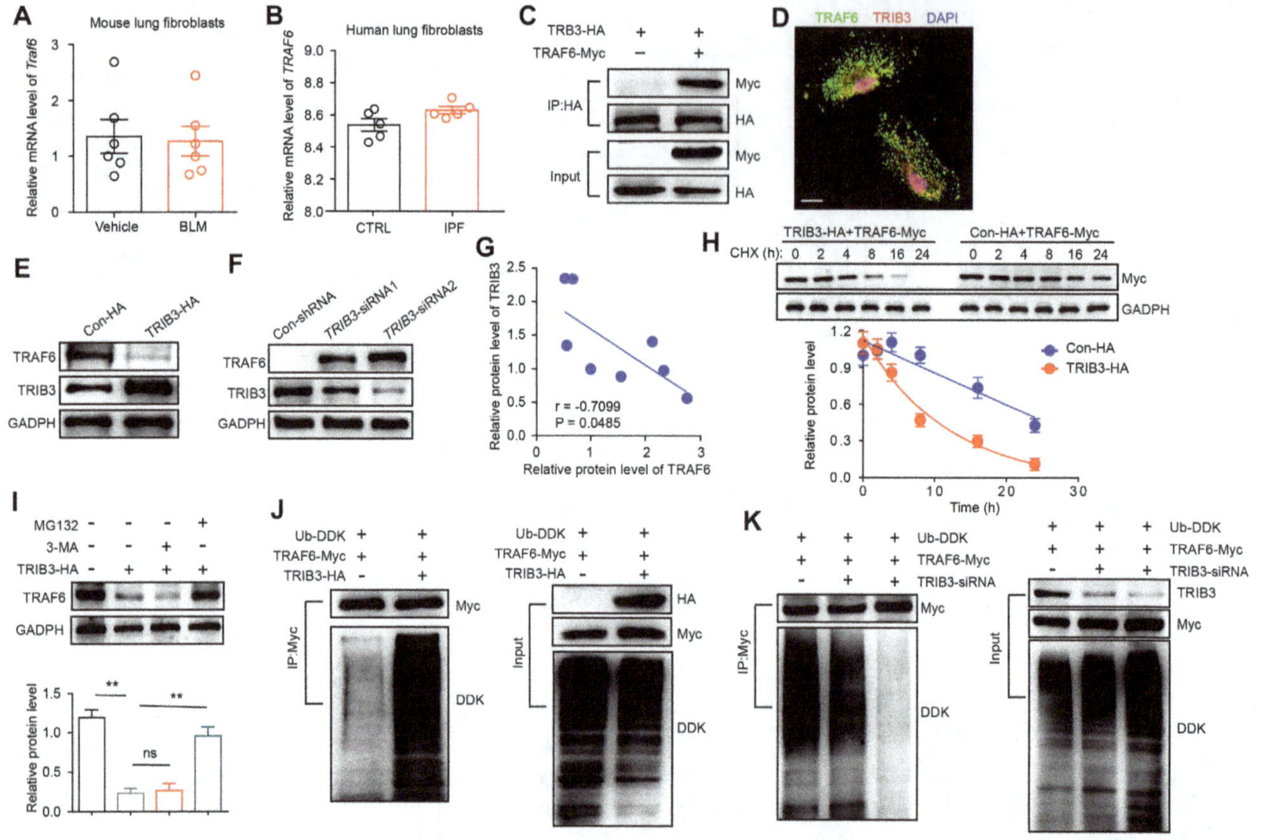

FIGURE 4 | TRIB3 decreases the expression of TRAF6 by promoting its degradation. **(A)** mRNA levels of *Traf6* as measured by qRT–PCR in lung fibroblasts from vehicle- and BLM-challenged mice. **(B)** *TRAF6* mRNA expression in lung fibroblasts of IPF patients compared with normal controls based on the reanalysis of a published dataset (GSE129164). **(C)** The interaction between TRAF6 and TRIB3 was evaluated by co-IP assays. HEK293T cell extracts were subjected to IP with an HA antibody and blotted with a Myc antibody. **(D)** Colocalization of TRAF6 and TRIB3 was evaluated in primary lung fibroblasts. Scale bars, 10 μm. **(E)** Sample immunoblot analyses of the expression of TRAF6 after TRIB3 overexpression in MRC5 cells. **(F)** Sample immunoblot analyses of the expression of TRAF6 after TRIB3 silencing in MRC5 cells. **(G)** Correlation analysis of TRAF6 protein expression and TRIB3 protein expression in mouse PF lung fibroblasts. **(H)** TRAF6 degradation in HEK293T cells with or without TRIB3 overexpression was determined by western blotting. **(I)** Analysis of the TRAF6 degradation pathway. Lung fibroblasts were incubated with CHX (20 μM), CHX plus 3-Methyladenine (3-MA, 5 mM), or MG132 (10 μM) for the indicated times. TRAF6 expression was detected by immunoblotting. **(J)** Immunoblots of ubiquitinated TRAF6 after TRIB3 overexpression. **(K)** Immunoblots of ubiquitinated TRAF6 after TRIB3 deletion. Data are representative of 3 independent experiments. Data represent means ± SEM Statistical significance: $^{**}p < 0.01$.

Cell Lines

MRC5 fibroblasts were cultured in minimal essential medium supplemented with 10% FCS, penicillin, streptomycin, and non-essential amino acid (NEAA) at 37°C in a humidified 5% CO_2 incubator.

Cell Transfection

Plasmids were transfected into cells with Lipofectamine 3,000 (Invitrogen) according to the manufacturer's instructions. siRNAs were transfected using Lipofectamine RNAiMAX (Invitrogen) according to the manufacturer's instructions.

Invasion Assays

Fibroblasts were cultured in serum-free DMEM for 24 h prior to cell invasion assays. Transwell invasion assays were performed using Transwell chambers with filter membranes of 8 μm pore size (Corning). The lower surface of the chambers was precoated with 10 μg ml^{-1} fibronectin, and the upper chambers were coated with BD Matrigel™ Basement Membrane Matrix (40 μl per well). Then, the chambers were inserted into 24-well culture plates. Single-cell suspensions were seeded into the upper chamber (1×10^4 cells per well in 0.4% FBS in DMEM), and the bottom chamber contained DMEM with 10% FBS. After 12 h, the medium was removed, and noninvasive cells were removed using cotton swabs. The invaded cells were fixed with 4% paraformaldehyde in PBS and stained with crystal violet staining solution. Invasive cells from 3 nonoverlapping fields of each membrane were imaged and counted using brightfield microscopy under 40x magnification.

RNA Extraction and Real-Time Polymerase Chain Reaction

Total RNA was isolated from cells and tissues using the Eastep® Super Total RNA Extraction Kit (Promega) according to the manufacturer's instructions. RNA was quantified using a

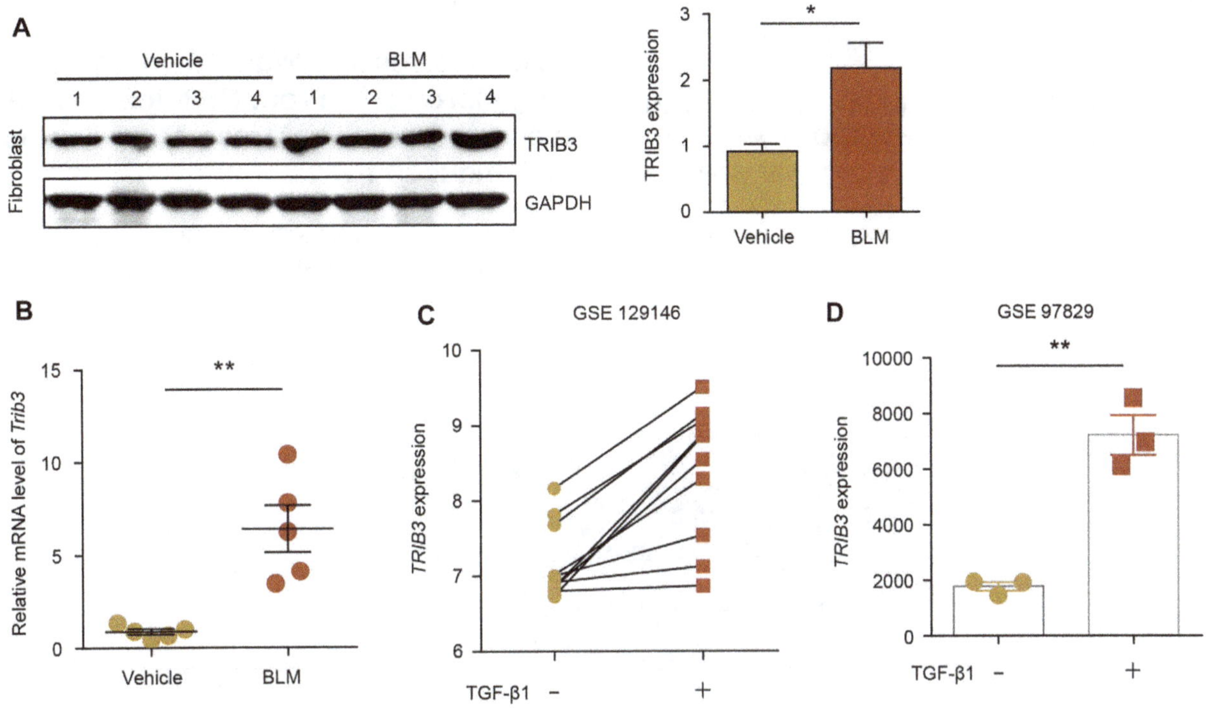

FIGURE 5 | TRIB3 expression is increased in PF lung fibroblasts. **(A)** Western blot analysis of TRIB3 expression in lung fibroblasts isolated from the lungs of mice following BLM induction. **(B)** mRNA levels of *Trib3* as measured by qRT–PCR in lung fibroblasts from vehicle- and BLM-challenged mice. **(C)** *TRIB3* mRNA expression in lung fibroblasts of IPF patients and normal controls treated with or without TGF-β1 based on the reanalysis of a published dataset (GSE129164). **(D)** *TRIB3* mRNA expression in lung fibroblasts treated with or without TGF- β1 based on the reanalysis of a published dataset (GSE97829). Data are representative of 3 independent experiments. Data represent means ± SEM Statistical significance: $^*p < 0.05$ or $^{**}p < 0.01$.

NanoDrop spectrophotometer. Reverse transcription was carried out with 1 mg of purified RNA using M-MLV reverse transcriptase (Transgen Biotech). Quantitative real-time PCR (qRT–PCR) was performed using the KAPA SYBR FAST RT-PCR Master Mix (2×) Kit (Kappa Biosystem, United States) and conducted by a LineGene 9,620 apparatus (Bioer). All primer details are listed in **Supplementary Table S1**.

Immunoblot

Tissues and cultured cells were lysed in RIPA buffer (Beyotime) containing protein inhibitors (Selleck). The protein concentration was determined by a BCA protein assay (Applygen Technologies Inc.). Proteins were mixed with 5× SDS sample loading buffer and incubated at 95°C for 10 min. Then, proteins were separated by SDS–PAGE gel, transferred to PVDF membranes (Millipore), and incubated with appropriate primary antibodies coupled with a horseradish peroxidase-conjugated secondary antibody. Images were visualized using ECL western blotting detection reagents (Tanon).

Coimmunoprecipitation (Co-IP)

Cells were washed twice in cold PBS and lysed in IP buffer (150 mmol/L NaCl, 25 mmol/L Tris-HCl (pH 7.4), 2.5 mmol/L $MgCl_2$, 0.5% NP-40, 0.5 mmol/L EDTA, and 5% glycerol) with protease inhibitors. Cell extracts were incubated with the indicated primary antibodies overnight at 4°C and then with Protein A/G Plus-Agarose (Santa Cruz, United States) at 4°C for 2 h. The beads were washed five times with wash buffer (IP buffer without NP-40), eluted in 2× SDS sample loading buffer, and then subjected to electrophoresis.

Immunostaining

For α-SMA immunostaining, cells cultured on coverslips were fixed with 4% (v/v) formaldehyde at room temperature for 10 min, permeabilized with 0.5% Triton X-100 at room temperature for 20 min, and blocked with 3% BSA at room temperature for 30 min. The slides were incubated with antibodies against α-SMA at 4°C overnight, followed by staining with Alexa Fluor 488-conjugated anti-mouse antibodies and CoraLite® 594-phalloidin for 2 h at room temperature. Finally, the slides were mounted with medium containing DAPI.

Luciferase Reporter Assay

For the luciferase reporter assay, MRC5 cells were cotransfected with TOP Flash or FOP Flash luciferase reporter. At 48 h post-transfection, the cells were collected and lysed with lysis buffer. The internal control used was pTK-Renilla. Firefly luciferase and Renilla luciferase activities were quantified using the dual-luciferase reporter assay system according to the manufacturer's instructions (Promega, Madison, WI).

Statistical Analysis

Statistical significance was calculated using GraphPad Prism 6 software. Data are representative and/or the mean ± SEM of 3 assays. An unpaired two-sided Student's t test was used to compare two groups, and one-way ANOVA was used to compare multiple groups unless otherwise indicated. Correlations between groups were determined by Pearson's correlation test. All experiments were conducted with at least 3 biological replicates. In all cases, $p < 0.05$ was considered statistically significant.

RESULTS

TRAF6 Expression Was Downregulated in Lung Fibroblasts From PF Mice and TRAF6 Overexpression Protected Mice Against BLM-Induced PF

To address the role of TRAF6 in PF, we first examined TRAF6 expression in the lungs of mice following BLM-induced PF. Western blot analysis showed decreased TRAF6 protein levels in the lungs of PF mice compared to those of controls (**Figure 1A**). Moreover,

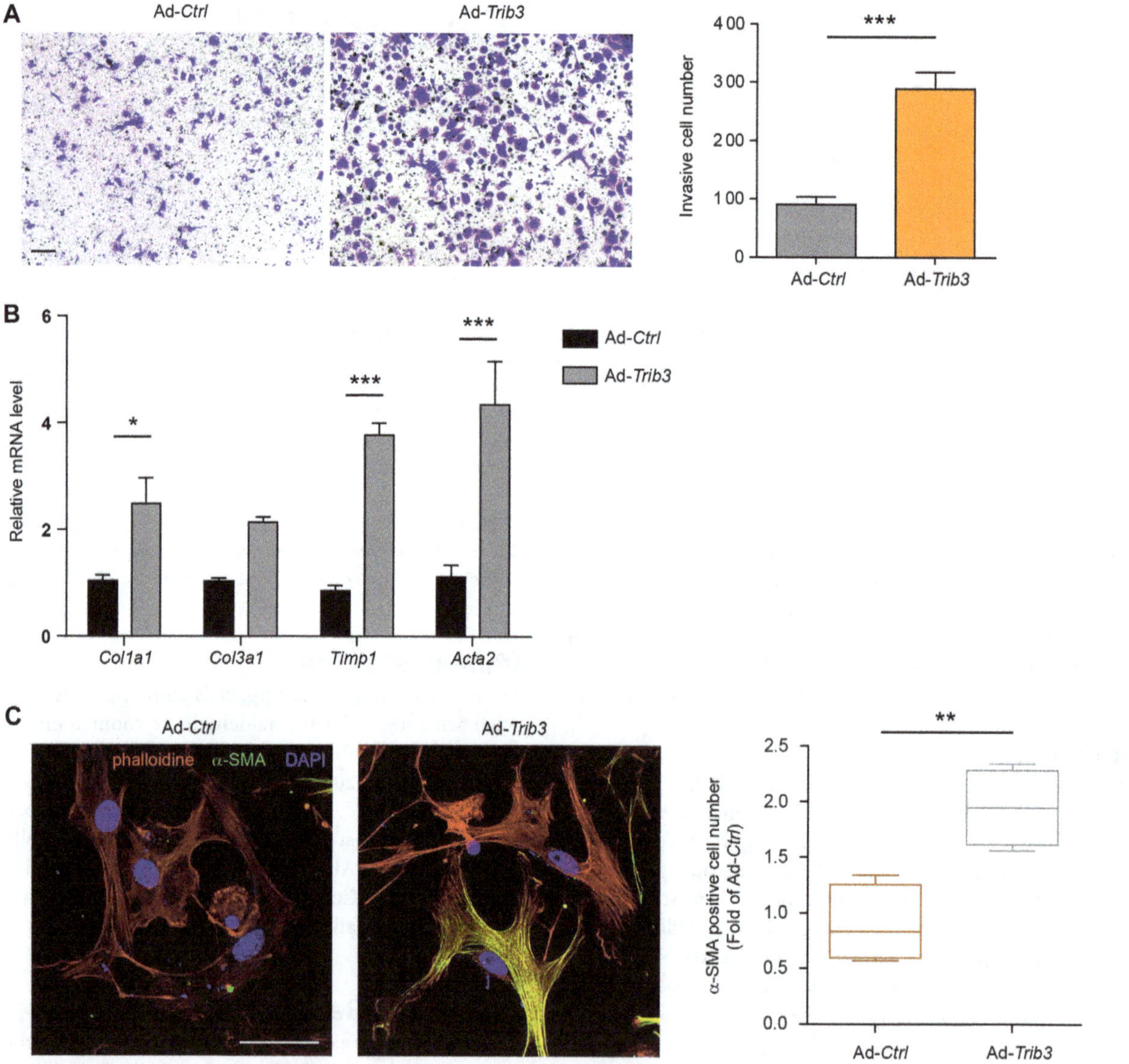

FIGURE 6 | Overexpression of TRIB3 activates lung fibroblasts. **(A)** Representative images and quantification of the invasion experiment results for mouse lung fibroblasts with or without TRIB3 overexpression. Scale bars, 100 μm. **(B)** mRNA expression of fibrosis genes in mouse lung fibroblasts with or without TRIB3 overexpression. **(C)** Representative images and quantification of α-SMA immunostaining in mouse lung fibroblasts with or without TRIB3 overexpression. Scale bars, 50 μm. Data are representative of 3 independent experiments. Data represent means ± SEM Statistical significance: $^{*}p < 0.05$, $^{**}p < 0.01$ or $^{***}p < 0.001$.

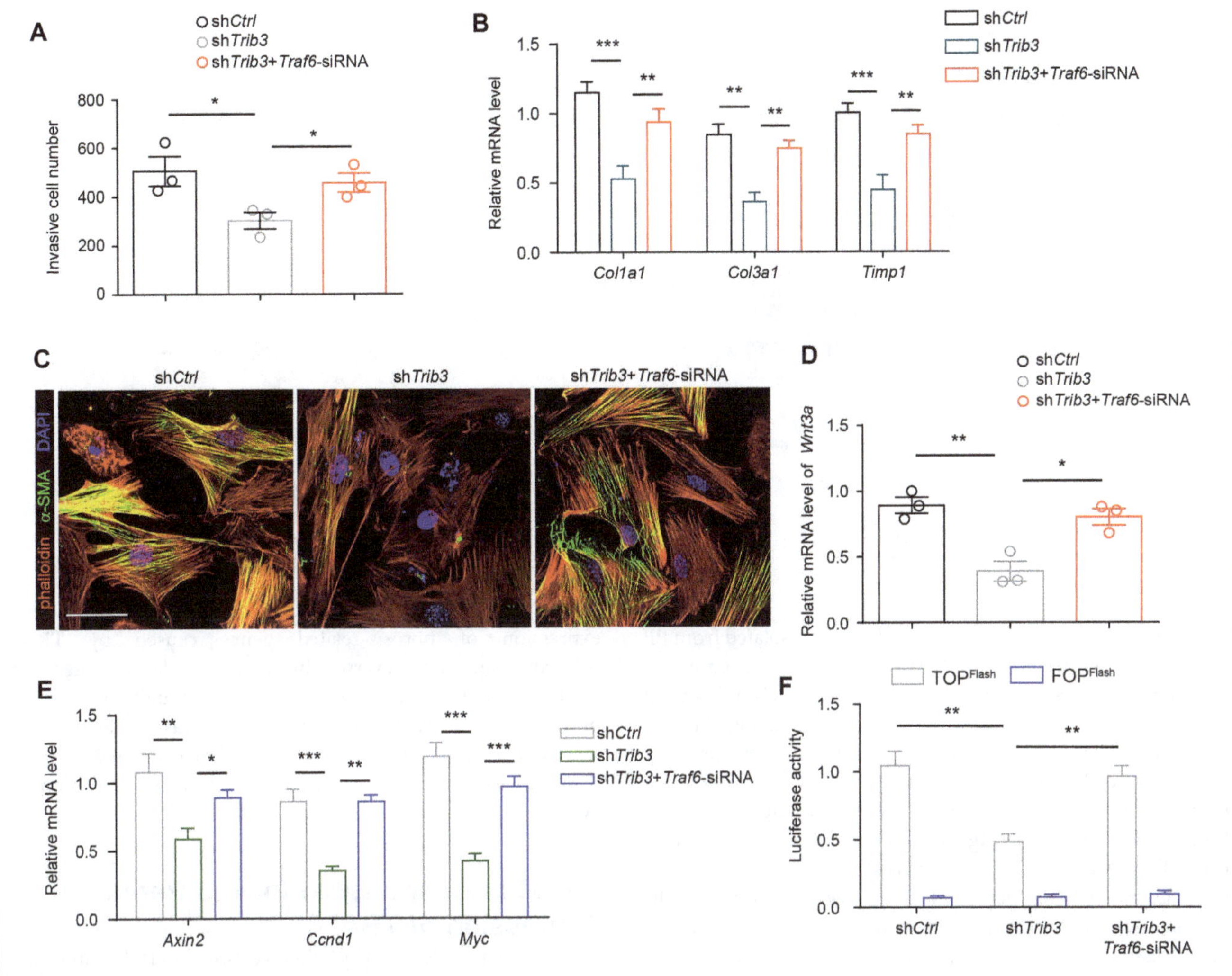

FIGURE 7 | TRIB3 activates lung fibroblasts by reducing TRAF6 expression. **(A)** Transwell assay for the evaluation of invasion of TRIB3-silenced PF lung fibroblasts with or without TRAF6 knockdown. **(B)** mRNA expression of fibrosis genes in TRIB3-silenced PF lung fibroblasts with or without TRAF6 knockdown. **(C)** Representative images of α-SMA immunostaining in TRIB3-silenced PF lung fibroblasts with or without TRAF6 knockdown. Scale bars, 50 μm. **(D)** mRNA expression of *Wnt3a* in TRIB3-silenced PF lung fibroblasts with or without TRAF6 knockdown. **(E)** mRNA expression of the β-catenin target genes in TRIB3-silenced PF lung fibroblasts with or without TRAF6 knockdown. **(F)** Wnt-reporter luciferase activity in TRIB3-silenced PF lung fibroblasts with or without TRAF6 knockdown. Data are representative of 3 independent experiments. Data represent means ± SEM Statistical significance: *$p < 0.05$, **$p < 0.01$ or ***$p < 0.001$.

decreased TRAF6 in PF lungs was associated with reduced pulmonary function (**Figure 1B**). The protein expression of TRAF6 was negatively correlated with the mRNA expression of *Acta2* (a marker of myofibroblasts) in fibrotic lungs (**Figure 1C**). These results prompted us to detect TRAF6 expression in lung fibroblasts, the effector cells in PF progression. Indeed, lower expression of TRAF6 was observed in lung fibroblasts from PF mice than in those from controls (**Figure 1D**). These findings demonstrate that TRAF6 in lung fibroblasts is negatively correlated with PF development.

To further confirm whether TRAF6 loss contributes to PF development *in vivo*, we instilled TRAF6-overexpressing lentivirus into lung tissue 10 days after BLM challenge. Overexpression of TRAF6 in lung tissue reduced BLM-induced PF changes, as revealed by the reduction in collagen deposition (**Figure 1E**), the improvement in lung function (**Figure 1F**), and the decreased hydroxyproline levels (an indicator of collagen content) in BLM mice (**Figure 1G**). Thus, TRAF6 may play an indispensable protective role in the progression of PF.

TRAF6 Overexpression Attenuates the Activation of Lung Fibroblasts From PF Mice

We next explored the functional relevance of TRAF6 in fibroblasts during PF progression. IHC staining showed that the expression of α-SMA was reduced in lung tissues from BLM-challenged mice under conditions of TRAF6 overexpression (**Figure 2A**), suggesting that TRAF6 overexpression suppressed fibroblast activation. To confirm

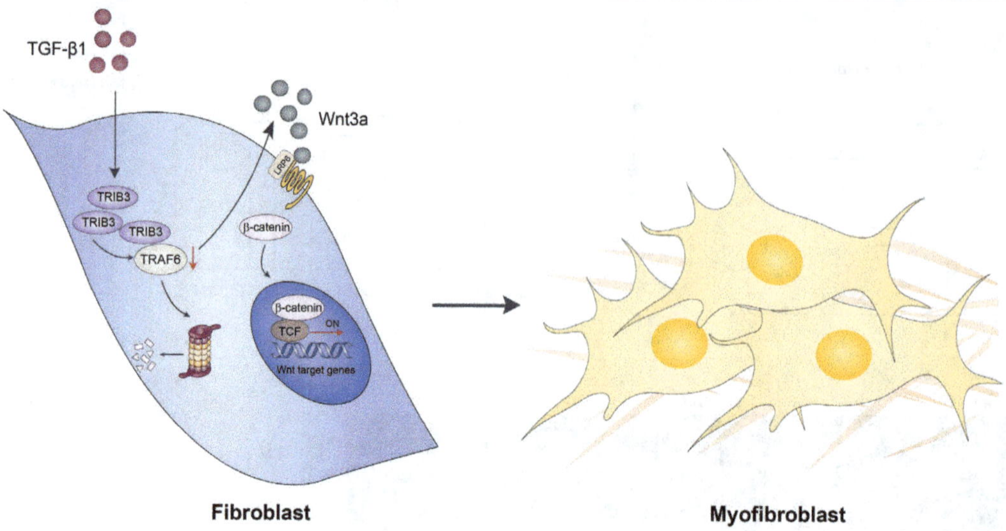

FIGURE 8 | Schematic diagram showing possible mechanisms by which TRAF6 involves in the development of pulmonary fibrosis.

this observation, primary mouse lung fibroblasts isolated from PF mice were transfected with a TRAF6-overexpressing adenovirus. PCR analysis revealed that the expression levels of several fibrosis-related genes and ECM proteins, including *Col1a1*, *Col3a1*, and *Timp1*, were reduced in fibroblasts overexpressing TRAF6 (**Figure 2B**). The matrigel invasion assay showed that the overexpression of TRAF6 decreased the invasive capacity of lung fibroblasts from PF mice (**Figure 2C**). In addition, the induction of TRAF6 overexpression in lung fibroblasts derived from PF mice decreased the percentages of α-SMA-positive cells (**Figure 2D**). Collectively, our data suggest that TRAF6 overexpression reverses the activation of myofibroblasts from PF mice and that TRAF6 deficiency during PF progression promotes the differentiation of lung fibroblasts into myofibroblasts.

TRAF6 Overexpression Decreases Wnt3a Expression

We explored how TRAF6 regulates the activation of lung fibroblasts. A previous study reported that TRAF6 overexpression in cardiac stem cells induced the downregulation of Wnt3a (Cao et al., 2015), which has been implicated in the pathogenesis of PF. We found that the overexpression of TRAF6 in lung fibroblasts from PF mice reduced the mRNA level of *Wnt3a* and that the depletion of TRAF6 in lung fibroblasts from control mice increased the mRNA level of *Wnt3a* (**Figures 3A,B**). TRAF6 depletion enhanced Wnt-reporter luciferase activity in PF lung fibroblasts (**Figure 3C**). In addition, western blot analysis demonstrated elevated expression of Wnt/β-catenin target genes in lung fibroblasts with TRAF6 depletion (**Figure 3D**). Moreover, the protein expression of TRAF6 was negatively correlated with the mRNA expression of *Wnt3a* in fibroblasts from PBS- and BLM-challenged mice (**Figure 3E**). The decreased expression of fibrosis-related genes caused by TRAF6 overexpression was reversed in lung fibroblasts treated with Wnt3a (**Figure 3F**). Furthermore, stimulation of lung fibroblasts with Wnt3a enhanced the invasive capacity that was suppressed by TRAF6 overexpression (**Figure 3G**). These data suggest that TRAF6 regulates fibroblast activation via Wnt3a.

TRIB3 Is Responsible for the Reduced Expression of TRAF6

We further investigated why TRAF6 expression is downregulated in fibroblasts during PF progression. PCR results showed that *Traf6* mRNA expression was comparable in lung fibroblasts from vehicle- and BLM-challenged mice (**Figure 4A**). We further analyzed TRAF6 gene expression in lung fibroblasts from IPF patients and healthy controls using a public microarray dataset (GSE129164). No difference in *TRAF6* mRNA expression was found between lung fibroblasts from IPF patients and healthy controls (**Figure 4B**). These data indicated that the decreased protein expression of TRAF6 in lung fibroblasts during PF progression might result from an alteration in its protein stability. Our group, along with others, has reported that TRIB3, a well-known stress sensor, is involved in regulating the stability of various proteins in the pathogenesis of chronic diseases (Lin et al., 2019; Yu J. M. et al., 2019; Liu S. et al., 2021). We then reasoned that TRIB3 might participate in regulating the altered protein expression of TRAF6. Indeed, an interaction between exogenous TRIB3 and TRAF6 was observed in HEK293T cells, and this was confirmed by the colocalization of TRIB3 and TRAF6 in primary mouse lung fibroblasts (**Figures 4C,D**). To map the interaction regions of TRAF6 and TRIB3, coIP assays were carried out using serial deletion mutants of either Myc-tagged TRAF6 or HA-tagged TRIB3. TRIB3 interacted with the ΔC domain but not with the ΔN domain of TRAF6 (**Supplementary Figure S1A**), and TRAF6 interacted with the KD and ΔN domains of TRIB3 (**Supplementary Figure S1B**). These data indicate that the ΔC domain of TRAF6 and the KD and ΔN domains of TRIB3 are required for the interaction between TRAF6 and TRIB3.

Overexpression of TRIB3 decreased the protein level of TRAF6, and depletion of TRIB3 increased the protein level of TRAF6 (**Figures 4E,F**). Moreover, the expression of TRAF6 was positively correlated with that of TRIB3 in lung fibroblasts from PBS- and BLM-challenged mice (**Figure 4G**). Indeed, the overexpression of TRIB3 reduced the half-life of TRAF6 (**Figure 4H**). Intracellular proteins are degraded by lysosomal autophagy pathways or the ubiquitin–proteasome system (UPS). We found that the UPS inhibitor MG132, but not the autophagy inhibitor 3-MA, reversed the TRIB3 overexpression-induced reduction in TRAF6 expression (**Figure 4I**). Furthermore, the overexpression and depletion of TRIB3 increased and blocked the ubiquitination of TRAF6, respectively (**Figures 4J,K**). These data indicate that the protein expression of TRAF6 can be regulated by TRIB3.

We then detected the expression of TRIB3 in lung fibroblasts during PF progression. TRIB3 exhibited markedly higher protein and mRNA expression levels in lung fibroblasts from PF mice than in those from control mice (**Figures 5A,B**). Based on the reanalysis of a published dataset (GSE129164), we found that stimulation of lung fibroblasts of IPF patients and normal controls with TGF-β1 (the principal profibrotic cytokines in lung fibrosis) increased *TRIB3* mRNA expression (**Figure 5C**). Another dataset also revealed higher *TRIB3* mRNA levels in human lung fibroblasts treated with TGF-β1 than in untreated cells (**Figure 5D**). Collectively, these data indicate that the enhanced expression of TRIB3 in lung fibroblasts results in a reduction in TRAF6 expression by promoting its ubiquitination and subsequent degradation.

TRAF6 Is Required for the Role of TRIB3 in Regulating Fibroblast Activation

Since the reduction in TRAF6 expression caused by TRIB3 contributes to the differentiation of fibroblasts to myofibroblasts, the above data prompted us to analyze the role of TRIB3 in regulating fibroblast activation. TRIB3 overexpression enhanced the invasive capacity of primary mouse lung fibroblasts (**Figure 6A**). Much higher levels of fibrosis-related genes were detected in TRIB3-overexpressing fibroblasts than in control fibroblasts (**Figure 6B**). Immunostaining analysis also indicated that TRIB3 overexpression in lung fibroblasts significantly increased the number of α-SMA-positive cells (**Figure 6C**), suggesting that TRIB3 induced the differentiation of fibroblasts into myofibroblasts. Consistently, we found that TRIB3 deficiency reversed the activation of myofibroblasts, as indicated by decreased invasive capacity, reduced expression of fibrosis-related genes, and fewer α-SMA-positive cells (**Figures 7A–C**). However, depletion of TRIB3 failed to inhibit the activation of TRAF6-silenced fibroblasts (**Figures 7A–C**). In addition, TRIB3 knockdown decreased the expression of *Wnt3a* and Wnt/β-catenin target genes in wild-type PF lung fibroblasts but not in fibroblasts with TRAF6 depletion (**Figures 7D,E**). Furthermore, TRIB3 depletion failed to reduce Wnt-reporter luciferase activity in lung fibroblasts with TRIB3 knockdown (**Figure 7F**). These results collectively demonstrate a TRIB3-TRAF6-Wnt3a signaling axis in regulating fibroblast activation.

DISCUSSION

TRAF6, a member of the TRAF family, plays a crucial role in immune signal transduction by acting as an adaptor protein downstream of multiple receptor families, including the interleukin-1 receptor (IL-1R) superfamily, the Toll-like receptor (TLR) family, and the TNFR superfamily. In recent years, TRAF6 has been extensively investigated in tumors, immunity, neurodegenerative diseases, ischemic stroke and osteoporosis (Li et al., 2017; Dou et al., 2018; Muto et al., 2022). Recent studies have also reported that TRAF6 is involved in the pathogenesis of NASH (Wang et al., 2020). They found that depletion of TRAF6 attenuated liver fibrosis in diet-induced NASH models, supporting a role for TRAF6 in promoting liver fibrosis. However, the role of TRAF6 in lung fibrosis remains unknown. In this study, we found that TRAF6 was downregulated in fibroblasts within the lung during the course of fibrotic processes. TRAF6 overexpression in fibroblasts from PF mice suppressed the activation of these cells. Furthermore, TRAF6 overexpression protected mice from BLM-induced lung fibrosis, with a decrease in the number of activated fibroblasts, also called myofibroblasts. Our data indicate that the downregulation of TRAF6 expression in fibroblasts contributes to PF progression by inducing the activation of those cells (**Figure 8**). This study selectively focused on the role of TRAF6 in fibroblasts. Given that TRAF6 is an intracellular protein widely expressed in epithelial cells, endothelial cells, and macrophages, future studies are needed to investigate the expression and role of TRAF6 in those cells during pulmonary fibrosis.

TRIB3, a stress sensor, is involved in the pathogenesis of various diseases, including obesity, diabetes, and tumors (Du et al., 2003; Oberkofler et al., 2010; Lin et al., 2019). Accumulating evidence has widely demonstrated that TRIB3 plays a vital role in organ fibrogenesis (Wang et al., 2014; Tomcik et al., 2016; Zhang et al., 2020). Our previous study, along with others, reported the key role of TRIB3 in promoting PF (Yu W. et al., 2019; Liu S. et al., 2021). We found that TRIB3 was substantially upregulated in alveolar macrophages (AMs) from patients with PF, inducing the profibrotic phenotype of AMs. Moreover, genetic knockout of TRIB3 specifically in AMs suppressed BLM-induced fibrotic changes in the lung. Another study found a central regulatory role of TRIB3 in fibroblast activation by stimulating canonical TGF-β1/Smad signaling in systemic sclerosis (Tomcik et al., 2016). Here, we found that elevated TRIB3 expression in fibroblasts from PF mice contributes to PF progression by enhancing the expression of Wnt3a, a crucial factor in the regulation of fibroblast activation (Li X. et al., 2020; Liu T. et al., 2021). Collectively, these data support that TRIB3 exerts profibrotic roles in different cell types during PF progression, demonstrating its potential value in the clinical treatment of PF.

As a member of the pseudokinase family, TRIB3 was found to regulate diverse processes in the progression of various diseases by interacting with functional proteins. For instance, the interaction of TRIB3 and the protein kinase GSK-3β interferes with the binding of GSK-3β to the E3 ligase UHRF1, thereby inhibiting the degradation of GSK-3β and leading to the profibrotic phenotype of Ams (Liu S. et al., 2021). TRIB3 interacted with MYC to suppress E3 ubiquitin ligase UBE3B-mediated MYC degradation, which induced the enhanced expression of MYC, causing the proliferation of lymphoma cells (Li K. et al., 2020). In the current study, the interaction of TRIB3 with TRAF6 in fibroblasts resulted in reduced TRAF6 expression. Intracellular proteins are degraded by the UPS or lysosomal autophagy pathway. We found that the UPS inhibitor MG132, but not the autophagy inhibitor 3-MA, reversed the TRIB3 overexpression-induced reduction in TRAF6 expression, indicating that the decrease in the protein level of TRAF6 caused by TRIB3 was related to its increased degradation through the UPS. This was consistent with previous studies showing that TRAF6 is degraded via the UPS (Li et al., 2014; Kim et al., 2017). Indeed, we observed increased ubiquitination and degradation of TRAF6 in TRIB3-overexpressing cells. We presumed that TRIB3, acting as a scaffolding protein, interacts with TRAF6 to recruit certain E3 ligases, thereby causing the ubiquitination and subsequent degradation of TRAF6. Obviously, further investigation of which kind of E3 ligase accounts for TRIB3 regulation of TRAF6 expression is warranted.

Increasing lines of evidence demonstrate that the aberrant activation of Wnt signaling is involved in the pathogenesis of PF (Morrisey, 2003; Skronska-Wasek et al., 2018). Attenuation of Wnt/β-catenin signaling can limit the development of fibrosis in mice. Wnt3a, the canonical ligand, is known to induce the activation of fibroblasts to myofibroblasts (Li X. et al., 2020). We found that depletion of TRAF6 in lung fibroblasts from control mice increased the expression of Wnt3a and Wnt/β-catenin target genes. A negative correlation was found between the expression of TRAF6 and Wnt3a in fibroblasts from PBS- and BLM-challenged mice. This was consistent with a prior study showing that TRAF6 overexpression induced the downregulation of Wnt3a in c-kit$^+$ cardiac stem cells. We also found that Wnt3a treatment reversed the suppressed activation of fibroblasts caused by TRAF6 overexpression. These results indicated that reduced expression of TRAF6 in lung fibroblasts induces the activation of fibroblasts by enhancing the expression of Wnt3a during PF progression. Thus, our work provides insight into the regulatory role of TRAF6 in Wnt3a expression in fibroblasts. Further investigation is necessary to determine the molecular mechanism by which TRAF6 controls Wnt3a expression.

Our findings revealed that the reduced expression of TRAF6 caused by TRIB3 overexpression in lung fibroblasts contributes to the progression of PF through upregulation of Wnt3a expression, which drives fibroblast differentiation into myofibroblasts. Accordingly, genetically enhancing TRAF6 expression or inhibiting the TRIB3-TRAF6 interaction may represent a novel therapeutic strategy for PF and other fibroproliferative lung diseases.

ETHICS STATEMENT

The animal study was reviewed and approved by The Second Xiangya Hospital of Central South University.

AUTHOR CONTRIBUTIONS

SL conceived the study. SL and JM designed the experiments. JM, QL, and MY performed the experiments. SL, QW, and YZ analyzed the data. BC and JY provided valuable suggestions and comments on the study design. JM and SL wrote and edited the manuscript.

REFERENCES

1. Cao, Q., Wang, Y., Huang, L., Wang, F., and Chen, S. (2015). TNF Receptor-Associated Factor 6 (TRAF6) Mediates the Angiotensin-Induced Non-canonical TGF-β Pathway Activation of C-Kit(+) Cardiac Stem Cells. *Am. J. Transl. Res.* 7 (11), 2233–43.
2. Cao, Z., Xiong, J., Takeuchi, M., Kurama, T., and Goeddel, D. V. (1996). TRAF6 Is a Signal Transducer for Interleukin-1. *Nature* 383 (6599), 443–446. doi:10.1038/383443a0
3. Dou, Y., Tian, X., Zhang, J., Wang, Z., and Chen, G. (2018). Roles of TRAF6 in Central Nervous System. *Curr. Neuropharmacol.* 16 (9), 1306–1313. doi:10.2174/1570159X16666180412094655
4. Du, K., Herzig, S., Kulkarni, R. N., and Montminy, M. (2003). TRB3: a Tribbles Homolog that Inhibits Akt/PKB Activation by Insulin in Liver. *Science* 300 (5625), 1574–1577. doi:10.1126/science.1079817
5. Frangogiannis, N. (2020). Transforming Growth Factor-β in Tissue Fibrosis. *J. Exp. Med.* 217 (3), e20190103. doi:10.1084/jem.20190103
6. George, P. M., Spagnolo, P., Kreuter, M., Altinisik, G., Bonifazi, M., Martinez, F. J., et al. (2020). Progressive Fibrosing Interstitial Lung Disease: Clinical Uncertainties, Consensus Recommendations, and Research Priorities. *Lancet Respir. Med.* 8 (9), 925–934. doi:10.1016/S2213-2600(20)30355-6
7. Hinz, B., and Lagares, D. (2020). Evasion of Apoptosis by Myofibroblasts: a Hallmark of Fibrotic Diseases. *Nat. Rev. Rheumatol.* 16 (1), 11–31. doi:10.1038/s41584-019-0324-5
8. Kim, E., Beon, J., Lee, S., Park, S. J., Ahn, H., Kim, M. G., et al. (2017). Inositol Polyphosphate Multikinase Promotes Toll-like Receptor-Induced Inflammation by Stabilizing TRAF6. *Sci. Adv.* 3 (4), e1602296. doi:10.1126/ sciadv.1602296
9. Li, K., Wang, F., Yang, Z. N., Zhang, T. T., Yuan, Y. F., Zhao, C. X., et al. (2020). TRIB3 Promotes MYC-Associated Lymphoma Development through Suppression of UBE3B-Mediated MYC Degradation. *Nat. Commun.* 11 (1), 6316. doi:10.1038/s41467-020-20107-1
10. Li, S., Shu, B., Zhang, Y., Li, J., Guo, J., Wang, Y., et al. (2014). Carboxyl Terminus of Hsp70-Interacting Protein Regulation of Osteoclast Formation in Mice through Promotion of Tumor Necrosis Factor Receptor-Associated Factor 6 Protein Degradation. *Arthritis Rheumato l.* 66 (7), 1854–1863. doi:10.1002/art.38521
11. Li, T., Qin, J. J., Yang, X., Ji, Y. X., Guo, F., Cheng, W. L., et al. (2017). The Ubiquitin E3 Ligase TRAF6 Exacerbates Ischemic Stroke by Ubiquitinating and Activating Rac1. *J. Neurosci.* 37 (50), 12123–12140. doi:10.1523/JNEUROSCI.1751-17.2017
12. Li, X., Liu, X., Deng, R., Gao, S., Yu, H., Huang, K., et al. (2020). Nintedanib Inhibits Wnt3a-Induced Myofibroblast Activation by Suppressing the Src/β-Catenin Pathway. *Front. Pharmacol.* 11, 310. doi:10.3389/fphar.2020.00310
13. Lin, J., Zhang, W., Niu, L. T., Zhu, Y. M., Weng, X. Q., Sheng, Y., et al. (2019). TRIB3 Stabilizes High TWIST1 Expression to Promote Rapid APL Progression and ATRA Resistance. *Clin. Cancer Res.* 25 (20), 6228–6242. doi:10.1158/1078- 0432.CCR-19-0510

14. Liu, G., Philp, A. M., Corte, T., Travis, M. A., Schilter, H., Hansbro, N. G., et al. (2021). Therapeutic Targets in Lung Tissue Remodelling and Fibrosis. *Pharmacol. Ther.* 225, 107839. doi:10.1016/j.pharmthera.2021.107839

15. Liu, S., Lv, X., Wei, X., Liu, C., Li, Q., Min, J., et al. (2021). TRIB3-GSK-3β Interaction Promotes Lung Fibrosis and Serves as a Potential Therapeutic Target. *Acta Pharm. Sin. B* 11 (10), 3105–3119. doi:10.1016/j.apsb.2021.06.017

16. Liu, S. S., Liu, C., Lv, X. X., Cui, B., Yan, J., Li, Y. X., et al. (2021). The Chemokine CCL1 Triggers an AMFR-SPRY1 Pathway that Promotes Differentiation of Lung Fibroblasts into Myofibroblasts and Drives Pulmonary Fibrosis. *Immunity* 54 (9), 2042–2048. doi:10.1016/j.immuni.2021.06.008

17. Liu, S. S., Lv, X. X., Liu, C., Qi, J., Li, Y. X., Wei, X. P., et al. (2019). Targeting Degradation of the Transcription Factor C/EBPβ Reduces Lung Fibrosis by Restoring Activity of the Ubiquitin-Editing Enzyme A20 in Macrophages. *Immunity* 51 (3), 522–e7. e527. doi:10.1016/j.immuni.2019.06.014

18. Liu, T., Gonzalez De Los Santos, F., Hirsch, M., Wu, Z., and Phan, S. H. (2021). Noncanonical Wnt Signaling Promotes Myofibroblast Differentiation in Pulmonary Fibrosis. *Am. J. Respir. Cell Mol. Biol.* 65 (5), 489–499. doi:10.1165/rcmb.2020-0499OC

19. Lo Re, S., Lecocq, M., Uwambayinema, F., Yakoub, Y., Delos, M., Demoulin, J. B., et al. (2011). Platelet-derived Growth Factor-Producing CD4+ Foxp3+ Regulatory T Lymphocytes Promote Lung Fibrosis. *Am. J. Respir. Crit. Care Med.* 184 (11), 1270–1281. doi:10.1164/rccm.201103-0516OC

20. Morrisey, E. E. (2003). Wnt Signaling and Pulmonary Fibrosis. *Am. J. Pathol.* 162 (5), 1393–1397. doi:10.1016/S0002-9440(10)64271-X

21. Muto, T., Guillamot, M., Yeung, J., Fang, J., Bennett, J., Nadorp, B., et al. (2022). TRAF6 Functions as a Tumor Suppressor in Myeloid Malignancies by Directly Targeting MYC Oncogenic Activity. *Cell Stem Cell* 29 (2), 298–e9. doi:10.1016/j. stem.2021.12.007

22. Naito, A., Azuma, S., Tanaka, S., Miyazaki, T., Takaki, S., Takatsu, K., et al. (1999). Severe Osteopetrosis, Defective Interleukin-1 Signalling and Lymph Node Organogenesis in TRAF6-Deficient Mice. *Genes Cells* 4 (6), 353–362. doi:10. 1046/j.1365-2443.1999.00265.x

23. Oberkofler, H., Pfeifenberger, A., Soyal, S., Felder, T., Hahne, P., Miller, K., et al. (2010). Aberrant Hepatic TRIB3 Gene Expression in Insulin-Resistant Obese Humans. *Diabetologia* 53 (9), 1971–1975. doi:10.1007/s00125-010-1772-2

24. Sgalla, G., Kulkarni, T., Antin-Ozerkis, D., Thannickal, V. J., and Richeldi, L. (2019). Update in Pulmonary Fibrosis 2018. *Am. J. Respir. Crit. Care Med.* 200 (3), 292–300. doi:10.1164/rccm.201903-0542UP

25. Skronska-Wasek, W., Gosens, R., Konigshoff, M., and Baarsma, H. A. (2018). WNT Receptor Signalling in Lung Physiology and Pathology. *Pharmacol. Ther.* 187, 150–166. doi:10.1016/j.pharmthera.2018.02.009

26. Tomcik, M., Palumbo-Zerr, K., Zerr, P., Sumova, B., Avouac, J., Dees, C., et al. (2016). Tribbles Homologue 3 Stimulates Canonical TGF-β Signalling to Regulate Fibroblast Activation and Tissue Fibrosis. *Ann. Rheum. Dis.* 75 (3), 609–616. doi:10.1136/annrheumdis-2014-206234

27. Walsh, M. C., Lee, J., and Choi, Y. (2015). Tumor Necrosis Factor Receptor-Associated Factor 6 (TRAF6) Regulation of Development, Function, and Homeostasis of the Immune System. *Immunol. Rev.* 266 (1), 72–92. doi:10. 1111/imr.12302

28. Wang, W., Sun, A., Lv, W., Cheng, J., Lv, S., Liu, X., et al. (2014). TRB3, Up-Regulated in Kidneys of Rats with Type1 Diabetes, Mediates Extracellular Matrix Accumulation *In Vivo* and *In Vitro*. *Diabetes Res. Clin. Pract.* 106 (1), 101–109. doi:10.1016/j.diabres.2014.07.015

29. Wang, Y., Wen, H., Fu, J., Cai, L., Li, P. L., Zhao, C. L., et al. (2020). Hepatocyte TNF Receptor-Associated Factor 6 Aggravates Hepatic Inflammation and Fibrosis by Promoting Lysine 6-Linked Polyubiquitination of Apoptosis Signal-Regulating Kinase 1. *Hepatology* 71 (1), 93–111. doi:10.1002/hep.30822

30. Wu, H., and Arron, J. R. (2003). TRAF6, a Molecular Bridge Spanning Adaptive Immunity, Innate Immunity and Osteoimmunology. *Bioessays* 25 (11), 1096–1105. doi:10.1002/bies.10352

31. Yang, W. L., Wang, J., Chan, C. H., Lee, S. W., Campos, A. D., Lamothe, B., et al. (2009). The E3 Ligase TRAF6 Regulates Akt Ubiquitination and Activation. *Science* 325 (5944), 1134–1138. doi:10.1126/science.1175065

32. Yu, J. M., Sun, W., Wang, Z. H., Liang, X., Hua, F., Li, K., et al. (2019). TRIB3 Supports Breast Cancer Stemness by Suppressing FOXO1 Degradation and Enhancing SOX2 Transcription. *Nat. Commun.* 10 (1), 5720. doi:10.1038/s41467-019-13700-6

33. Yu, W., Song, X., and Liu, Y. (2019). TRB3 Regulates Pulmonary Interstitial Fibrosis through the MAPK Signaling Pathway. *Int. J. Clin. Exp. Pathol.* 12 (9), 3247–3257.

34. Zhang, J. L., Du, B. B., Zhang, D. H., Li, H., Kong, L. Y., Fan, G. J., et al. (2021). OTUB1 Alleviates NASH through Inhibition of the TRAF6-ASK1 Signaling Pathways. *Hepatology* 75, 1218–1234. doi:10.1002/hep.32179

35. Zhang, X. W., Zhou, J. C., Peng, D., Hua, F., Li, K., Yu, J. J., et al. (2020). Disrupting the TRIB3-SQSTM1 Interaction Reduces Liver Fibrosis by Restoring Autophagy and Suppressing Exosome-Mediated HSC Activation. *Autophagy* 16 (5), 782–796. doi:10.1080/15548627.2019.1635383

10

Investigation of a Hypoxia-Immune-Related Microenvironment Gene Signature and Prediction Model for Idiopathic Pulmonary Fibrosis

Xinyu Li[1,2†], Haozheng Cai[1†], Yufeng Cai[3†], Quyan Zhang[1,2], Yinghe Ding[1,2] and Quan Zhuang[1,4]*

[1] Transplantation Center, The 3rd Xiangya Hospital, Central South University, Changsha, China, [2] Xiangya School of Medicine, Central South University, Changsha, China, [3] School of Life Science, Central South University, Changsha, China, [4] Research Center of National Health Ministry on Transplantation Medicine, Changsha, China

***Correspondence:**
Quan Zhuang
zhuangquansteven@163.com

[†]These authors have contributed equally to this work

Background: There is growing evidence found that the role of hypoxia and immune status in idiopathic pulmonary fibrosis (IPF). However, there are few studies about the role of hypoxia and immune status in the lung milieu in the prognosis of IPF. This study aimed to develop a hypoxia-immune-related prediction model for the prognosis of IPF.

Methods: Hypoxia and immune status were estimated with microarray data of a discovery cohort from the GEO database using UMAP and ESTIMATE algorithms respectively. The Cox regression model with the LASSO method was used for identifying prognostic genes and developing hypoxia-immune-related genes. Cibersort was used to evaluate the difference of 22 kinds of immune cell infiltration. Three independent validation cohorts from GEO database were used for external validation. Peripheral blood mononuclear cell (PBMC) and bronchoalveolar lavage fluid (BALF) were collected to be tested by Quantitative reverse transcriptase-PCR (qRT-PCR) and flow cytometry from 22 clinical samples, including 13 healthy controls, six patients with non-fibrotic pneumonia and three patients with pulmonary fibrosis.

Results: Hypoxia and immune status were significantly associated with the prognosis of IPF patients. High hypoxia and high immune status were identified as risk factors for overall survival. CD8+ T cell, activated CD4+ memory T cell, NK cell, activated mast cell, M1 and M0 macrophages were identified as key immune cells in hypoxia-immune-related microenvironment. A prediction model for IPF prognosis was established based on the hypoxia-immune-related one protective and nine risk DEGs. In the independent validation cohorts, the prognostic prediction model performed the significant applicability in peripheral whole blood, peripheral blood mononuclear cell, and lung tissue of IPF patients. The preliminary clinical specimen validation suggested the reliability of most conclusions.

Conclusions: The hypoxia-immune-based prediction model for the prognosis of IPF provides a new idea for prognosis and treatment.

Keywords: idiopathic pulmonary fibrosis, microenvironment, hypoxia, immune, prognosis

INTRODUCTION

Idiopathic pulmonary fibrosis (IPF) is a chronic, progressive interstitial lung disease. The prognosis of patients with IPF is poor, with a median survival of 3 to 5 years (1). Several prognostic staging systems for IPF have been established by clinical and physiologic variables (2–5). Biomarkers in peripheral blood are also evaluated as a tool for prognosis (6–8). A recent study also revealed the role of genetic variability in the survival of IPF (9). In addition, molecular markers of IPF patients could also be identified by bronchoalveolar lavage (BAL) cells, and the collection of BAL cells is non-invasive compared with lung biopsy (10). However, very little is known whether molecular events in the lung milieu are predictive of outcome in IPF. Considering accurate diagnosis and personalized treatment, there is still a critical need for a way to predict the progression of IPF.

As a chronic lung disorder, the central processes in IPF are inflammation and fibrosis (11). Immune dysregulation has been considered as a promoting factor in the development of IPF, including several biomarkers associated with the prognosis of IPF (12). Inflammatory cytokines released by immune cells may activate fibroblasts, connective tissue cell proliferation, angiogenesis (11). Furthermore, hypoxia is common in the process of fibrosis in many diseases (13, 14). Excessive collagen synthesized by fibroblasts deteriorate oxygen supply and accelerate the pathological process. Studies showed the relationship between immune response and hypoxia and lung function (15). However, the underlying mechanisms have not been discussed.

With a series of genetic and bioinformatics analyses, we associated immune status with hypoxia and explore its value for the prognosis of patients with IPF. Here, we developed a hypoxia-immune-related prediction model for the prognosis of IPF, intended to provide novel ideas for accurate diagnosis and treatment at the gene level. Better knowledge of the oxygen balance control and the immune regulation involved is important to advance the development of IPF.

MATERIALS AND METHODS

Patient Cohort and Data Preparation

The discovery cohort of the study contained 176 IPF patients from the Gene Expression Omnibus (GEO, available at: https://www.ncbi.nlm.nih.gov/geo/) database (GSE70866). The tissue source of sequencing samples is the patients' BAL cells. The microarray data of GSE70866 was based on GPL14550 Platform (Agilent-028004 SurePrint G3 Human GE 8x60K Microarray, Agilent Technologies) and GPL17077 Platform (Agilent-039494 SurePrint G3 Human GE v2 8 × 60K Microarray, Agilent Technologies), including 176 IPF patients' BAL cells. Three validation cohorts were used for external validations (GSE93606, GSE28221, and GSE32537) to examine the predictive effect of the prediction method. The microarray data of GSE93606 was based on GPL11532 Platforms (Affymetrix Human Gene 1.1 ST Array, Affymetrix, Santa Clara, CA, USA), including 57 IPF patients' peripheral whole blood. The microarray data of GSE28221 was based on GPL5175 Platforms (Affymetrix Human Exon 1.0 ST Array, Affymetrix, Santa Clara, CA, USA) and GPL6480 Platforms (Agilent-014850 Whole Human Genome Microarray 4x44K G4112F, Agilent Technologies), including 120 IPF patients' peripheral blood mononuclear cell. The microarray data of GSE32537 based on GPL6244 (Affymetrix Human Gene 1.0 ST Array, Affymetrix, Santa Clara, CA, USA) included 119 lung tissues with IPF. The batch effect was eliminated by sva package, which contains functions for identifying and building surrogate variables for high-dimensional data sets.

All procedures of this study complied with the protocol. For analyses of data from a public database, approval and informed consent from the local ethics committee were not required.

Identification of Hypoxia Status and Hypoxia-Related DEGs

To identify the hypoxia status, a non-linear dimensionality reduction algorithm of Uniform Manifold Approximation and Projection (UMAP) was applied, which could divide or condense a group of patients into a series of distinct clusters, according to the given hallmarks or signatures. The hallmark gene sets of hypoxia include 200 genes and were downloaded from the Molecular Signatures Database (MSigDB version 6.0). Based on the clusters, two groups including "hypoxia^{low}" and "hypoxia^{high}" were identified to identify the hypoxia status. The limma algorithm was applied to identify differentially expressed genes (DEGs) between the two groups (16). Genes with a false discovery rate (FDR) adjusted p-value <0.0001 and an absolute value of log2 (fold change) >1 were considered as hypoxia-related DEGs.

Identification of Immune Status and Immune-Related DEGs

To identify the immune status, the Estimation of Stromal and Immune cells in MAlignant Tumours using Expression data (ESTIMATE) algorithm was applied to identity the infiltration degree of immune cells and predict the immune status (17). Based on the immune status, patients were classified into two groups. Maximally selected rank statistics was applied by using an R package "survival", and "survminer" to identify the optimal cutting point to divide patients. Based on the optimal cutting point, patients with high immune scores were attributed to "immune^{high}" group and "immune^{low}" group. The limma algorithm was applied to identify DEGs between the two groups. Genes with a FDR adjusted p-value <0.0001 and an absolute value of log2 (fold change) >1 were considered as immune-related DEGs.

To further identify the abundance of 22 immune cells, CIBERSORT is a deconvolution algorithm based on the gene expression data to resolve immune cell composition (18). Those with p <0.05 were included.

Identification of Hypoxia-Immune-Related Prognostic DEGs

According to the above hypoxia and immune grouping, patients were divided into three groups, *i.e.*, hypoxia^{high}/immune^{high}, hypoxia^{low}/immune^{low}, and mix groups. The limma algorithm was applied to identify DEGs between "hypoxia^{high}/immune^{high} group and hypoxia^{low}/immune^{low} group. Genes with a FDR adjusted p-value <0.0001 and an absolute value of log2 (fold change) >1 were considered as hypoxia-immune-related DEGs. DEGs were then divided into protective and risk DEGs. The risk DEGs contained all EDGs highly expressed in hypoxia^{high}/immune^{high} group and the rest were protective DEGs. To obtain hypoxia-immune-related prognostic DEGs, univariate Cox analyses were further performed to screen all protective and risk DEGs. Those with a p <0.001 were considered as significant.

Prognosis Prediction Model of IPF Based On Hypoxia-Immune-Related DEGs

The Least Absolute Shrinkage and Selection Operator (LASSO) is a kind of linear regression using shrinkage, which is applied to survival analysis with high-dimensional data (19). In this study, the LASSO Cox regression model was applied to select the optimal variables from all identified hypoxia-immune-related prognostic DEGs in the discovery cohort. Three-fold cross-validation and 1,000 iterations were conducted to reduce the potential instability of the results. The optimal tuning parameter λ was identified *via* 1-SE (standard error) criterion. Then we create the prognosis prediction model of IPF using the selected prognostic gene signature. For each patient, the risk score was the sum of the expression of the characteristic DEGs and the corresponding coefficients derived from the multivariate Cox regression model. According to the risk scores, the optimal cutting point was identified using the maximally selected rank method, and the prognosis prediction model of IPF was formed.

Functional and Pathway Enrichment Analysis

Database for Annotation, Visualization and Integrated Discovery was used for Gene Ontology (GO) enrichment analysis (20). The risk DEGs of IPF patients were screened for functional enrichment. GO analysis was used to evaluate the degree of enrichment of the DEGs in biological processes, cellular components, and molecular functions. Those with p-value <0.05 and count (the number of enriched genes) ≥3 were considered as the cutoff criterion.

Preliminary Validation of Clinical Specimens

Peripheral blood mononuclear cell (PBMC) and bronchoalveolar lavage fluid (BALF) were collected from 22 clinical samples, including 13 healthy controls, six with non-fibrotic pneumonia and three with pulmonary fibrosis. The clinical information such as age, gender, alveolar-arterial oxygen gradient (A-aDO2), and hospital day was shown in **Supplementary Materials**. The study was reviewed and approved by the institutional review board (Ethics Committee) of the 3rd Xiangya Hospital, Central South University (No. 21028).

Quantitative reverse transcriptase-PCR (qRT-PCR) was used to quantitative expression of key DEGs. Total RNA was extracted from the tissues using TRIzol Reagent (Thermo Fisher Scientific). PCR was performed using an Thermo Scientific PikoReal PCR cycler. The cycle threshold (CT) data were determined, and the mean CT was determined from triplicate PCRs. Relative gene expression was calculated with the equation $2^{-\Delta CT}$.

Flow cytometry analysis was used to determine the proportion of immune cells. The cell suspension was counted and mixed with ACK Lysis Buffer (Thermo Fisher Scientific) to remove red blood cells. Then 1×10^6 cells were resuspended in 100 μl staining buffer and incubated with monoclonal antibodies in dark for 15 min at 4°C. Our flow cytometric staining strategy consisted of the following fluorochrome-conjugated monoclonal antibodies: anti-CD3-Alexa-Flour700 (Biolegend), anti-CD4-eFlour450 (eBioscience), anti-CD45RA-APC-eFluor 780 (eBioscience), anti-CCR7-PerCP-eFluor 710 (eBioscience), anti-CD16-eFluor506 (eBioscience), anti-CD56-PE (eBioscience), anti-CD206- PE-Cyanine7 (eBioscience), anti-CD68-FITC (eBioscience), anti-CD107a-eFluor660 (eBioscience). CD3 and CD4 were used to identify T cells. $CD3^+CD4^+CD45RA^-CCR7^-$ cells were defined as activated $CD4^+$ memory T cells. CD56 and CD16 were used to identify NK cells. $CD107a^+$ NK cells were defined as activated NK cells. $CD68^+CD16^-CD206^-$ cells were defined as M1-like macrophages and $CD68^+CD16^-CD206^+$ cells were defined as M0-like macrophages. After washing and resuspending, samples were detected using BD FACSDiva software and performed using BD FACSCanto II.

Statistical Analysis

All analyses were performed with R version 4.0.2 (www.r-project.org/) and the corresponding packages. UMAP algorithm was performed by using R package "umapr" for non-linear dimensionality reduction. Immune score was performed by using R package "estimate". The Lasso Cox regression model was performed by using R package "glmnet". Data were analyzed with standard statistical tests as appropriate. Multiple testing was adjusted by the FDR method. Multivariate Cox regression analysis was performed to identify optimal signatures. Flowjo V 10.62 was used to analyzed flow cytometric data. Original data from PCR and flow cytometry were presented as the mean ± standard deviation (SD) and were compared using Student's t-test, Welch's t-test or the Mann–Whitney U test, where appropriate. GraphPad Prism 7.0 (GraphPad Software Inc., La

Jolla, CA, USA) was used to perform the statistical analyses. Values of $p < 0.05$ were considered statistically significant.

The general idea and methodologies used in this study were drawn as a flow chart (**Figure 1**).

RESULTS

Hypoxia Status and Hypoxia-Related DEGs in IPF

The discovery cohort contained 176 IPF patients from the GEO databases. The batch effect was eliminated by sva package (**Figures 2A, B**). Patient clinical information is shown in **Table 1**. With the expression matrix constructed by 200 hypoxia marker genes from MSigDB, the non-linear dimensionality reduction algorithm UMAP was used to determine two clusters, and each patient is assigned to the nearest clusters (**Figure 2C**). Cluster 1 and Cluster 2 contained 95 and 81 patients respectively. Expression profiles were compared between the two clusters, and 239 DEGs related to hypoxia were obtained. Enrichment analysis showed overexpressed genes in Cluster 2 were enriched in "oxygen transport (GO:0015671)" and "response to hypoxia (GO:0001666)" (**Figure 2D**). This indicated that the level of hypoxia in Cluster2 was at high status. Thereby, the patients in Clusterl and Cluster2 were determined as hypoxia^{low} and hypoxia^{high} groups. In addition, overexpressed genes in Cluster2 were also enriched in positive regulation of GTPase activity and cell adhesion. Patients' clinical information of each cluster is shown in **Table 2**. The survival status of patients in different groups was further analyzed (**Figure 2E**). There was a significant difference in survival between two clusters (log rank test, $p < 0.0001$), and the prognosis of patients with a high level of hypoxia is worse. Among 239 DEGs, 232 DEGs were overexpressed in the hypoxia^{high} cluster, which were regarded as hypoxia-associated risk DEGs. The other seven genes overexpressed in the hypoxia^{low} cluster, which are regarded as hypoxia-associated protective DEGs. In a word, most of the hypoxia-related DEGs are regarded as risk factors.

Immune Status and Immune-Related DEGs in IPF

The immune score was calculated by ESTIMATE to identity the infiltration degree of immune cells. The optimal cutting point "2,959.22" was determined based on maximally selected rank statistics (**Figures 2F, G**). Then the immune^{high} group and immune^{low} group were divided, containing 108 and 68 patients respectively. Patients' clinical information of each cluster is shown in **Table 3**. Further survival analysis showed a significant difference between two groups (log rank test, $p < 0.05$), and the survival of patients with a high level of immune infiltration is worse (**Figure 2I**). Therefore, high immune infiltration is also a risk factor for bad prognosis. This conclusion is also supported by the highly enriched immune-related pathways in the hypoxia^{high} group with a poor prognosis. Expression profiles were compared between the two groups, and 196 DEGs related to immune status were obtained (**Figure 2H**). Among them, 191 genes were overexpressed in the immune^{high}

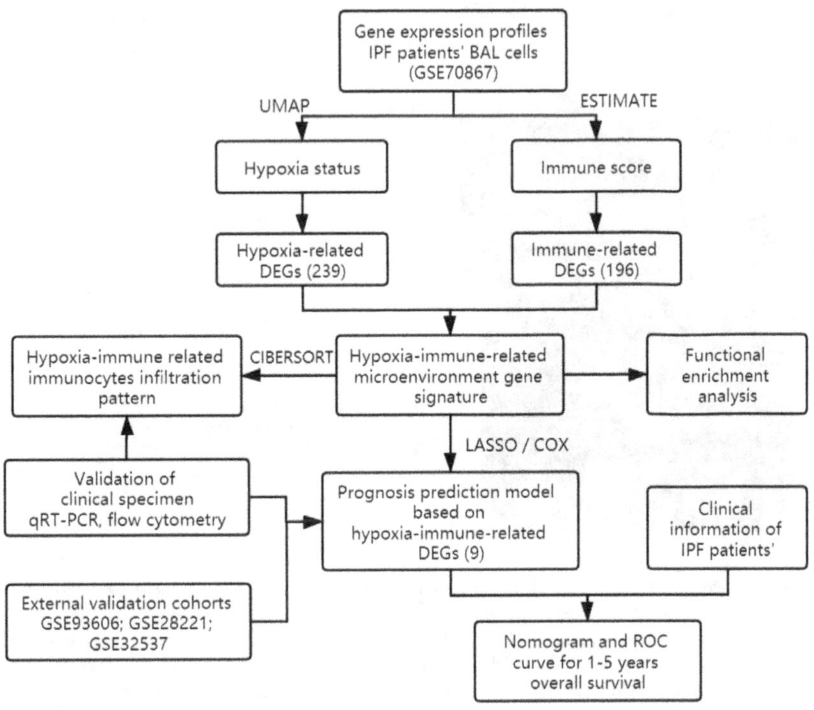

FIGURE 1 | Flow chart of methodologies used in this study.

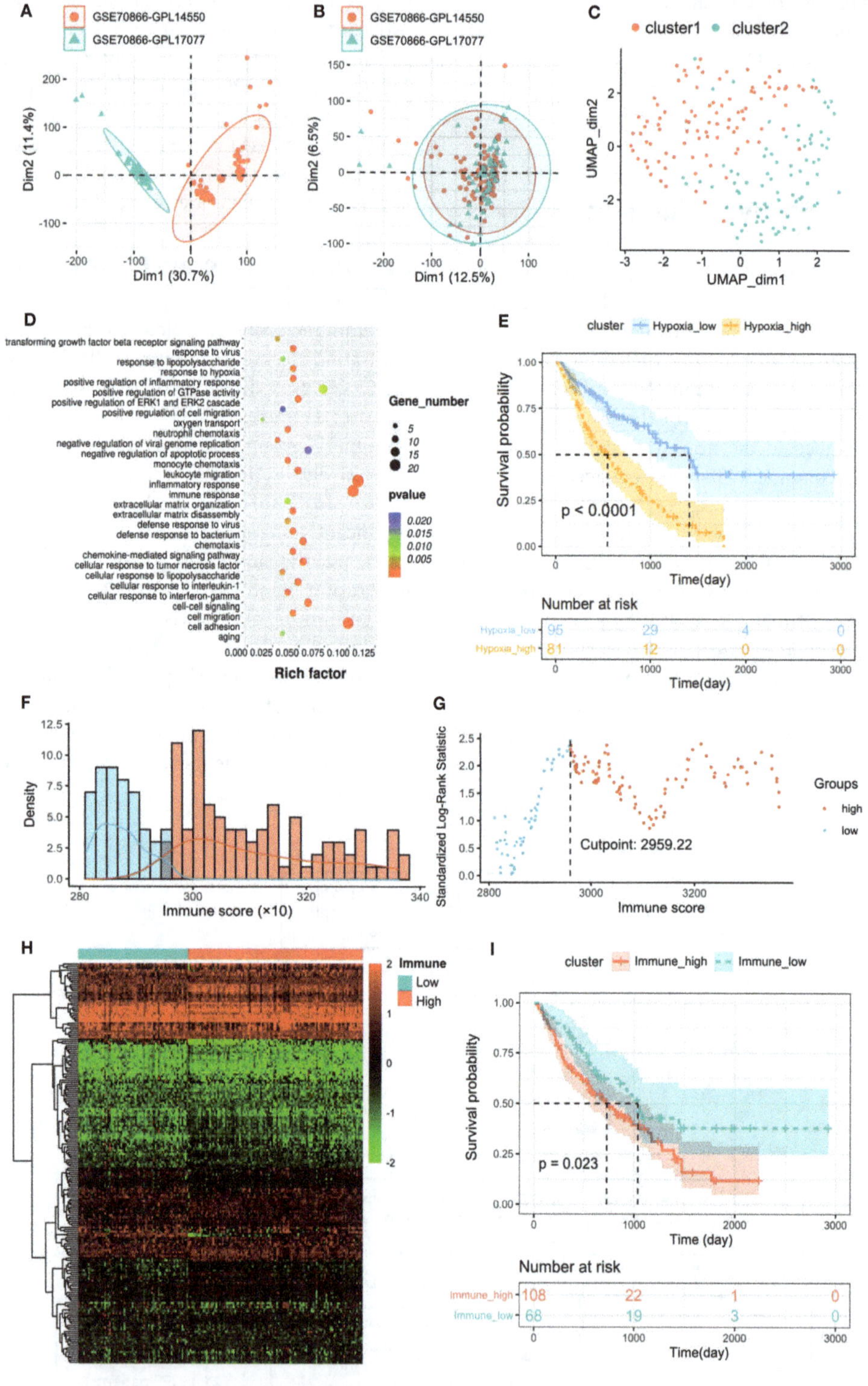

FIGURE 2 | **(A, B)** Eliminating the batch effect between different sequencing platforms. **(A)** The PCA plot before elimination of batch effect, and **(B)** is the PCA plot after elimination. The distance of sample point clusters indicates that they come from different batches and sequencing platforms. While in B, after eliminating the batch effect, the difference in distance between batches is reduced. **(C)** UMAP clustering plot based on marker gene set of hypoxia. **(D)** Biological process functional enrichment analysis of differentially expressed genes between hypoxia^{high} and hypoxia^{low} groups. **(E)** Kaplan–Meier plot of overall survival in two clusters. **(F)** Histogram based on maximally selected rank grouping. **(G)** The cut-off point with the maximum standard log-rank statistic was marked with a vertical dashed line. **(H)** The differential gene expression profiles between hypoxia^{high} and hypoxia^{low} groups were visualized in heatmap. **(I)** Kaplan–Meier plot of overall survival between immune^{high} and immune^{low} groups.

TABLE 1 | Basic information of IPF patients in discovery cohort.

Characteristics	Whole cohort (176)	Low risk (55)	High risk (121)
Gender			
Male	117 (0.665)	31 (0.564)	86 (0.711)
Female	59 (0.335)	24 (0.436)	35 (0.289)
Age			
≥65 years	86 (0.489)	30 (0.545)	56 (0.463)
<65 years	90 (0.511)	25 (0.455)	65 (0.537)
UMAP clustering			
Cluster1	95 (0.540)	47(0.855)	48 (0.397)
Cluster2	81 (0.460)	8 (0.145)	73 (0.603)
Hypoxia status			
High	81 (0.460)	8 (0.145)	73 (0.603)
Low	95 (0.540)	47(0.855)	48 (0.397)
Immune status			
High	108 (0.614)	21 (0.382)	87 (0.719)
Low	68 (0.386)	34 (0.618)	34 (0.281)
Risk group			
High	121 (0.688)	0	121 (1.000)
Low	55 (0.312)	55 (1.000)	0

TABLE 2 | Basic information of IPF patients in different hypoxia-based clusters.

Characteristics	Whole cohort (176)	$hypoxia^{low}$ (95)	$hypoxia^{high}$ (81)
Gender			
Male	117 (0.665)	58 (0.610)	59 (0.728)
Female	59 (0.335)	37 (0.390)	22 (0.272)
Age			
≥65 years	86 (0.489)	48 (0.505)	38 (0.470)
<65 years	90 (0.511)	47 (0.495)	43 (0.530)

TABLE 3 | Basic information of IPF patients in different immune-based clusters.

Characteristics	Whole cohort (176)	$immune^{low}$ (68)	$immune^{high}$ (108)
Gender			
Male	117 (0.665)	44 (0.647)	72 (0.667)
Female	59 (0.335)	24 (0.353)	36 (0.333)
Age			
≥65 years	86 (0.489)	38 (0.559)	48 (0.445)
<65 years	90 (0.511)	30 (0.441)	60 (0.555)

cluster, which were regarded as immune-associated risk DEGs. The other five genes overexpressed in the $immune^{low}$ cluster, which are regarded as immune-associated protective DEGs.

Hypoxia–Immune-Related DEGs in IPF

According to the above hypoxia and immune grouping, we further combined to form three groups: $hypoxia^{high}$/$immune^{high}$, $hypoxia^{low}$/$immune^{low}$, and mix groups. The survival status of patients in different groups was further analyzed (**Figure 3A**). There was a significant difference in survival among three groups (log rank test, $p < 0.0001$). Survival in mix group is at an intermediate level. As we expected, a high level of hypoxia and immune activity is the most dangerous factor while patients in group $hypoxia^{low}$/$immune^{low}$ have the best prognosis.

The differential gene expression profiles between $hypoxia^{high}$/$immune^{high}$ and $hypoxia^{low}$/$immune^{low}$ groups were visualized in heatmap (**Figure 3B**). We further intersect the hypoxia-related DEGs and the immune-related DEGs to identify the hypoxia–immune-related DEGs in IPF. We obtained a total of 62 DEGs, of which 61 were highly expressed in $hypoxia^{high}$ and $immune^{high}$ groups, so they were defined as hypoxia-immune-related risk DEGs (**Figure 3C**). Correspondingly, the remaining DEG is defined as hypoxia-immune-related protective DEG (**Figure 3D**). The GO enrichment analysis showed that "immune response", "inflammatory response", and "positive regulation of ERK1/2 cascade" are main biological process (**Figure 3E**).

Prognosis Prediction Model of IPF Based on Hypoxia-Immune-Related DEGs

To further determine the DEGs significantly related to the prognosis, we used univariate Cox analysis for screening and 29 DEGs with $p < 0.001$ were retained (**Figure 4A**). Among them, one protective and 28 risk DEGs were included.

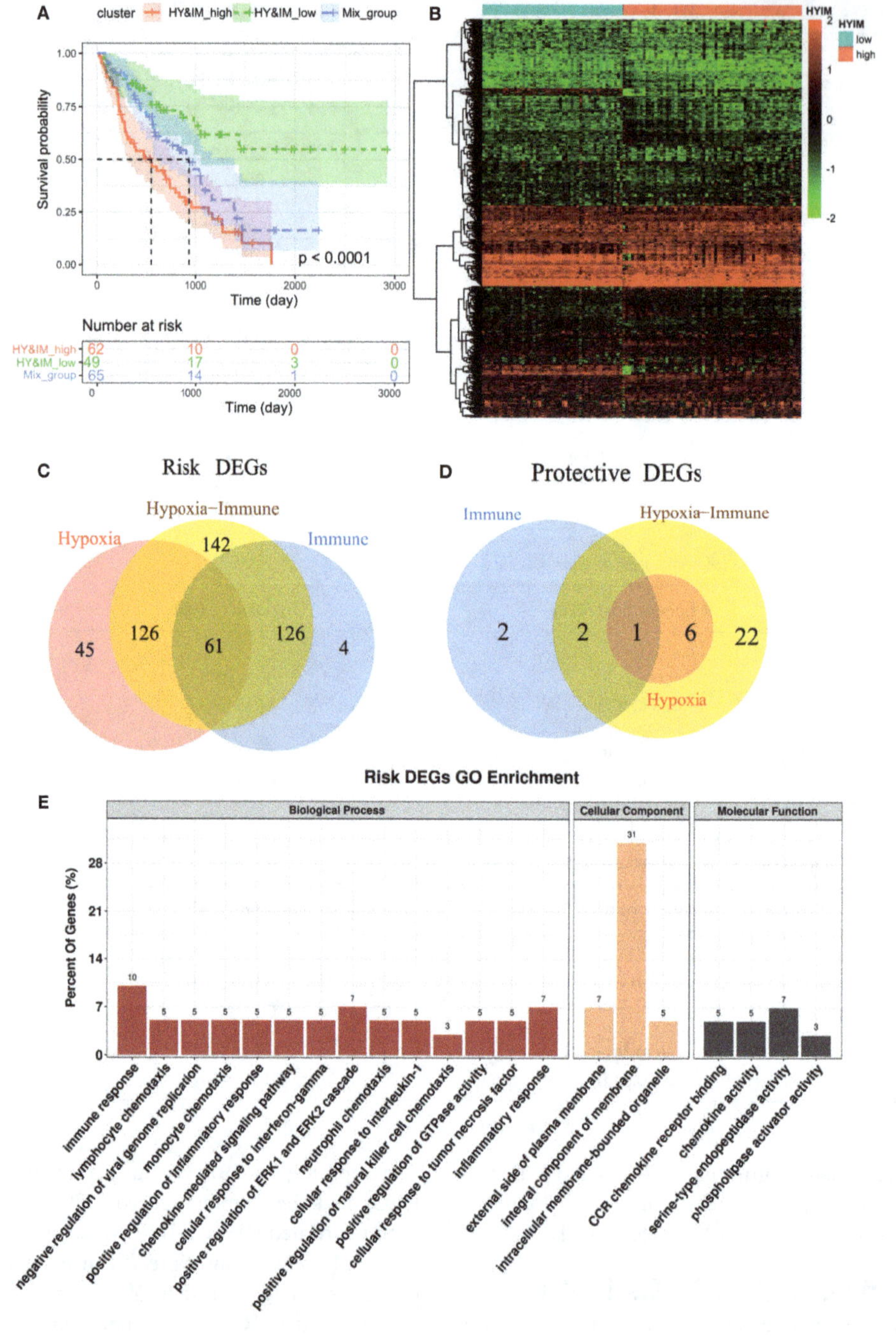

FIGURE 3 | **(A)** Kaplan–Meier plot of overall survival between hypoxia^{high}/immune^{high}, hypoxia^{low}/immune^{low}, and mix groups. **(B)** Heatmap shows the differential gene expression profiles between hypoxia^{high}/immune^{high} and hypoxia^{low}/immune^{low} groups **(C,D)** Venn diagrams show the hypoxia-immune related risk DEGs (61) and protective DEG (1). € GO enrichment analysis of risk DEGs.

Using lasso regression method, nine optimal variables were obtained from the above 29 hypoxia-immune-prognostic-related DEGs (**Figures 4B, C**). Then we use the expression levels of nine characteristic DEGs and the corresponding coefficients derived from the multivariate Cox regression model to estimate the risk score for each patient: risk score = −0.13307 × expression of NALCN + 0.09893 × expression of IL1R2 + 0.06226 × expression of S100A12 + 0.06890 × expression of PROK2 + 0.04883 × expression of CCL8 + 0.05654 × expression of RAB15 + 0.10671 × expression of MARCKSL1 + 0.09986 × expression of TPCN1 + 0.05696 × expression of HS3ST3B1.

By calculating the risk score of each patient, we divided the patients into two groups through the maximally selected rank method: high-risk group and low-risk group (**Figure 4D**). The

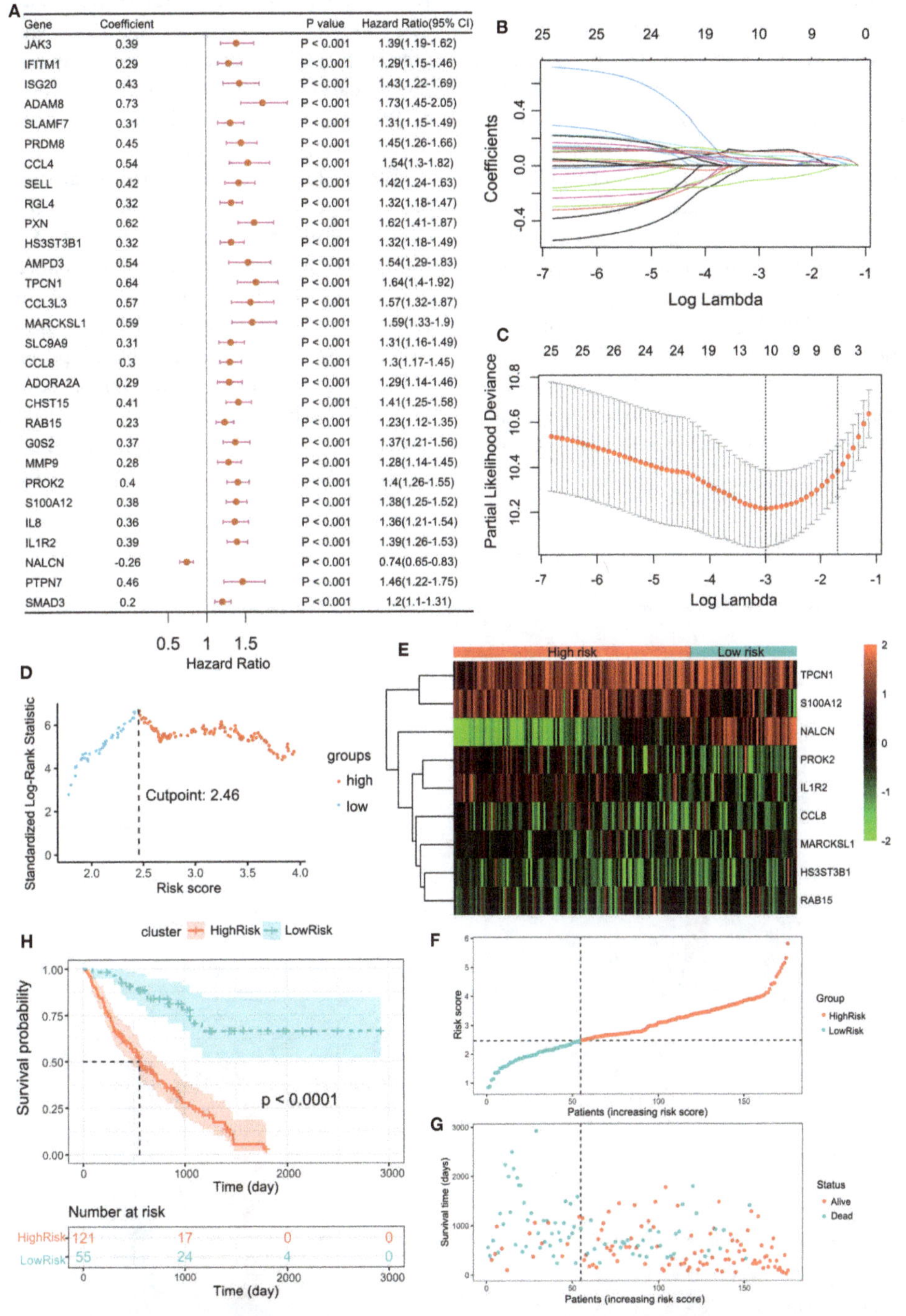

FIGURE 4 | **(A)** Forest plot of 29 DEGs with P <0.001 by univariate Cox regression. **(B)** LASSO coefficient profiles of 29 screened DEGs. **(C)** Three-fold cross-validation of lasso analysis. Error bars represented the SE. The dotted vertical lines showed the optimal values. **(D)** The cut-off point with the maximum standard log-rank statistic was marked with a vertical dashed lines. **(E)** The expression profiles of DEGs involved in multivariate Cox regression model. **(F)** The distribution of patients with increased risk score in two groups. **(G)** Scatter plot showed the survival of patients with increased risk score. **(H)** Kaplan–Meier plot of overall survival between high-risk and low-risk groups.

nine optimal DEG expression profiles between high-risk and low-risk groups were visualized in heatmap (**Figure 4E**). Survival analysis showed that there was a significant difference between the two groups (log rank test, $p < 0.0001$). Compared with the low-risk group, the prognosis of the high-risk group is significantly worse (**Figures 4F–H**).

Hypoxia-Immune Related Immunocyte Infiltration Pattern

In addition, CIBERSORT was used to estimate the infiltration of 22 kinds of immune cells in the samples. Correlation analysis showed a general association in different immune cells (**Figure 5A**). Among them, the infiltration of six specific immune cells was significantly different in hypoxia^{high}/immune^{high} and hypoxia^{low}/immune^{low} group, that is, CD8+ T cell, activated CD4+ memory T cell, activated natural killer (NK) cell, activated mast cell, M0 macrophage, M1 macrophage (**Figure 5B**). Further correlation analysis showed the relationship between six specific immune cells and risk score. Among them, most infiltration degree is positively correlated with risk DEGs expression and risk score, but the infiltration of M0 cells was negatively correlated with the risk DEGs expression and risk score (**Figure 5C**). Among them, M0 macrophages and NK cells had the most significant correlation with key DEGs and risk score.

Validation of the Prognostic Prediction Model in External Independent Cohorts

The ROC curve showed that the AUCs within 1-5 years were all greater than 0.75 in discovery cohort (**Figure 6A**). This suggested the evaluation model had a good predictive value for the prognosis of IPF patients. We also developed a nomogram for 1-5 years overall survival prediction based on Cox model (**Figure 6B**).

We further verify the above prediction method in external data sets" GSE93606", "GSE28221", and "GSE32537". Patient clinical information is shown in **Table 4**. In each independent validation cohort, we divided the IPF patients into high-risk and low-risk groups based on the risk score. In GSE28221 and GSE93606 IPF cohorts, survival comparison showed that low-risk group had significantly better prognosis outcomes than high-risk group (**Figures 6C, D**). In addition, we focused on the clinicopathologic features of IPF in GSE32537 cohort. The patients in low-risk group generally had higher forced vital capacity (FVC) and carbon monoxide diffusing capacity

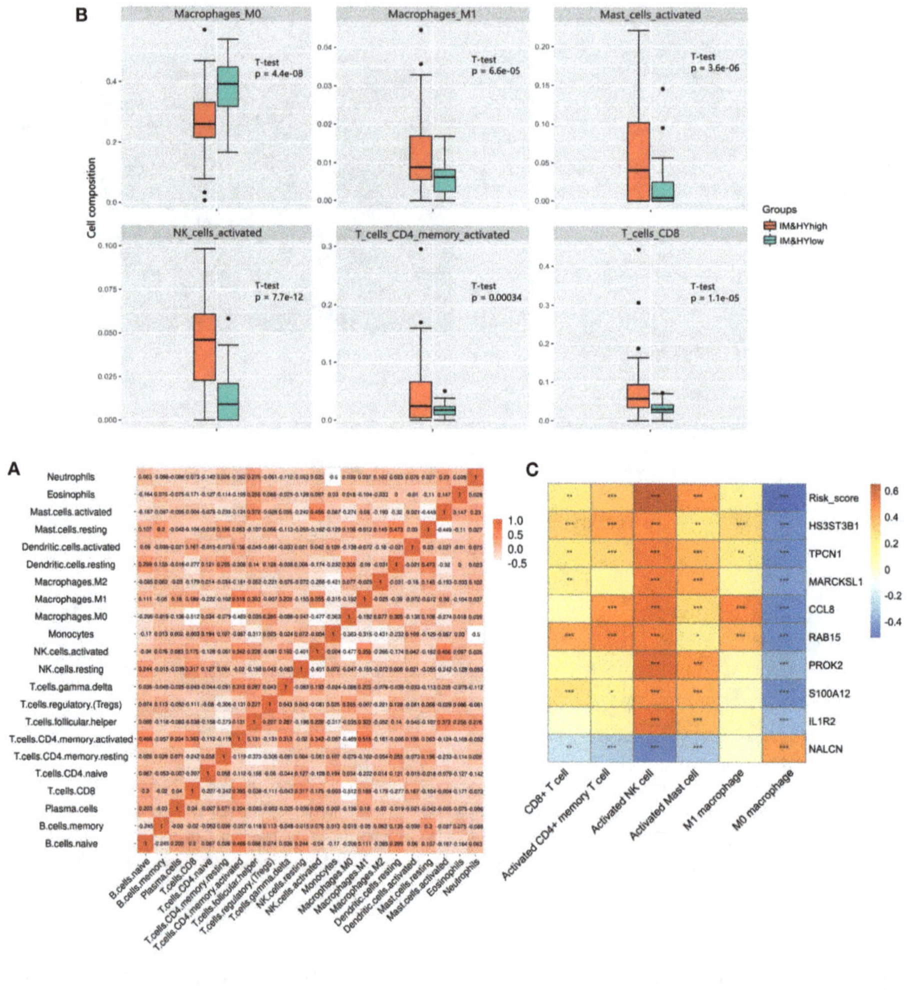

FIGURE 5 | (A) Heatmap showed the correlation coefficient between different immune cells. **(B)** The box plot showed the significant difference of immune cells' infiltration between two groups. **(C)** Heatmap showed the correlation coefficient between immune cells and DEGs involved in Cox model (*** means P < 0.01, ** means P < 0.05, and * means P < 0.1).

(DLCO) ($P < 0.05$), which meant better lung function (**Figures 6E, F**). While the patients in high-risk group had higher St. George's total score ($P < 0.05$), which suggested worse lung function and quality of life (**Figure 6G**).

In a word, these results suggest that our prognostic prediction model is also of great significance based on peripheral whole blood, peripheral blood mononuclear cell, and lung tissue.

Preliminary Validation of Clinical Specimens

The results of qRT-PCR in PBMC suggested that DEGs of CCL8, IL1R2, NALCN, S100A12, and PROK2 were significantly different between the patients and healthy controls (**Figure 7A**). Among the patients, CCL8, IL1R2, and PROK2 were significantly up-expressed in fibrotic samples than non-

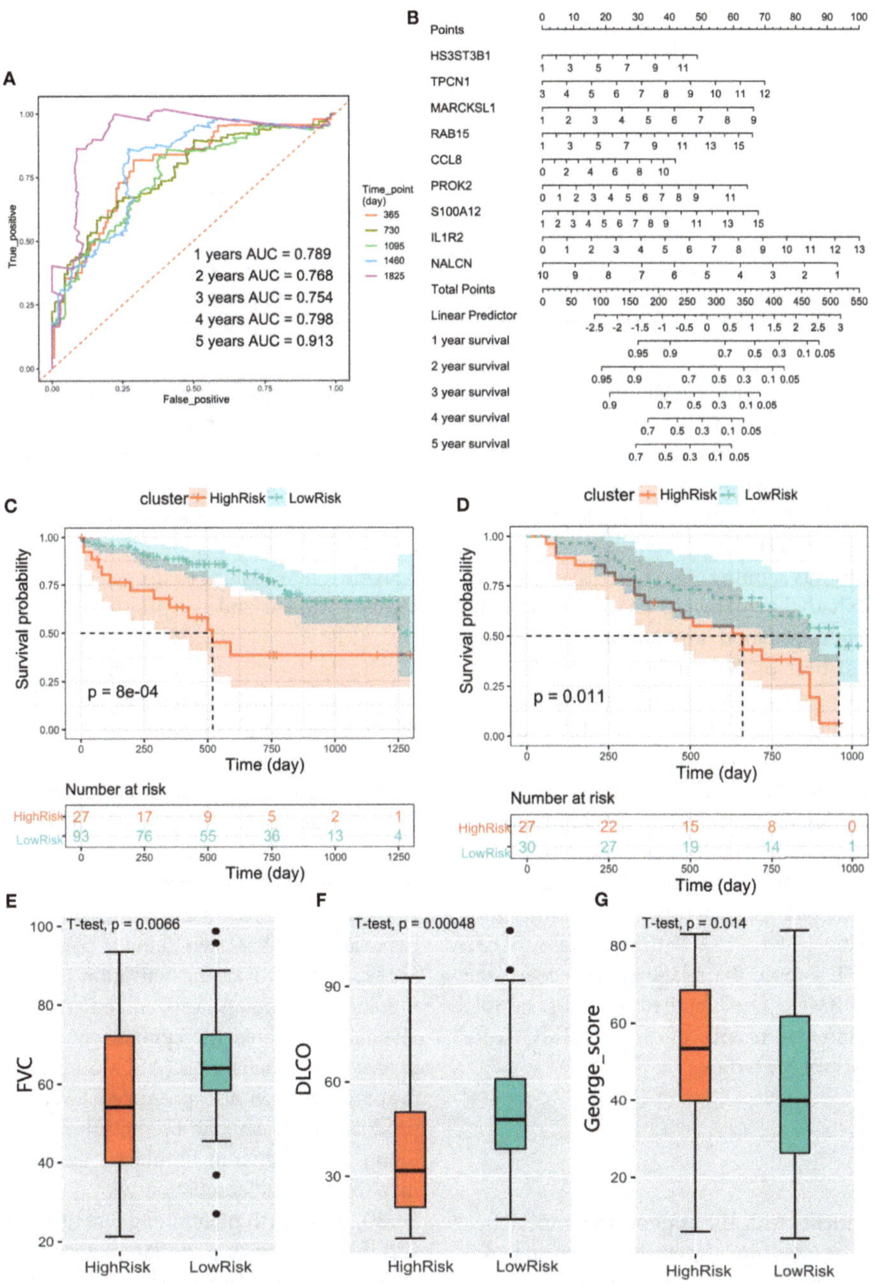

FIGURE 6 | **(A)** ROC curve evaluated the predictive value of the model for the prognosis of patients in discovery cohort within 1–5 years. **(B)** The nomogram for 1–5 years overall survival based on Cox model. **(C)** Kaplan–Meier plot of overall survival between high-risk and low-risk groups in GSE28221 validation cohort. **(D)** Kaplan–Meier plot of overall survival between high-risk and low-risk groups in GSE93606 validation cohort. **(E–G)** The box plot showed the difference of FVC, DLCO, and George's score between low-risk group and high-risk groups in GSE32537 validation cohort.

TABLE 4 | Basic information of IPF patients in validation cohort.

Characteristics	Whole cohort (296)	Low risk (182)	High risk (114)
GSE93606	Whole cohort (57)	Low risk (30)	High risk (27)
Gender			
Male	38 (0.667)	18 (0.600)	20 (0.741)
Female	19 (0.333)	12 (0.400)	7 (0.259)
Age			
≥65 years	35 (0.614)	18 (0.600)	17 (0.630)
<65 years	22 (0.386)	12 (0.400)	10 (0.370)
GSE32537	Whole cohort (119)	Low risk (59)	High risk (60)
Gender			
Male	42 (0.353)	25 (0.424)	17 (0.283)
Female	77 (0.647)	34 (0.576)	43 (0.717)
Age			
≥65 years	53 (0.445)	31 (0.525)	22 (0.367)
<65 years	66 (0.555)	28 (0.475)	38 (0.633)
GSE28221	Whole cohort (120)	Low risk (93)	High risk (27)
Gender			
Male	92 (0.767)	71 (0.763)	21 (0.778)
Female	28 (0.233)	22 (0.237)	6 (0.222)
Age			
≥65 years	76 (0.633)	55 (0.591)	21 (0.778)
<65 years	44 (0.367)	38 (0.409)	6 (0.222)

fibrotic samples (**Figure 7B**). The PBMC results of flow cytometry showed that the proportion of NK cells was increased significantly in the patients than healthy controls (**Figure 7C**), and among the patients' BALF, the proportion of NK cells was also increased significantly in fibrotic samples than in non-fibrotic ones (**Figure 7D**). The proportion of activated NK cells in BALF samples was significantly higher than those in PBMC samples, and it had the following characteristics: the increasing trend of peripheral blood to pulmonary bronchus (**Figure 7E**). The proportion of NK or activated NK cells' infiltration in BALF was positively correlated with patients A-aDO2 and hospital day, suggesting that high NK infiltration is a risk factor for poor prognosis (**Figures 7F, G**). In addition, the flow cytometry showed that the increasing CD4+ T cells in peripheral blood might promote the macrophage infiltration in pulmonary bronchus and promoted their polarization to M1-like phenotype (**Figure 7H**). The proportion of CD4+ T, activated CD4+ memory T cells, and M1-like macrophages infiltration in BALF or PBMC was positively correlated with patients' A-aDO2 (**Figures 7I–K**). **Figure 7L** showed the relationship between the results of BALF and PBMC. The detailed data of sample information and experimental results of BALF/PBMC were shown in the **Supplementary Materials**.

DISCUSSION

Since the prognosis of patients with IPF is poor, the importance of building a prognostic staging system for personalized treatment is self-evident. The prognostic staging system could divide the patients into several groups according to the given markers. In this study, we used the transcriptional profiles of the bronchoalveolar lavage fluid (BALF) to analyze the relationship between the level of biomarkers and the prognosis of patients. We found that both hypoxia and immune status were related to the survival and even respiratory function of patients with IPF. Furthermore, we established a new prognostic classifier including nine-gene signature for patients with IPF. It is effective in the prognosis of patients with IPF in the discovery cohort and three independent validation cohorts. These findings provide a new insight to the relationship between biomarkers in the lung milieu and the prognosis and stratification of patients with IPF.

Several articles reported the role of immune and hypoxia microenvironment in lung diseases (15). On one hand, immune dysregulation and inflammation are regarded as the basis of chronic lung diseases, including IPF (11). Bioinformatics analysis of RNA network and immune infiltration showed that immune cells were associated with the severity of IPF (21). Both innate and adaptive immunity were activated in fibrogenesis (22). On the other hand, hypoxia is common in lung disease. Hypoxia-inducible factor-1α (HIF-1α) is a key regulating factor in cell response to hypoxia, which has been found to participate in many lung diseases (23–25). In hypoxia, the activation of HIF-1α mediates glycolysis modification, angiogenesis, and other adaptive mechanism (26, 27). Hypoxia promoted the epithelia–mesenchymal transition (EMT) of alveolar epithelial cells (AECs) in IPF, and transforming growth factor β (TGF-β) also promoted EMT with increased lactic acid produced by metabolic modification (24, 28). Also, HIF-1α was found to be active in fibroblasts from IPF patients and induced myofibroblast differentiation with the existence of TGF-β (24, 26, 29, 30). It is worth mentioning that hypoxia facilitated proliferation and the secretion of proinflammatory cytokines in mast cells, and thus influenced fibrogenesis (31). In IPF, alveolar macrophages showed a perturbation of mitochondria homeostasis, including increased mitochondria reactive oxygen species (mtROS), in which HIF-1α may have participated (32). These findings were in accordance with the results. The result of infiltration of different

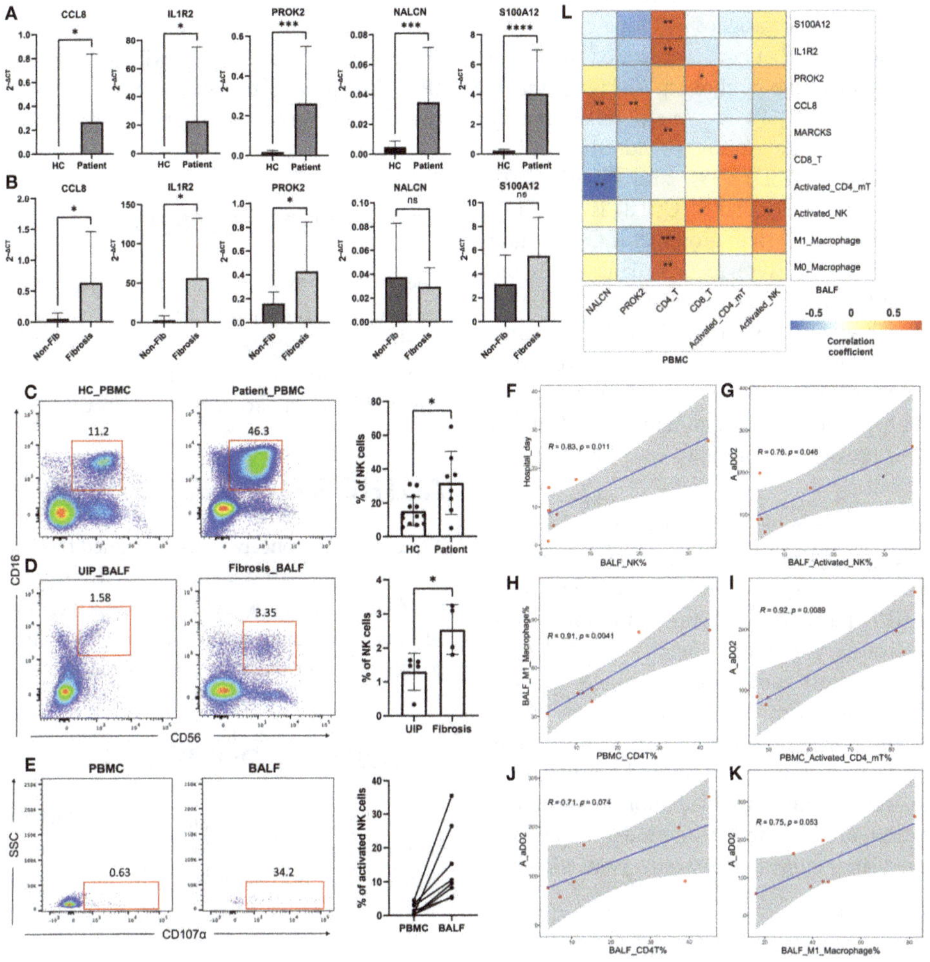

FIGURE 7 | (A, B) The plots showed the results of qRT-PCR. Plot A showed the difference of DEGs expression in PBMC between healthy controls (HC) and patients. Plot B showed the difference of DEGs expression in PBMC between non-fibrotic pneumonia group (Non-Fib) and pulmonary fibrosis group (Fibrosis). **(C–E)** CD56 and CD16 were used to identify NK cells in flow cytometry. CD56$^+$CD16$^+$CD107a$^+$ cells were defined as activated NK cells. Plot C showed the difference of NK% in PBMC between healthy controls (HC) and patients. Plot D showed the difference of NK% in BALF between usual interstitial pneumonitis (UIP, from Non-Fib group) and pulmonary fibrosis group (Fibrosis). **(F–K)** Pearson analysis showed the correlation between cell proportion and clinical features. **(L)** Pearson analysis showed the correlation between the results of BALF and PBMC. *, **, ***, **** respectively represent P values of t-test < 0.05, < 0.01, < 0.001, < 0.0001.

types of immune cells showed that both innate immunity and adaptive immunity were activated in hypoxia^{high}/immune^{high} group, presenting poorer prognosis. In a word, hypoxia, as the inducement of immune activation, mediates chronic airway inflammation and leads to fibrosis. Then, cell and organ dysfunction caused by fibrosis aggravates the formation of hypoxic inflammatory microenvironment, which forms a feedback loop.

The result of CIBERSORT showed that the infiltration of M0 macrophage in hypoxia^{low}/immune^{low} group was higher than hypoxia^{high}/immune^{high} group. As inactive and naive macrophages, the low proportion of M0 macrophages in the low-risk group suggested a lower level of inflammatory activation (33). At the same time, the infiltration of CD8+ T cell, activated CD4+ memory T cell, activated NK cell, activated mast cell, and M1 macrophage in hypoxia^{high}/immune^{high} group was higher than that in hypoxia^{low}/immune^{low} group, presenting a higher level of inflammation. As was discussed above, the role of CD4+ T cell, mast cell, and M1 macrophage in fibrosis was widely reported. It is worth noting that M0 macrophage and NK cell had the most significant correlation with key hypoxia-immune DEGs and risk score. However, the role of CD8+ T cell, NK cell, and M0 macrophage in fibrosis has not been fully verified. These may provide a new idea to understand the characteristic immune cells in fibrotic infiltration.

Also, we found that hypoxia-immune DEGs were mainly risk DEGs, taking part in the integral component of membrane and immune response, and the protective DEG was a gene encoding voltage-independent, non-selective cation channel. The roles of these predictive signature genes have been reported previously in lung diseases. Interleukin-1 receptor 2 (IL-1R2) is an anti-inflammatory cytokine. The increase level of IL-1R2 has been reported to be associated with poor prognosis in lung cancer (34, 35), and the increase level of IL-1 was associated with the development of chronic obstructive pulmonary disease (COPD) (36, 37). Another risk gene S100A12 is a novel inflammatory disease biomarker in acute respiratory distress syndrome (ARDS) (38), interstitial lung disease (ILD) (39), and COPD (40). Moreover, C-C Motif Chemokine Ligand 8 (CCL8) is a kind of monocyte chemoattractant, regulating group 2 ILCs in lung inflammation (41). These results were in accordance with the results in this article that the overexpression of IL-1R2, S100A12, and ILC2s may be predictive for poor diagnosis of IPF patients. NALCN gene encodes a voltage-independent, non-selective cation channel. Other signature genes are rarely reported in lung diseases. In this study, combing hypoxia and immune status, we identified these signature genes to provide new insights into the prognosis of IPF.

In particular, in the independent external validations of this study, the prognostic prediction model was performed in peripheral whole blood, peripheral blood mononuclear cell, and lung tissue of IPF patients, and the outcomes were significant. The preliminary clinical specimen validation suggested the reliability of most conclusions, but there are still limitations, such as insufficient sample size. And because of the individual differences and other confounding factors, the results based on the existing database must have some deviation from the reality. Although these results provided more possibilities and a wider application of this predictive model in clinical setting, a well-designed and multi-center study is needed for further exploration.

CONCLUSIONS

The immune and hypoxia status in alveolar molecular environment is associated with the prognosis of patients with IPF. The prognostic model based on several signature genes raised a new way to predict the progression and prognosis of IPF.

ETHICS STATEMENT

The studies involving human participants were reviewed and approved by the institutional review board (Ethics Committee) of the 3rd Xiangya Hospital, Central South University (No. 21028). The patients/participants provided their written informed consent to participate in this study.

AUTHOR CONTRIBUTIONS

The study was conceived and designed by QZhu. Statistical analyses were performed by XL and YC. Software package was prepared by QYZ and YD. Flow cytometry was performed by XL and HC. Manuscript was written by XL, HC, and QZhu. All authors contributed to the article and approved the submitted version.

ACKNOWLEDGMENTS

We thanked Ms. Hanying Liu from Department of Pulmonary Disease. the 3rd Xiangya Hospital of Central South University for supplying clinical samples.

REFERENCES

1. Martinez FJ, Collard HR, Pardo A, Raghu G, Richeldi L, Selman M, et al. Idiopathic Pulmonary Fibrosis. *Nat Rev Dis Primers* (2017) 3:17074. doi: 10.1038/nrdp.2017.74
2. du Bois RM, Weycker D, Albera C, Bradford WZ, Costabel U, Kartashov A, et al. Ascertainment of Individual Risk of Mortality for Patients With Idiopathic Pulmonary Fibrosis. *Am J Respir Crit Care Med* (2011) 184 (4):459–66. doi: 10.1164/rccm.201011-1790OC
3. Ley B, Ryerson CJ, Vittinghoff E, Ryu JH, Tomassetti S, Lee JS, et al. A Multidimensional Index and Staging System for Idiopathic Pulmonary Fibrosis. *Ann Intern Med* (2012) 156(10):684–91. doi: 10.7326/0003-4819-156-10-201205150-00004
4. Ley B, Bradford WZ, Weycker D, Vittinghoff E, du Bois RM, Collard HR. Unified Baseline and Longitudinal Mortality Prediction in Idiopathic Pulmonary Fibrosis. *Eur Respir J* (2015) 45(5):1374–81. doi: 10.1183/09031936.00146314
5. Kamiya H, Panlaqui OM. Systematic Review and Meta-Analysis of Prognostic Factors of Acute Exacerbation of Idiopathic Pulmonary Fibrosis. *BMJ Open* (2020) 10(6):e035420. doi: 10.1136/bmjopen-2019-035420
6. Richards TJ, Kaminski N, Baribaud F, Flavin S, Brodmerkel C, Horowitz D, et al. Peripheral Blood Proteins Predict Mortality in Idiopathic Pulmonary Fibrosis. *Am J Respir Crit Care Med* (2012) 185(1):67–76. doi: 10.1164/rccm.201101-0058OC
7. Li X, Zhou Y, Zou R, Chen H, Liu X, Qiu X, et al. Associations of Serological Biomarkers of Sicam-1, IL-1, MIF, and su-PAR With 3-Month Mortality in Acute Exacerbation of Idiopathic Pulmonary Fibrosis. *Mediators Inflamm* (2020) 2020:4534272. doi: 10.1155/2020/4534272
8. Ramírez-Aragón M, Hernández-Sánchez F, Rodríguez-Reyna TS, Buendía-Roldán I, Güitrón-Castillo G, Núñez-Alvarez CA, et al. The Transcription Factor SCX is a Potential Serum Biomarker of Fibrotic Diseases. *Int J Mol Sci* (2020) 21(14):5012. doi: 10.3390/ijms21145012
9. Wiertz IA, Moll SA, Seeliger B, Barlo NP, van der Vis JJ, Korthagen NM, et al. Genetic Variation in CCL18 Gene Influences Ccl18 Expression and Correlates With Survival in Idiopathic Pulmonary Fibrosis: Part a. *J Clin Med* (2020) 9 (6):1940. doi: 10.3390/jcm9061940
10. Prasse A, Binder H, Schupp JC, Kayser G, Bargagli E, Jaeger B, et al. Bal Cell Gene Expression is Indicative of Outcome and Airway Basal Cell Involvement in Idiopathic Pulmonary Fibrosis. *Am J Respir Crit Care Med* (2019) 199 (5):622–30. doi: 10.1164/rccm.201712-2551OC
11. Jee AS, Sahhar J, Youssef P, Bleasel J, Adelstein S, Nguyen M, et al. Review: Serum Biomarkers in Idiopathic Pulmonary Fibrosis and Systemic Sclerosis Associated Interstitial Lung Disease - Frontiers and Horizons. *Pharmacol Ther* (2019) 202:40–52. doi: 10.1016/j.pharmthera.2019.05.014
12. Harrell CR, Sadikot R, Pascual J, Fellabaum C, Jankovic MG, Jovicic N, et al. Mesenchymal Stem Cell-Based Therapy of Inflammatory Lung Diseases: Current Understanding and Future Perspectives. *Stem Cells Int* (2019) 2019:4236973. doi: 10.1155/2019/4236973
13. Landi C, Bargagli E, Carleo A, Bianchi L, Gagliardi A, Prasse A, et al. A System Biology Study of BALF From Patients Affected by Idiopathic Pulmonary Fibrosis (IPF) and Healthy Controls. *Proteomics Clin Appl* (2014) 8(11-12):932–50. doi: 10.1002/prca.201400001
14. Ornatowski W, Lu Q, Yegambaram M, Garcia AE, Zemskov EA, Maltepe E, et al. Complex Interplay Between Autophagy and Oxidative Stress in the Development of Pulmonary Disease. *Redox Biol* (2020) 36:101679. doi: 10.1016/j.redox.2020.101679
15. Steele MP, Luna LG, Coldren CD, Murphy E, Hennessy CE, Heinz D, et al. Relationship Between Gene Expression and Lung Function in Idiopathic Interstitial Pneumonias. *BMC Genomics* (2015) 16:869. doi: 10.1186/s12864-015-2102-3

16. Ritchie ME, Phipson B, Wu D, Hu Y, Law CW, Shi W, et al. Limma Powers Differential Expression Analyses for RNA-sequencing and Microarray Studies. *Nucleic Acids Res* (2015) 43(7):e47. doi: 10.1093/nar/gkv007
17. Yoshihara K, Shahmoradgoli M, Martínez E, Vegesna R, Kim H, Torres-Garcia W, et al. Inferring Tumour Purity and Stromal and Immune Cell Admixture From Expression Data. *Nat Commun* (2013) 4:2612. doi: 10.1038/ncomms3612
18. Newman AM, Liu CL, Green MR, Gentles AJ, Feng W, Xu Y, et al. Robust Enumeration of Cell Subsets From Tissue Expression Profiles. *Nat Methods* (2015) 12(5):453–7. doi: 10.1038/nmeth.3337
19. Liu X-Y, Liang Y, Xu Z-B, Zhang H, Leung K-S. Adaptive $L_1/_2$ Shooting Regularization Method for Survival Analysis Using Gene Expression Data. *ScientificWorldJournal* (2013) 2013:475702. doi: 10.1155/2013/475702
20. Huang da W, Sherman BT, Lempicki RA. Systematic and Integrative Analysis of Large Gene Lists Using DAVID Bioinformatics Resources. *Nat Protoc* (2009) 4(1):44–57. doi: 10.1038/nprot.2008.211
21. Wang Z, Qu S, Zhu J, Chen F, Ma L. Comprehensive Analysis of lncRNA-associated Competing Endogenous RNA Network and Immune Infiltration in Idiopathic Pulmonary Fibrosis. *J Thoracic Dis* (2020) 12(5):1856–65. doi: 10.21037/jtd-19-2842
22. Zhang M, Zhang S. T Cells in Fibrosis and Fibrotic Diseases. *Front Immunol* (2020) 11:1142. doi: 10.3389/fimmu.2020.01142
23. Shukla SD, Walters EH, Simpson JL, Keely S, Wark PAB, O'Toole RF, et al. Hypoxia-Inducible Factor and Bacterial Infections in Chronic Obstructive Pulmonary Disease. *Respirol (Carlton Vic)* (2020) 25(1):53–63. doi: 10.1111/resp.13722
24. Chen Z, Liu M, Li L, Chen L. Involvement of the Warburg Effect in non-Tumor Diseases Processes. *J Cell Physiol* (2018) 233(4):2839–49. doi: 10.1002/jcp.25998
25. Tzouvelekis A, Harokopos V, Paparountas T, Oikonomou N, Chatziioannou A, Vilaras G, et al. Comparative Expression Profiling in Pulmonary Fibrosis Suggests a Role of Hypoxia-Inducible factor-1alpha in Disease Pathogenesis. *Am J Respir Crit Care Med* (2007) 176(11):1108–19. doi: 10.1164/rccm.200705-683OC
26. Bargagli E, Refini RM, d'Alessandro M, Bergantini L, Cameli P, Vantaggiato L, et al. Metabolic Dysregulation in Idiopathic Pulmonary Fibrosis. *Int J Mol Sci* (2020) 21(16):5663. doi: 10.3390/ijms21165663
27. Contreras-Lopez R, Elizondo-Vega R, Paredes MJ, Luque-Campos N, Torres MJ, Tejedor G, et al. Hif1α-Dependent Metabolic Reprogramming Governs Mesenchymal Stem/Stromal Cell Immunoregulatory Functions. *FASEB J* (2020) 34(6):8250–64. doi: 10.1096/fj.201902232R
28. Delbrel E, Uzunhan Y, Soumare A, Gille T, Marchant D, Planès C, et al. Er Stress is Involved in Epithelial-To-Mesenchymal Transition of Alveolar Epithelial Cells Exposed to a Hypoxic Microenvironment. *Int J Mol Sci* (2019) 20(6):1299. doi: 10.3390/ijms20061299
29. Zhao X, Kwan JYY, Yip K, Liu PP, Liu FF. Targeting Metabolic Dysregulation for Fibrosis Therapy. *Nat Rev Drug Discov* (2020) 19(1):57–75. doi: 10.1038/s41573-019-0040-5
30. Aquino-Gálvez A, González-Ávila G, Jiménez-Sánchez LL, Maldonado-Martínez HA, Cisneros J, Toscano-Marquez F, et al. Dysregulated Expression of Hypoxia-Inducible Factors Augments Myofibroblasts Differentiation in Idiopathic Pulmonary Fibrosis. *Respir Res* (2019) 20 (1):130. doi: 10.1186/s12931-019-1100-4
31. Wang X, Lin L, Chai X, Wu Y, Li Y, Liu X. Hypoxic Mast Cells Accelerate the Proliferation, Collagen Accumulation and Phenotypic Alteration of Human Lung Fibroblasts. *Int J Mol Med* (2020) 45(1):175–85. doi: 10.3892/ijmm.2019.4400
32. Tsitoura E, Vasarmidi E, Bibaki E, Trachalaki A, Koutoulaki C, Papastratigakis G, et al. Accumulation of Damaged Mitochondria in Alveolar Macrophages With Reduced OXPHOS Related Gene Expression in IPF. *Respir Res* (2019) 20(1):264. doi: 10.1186/s12931-019-1196-6
33. Li C, Xu MM, Wang K, Adler AJ, Vella AT, Zhou B. Macrophage Polarization and Meta-Inflammation. *Trans Res J Lab Clin Med* (2018) 191:29–44. doi: 10.1016/j.trsl.2017.10.004
34. Wang C, Zhang C, Xu J, Li Y, Wang J, Liu H, et al. Association Between IL-1R2 Polymorphisms and Lung Cancer Risk in the Chinese Han Population: A Case-Control Study. *Mol Genet Genom Med* (2019) 7(5):e644. doi: 10.1002/mgg3.644
35. Zhang M, Zhu K, Pu H, Wang Z, Zhao H, Zhang J, et al. An Immune-Related Signature Predicts Survival in Patients With Lung Adenocarcinoma. *Front Oncol* (2019) 9:1314. doi: 10.3389/fonc.2019.01314
36. Yi G, Liang M, Li M, Fang X, Liu J, Lai Y, et al. A Large Lung Gene Expression Study Identifying IL1B as a Novel Player in Airway Inflammation in COPD Airway Epithelial Cells. *Inflammation Res* (2018) 67(6):539–51. doi: 10.1007/s00011-018-1145-8
37. Baines KJ, Fu JJ, McDonald VM, Gibson PG. Airway Gene Expression of IL-1 Pathway Mediators Predicts Exacerbation Risk in Obstructive Airway Disease. *Int J Chronic Obstructive Pulmonary Dis* (2017) 12:541–50. doi: 10.2147/copd.S119443
38. Zhang Z, Han N, Shen Y. S100A12 Promotes Inflammation and Cell Apoptosis in Sepsis-Induced ARDS Via Activation of NLRP3 Inflammasome Signaling. *Mol Immunol* (2020) 122:38–48. doi: 10.1016/j.molimm.2020.03.022
39. Lou Y, Zheng Y, Fan B, Zhang L, Zhu F, Wang X, et al. Serum S100A12 Levels are Correlated With Clinical Severity in Patients With Dermatomyositis-Associated Interstitial Lung Disease. *J Int Med Res* (2019) 48(4). doi: 10.1177/0300060519887841. 300060519887841.
40. Dai J, Huang YJ, He X, Zhao M, Wang X, Liu ZS, et al. Acetylation Blocks Cgas Activity and Inhibits Self-DNA-Induced Autoimmunity. *Cell* (2019) 176 (6):1447–60. doi: 10.1016/j.cell.2019.01.016. e14.
41. Mindt BC, Fritz JH. Next Stop: Perivasculature! ILC2s Hitch a Ride on the CCL8 Express. *Sci Immunol* (2019) 4(36). doi: 10.1126/sciimmunol.aax4583

11

Comorbid Conditions in Idiopathic Pulmonary Fibrosis: Recognition and Management

Justin M. Oldham[1] and Harold R. Collard[2]*

[1] Department of Medicine, Division of Pulmonary, Critical Care and Sleep Medicine, University of California at Davis, Davis, CA, United States, [2] Department of Medicine, Division of Pulmonary and Critical Care Medicine, University of California at San Francisco, San Francisco, CA, United States

***Correspondence:**
Justin M. Oldham
joldham@ucdavis.edu

Idiopathic pulmonary fibrosis (IPF), a fibrosing interstitial pneumonia of unknown etiology, primarily affects older adults and leads to a progressive decline in lung function and quality of life. With a median survival of 3–5 years, IPF is the most common and deadly of the idiopathic interstitial pneumonias. Despite the poor survivorship, there exists substantial variation in disease progression, making accurate prognostication difficult. Lung transplantation remains the sole curative intervention in IPF, but two anti-fibrotic therapies were recently shown to slow pulmonary function decline and are now approved for the treatment of IPF in many countries around the world. While the approval of these therapies represents an important first step in combatting of this devastating disease, a comprehensive approach to diagnosing and treating patients with IPF remains critically important. Included in this comprehensive assessment is the recognition and appropriate management of comorbid conditions. Though IPF is characterized by single organ involvement, many comorbid conditions occur within other organ systems. Common cardiovascular processes include coronary artery disease and pulmonary hypertension (PH), while gastroesophageal reflux and hiatal hernia are the most commonly encountered gastrointestinal disorders. Hematologic abnormalities appear to place patients with IPF at increased risk of venous thromboembolism, while diabetes mellitus (DM) and hypothyroidism are prevalent metabolic disorders. Several pulmonary comorbidities have also been linked to IPF, and include emphysema, lung cancer, and obstructive sleep apnea. While the treatment of some comorbid conditions, such as CAD, DM, and hypothyroidism is recommended irrespective of IPF, the benefit of treating others, such as gastroesophageal reflux and PH, remains unclear. In this review, we highlight common comorbid conditions encountered in IPF, discuss disease-specific diagnostic modalities, and review the current state of treatment data for several key comorbidities.

Keywords: idiopathic pulmonary fibrosis, idiopathic interstitial pneumonia, interstitial lung disease, pulmonary fibrosis, co-morbidity

INTRODUCTION

Idiopathic Pulmonary Fibrosis (IPF), a fibrosing interstitial lung disease (ILD) of unknown etiology, primarily affects older adults and leads to a progressive decline in lung function and quality of life (1–4). With an estimated prevalence of 18–63 cases per 100,000 and median survival of 3–5 years (5, 6), IPF remains the most common and deadly of the idiopathic interstitial pneumonias (IIPs).

Despite poor survivorship, there exists substantial variability in disease progression, whereby most patients experience a steady clinical decline, some remain stable over many years and others die from rapidly progressive disease (3, 7, 8). Lung transplantation remains the sole curative intervention for IPF, but two anti-fibrotic therapies were recently shown to slow pulmonary function decline in phase III clinical trials (9–11). *Post hoc* analyses of clinical trial datasets also suggest that anti-fibrotic therapy may reduce the risk of acute exacerbations and improve overall survival in those with IPF (12–14).

While the identification of therapies that effectively slow IPF progression represents a monumental step forward in the care of patients with IPF, pharmacotherapy is but one component of the multi-pronged approach necessary to optimally manage patients with IPF. Other equally important pieces include evidence-based prognostication (15) improvement of functional status with formal pulmonary rehabilitation and supplemental oxygen (where appropriate), patient education with regard to IPF pathobiology, natural history, and clinical trial availability, and management of common comorbidities (4, 16). In this review, we highlight common comorbidities encountered in IPF, discuss diagnostic and screening modalities, and review the current state of treatment data for such conditions.

PULMONARY COMORBIDITIES

Emphysema

Roughly 70–80% of individuals with IPF endorse a history of cigarette smoking, which has long been an established IPF risk factor (17–20). Not surprisingly, about 30% of IPF patients have concurrent pulmonary emphysema (21, 22), including 8–27% with ≥10% emphysematous involvement throughout the lungs (**Figure 1**) (22, 23). The syndrome of combined pulmonary fibrosis and emphysema (CPFE) has recently gained recognition as a potentially unique IPF phenotype (24). Individuals with CPFE tend to be males with an extensive smoking history and increased oxygen requirement (21–24). Pulmonary function testing in these individuals often shows relatively preserved total lung capacity and forced vital capacity (FVC), with a disproportionate reduction in diffusion capacity (DLCO) (**Figure 2**) (21, 22, 24). These physiologic hallmarks of CPFE likely reflect the opposing impact of parenchymal fibrosis and parenchymal destruction on airflow and lung volumes, along with additive impact on gas exchange.

High-resolution computed tomography (HRCT) is part of the routine diagnostic evaluation of all patients with suspected IPF (4), and routine semi-quantitative assessment of emphysematous involvement may help readily identify those with CPFE once a diagnostic consensus is established. The recognition of CPFE has potential management implications. Some studies suggest that CPFE is associated with reduced survival (21, 23, 25), but others have not replicated this observation (22, 26). Paradoxically, patients with CPFE appear to have a slower rate of FVC decline, perhaps due to the impact of emphysema on the manner in which FVC reflects progressive fibrosis (27). An increased prevalence of pulmonary hypertension (PH) has also been demonstrated among those with CPFE (22, 23), which may also impact survival (23, 24). Treatment of patients with IPF and CPFE with inhaled long-acting anti-cholinergic, inhaled long-acting beta-agonist and/or inhaled corticosteroids is of unclear benefit (21, 24). We believe that clinicians should consider the addition of these therapies according to chronic obstructive pulmonary disease consensus guidelines (28).

Lung Cancer

Compared to those in the general population, individuals with IPF have a nearly 5-fold increased risk of developing lung cancer, with 3–22% of patients affected and an estimated incidence of 11 cases per 100,000 person-years (29–32). The annual lung cancer risk also appears to rise in the years following IPF diagnosis (32), which was supported by an autopsy study that identified concurrent pulmonary malignancy in nearly 50% of cases with histologic UIP (33). The strong link between IPF and cigarette smoking history (17) likely explains a portion of the increased lung cancer risk, as the overwhelming majority of patients with IPF who develop lung cancer endorse such a history (32–34). The higher prevalence of lung cancer among those with CPFE compared to lone IPF also supports this observation (34–36).

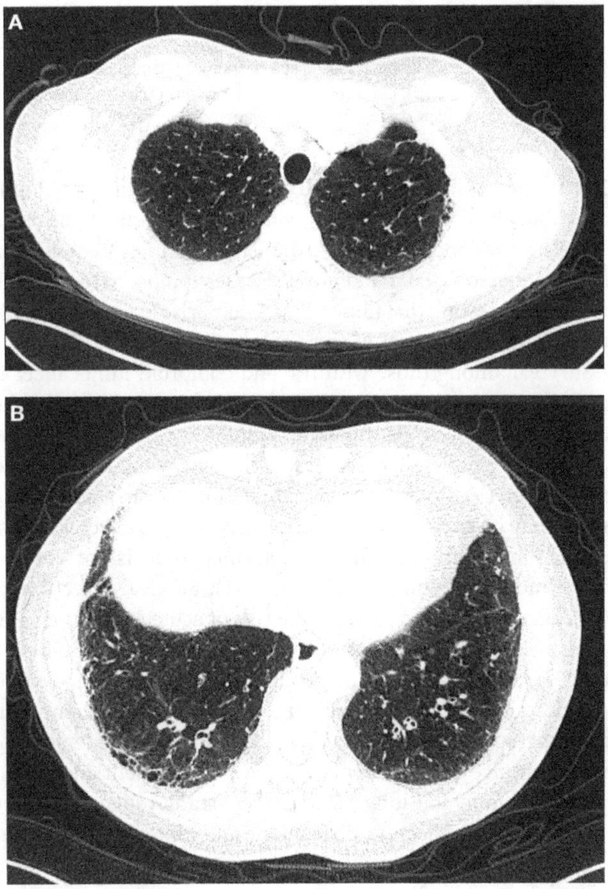

FIGURE 1 | High-resolution computed tomography findings in a patient, with combined pulmonary fibrosis and emphysema. Centrilobular emphysema is observed on apical views **(A)** and basilar predominant sub-pleural reticulation and honeycombing characteristic of UIP is observed on basilar views **(B)**.

A

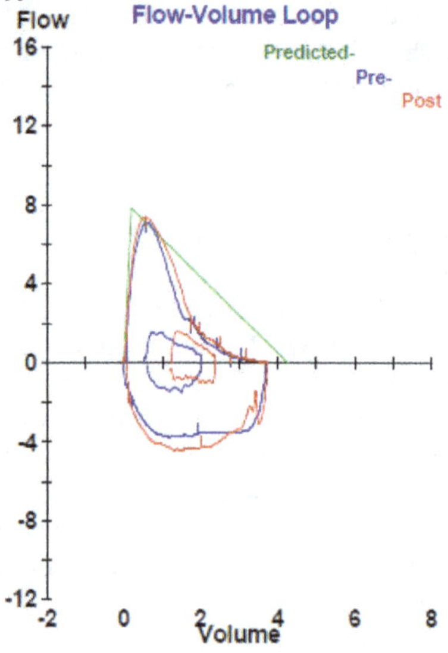

B

		Ref	C.I. (95)	Pre	% Ref	Post	% Ref
Spirometry							
FVC	Liters	4.27	(3.3 - 5.2)	3.70	87	3.74	87
FEV1	Liters	3.09	(2.3 - 3.9)	2.44	79	2.57	83
FEV1/FVC	%	72	(62.7 - 82.0)	66		69	
FEV3	Liters			3.07		3.19	
FEV3/FVC	%			83		85	
FEV6	Liters	4.01	(3.1 - 4.9)	3.41	85	3.52	88
FEV1/FEV6	%	77	(67.9 - 85.8)	72		73	
FEF25-75%	L/sec	2.22	(0.6 - 3.8)	1.16	52	1.42	64
PEF	L/sec	7.82	(5.5 - 10.2)	7.13	91	7.46	95
FET100%	Sec			12.30		11.16	
FIVC	Liters			3.71		3.67	
PIF	L/sec			3.75		4.40	
Lung Volumes							
TLC	Liters	7.14	(5.5 - 8.7)	5.77	81		
VC	Liters	4.27	(3.3 - 5.2)	3.73	87		
IC	Liters	2.95	(2.2 - 3.7)	2.35	80		
FRC PL	Liters	3.84	(2.4 - 5.3)	3.42	89		
ERV	Liters	1.47	(1.1 - 1.8)	1.38	94		
RV	Liters	2.60	(1.8 - 3.4)	2.04	78		
RV/TLC	%	38	(28.7 - 46.3)	35			
Diffusing Capacity							
DLCO	mL/mmHg/min	26.4	(19.5 - 33.3)			4.9	18
DL Adj	mL/mmHg/min	26.4	(19.5 - 33.4)			4.9	18
DL/VA Adj	mL/mHg/min/L	3.66				1.03	28
VA	Liters	7.22	(6.1 - 8.4)			4.75	66

FIGURE 2 | Pulmonary function testing in a patient with combined pulmonary fibrosis and emphysema. Flow volume loop **(A)** shows mild obstructive morphology, but normal spirometry **(B)**. Lung volumes **(B)** are normal. Diffusion capacity **(B)** is markedly reduced.

Most studies show squamous cell carcinoma to slightly predominate over adenocarcinoma (37), while a recent investigation of IPF-related adenocarcinomas demonstrated a high frequency of bronchiole-associated markers in IPF cases compared to non-IPF controls, suggesting that these tumors may arise from abnormally proliferating bronchioles in areas of honeycomb cyst (38).

Survival among those with IPF and comorbid lung cancer is poor (34, 39) and often stems from malignancy-related clinical deterioration, as similar rates of pulmonary function decline have been demonstrated in those with and without comorbid lung cancer (34). While surgical resection of early stage lung cancer may be curative, IPF severity and disease trajectory must be taken into consideration, given an increased risk of postoperative morbidity and mortality (40, 41). Surgical resection of lung cancer appears to increase the risk of acute exacerbation in patients with IPF, which has been reported in 7–32% of patients (42–45). Acute exacerbation and clinical deterioration have also been described in patients with IPF undergoing treatment with chemotherapy (46, 47) and radiation therapy (48), underscoring the importance of patient education and risk/benefit analysis in those with inoperable lung cancer. Recent studies suggest that the anti-proliferative effects of pirfenidone and nintedanib may synergize with current chemotherapeutic regimens, but additional research is needed (37, 49, 50).

As for emphysema, HRCT serves as a reasonable modality for lung cancer screening, but many HRCT protocols still perform non-contiguous imaging, which can miss early nodules and other local changes; contiguous imaging is required (4). Most lung cancers identified are incidental, with a large minority having a potential surgical cure (34, 39). As such, we believe clinicians should consider annual lung cancer screening with low-dose computed tomography (51) in high-risk patients with IPF, including those with CPFE and/or longstanding smoking history. Clinicians should also maintain a low threshold for repeat imaging in those who experience clinical worsening despite stable pulmonary function or develop symptoms atypical for IPF.

Obstructive Sleep Apnea (OSA)

Preliminary studies suggest that OSA may be an underappreciated comorbid condition in those with IPF. Three investigations have shown OSA to be present in 58–88% of patients with IPF, with up to 68% having moderate-to-severe OSA based on an apnea–hypopnea index ≥15 events/hour (52–54). In addition, severe sleep apnea was recently shown to be strongly associated with ischemic heart disease in patients with IPF (54). Despite this potential high prevalence, few IPF patients are evaluated for OSA. A retrospective investigation of IPF patients showed that less than 3% of patients were referred for polysomnography (55). Untreated OSA can result in nocturnal hypoxemia, the presence of which was recently shown to predict worsened survival in patients with IPF (56). Nocturnal hypoxemia strongly correlates with an increased right ventricular systolic pressure (RVSP) (56), which may reflect PH (57).

As with the general population, moderate-to-severe OSA is generally treated with continuous positive airway pressure (CPAP). CPAP initiation has been shown to improve quality of life measures and sleep instruments in those with IPF and comorbid moderate-to-severe OSA, though CPAP non-adherence was common (58). The optimal tool for OSA screening in patients with IPF has yet to be determined, as commonly utilized OSA screening tools, including the Epworth sleepiness scale and Sleep Apnea Scale for Sleep Disorders Questionnaire, did not differentiate IPF patients with and without OSA in a recent prospective investigation (52). Until an effective screening tool is established, clinicians should maintain a low threshold for polysomnography referral in patients with IPF.

CARDIOVASCULAR COMORBIDITIES

Coronary Artery Disease (CAD)

Idiopathic pulmonary fibrosis and CAD share several risk factors, including increasing age, male gender, and smoking history. Among the largest retrospective studies conducted to date, the estimated prevalence of CAD in those with IPF ranges from 4 to 25% (59–63). A prevalence of up to 68% was described in a cohort of 73 IPF patients who underwent cardiac catheterization as part of a lung transplant work-up (64). Among these individuals, 18% of patients had significant CAD, defined as >50% stenosis of a major coronary vessel on cardiac catheterization or need for percutaneous coronary intervention. Longitudinal analyses have suggested that 7% of patients will develop CAD in the years following IPF diagnosis (63) and that such patients have a 3-fold higher risk of experiencing acute coronary syndrome compared to non-IPF control subjects (61).

The U.S. Preventative Services Task Force concluded that there was insufficient evidence to recommend for or against routine CAD screening in asymptomatic, high-risk individuals in the general population (65). Among symptomatic patients, the American Heart Association suggests that cardiac CT may be a reasonable modality for CAD screening, as the presence of coronary calcifications is a reliable predictor of CAD (66). Because HRCT is recommended for all patients with IPF, the assessment of coronary artery calcification may provide a reliable tool for non-invasive CAD screening in this high-risk population. A study of 57 patients with IPF who underwent cardiac catheterization showed that the presence of moderate-to-severe coronary calcifications had a sensitivity and specificity of >80% for detecting CAD (67). Because significant CAD has been associated with worse survival in patients with IPF (64), clinicians should consider a cardiology referral in patients with angina or moderate-to-severe coronary calcifications on HRCT.

Pulmonary Hypertension

Pulmonary hypertension defined as mean pulmonary artery pressure (mPAP) ≥25 mm Hg (68), commonly complicates IPF, especially as the disease progresses. The true prevalence of PH in those with IPF is difficult to ascertain, as estimates vary widely based on case finding methodology and the IPF population under consideration. A PH prevalence as low as 3% has been reported in patients with IPF using insurance claims data (62) and as high as 84% using transthoracic echocardiogram (TTE) (69). A prevalence of 29–46% has been reported in studies utilizing right heart catheterization, which remains the gold standard for PH detection (60, 68, 70–75). However, these studies may overestimate the true prevalence, as the majority of patients included in these studies underwent right heart catheterization as part of a lung transplant evaluation, suggesting that many had advanced disease.

Pulmonary hypertension should be suspected in patients with dyspnea or oxygen desaturation out of proportion to pulmonary function, disproportionately low DLCO, evidence of right heart failure on physical exam, or evidence of pulmonary artery enlargement and/or right ventricular hypertrophy on imaging studies. TTE, which estimates RVSP as a surrogate for mPAP, is perhaps the most commonly utilized modality to screen for PH. Although TTE-estimated RVSP has been shown to correlate poorly with mPAP determined by right heart catheterization (73, 76), an RVSP >35 mm Hg has been shown to have a sensitivity of >85% for detecting PH in patients with IPF (73). Unfortunately, the specificity of this RVSP cut-off is only 29%, so clinicians should expect a large number of false positives if using this threshold for triggering right heart catheterization. The decision to refer a patient for cardiac catheterization when TTE suggests the presence of PH should be made on a case-by-case basis.

There are currently no approved therapies for the treatment of PH in patients with IPF and the last decade has seen a disappointing number of negative clinical trials using vasodilator therapies. Several studies have investigated the use of PH therapies for IPF in general (regardless of the presence of PH) and failed to demonstrate efficacy in slowing IPF progression (77–79), and did not alter cardiovascular hemodynamics in those with concurrent PH (80, 81). A small trial of ambrisentan in patients with IPF and right heart catheterization-proven PH (NCT00879229) was stopped after a parent trial of ambrisentan showed no benefit in the subgroup of IPF patients with known PH (78). A similar trial of riociguat (NCT02138825), a soluble guanylate cyclase stimulator, was also terminated after interim analysis showed that those in the intervention arm had an increased risk of death and other serious adverse events.

The phosphodiesterase-5 inhibitor sildenafil was studied in patients with advanced IPF (defined by a baseline DLCO of less than 35%). While it did not significantly alter the primary functional endpoint of walk distance, it did show improvements in dyspnea score, oxygenation, and quality of life (82). A *post hoc* subgroup analysis of patients with evidence of PH by TTE showed that sildenafil therapy did improve walk distance as well (83). Based on these data, clinical trials investigating sildenafil in combination with anti-fibrotic therapy for patients with IPF-associated PH (NCT02951429, NCT02802345) are currently enrolling. The most recent evidence-based guidelines conditionally recommend against the routine use of sildenafil in patients with IPF until randomized controlled trials provide more definitive data (16).

Pulmonary Embolism (PE)/Venous Thromboembolism (VTE)

Relatively few studies have assessed the epidemiology and clinical consequences of PE and more broadly VTE in patients with IPF. A study utilizing U.S. insurance claims data suggested that 2.7% of individuals with a diagnosis code for IPF also carried a diagnosis of PE (62). Another U.S. insurance claims-based investigation showed that among decedents with a diagnosis of IPF, 1.7% had concurrent VTE (84). These estimates were supported by a case–control analysis conducted in the U.K., which reported a VTE prevalence of 2% in their IPF population, which was 2-fold higher than that observed among non-IPF control subjects (61). Danish investigators showed that individuals previously diagnosed with a VTE were at increased risk of developing incident IIP, suggesting that VTE may be a risk factor for IPF and other IIPs (85).

Longitudinal analyses of patients with IPF suggest that the risk of incident VTE is 3–6 times higher among patients with IPF compared to control subjects, with an estimated 6–9 new events per 1,000 person-years (61, 86). As such, clinicians should maintain a low threshold for PE evaluation in patients with progressive symptoms in the setting of stable pulmonary function metrics. PE should also be excluded in patients with acute or subacute clinical worsening, as this often indicates an acute exacerbation (87). A multi-phase HRCT with and without contrast enhancement should be considered to optimally assess the pulmonary vasculature and parenchyma. Lower extremity duplex ultrasound can be considered for patients with a contrast allergy and in those too unstable to undergo HRCT.

The treatment of PE/VTE requires prolonged blockade of the coagulation cascade, which facilitates clot resolution. The American College of Chest Physicians recommend 3 months of anticoagulant therapy in those with VTE provoked by surgery or other known VTE risk factor. These guidelines also recommend at least 3 months of anticoagulant therapy in patients with a first-time unprovoked VTE, after which time the risk–benefit ratio for extended therapy should be considered (88). This assessment is of particular importance in patients with IPF, as warfarin therapy was shown to increase the risk of death in a general population of IPF patients (excluding those who required anticoagulation for a non-IPF indication) (89). Warfarin therapy has also been linked to worse outcomes in uncontrolled studies, including a recent *post hoc* analysis of IPF clinical trial datasets (90, 91). These findings raise the question of whether warfarin therapy should be used in patients with IPF who require anticoagulation for comorbid diseases (e.g. PE, atrial fibrillation). More research is needed to determine the optimal therapy and duration of therapy for patients with IPF with an indication for anticoagulation.

GASTROINTESTINAL COMORBIDITIES

Gastro-Esophageal Reflux (GER)

Gastro-esophageal reflux is another common comorbid condition in patients with IPF (92), but the true prevalence of GER in patients with IPF is difficult to ascertain. Several large epidemiological studies have suggested a prevalence of 30–50% (19, 93, 94), but studies that utilized esophageal pH monitoring suggest that GER may affect over 80% of individuals with IPF (95, 96). Complicating estimates further is the fact that some individuals have silent GER (95) and other primarily non-acid GER (97).

The ideal modality for diagnosing GER remains unclear. While all patients should be screened for GER-associated symptoms, including heartburn, choking, and regurgitation, symptom-based screening has a low sensitivity for detecting pathologic GER (95, 98). Fluoroscopic barium swallow testing can detect GER and microaspiration, but this also suffers from poor sensitivity (99, 100). Gastro-esophageal scintigraphy can detect GER with 80% sensitivity but is not a widely available (101). Esophageal pH monitoring remains the gold standard for diagnosing acid GER, with a reported sensitivity and specificity of over 80% (102, 103). Recent studies suggest that multi-channel intraluminal esophageal impedance testing may be a superior modality for detecting both acid and non-acid GER, but this modality is not widely available at present (103, 104).

It has been hypothesized that GER may contribute to the progression of IPF in some patients. Several studies, with mixed results, have explored the influence of anti-acid therapy on IPF disease course. GER therapy was associated with improved survival in a retrospective, multi-center cohort analysis (19) and less pulmonary function decline in a *post hoc* analysis of three clinical trial datasets (105). These findings were not replicated in a recent *post hoc* analysis of a separate clinical trial dataset (106). Additional data evaluating the efficacy of both medical and surgical GER therapy in patients with IPF are expected in the near future as two phase II clinical trials are underway (NC02085018; NCT01982968).

Hiatal Hernia (HH)

A likely contributor to the high prevalence of GER in patients with IPF is HH, which has been described in 40–53% of patients with IPF (107, 108). While an increasing degree of HH is likely to result in GER symptoms, mild HH can be asymptomatic (108). HH can be identified on HRCT mediastinal views and does not require dedicated imaging. HH treatment largely focuses on GER-associated symptom control, but surgical correction should be considered in patients with refractory symptoms. A retrospective investigation of patients awaiting lung transplantation showed that Nissen fundoplication was well tolerated and was associated with stabilization of oxygen levels in this patient population (109).

ENDOCRINE/METABOLIC COMORBIDITIES

Hypothyroidism

While 1–2% of men and 5–9% of women in the general population carry a diagnosis of hypothyroidism (110–112), a recent case–control analysis demonstrated a substantially higher prevalence among individuals with IPF, with 13% of men and 28% of women affected (20). Furthermore, those with combined IPF and hypothyroidism had reduced survival compared to those with IPF alone. The biology underpinning an increased prevalence of hypothyroidism in IPF remains unclear, but because autoimmune thyroiditis is the most common cause of hypothyroidism in developed nations (110–112), aberrant immune activation in IPF may play a role.

Diabetes Mellitus (DM)

Case–control analyses performed in Japan, Mexico, and the U.K. estimated the prevalence of DM type 2 to be 10–33%, among

TABLE 1 | Common comorbidities in patients with idiopathic pulmonary fibrosis.

Comorbidity	Prevalence (%)	Outcome association
Emphysema	8–34	Mixed results; may increase mortality risk Increased prevalence of pulmonary hypertension (PH)
Lung cancer	3–22	Increased mortality risk Surgical resection may increase mortality and acute exacerbation risk Chemotherapy may increase acute exacerbation risk
Obstructive sleep apnea	58–88	May increase mortality risk through worsening nocturnal hypoxemia
Coronary artery disease	4–68	May increase mortality risk
PH	3–84	Increases mortality risk
Pulmonary embolism/venous thromboembolism	2–3	Treatment with anti-coagulation may increase mortality risk
Gastro-esophageal reflux	30–80	Mixed results; treatment with antacid therapy may improve survival and reduce disease progression
Hiatal hernia	40–53	Surgical correction may improve survival and stabilize oxygenation in patients awaiting transplant
Hypothyroidism	13–28	May increase mortality risk
Diabetes mellitus type 2	10–33	Unknown
Depression	12–49	Unknown
Anxiety	10	Unknown

individuals with IPF, which was significantly higher than that of matched control populations (18, 93, 113). These findings persisted after exclusion of individuals treated with systemic corticosteroid therapy, which is known to alter glucose levels (18, 93). Outcome data were not reported in these studies, so it remains unclear whether the presence of DM influences survival in patients with IPF.

MENTAL HEALTH COMORBIDITIES

Depression and Anxiety

Idiopathic pulmonary fibrosis progression commonly manifests as worsening dyspnea, declining pulmonary function, and hypoxemia. While these manifestations undoubtedly impact quality of life, they have been shown to correlate with depression and anxiety (114–116). Despite these findings, few epidemiologic studies of mental health comorbidities have been performed in IPF. While 3.4% of patients with a diagnosis code for IPF also had a diagnosis code for depression in an investigation of insurance claims (62), IPF cohort studies suggest a prevalence of 12–49% (115, 116). Anxiety was shown to affect approximately 10% of IPF patients in a single center study (116).

A small IPF cohort study based in Europe suggested that increasing duration of disease correlates with standardized depression scores (117), while an ILD cohort study based in Australia showed that an increasing number of comorbid conditions also correlates with increasing depression scores (116). The impact of depression and anxiety on outcomes remains unclear in IPF. In addition, the ideal screening tool to detect depression and anxiety in this patient population has yet to be validated.

CONCLUSION

Idiopathic pulmonary fibrosis remains a devastating diagnosis for patients and their families, and its management requires a multi-pronged approach. Comorbidity assessment and management is a cornerstone of comprehensive management of IPF and we have reviewed the most commonly associated comorbidities that clinicians should consider (**Table 1**). Aggressive management of comorbidities is promoted by IPF centers of excellence across the country and may explain some of the improved survival associated with these centers (118). We strongly believe that proper comorbidity assessment and management can improve quality of life and has the potential to improve patient survival in IPF.

AUTHOR CONTRIBUTIONS

JO and HC contributed to the conception and writing of this review. Both authors have reviewed and approved the submitted work.

REFERENCES

1. De Vries J, Kessels BL, Drent M. Quality of life of idiopathic pulmonary fibrosis patients. *Eur Respir J* (2001) 17(5):954–61. doi:10.1183/09031936.01.17509540
2. Tomioka H, Imanaka K, Hashimoto K, Iwasaki H. Health-related quality of life in patients with idiopathic pulmonary fibrosis – cross-sectional and longitudinal study. *Intern Med* (2007) 46(18):1533–42. doi:10.2169/internalmedicine.46.6218
3. Nathan SD, Shlobin OA, Weir N, Ahmad S, Kaldjob JM, Battle E, et al. Long-term course and prognosis of idiopathic pulmonary fibrosis in the new millennium. *Chest* (2011) 140(1):221–9. doi:10.1378/chest.10-2572
4. Raghu G, Collard HR, Egan JJ, Martinez FJ, Behr J, Brown KK, et al. An official ATS/ERS/JRS/ALAT statement: idiopathic pulmonary fibrosis: evidence-based guidelines for diagnosis and management. *Am J Respir Crit Care Med* (2011) 183(6):788–824. doi:10.1164/rccm.2009-040GL
5. Fernandez Perez ER, Daniels CE, Schroeder DR, St Sauver J, Hartman TE, Bartholmai BJ, et al. Incidence, prevalence, and clinical course of idiopathic pulmonary fibrosis: a population-based study. *Chest* (2010) 137(1):129–37. doi:10.1378/chest.09-1002
6. Raghu G, Chen SY, Hou Q, Yeh WS, Collard HR. Incidence and prevalence of idiopathic pulmonary fibrosis in US adults 18-64 years old. *Eur Respir J* (2016) 48(1):179–86. doi:10.1183/13993003.01653-2015
7. Selman M, Carrillo G, Estrada A, Mejia M, Becerril C, Cisneros J, et al. Accelerated variant of idiopathic pulmonary fibrosis: clinical behavior and gene expression pattern. *PLoS One* (2007) 2(5):e482. doi:10.1371/journal.pone.0000482
8. Ley B, Collard HR, King TE Jr. Clinical course and prediction of survival in idiopathic pulmonary fibrosis. *Am J Respir Crit Care Med* (2011) 183(4):431–40. doi:10.1164/rccm.201006-0894CI
9. Noble PW, Albera C, Bradford WZ, Costabel U, Glassberg MK, Kardatzke D, et al. Pirfenidone in patients with idiopathic pulmonary fibrosis (CAPACITY):

two randomised trials. *Lancet* (2011) 377(9779):1760–9. doi:10.1016/S0140-6736(11)60405-4

10. King TE Jr, Bradford WZ, Castro-Bernardini S, Fagan EA, Glaspole I, Glassberg MK, et al. A phase 3 trial of pirfenidone in patients with idiopathic pulmonary fibrosis. *N Engl J Med* (2014) 370(22):2083–92. doi:10.1056/NEJMoa1402582
11. Richeldi L, du Bois RM, Raghu G, Azuma A, Brown KK, Costabel U, et al. Efficacy and safety of nintedanib in idiopathic pulmonary fibrosis. *N Engl J Med* (2014) 370(22):2071–82. doi:10.1056/NEJMoa1402584
12. Noble PW, Albera C, Bradford WZ, Costabel U, du Bois RM, Fagan EA, et al. Pirfenidone for idiopathic pulmonary fibrosis: analysis of pooled data from three multinational phase 3 trials. *Eur Respir J* (2016) 47(1):243–53. doi:10.1183/13993003.00026-2015
13. Richeldi L, Cottin V, du Bois RM, Selman M, Kimura T, Bailes Z, et al. Nintedanib in patients with idiopathic pulmonary fibrosis: combined evidence from the TOMORROW and INPULSIS((R)) trials. *Respir Med* (2016) 113:74–9. doi:10.1016/j.rmed.2016.02.001
14. Nathan SD, Albera C, Bradford WZ, Costabel U, Glaspole I, Glassberg MK, et al. Effect of pirfenidone on mortality: pooled analyses and meta-analyses of clinical trials in idiopathic pulmonary fibrosis. *Lancet Respir Med* (2017) 5(1):33–41. doi:10.1016/S2213-2600(16)30326-5
15. Ley B, Ryerson CJ, Vittinghoff E, Ryu JH, Tomassetti S, Lee JS, et al. A multidimensional index and staging system for idiopathic pulmonary fibrosis. *Ann Intern Med* (2012) 156(10):684–91. doi:10.1059/0003-4819-156-10-201205150-00004
16. Raghu G, Rochwerg B, Zhang Y, Garcia CA, Azuma A, Behr J, et al. An official ATS/ERS/JRS/ALAT clinical practice guideline: treatment of idiopathic pulmonary fibrosis. An update of the 2011 clinical practice guideline. *Am J Respir Crit Care Med* (2015) 192(2):e3–19. doi:10.1164/rccm.201506-1063ST
17. Baumgartner KB, Samet JM, Stidley CA, Colby TV, Waldron JA. Cigarette smoking: a risk factor for idiopathic pulmonary fibrosis. *Am J Respir Crit Care Med* (1997) 155(1):242–8. doi:10.1164/ajrccm.155.1.9001319
18. Enomoto T, Usuki J, Azuma A, Nakagawa T, Kudoh S. Diabetes mellitus may increase risk for idiopathic pulmonary fibrosis. *Chest* (2003) 123(6):2007–11. doi:10.1378/chest.123.6.2007
19. Lee JS, Ryu JH, Elicker BM, Lydell CP, Jones KD, Wolters PJ, et al. Gastroesophageal reflux therapy is associated with longer survival in patients with idiopathic pulmonary fibrosis. *Am J Respir Crit Care Med* (2011) 184(12):1390–4. doi:10.1164/rccm.201101-0138OC
20. Oldham JM, Kumar D, Lee C, Patel SB, Takahashi-Manns S, Demchuk C, et al. Thyroid disease is prevalent and predicts survival in patients with idiopathic pulmonary fibrosis. *Chest* (2015) 148(3):692–700. doi:10.1378/chest.14-2714
21. Kurashima K, Takayanagi N, Tsuchiya N, Kanauchi T, Ueda M, Hoshi T, et al. The effect of emphysema on lung function and survival in patients with idiopathic pulmonary fibrosis. *Respirology* (2010) 15(5):843–8. doi:10.1111/j.1440-1843.2010.01778.x
22. Ryerson CJ, Hartman T, Elicker BM, Ley B, Lee JS, Abbritti M, et al. Clinical features and outcomes in combined pulmonary fibrosis and emphysema in idiopathic pulmonary fibrosis. *Chest* (2013) 144(1):234–40. doi:10.1378/chest.12-2403
23. Mejia M, Carrillo G, Rojas-Serrano J, Estrada A, Suarez T, Alonso D, et al. Idiopathic pulmonary fibrosis and emphysema: decreased survival associated with severe pulmonary arterial hypertension. *Chest* (2009) 136(1):10–5. doi:10.1378/chest.08-2306
24. Cottin V, Nunes H, Brillet PY, Delaval P, Devouassoux G, Tillie-Leblond I, et al. Combined pulmonary fibrosis and emphysema: a distinct underrecognised entity. *Eur Respir J* (2005) 26(4):586–93. doi:10.1183/09031936.05.00021005
25. Kohashi Y, Arai T, Sugimoto C, Tachibana K, Akira M, Kitaichi M, et al. Clinical impact of emphysema evaluated by high-resolution computed tomography on idiopathic pulmonary fibrosis diagnosed by surgical lung biopsy. *Respiration* (2016) 92(4):220–8. doi:10.1159/000448118
26. Jankowich MD, Rounds S. Combined pulmonary fibrosis and emphysema alters physiology but has similar mortality to pulmonary fibrosis without emphysema. *Lung* (2010) 188(5):365–73. doi:10.1007/s00408-010-9251-6
27. Cottin V, Hansell DM, Sverzellati N, Weycker D, Antoniou KM, Atwood M, et al. Effect of emphysema extent on serial lung function in patients with idiopathic pulmonary fibrosis. *Am J Respir Crit Care Med* (2017). doi:10.1164/rccm.201612-2492OC
28. Qaseem A, Wilt TJ, Weinberger SE, Hanania NA, Criner G, van der Molen T, et al. Diagnosis and management of stable chronic obstructive pulmonary disease: a clinical practice guideline update from the American College of Physicians, American College of Chest Physicians, American Thoracic Society, and European Respiratory Society. *Ann Intern Med* (2011) 155(3):179–91. doi:10.7326/0003-4819-155-3-201108020-00008
29. Hubbard R, Venn A, Lewis S, Britton J. Lung cancer and cryptogenic fibrosing alveolitis. A population-based cohort study. *Am J Respir Crit Care Med* (2000) 161(1):5–8. doi:10.1164/ajrccm.161.1.9906062
30. Park J, Kim DS, Shim TS, Lim CM, Koh Y, Lee SD, et al. Lung cancer in patients with idiopathic pulmonary fibrosis. *Eur Respir J* (2001) 17(6):1216–9. doi:10.1183/09031936.01.99055301
31. Le Jeune I, Gribbin J, West J, Smith C, Cullinan P, Hubbard R. The incidence of cancer in patients with idiopathic pulmonary fibrosis and sarcoidosis in the UK. *Respir Med* (2007) 101(12):2534–40. doi:10.1016/j.rmed.2007.07.012
32. Ozawa Y, Suda T, Naito T, Enomoto N, Hashimoto D, Fujisawa T, et al. Cumulative incidence of and predictive factors for lung cancer in IPF. *Respirology* (2009) 14(5):723–8. doi:10.1111/j.1440-1843.2009.01547.x
33. Matsushita H, Tanaka S, Saiki Y, Hara M, Nakata K, Tanimura S, et al. Lung cancer associated with usual interstitial pneumonia. *Pathol Int* (1995) 45(12):925–32. doi:10.1111/j.1440-1827.1995.tb03417.x
34. Tomassetti S, Gurioli C, Ryu JH, Decker PA, Ravaglia C, Tantalocco P, et al. The impact of lung cancer on survival of idiopathic pulmonary fibrosis. *Chest* (2015) 147(1):157–64. doi:10.1378/chest.14-0359
35. Usui K, Tanai C, Tanaka Y, Noda H, Ishihara T. The prevalence of pulmonary fibrosis combined with emphysema in patients with lung cancer. *Respirology* (2011) 16(2):326–31. doi:10.1111/j.1440-1843.2010.01907.x
36. Koo HJ, Do KH, Lee JB, Alblushi S, Lee SM. Lung cancer in combined pulmonary fibrosis and emphysema: a systematic review and meta-analysis. *PLoS One* (2016) 11(9):e0161437. doi:10.1371/journal.pone.0161437
37. Karampitsakos T, Tzilas V, Tringidou R, Steiropoulos P, Aidinis V, Papiris SA, et al. Lung cancer in patients with idiopathic pulmonary fibrosis. *Pulm Pharmacol Ther* (2017). doi:10.1016/j.pupt.2017.03.016
38. Calio A, Lever V, Rossi A, Gilioli E, Brunelli M, Dubini A, et al. Increased frequency of bronchiolar histotypes in lung carcinomas associated with idiopathic pulmonary fibrosis. *Histopathology* (2017). doi:10.1111/his.13269
39. Aubry MC, Myers JL, Douglas WW, Tazelaar HD, Washington Stephens TL, Hartman TE, et al. Primary pulmonary carcinoma in patients with idiopathic pulmonary fibrosis. *Mayo Clin Proc* (2002) 77(8):763–70. doi:10.4065/77.8.763
40. Kushibe K, Kawaguchi T, Takahama M, Kimura M, Tojo T, Taniguchi S. Operative indications for lung cancer with idiopathic pulmonary fibrosis. *Thorac Cardiovasc Surg* (2007) 55(8):505–8. doi:10.1055/s-2007-965645
41. Omori T, Tajiri M, Baba T, Ogura T, Iwasawa T, Okudela K, et al. Pulmonary resection for lung cancer in patients with idiopathic interstitial pneumonia. *Ann Thorac Surg* (2015) 100(3):954–60. doi:10.1016/j.athoracsur.2015.03.094
42. Watanabe A, Higami T, Ohori S, Koyanagi T, Nakashima S, Mawatari T. Is lung cancer resection indicated in patients with idiopathic pulmonary fibrosis? *J Thorac Cardiovasc Surg* (2008) 136(5):1357–63.e1351–2. doi:10.1016/j.jtcvs.2008.07.016
43. Suzuki H, Sekine Y, Yoshida S, Suzuki M, Shibuya K, Yonemori Y, et al. Risk of acute exacerbation of interstitial pneumonia after pulmonary resection for lung cancer in patients with idiopathic pulmonary fibrosis based on preoperative high-resolution computed tomography. *Surg Today* (2011) 41(7):914–21. doi:10.1007/s00595-010-4384-z
44. Mizuno Y, Iwata H, Shirahashi K, Takamochi K, Oh S, Suzuki K, et al. The importance of intraoperative fluid balance for the prevention of postoperative acute exacerbation of idiopathic pulmonary fibrosis after pulmonary resection for primary lung cancer. *Eur J Cardiothorac Surg* (2012) 41(6):e161–5. doi:10.1093/ejcts/ezs147
45. Choi SM, Lee J, Park YS, Cho YJ, Lee CH, Lee SM, et al. Postoperative pulmonary complications after surgery in patients with interstitial lung disease. *Respiration* (2014) 87(4):287–93. doi:10.1159/000357046
46. Isobe K, Hata Y, Sakamoto S, Takai Y, Shibuya K, Homma S. Clinical characteristics of acute respiratory deterioration in pulmonary fibrosis associated with lung cancer following anti-cancer therapy. *Respirology* (2010) 15(1):88–92. doi:10.1111/j.1440-1843.2009.01666.x
47. Kenmotsu H, Naito T, Kimura M, Ono A, Shukuya T, Nakamura Y, et al. The risk of cytotoxic chemotherapy-related exacerbation of interstitial lung

disease with lung cancer. *J Thorac Oncol* (2011) 6(7):1242–6. doi:10.1097/JTO.0b013e318216ee6b
48. Ono T, Hareyama M, Nakamura T, Kimura K, Hayashi Y, Azami Y, et al. The clinical results of proton beam therapy in patients with idiopathic pulmonary fibrosis: a single center experience. *Radiat Oncol* (2016) 11:56. doi:10.1186/s13014-016-0637-3
49. Reck M, Kaiser R, Mellemgaard A, Douillard JY, Orlov S, Krzakowski M, et al. Docetaxel plus nintedanib versus docetaxel plus placebo in patients with previously treated non-small-cell lung cancer (LUME-Lung 1): a phase 3, double-blind, randomised controlled trial. *Lancet Oncol* (2014) 15(2):143–55. doi:10.1016/S1470-2045(13)70586-2
50. Mediavilla-Varela M, Boateng K, Noyes D, Antonia SJ. The anti-fibrotic agent pirfenidone synergizes with cisplatin in killing tumor cells and cancer-associated fibroblasts. *BMC Cancer* (2016) 16:176. doi:10.1186/s12885-016-2162-z
51. National Lung Screening Trial Research Team, Aberle DR, Adams AM, Berg CD, Black WC, Clapp JD, et al. Reduced lung-cancer mortality with low-dose computed tomographic screening. *N Engl J Med* (2011) 365(5):395–409. doi:10.1056/NEJMoa1102873
52. Lancaster LH, Mason WR, Parnell JA, Rice TW, Loyd JE, Milstone AP, et al. Obstructive sleep apnea is common in idiopathic pulmonary fibrosis. *Chest* (2009) 136(3):772–8. doi:10.1378/chest.08-2776
53. Mermigkis C, Stagaki E, Tryfon S, Schiza S, Amfilochiou A, Polychronopoulos V, et al. How common is sleep-disordered breathing in patients with idiopathic pulmonary fibrosis? *Sleep Breath* (2010) 14(4):387–90. doi:10.1007/s11325-010-0336-5
54. Gille T, Didier M, Boubaya M, Moya L, Sutton A, Carton Z, et al. Obstructive sleep apnoea and related comorbidities in incident idiopathic pulmonary fibrosis. *Eur Respir J* (2017) 49(6). doi:10.1183/13993003.01934-2016
55. Mermigkis C, Chapman J, Golish J, Mermigkis D, Budur K, Kopanakis A, et al. Sleep-related breathing disorders in patients with idiopathic pulmonary fibrosis. *Lung* (2007) 185(3):173–8. doi:10.1007/s00408-007-9004-3
56. Kolilekas L, Manali E, Vlami KA, Lyberopoulos P, Triantafillidou C, Kagouridis K, et al. Sleep oxygen desaturation predicts survival in idiopathic pulmonary fibrosis. *J Clin Sleep Med* (2013) 9(6):593–601. doi:10.5664/jcsm.2758
57. Song JW, Song JK, Kim DS. Echocardiography and brain natriuretic peptide as prognostic indicators in idiopathic pulmonary fibrosis. *Respir Med* (2009) 103(2):180–6. doi:10.1016/j.rmed.2008.11.012
58. Mermigkis C, Bouloukaki I, Antoniou K, Papadogiannis G, Giannarakis I, Varouchakis G, et al. Obstructive sleep apnea should be treated in patients with idiopathic pulmonary fibrosis. *Sleep Breath* (2015) 19(1):385–91. doi:10.1007/s11325-014-1033-6
59. Miyake Y, Sasaki S, Yokoyama T, Chida K, Azuma A, Suda T, et al. Case-control study of medical history and idiopathic pulmonary fibrosis in Japan. *Respirology* (2005) 10(4):504–9. doi:10.1111/j.1440-1843.2005.00742.x
60. Lederer DJ, Arcasoy SM, Wilt JS, D'Ovidio F, Sonett JR, Kawut SM. Six-minute-walk distance predicts waiting list survival in idiopathic pulmonary fibrosis. *Am J Respir Crit Care Med* (2006) 174(6):659–64. doi:10.1164/rccm.200604-520OC
61. Hubbard RB, Smith C, Le Jeune I, Gribbin J, Fogarty AW. The association between idiopathic pulmonary fibrosis and vascular disease: a population-based study. *Am J Respir Crit Care Med* (2008) 178(12):1257–61. doi:10.1164/rccm.200805-725OC
62. Collard HR, Ward AJ, Lanes S, Cortney Hayflinger D, Rosenberg DM, Hunsche E. Burden of illness in idiopathic pulmonary fibrosis. *J Med Econ* (2012) 15(5):829–35. doi:10.3111/13696998.2012.680553
63. Kim WY, Mok Y, Kim GW, Baek SJ, Yun YD, Jee SH, et al. Association between idiopathic pulmonary fibrosis and coronary artery disease: a case-control study and cohort analysis. *Sarcoidosis Vasc Diffuse Lung Dis* (2015) 31(4):289–96.
64. Nathan SD, Basavaraj A, Reichner C, Shlobin OA, Ahmad S, Kiernan J, et al. Prevalence and impact of coronary artery disease in idiopathic pulmonary fibrosis. *Respir Med* (2010) 104(7):1035–41. doi:10.1016/j.rmed.2010.02.008
65. Moyer VA; U.S. Preventive Services Task Force. Screening for coronary heart disease with electrocardiography: U.S. Preventive Services Task Force recommendation statement. *Ann Intern Med* (2012) 157(7):512–8. doi:10.7326/0003-4819-157-7-201210020-00514
66. Budoff MJ, Achenbach S, Blumenthal RS, Carr JJ, Goldin JG, Greenland P, et al. Assessment of coronary artery disease by cardiac computed tomography: a scientific statement from the American Heart Association Committee on Cardiovascular Imaging and Intervention, Council on Cardiovascular Radiology and Intervention, and Committee on Cardiac Imaging, Council on Clinical Cardiology. *Circulation* (2006) 114(16):1761–91. doi:10.1161/CIRCULATIONAHA.106.178458
67. Nathan SD, Weir N, Shlobin OA, Urban BA, Curry CA, Basavaraj A, et al. The value of computed tomography scanning for the detection of coronary artery disease in patients with idiopathic pulmonary fibrosis. *Respirology* (2011) 16(3):481–6. doi:10.1111/j.1440-1843.2010.01919.x
68. Galie N, Humbert M, Vachiery JL, Gibbs S, Lang I, Torbicki A, et al. 2015 ESC/ERS Guidelines for the diagnosis and treatment of pulmonary hypertension: the Joint Task Force for the Diagnosis and Treatment of Pulmonary Hypertension of the European Society of Cardiology (ESC) and the European Respiratory Society (ERS): endorsed by: Association for European Paediatric and Congenital Cardiology (AEPC), International Society for Heart and Lung Transplantation (ISHLT). *Eur Heart J* (2016) 37(1):67–119. doi:10.1093/eurheartj/ehv317
69. Nadrous HF, Pellikka PA, Krowka MJ, Swanson KL, Chaowalit N, Decker PA, et al. Pulmonary hypertension in patients with idiopathic pulmonary fibrosis. *Chest* (2005) 128(4):2393–9. doi:10.1378/chest.128.4.2393
70. Nathan SD, Shlobin OA, Ahmad S, Urbanek S, Barnett SD. Pulmonary hypertension and pulmonary function testing in idiopathic pulmonary fibrosis. *Chest* (2007) 131(3):657–63. doi:10.1378/chest.06-2485
71. Shorr AF, Wainright JL, Cors CS, Lettieri CJ, Nathan SD. Pulmonary hypertension in patients with pulmonary fibrosis awaiting lung transplant. *Eur Respir J* (2007) 30(4):715–21. doi:10.1183/09031936.00107206
72. Nathan SD, Shlobin OA, Ahmad S, Koch J, Barnett SD, Ad N, et al. Serial development of pulmonary hypertension in patients with idiopathic pulmonary fibrosis. *Respiration* (2008) 76(3):288–94. doi:10.1159/000114246
73. Nathan SD, Shlobin OA, Barnett SD, Saggar R, Belperio JA, Ross DJ, et al. Right ventricular systolic pressure by echocardiography as a predictor of pulmonary hypertension in idiopathic pulmonary fibrosis. *Respir Med* (2008) 102(9):1305–10. doi:10.1016/j.rmed.2008.03.022
74. Minai OA, Santacruz JF, Alster JM, Budev MM, McCarthy K. Impact of pulmonary hemodynamics on 6-min walk test in idiopathic pulmonary fibrosis. *Respir Med* (2012) 106(11):1613–21. doi:10.1016/j.rmed.2012.07.013
75. Rivera-Lebron BN, Forfia PR, Kreider M, Lee JC, Holmes JH, Kawut SM. Echocardiographic and hemodynamic predictors of mortality in idiopathic pulmonary fibrosis. *Chest* (2013) 144(2):564–70. doi:10.1378/chest.12-2298
76. Arcasoy SM, Christie JD, Ferrari VA, Sutton MS, Zisman DA, Blumenthal NP, et al. Echocardiographic assessment of pulmonary hypertension in patients with advanced lung disease. *Am J Respir Crit Care Med* (2003) 167(5):735–40. doi:10.1164/rccm.200210-1130OC
77. King TE Jr, Brown KK, Raghu G, du Bois RM, Lynch DA, Martinez F, et al. BUILD-3: a randomized, controlled trial of bosentan in idiopathic pulmonary fibrosis. *Am J Respir Crit Care Med* (2011) 184(1):92–9. doi:10.1164/rccm.201011-1874OC
78. Raghu G, Behr J, Brown KK, Egan JJ, Kawut SM, Flaherty KR, et al. Treatment of idiopathic pulmonary fibrosis with ambrisentan: a parallel, randomized trial. *Ann Intern Med* (2013) 158(9):641–9. doi:10.7326/0003-4819-158-9-201305070-00003
79. Raghu G, Million-Rousseau R, Morganti A, Perchenet L, Behr J, Group MS. Macitentan for the treatment of idiopathic pulmonary fibrosis: the randomised controlled MUSIC trial. *Eur Respir J* (2013) 42(6):1622–32. doi:10.1183/09031936.00104612
80. Corte TJ, Keir GJ, Dimopoulos K, Howard L, Corris PA, Parfitt L, et al. Bosentan in pulmonary hypertension associated with fibrotic idiopathic interstitial pneumonia. *Am J Respir Crit Care Med* (2014) 190(2):208–17. doi:10.1164/rccm.201403-0446OC
81. Raghu G, Nathan SD, Behr J, Brown KK, Egan JJ, Kawut SM, et al. Pulmonary hypertension in idiopathic pulmonary fibrosis with mild-to-moderate restriction. *Eur Respir J* (2015) 46(5):1370–7. doi:10.1183/13993003.01537-2014
82. Zisman DA, Schwarz M, Anstrom KJ, Collard HR, Flaherty KR, Hunninghake GW. A controlled trial of sildenafil in advanced idiopathic pulmonary fibrosis. *N Engl J Med* (2010) 363(7):620–8. doi:10.1056/NEJMoa1002110
83. Han MK, Bach DS, Hagan PG, Yow E, Flaherty KR, Toews GB, et al. Sildenafil preserves exercise capacity in patients with idiopathic pulmonary fibrosis and right-sided ventricular dysfunction. *Chest* (2013) 143(6):1699–708. doi:10.1378/chest.12-1594

84. Sprunger DB, Olson AL, Huie TJ, Fernandez-Perez ER, Fischer A, Solomon JJ, et al. Pulmonary fibrosis is associated with an elevated risk of thromboembolic disease. *Eur Respir J* (2012) 39(1):125–32. doi:10.1183/09031936.00041411
85. Sode BF, Dahl M, Nielsen SF, Nordestgaard BG. Venous thromboembolism and risk of idiopathic interstitial pneumonia: a nationwide study. *Am J Respir Crit Care Med* (2010) 181(10):1085–92. doi:10.1164/rccm.200912-1951OC
86. Dalleywater W, Powell HA, Fogarty AW, Hubbard RB, Navaratnam V. Venous thromboembolism in people with idiopathic pulmonary fibrosis: a population-based study. *Eur Respir J* (2014) 44(6):1714–5. doi:10.1183/09031936.00099614
87. Collard HR, Ryerson CJ, Corte TJ, Jenkins G, Kondoh Y, Lederer DJ, et al. Acute exacerbation of idiopathic pulmonary fibrosis. An International Working Group Report. *Am J Respir Crit Care Med* (2016) 194(3):265–75. doi:10.1164/rccm.201604-0801CI
88. Kearon C, Akl EA, Ornelas J, Blaivas A, Jimenez D, Bounameaux H, et al. Antithrombotic therapy for VTE disease: CHEST guideline and expert panel report. *Chest* (2016) 149(2):315–52. doi:10.1016/j.chest.2015.11.026
89. Noth I, Anstrom KJ, Calvert SB, de Andrade J, Flaherty KR, Glazer C, et al. A placebo-controlled randomized trial of warfarin in idiopathic pulmonary fibrosis. *Am J Respir Crit Care Med* (2012) 186(1):88–95. doi:10.1164/rccm.201202-0314OC
90. Tomassetti S, Ruy JH, Gurioli C, Ravaglia C, Buccioli M, Tantalocco P, et al. The effect of anticoagulant therapy for idiopathic pulmonary fibrosis in real life practice. *Sarcoidosis Vasc Diffuse Lung Dis* (2013) 30(2):121–7.
91. Kreuter M, Wijsenbeek MS, Vasakova M, Spagnolo P, Kolb M, Costabel U, et al. Unfavourable effects of medically indicated oral anticoagulants on survival in idiopathic pulmonary fibrosis. *Eur Respir J* (2016) 47(6):1776–84. doi:10.1183/13993003.02087-2015
92. Lee JS, Collard HR, Raghu G, Sweet MP, Hays SR, Campos GM, et al. Does chronic microaspiration cause idiopathic pulmonary fibrosis? *Am J Med* (2010) 123(4):304–11. doi:10.1016/j.amjmed.2009.07.033
93. Gribbin J, Hubbard R, Smith C. Role of diabetes mellitus and gastro-oesophageal reflux in the aetiology of idiopathic pulmonary fibrosis. *Respir Med* (2009) 103(6):927–31. doi:10.1016/j.rmed.2008.11.001
94. Ryerson CJ, Abbritti M, Ley B, Elicker BM, Jones KD, Collard HR. Cough predicts prognosis in idiopathic pulmonary fibrosis. *Respirology* (2011) 16(6):969–75. doi:10.1111/j.1440-1843.2011.01996.x
95. Raghu G, Freudenberger TD, Yang S, Curtis JR, Spada C, Hayes J, et al. High prevalence of abnormal acid gastro-oesophageal reflux in idiopathic pulmonary fibrosis. *Eur Respir J* (2006) 27(1):136–42. doi:10.1183/09031936.06.00037005
96. Savarino E, Carbone R, Marabotto E, Furnari M, Sconfienza L, Ghio M, et al. Gastro-oesophageal reflux and gastric aspiration in idiopathic pulmonary fibrosis patients. *Eur Respir J* (2013) 42(5):1322–31. doi:10.1183/09031936.00101212
97. Gavini S, Finn RT, Lo WK, Goldberg HJ, Burakoff R, Feldman N, et al. Idiopathic pulmonary fibrosis is associated with increased impedance measures of reflux compared to non-fibrotic disease among pre-lung transplant patients. *Neurogastroenterol Motil* (2015) 27(9):1326–32. doi:10.1111/nmo.12627
98. Sweet MP, Patti MG, Leard LE, Golden JA, Hays SR, Hoopes C, et al. Gastroesophageal reflux in patients with idiopathic pulmonary fibrosis referred for lung transplantation. *J Thorac Cardiovasc Surg* (2007) 133(4):1078–84. doi:10.1016/j.jtcvs.2006.09.085
99. Chen MY, Ott DJ, Sinclair JW, Wu WC, Gelfand DW. Gastroesophageal reflux disease: correlation of esophageal pH testing and radiographic findings. *Radiology* (1992) 185(2):483–6. doi:10.1148/radiology.185.2.1410359
100. Thompson JK, Koehler RE, Richter JE. Detection of gastroesophageal reflux: value of barium studies compared with 24-hr pH monitoring. *AJR Am J Roentgenol* (1994) 162(3):621–6. doi:10.2214/ajr.162.3.8109509
101. Falk GL, Beattie J, Ing A, Falk SE, Magee M, Burton L, et al. Scintigraphy in laryngopharyngeal and gastroesophageal reflux disease: a definitive diagnostic test? *World J Gastroenterol* (2015) 21(12):3619–27. doi:10.3748/wjg.v21.i12.3619
102. Madan K, Ahuja V, Gupta SD, Bal C, Kapoor A, Sharma MP. Impact of 24-h esophageal pH monitoring on the diagnosis of gastroesophageal reflux disease: defining the gold standard. *J Gastroenterol Hepatol* (2005) 20(1):30–7. doi:10.1111/j.1440-1746.2004.03530.x
103. Rosen R, Lord C, Nurko S. The sensitivity of multichannel intraluminal impedance and the pH probe in the evaluation of gastroesophageal reflux in children. *Clin Gastroenterol Hepatol* (2006) 4(2):167–72. doi:10.1016/S1542-3565(05)00854-2
104. Hila A, Agrawal A, Castell DO. Combined multichannel intraluminal impedance and pH esophageal testing compared to pH alone for diagnosing both acid and weakly acidic gastroesophageal reflux. *Clin Gastroenterol Hepatol* (2007) 5(2):172–7. doi:10.1016/j.cgh.2006.11.015
105. Lee JS, Collard HR, Anstrom KJ, Martinez FJ, Noth I, Roberts RS, et al. Anti-acid treatment and disease progression in idiopathic pulmonary fibrosis: an analysis of data from three randomised controlled trials. *Lancet Respir Med* (2013) 1(5):369–76. doi:10.1016/S2213-2600(13)70105-X
106. Kreuter M, Wuyts W, Renzoni E, Koschel D, Maher TM, Kolb M, et al. Antacid therapy and disease outcomes in idiopathic pulmonary fibrosis: a pooled analysis. *Lancet Respir Med* (2016) 4(5):381–9. doi:10.1016/S2213-2600(16)00067-9
107. Noth I, Zangan SM, Soares RV, Forsythe A, Demchuk C, Takahashi SM, et al. Prevalence of hiatal hernia by blinded multidetector CT in patients with idiopathic pulmonary fibrosis. *Eur Respir J* (2012) 39(2):344–51. doi:10.1183/09031936.00099910
108. Tossier C, Dupin C, Plantier L, Leger J, Flament T, Favelle O, et al. Hiatal hernia on thoracic computed tomography in pulmonary fibrosis. *Eur Respir J* (2016) 48(3):833–42. doi:10.1183/13993003.01796-2015
109. Linden PA, Gilbert RJ, Yeap BY, Boyle K, Deykin A, Jaklitsch MT, et al. Laparoscopic fundoplication in patients with end-stage lung disease awaiting transplantation. *J Thorac Cardiovasc Surg* (2006) 131(2):438–46. doi:10.1016/j.jtcvs.2005.10.014
110. Sawin CT, Castelli WP, Hershman JM, McNamara P, Bacharach P. The aging thyroid. Thyroid deficiency in the Framingham Study. *Arch Intern Med* (1985) 145(8):1386–8. doi:10.1001/archinte.1985.00360080056006
111. Vanderpump MP, Tunbridge WM, French JM, Appleton D, Bates D, Clark F, et al. The incidence of thyroid disorders in the community: a twenty-year follow-up of the Whickham Survey. *Clin Endocrinol (Oxf)* (1995) 43(1):55–68. doi:10.1111/j.1365-2265.1995.tb01894.x
112. Garber JR, Cobin RH, Gharib H, Hennessey JV, Klein I, Mechanick JI, et al. Clinical practice guidelines for hypothyroidism in adults: cosponsored by the American Association of Clinical Endocrinologists and the American Thyroid Association. *Endocr Pract* (2012) 18(6):988–1028. doi:10.4158/EP12280.GL
113. Garcia-Sancho Figueroa MC, Carrillo G, Perez-Padilla R, Fernandez-Plata MR, Buendia-Roldan I, Vargas MH, et al. Risk factors for idiopathic pulmonary fibrosis in a Mexican population. A case-control study. *Respir Med* (2010) 104(2):305–9. doi:10.1016/j.rmed.2009.08.013
114. Ryerson CJ, Donesky D, Pantilat SZ, Collard HR. Dyspnea in idiopathic pulmonary fibrosis: a systematic review. *J Pain Symptom Manage* (2012) 43(4):771–82. doi:10.1016/j.jpainsymman.2011.04.026
115. Akhtar AA, Ali MA, Smith RP. Depression in patients with idiopathic pulmonary fibrosis. *Chron Respir Dis* (2013) 10(3):127–33. doi:10.1177/1479972313493098
116. Holland AE, Fiore JF Jr, Bell EC, Goh N, Westall G, Symons K, et al. Dyspnoea and comorbidity contribute to anxiety and depression in interstitial lung disease. *Respirology* (2014) 19(8):1215–21. doi:10.1111/resp.12360
117. Tzanakis N, Samiou M, Lambiri I, Antoniou K, Siafakas N, Bouros D. Evaluation of health-related quality-of-life and dyspnea scales in patients with idiopathic pulmonary fibrosis. Correlation with pulmonary function tests. *Eur J Intern Med* (2005) 16(2):105–12. doi:10.1016/j.ejim.2004.09.013
118. Lamas DJ, Kawut SM, Bagiella E, Philip N, Arcasoy SM, Lederer DJ. Delayed access and survival in idiopathic pulmonary fibrosis: a cohort study. *Am J Respir Crit Care Med* (2011) 184(7):842–7. doi:10.1164/rccm.201104-0668OC

12

Prognostic Predictive Characteristics in Patients with Fibrosing Interstitial Lung Disease

Yuanying Wang[1], *Ziyun Guo*[1], *Ruimin Ma*[1], *Jingwei Wang*[1], *Na Wu*[1,2], *Yali Fan*[1] *and Qiao Ye*[1,2]*

[1]*Clinical Center for Interstitial Lung Diseases, Beijing Institute of Respiratory Medicine, Beijing Chaoyang Hospital, Capital Medical University, Beijing, China,* [2]*Department of Occupational Medicine and Toxicology, Beijing Chaoyang Hospital, Capital Medical University, Beijing, China*

***Correspondence:**
Qiao Ye
yeqiao_chaoyang@sina.com

Background: Limited data are available regarding the entire spectrum of interstitial lung disease with a progressive fibrosing feature. We investigated the prevalence and prognostic predictive characteristics in patients with PF-ILD.

Methods: This retrospective cohort study included patients with fibrosing ILD who were investigated between 1 January 2015 and 30 April 2021. We recorded clinical features and outcomes to identify the possible risk factors for fibrosing progression as well as mortality.

Results: Of the 579 patients with fibrosing ILD, 227 (39.21%) met the criteria for progression. Clubbing of fingers [odds ratio (OR) 1.52, 95% confidence interval (CI) 1.03 to 2.24, p = 0.035] and a high-resolution computed tomography (HRCT)-documented usual interstitial pneumonia (UIP)-like fibrotic pattern (OR 1.95, 95% CI 1.33 to 2.86, p = 0.001) were risk factors for fibrosis progression. The mortality was worse in patients with PF with hypoxemia [hazard ratio (HR) 2.08, 95% CI 1.31 to 3.32, p = 0.002], in those with baseline diffusion capacity of the lung for carbon monoxide (DLCO) % predicted <50% (HR 2.25, 95% CI 1.45 to 3.50, p < 0.001), or in those with UIP-like fibrotic pattern (HR 1.68, 95% CI 1.04 to 2.71, p < 0.001).

Conclusion: Clubbing of fingers and an HRCT-documented UIP-like fibrotic pattern were more likely to be associated with progressive fibrosing with varied prevalence based on the specific diagnosis. Among patients with progressive fibrosing, those with hypoxemia, lower baseline DLCO% predicted, or UIP-like fibrotic pattern showed poor mortality.

Keywords: progressive fibrosing interstitial lung disease, prognosis, lung function test, blood count values, anti-fibrotic treatment

---

Abbreviations: AISI, aggregate index of systemic inflammation; BMI, body mass index; CI, confidence interval; CTD, connective tissue disease; DLCO, diffusion capacity of the lung for carbon monoxide; FHP, fibrotic hypersensitivity pneumonitis; FVC, forced vital capacity; HR, hazard ratio; HRCT, high-resolution computed tomography; iNSIP, idiopathic non-specific interstitial pneumonia; IIP, idiopathic interstitial pneumonia; ILD, interstitial lung disease; IPF, idiopathic pulmonary fibrosis; IQR, interquartile range; MLR, monocyte-to-lymphocyte ratio; NLR, neutrophil-to-lymphocyte ratio; OR, hazard ratio; PF, progressive fibrosing; PFT, pulmonary function testing; PLR, platelet-to-lymphocyte ratio; pSS-ILD, primary Sjögren syndrome-associated ILD; SD, standard deviation; RDW: red cell distribution width; SIRI, systemic inflammatory response index; SSc-ILD, sclerosis-associated ILD; UIP, usual interstitial pneumonia; WBC, white blood cell.

INTRODUCTION

The disease course in fibrosing interstitial lung disease (ILD) is highly heterogeneous and difficult to predict. Some patients experience a stable course or slowly functional decline while other patients may experience a rapidly progressive change (Cottin et al., 2018). Progressive fibrosing interstitial lung disease (PF-ILD) is a term referring to a group of diseases characterized by a high-resolution computed tomography (HRCT)-documented increase in the extent of pulmonary fibrosis, a decline in lung function, worsening respiratory symptoms and quality of life, and a high risk of early mortality despite available treatments, with a clinical course similar to that of idiopathic pulmonary fibrosis (IPF) (Cottin et al., 2018). PF-ILDs include a heterogeneous group of disorders associated with multifactorial etiology, including IPF, connective tissue disease-associated ILD (CTD-ILD), fibrotic hypersensitivity pneumonitis (FHP), unclassifiable idiopathic interstitial pneumonia (uIIP), and idiopathic non-specific interstitial pneumonia (Cottin et al., 2019). Reportedly, PF-ILDs may develop in approximately 33.0% of patients with fibrosing ILDs other than IPF (Olson et al., 2018; Nasser et al., 2021a; Ruaro et al., 2021; Lee et al., 2022). The estimated incidence of PF-ILD ranged from 4.0 to 4.7/100,000 person-years and the estimated prevalence from 6.6 to 19.4/100,000 individuals (Nasser et al., 2021a; Nasser et al., 2021b).

Several clinical trials have encompassed patients with progressive fibrosing, with the eligibility criteria for these studies helping to guide a standardized diagnosis of PF-ILD (Wongkarnjana et al., 2020). Although no uniform criteria were established, guidelines recommended monitoring of fibrosis progression based on evaluation of multiple components, such as a decline in lung function, increase in chest imaging-documented fibrosis, symptomatic worsening, and composite measures of these variables (George et al., 2020; Wongkarnjana et al., 2020; Raghu et al., 2022).

In view of the clinical and underlying physiological similarities between IPF and other PF-ILDs, anti-fibrotic agents, such as nintedanib or pirfenidone, are considered to be effective against progressive fibrosis (Flaherty et al., 2019; Gibson et al., 2020). However, watchful observation until the onset of HRCT-documented lung function decline and extensive fibrosis delays initiation of early anti-fibrotic therapy, and patients invariably present with clinically significant and irreversible injury. Several studies have investigated the clinical features and likely predictors in patients at high risk of PF-ILD at baseline (Kolb and Vašáková, 2019). Certain conditions, such as FHP (which is not associated with any specific antigen) and increasing age predispose to PF-ILD (Sharma et al., 2021; Churg, 2022). Smoking status was a risk factor for rheumatoid arthritis-ILD (RA-ILD) or primary Sjögren syndrome associated with ILD (Johnson, 2017; Wang et al., 2018). Male sex and a high baseline modified Rodnan skin score were strong predictors of forced vital capacity (FVC) decline in patients with systemic sclerosis-ILD (SSc-ILD) (Hoffmann-Vold et al., 2021). Risk factors for mortality have also been identified. Regardless of a specific diagnosis of ILD, patients with an HRCT-documented usual interstitial pneumonia (UIP) pattern or extensive traction bronchiectasis, FVC decline, or older age showed the highest mortality risk (Walsh et al., 2018; Yang et al., 2022). In addition, peripheral blood monocyte counts have been investigated in IPF and other ILDs as a predictor of prognosis (Misharin et al., 2017; Barratt et al., 2021). Although studies have reported findings for individual types of PF-ILDs (for example, SSc-ILD, RA-ILD, other CTD-ILDs, and FHP), limited data are available regarding the PF-ILDs as a whole group (Khanna et al., 2020; Skibba et al., 2020; Orlandi et al., 2022). Early accurate diagnosis of most ILDs was difficult. Studying clinical courses for the heterogeneous group of fibrosing ILDs as a whole group was essential to identify patients with the most rapidly progressive feature or poor prognosis and initiate early anti-fibrotic treatment.

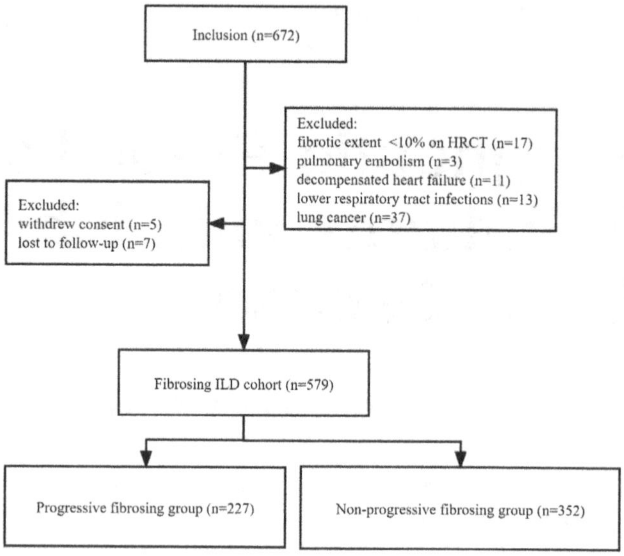

FIGURE 1 | Patient flowchart. ILD, interstitial lung disease; PFT, pulmonary function test; HRCT, high-resolution computed tomography.

The aims of this study were: 1) to investigate the prevalence and clinical features of the PF-ILDs and 2) to explore the potential factors associated with progression or mortality.

MATERIALS AND METHODS

Study Design and Participants

This observational retrospective cohort study was performed at Beijing Chao-Yang Hospital, China, a regional tertiary referral center specialized in the management of ILDs. We retrospectively screened all patients aged ≥18 years with a multidisciplinary diagnosis of fibrosing ILDs between 1 January 2015 and 30 April 2021. Multidisciplinary diagnoses were conducted between pulmonologists (QY, NW, and YW), radiologists (YF and JW), a rheumatologist (ZG), and a pathologist (RM) experienced in the diagnosis of ILD based on clinical characteristics, HRCT, and lung biopsy if appropriate. Patients whose results of baseline pulmonary function tests (PFTs) and

HRCT were available were enrolled in the study. Following were the exclusion criteria: 1) <10% fibrosis documented on baseline HRCT, 2) diagnosis of pulmonary embolism, decompensated heart failure, or lower respiratory tract infections associated with disease progression, 3) lung cancer at baseline, 4) withdrawal of consent for study participation, and 5) loss to follow-up (**Figure 1**). The study was registered at www.chictr.org.cn ChiCTR2100049247 and was approved by the Ethics Committee of Beijing Chao-Yang Hospital (2020-KY-437). All procedures were performed in accordance with the principles of the Declaration of Helsinki.

Data Collection

We reviewed patients' medical records to uniformly extract clinical data at the first clinical visit, including demographic information, physical examination, and routine clinical laboratory test results. Clinical and survival data were obtained from medical records, outpatient follow-up records (usually every 6–12 months), hospitalization details, and telephone interviews. Hypoxemia was defined as the partial pressure of oxygen in the arterial blood (PaO2) of less than 80 mm Hg obtained from the arterial blood gas (ABG) test at rest. The derivative blood cell count inflammation indexes included the neutrophil-to-lymphocyte ratio (NLR: neutrophils/lymphocytes), monocyte-to-lymphocyte ratio (MLR: monocytes/lymphocytes), platelet-to-lymphocyte ratio (PLR: platelet/lymphocyte), systemic inflammatory index (SII: neutrophils × platelets/lymphocytes), systemic inflammatory response index (SIRI: neutrophils × monocytes/lymphocytes), and aggregate index of systemic inflammation (AISI: neutrophils × platelets × monocytes/ lymphocytes). The HRCT-documented UIP-like pattern included definitive UIP or a probable UIP pattern according to the Clinical Practice Guideline of IPF (Raghu et al., 2011; Raghu et al., 2018). Two thoracic radiologists (YF and JW) blinded to the clinical data independently determined whether the fibrosis involved >10% of the total lung and reviewed the HRCT scans by visual assessment. The disagreements were resolved *via* consensus. The kappa value for the interobserver correlation was 0.84.

The follow-up period ended on 30 April 2021. The primary outcome was progressive fibrosing. Patients who fulfilled any of the following criteria within 24 months despite administration of standard treatment were considered experiencing progressive fibrosis (Cottin et al., 2018; Flaherty et al., 2019): 1) a relative decline of ≥10% in FVC, 2) relative decline of ≥15% in diffusion capacity of the lung for carbon monoxide (DLCO), and 3) worsening symptoms and/or worsening radiological findings accompanied by a ≥5% to <10% relative decrease in FVC. The secondary outcome was all-cause mortality during the follow-up period. Survival was calculated from the time of the first visit to the outcome or the end of follow-up.

Sample Size Calculation

PASS software, version 11.0 (NCSS, LLC. Kaysville, Utah, United States) was used to calculate the sample size. The sample allocation ratio was 1: 2 (PF: non-PF), given the estimated prevalence of PF-ILD among patients with fibrosing ILDs was 33.0% (Nasser et al., 2021a). We used a two-sided log-rank test for the 6-year all-cause mortality with 1-year accrual periods and an estimated 10.0% proportion of dropping out for both groups. An overall sample size of 260 patients (174 in the non-PF-ILD group and 86 in the PF-ILD group) was deemed sufficient to achieve >90% power at a 0.05% significance level to detect a hazard ratio (HR) of death with the 6-year mortality rate considered to be 40.0% for the PF group and 18.0% for the non-PF group (Adegunsoye et al., 2018). However, we attempted to enroll as many patients as possible within the study period. The final cohort included 579 patients, of which 227 patients were diagnosed with PF-ILD (85 deaths), fulfilling the 10-events-per-variable criterion of multivariable logistic regression and Cox analysis.

Statistical Analysis

Statistical analyses were performed using SPSS Statistics software, version 26 (IBM, Inc., Chicago, IL, United States). Missing data were imputed using mean/median or removed for a complete case analysis. Data were expressed as means (SD) or medians (range), depending on the distribution. The Mann–Whitney U or *t*-test was used for continuous variables for comparison of intergroup differences and the chi-squared test or Fisher's exact test for categorical variables. Linear mixed-effects analysis was applied to analyze disease behavior over time, with random terms for intercept and slope (for time-from-diagnosis). The covariance for the repeated measures was left autoregressive 1: heterogeneous, which yielded the best fit. Multicollinearity diagnostic tests were performed. Logistic regression analyses were used to investigate risk factors for the PF-ILD, and continuous variables were converted into dichotomous variables mainly through the median cut-off. The cut-off value was 70.0% for FVC% predicted and 50.0% for DLCO% predicted (Abe et al., 2021; Lacedonia et al., 2022). Survival curves were obtained using the Kaplan–Meier method, and Cox proportional analyses were performed to identify prognostic factors for mortality. Proportional hazards in the Cox analysis were checked using the Schoenfeld residual test. A p-value < 0.05 was considered statistically significant.

RESULTS

Demographic and Clinical Characteristics

In this study, 277 (39.21%) out of 579 ILD patients met the criteria for PF-ILD; 64, 88, and 108 patients met criteria 1, 2, and 3, respectively; 28 patients met both the criteria 1 and 2, and 16 patients met both the criteria 2 and 3 (**Supplementary Figure S1**). Statistically significant baseline differences were observed in age ($p = 0.001$), underlying diagnosis ($p < 0.001$), clubbing of fingers ($p = 0.005$), and HRCT-documented UIP-like fibrotic pattern ($p < 0.001$) between the PF-ILD and non-PF-ILD groups (**Table 1**). Baseline blood count values did not differ significantly between patients with PF and non-PF. Within the PF-ILD group, gender, age, smoking status, UIP-like fibrotic pattern, FVC, GAP stage distribution, and anti-fibrotic treatment were statistically significant between IPF and non-IPF patients (**Table 2**).

TABLE 1 | Demographics and clinical characteristics of the cohort.

	All	PF-ILD group	Non-PF-ILD group	*p*-value
Number	579	227 (39.21)	352 (60.79)	
Male, *n* (%)	296 (51.12)	121 (53.30)	175 (49.72)	0.399
Age, years (IQR)	62 (55–68)	64 (57–70)	62 (54–68)	0.001
BMI, kg/m^2 (SD)	25.90 (3.31)	25.92 (3.50)	25.89 (3.19)	0.907
Ever smoker, *n* (%)	233 (40.24)	98 (43.17)	135 (38.40)	0.248
Diagnosis, *n* (%)				<0.001
IPF	145 (25.04)	77 (33.92)	68 (19.32)	
CTD-ILD	297 (51.30)	109 (48.02)	188 (53.41)	
FHP	56 (9.67)	16 (7.05)	40 (11.36)	
uIIP	81 (13.99)	25 (11.01)	56 (15.91)	
Signs, *n* (%)				
Velcro crackles	531 (91.71)	214 (94.27)	317 (90.06)	0.072
Clubbing of fingers	154 (26.60)	75 (33.04)	79 (22.44)	0.005
Blood count values				
WBC ($n * 10^9$/L)	7.60 (5.98–8.53)	7.40 (5.69–8.63)	7.77 (6.28–8.52)	0.132
Neutrophils ($n * 10^9$/L)	4.87 (3.46–8.50)	4.54 (3.23–5.97)	5.06 (3.68–5.66)	0.156
Lymphocytes ($n * 10^9$/L)	1.91 (1.42–2.30)	1.91 (1.35–2.29)	1.91 (1.46–2.30)	0.622
Monocyte ($n * 10^9$/L)	0.47 (0.37–0.54)	0.47 (0.35–0.55)	0.48 (0.38–0.54)	0.293
RDW	13.20 (12.60–13.99)	13.20 (12.70–13.99)	13.20 (12.52–13.99)	0.570
LMR	3.90 (3.22–5.26)	3.90 (3.14–5.07)	3.90 (3.27–5.27)	0.393
NLR	2.68 (1.84–3.42)	2.60 (1.74–3.46)	2.68 (1.88–3.40)	0.914
PLR	121.68 (92.16–159.01)	121.68 (90.36–157.86)	121.68 (94.10–163.73)	0.214
SIRI	1.31 (0.76–1.65)	1.25 (0.73–1.85)	1.31 (0.77–1.55)	0.265
AISI	305.26 (145.40–396.00)	286.60 (139.56–433.36)	305.26 (156.84–377.23)	0.947
Pulmonary function (SD)				
FVC (L)	2.64 (0.80)	2.64 (0.79)	2.64 (0.82)	0.932
FVC% pred	85.45 (19.72)	85.94 (19.53)	85.15 (19.86)	0.633
DLCO% pred	60.26 (18.61)	58.94 (18.82)	61.11 (18.46)	0.171
UIP-like fibrotic pattern on HRCT, n (%)	163 (28.15)	86 (37.89)	77 (21.88)	<0.001
Hypoxemia, *n* (%)	119 (20.55)	54 (23.80)	65 (18.50)	0.122
Hospitalization at baseline, n (%)	162 (27.98)	70 (30.84)	92 (26.14)	0.219
Hospitalization frequency, n (IQR)	0 (0.1)	1 (0.1)	0 (0.1)	<0.001
Hospitalization frequency, *n* (%)				0.002
0	298 (51.47)	101 (44.49)	197 (55.97)	
1–2	236 (40.76)	99 (43.61)	137 (38.92)	
≥3	45 (7.77)	27 (11.89)	18 (5.11)	
Death, *n* (%)	128 (22.11)	85 (37.45)	43 (12.22)	<0.001
Median duration of follow-up, years (IQR)	3 (2.4)	3 (2.5.4)	3 (2.4)	0.054

Data were presented as mean ± SD or n (%) or median (IQR).

AISI, aggregate index of systemic inflammation; BMI, body mass index; CTD, connective tissue disease; DLCO, diffusion capacity of the lung for carbon monoxide; FHP, fibrotic hypersensitivity pneumonitis; FVC, forced vital capacity; HRCT, high-resolution computed tomography; iNSIP, idiopathic non-specific interstitial pneumonia; IPF, idiopathic pulmonary fibrosis; MLR, monocyte-to-lymphocyte ratio; NLR, neutrophil-to-lymphocyte ratio; PF, progressive fibrosing; PLR, platelet-to-lymphocyte ratio; RDW: red cell distribution width; SIRI, systemic inflammatory response index; uIIP, unclassifiable idiopathic interstitial pneumonia; UIP, usual interstitial pneumonia; WBC, white blood cell.

Comorbidity information for the whole cohort is shown in **Supplementary Figure S2**. The prevalence for pulmonary hypertension was 8.81% in the PF group and 5.11% in the non-PF group.

Prevalence of Progressive Fibrosing Interstitial Lung Disease

The most frequent diagnoses included CTD-ILD (*n* = 297%, 51.30%), IPF (*n* = 145%, 25.04%), uIIP (*n* = 81%, 13.99%), and FHP (*n* = 56%, 9.67%) (**Table 1**). The prevalence of PF-ILD in patients with ILDs, including those with IPF (*n* = 77), CTD-ILD (*n* = 109), FHP (*n* = 16), and uIIP (*n* = 25) was 53.10%, 36.70%, 28.57%, and 30.86%, respectively (**Supplementary Figure S3**).

Treatments and Hospitalization

In the entire cohort, 74.96% of patients (*n* = 434) received at least one of the following treatments: administration of glucocorticoids, immunosuppressive agents, anti-fibrotic treatment, and oxygen therapy. Anti-fibrotic treatment was administered to 32.16% of patients with PF-ILD (*n* = 73) (**Supplementary Table S1**). In the PF group, 42 (54.50%) of IPF patients and 31 (20.70%) of non-IPF patients (29 CTD-ILD, 1 FHP, and 1 uIIP) received anti-fibrotic treatment (**Table 2**). Patients hospitalized within 1 month of the first visit were considered hospitalized at baseline. We observed that 298 (51.47%) patients underwent hospitalization at least once during follow-up, and 27 (11.89%) of 227 patients in the PF-ILD group vs. 18 (5.11%) of the 352 patients in the non-PF group underwent hospitalization at least thrice (**Table 1**).

TABLE 2 | Demographics and clinical characteristics of patients within the PF group.

	IPF	Non-IPF	*p*-value
Number	77	150	
Male, *n* (%)	60 (77.92)	61 (40.67)	<0.001
Age, years (IQR)	66 (60–74)	63 (55–68)	<0.001
BMI, kg/m^2 (SD)	26.29 (3.19)	25.73 (3.65)	0.255
Ever smoker, *n* (%)	55 (71.43)	43 (28.67)	<0.001
Signs, *n* (%)			
Velcro crackles	29 (37.70)	46 (30.67)	0.337
Clubbing of fingers	71 (92.20)	143 (95.33)	0.289
Pulmonary function (SD)			
FVC (L)	2.80 (0.66)	2.45 (0.81)	0.001
FVC% pred	82.96 (16.86)	87.46 (20.67)	0.100
DLCO% pred	56.61 (19.47)	60.14 (18.43)	0.180
UIP-like fibrotic pattern on HRCT, n (%)	65 (84.42)	21 (14.00)[#]	<0.001
Hypoxemia, *n* (%)	19 (24.68)	35 (23.33)	0.822
GAP score	3 (1–2)	2 (1–3)	
Stage I (%)	55 (71.43)	123 (82.00)	
Stage II (%)	19 (24.68)	26 (17.33)	
Stage III (%)	3 (3.90)	1 (0.67)	0.077
Anti-fibrotic treatment (%)	42 (54.55)	31 (20.67)	<0.001

Data were presented as mean ± SD or n (%) or median (IQR).
#: 29 patients with CTD-ILD, 1 patient with FHP, and 1 patient with uIIP were included.
BMI, body mass index; DLCO, diffusion capacity of the lung for carbon monoxide; FVC, forced vital capacity; HRCT, high-resolution computed tomography; IPF, idiopathic pulmonary fibrosis; PF, progressive fibrosing; UIP, usual interstitial pneumonia.

Lung Function Changes

Figure 2 showed the mean lung function measures across different time intervals. The slope of FVC differed between the PF-ILD (−0.07 L/6 months, 95% CI −0.09 to −0.05) and non-PF-ILD (0.01 L/6 months, 95% CI 0.01–0.05) subgroups ($p = 0.001$) (**Figure 2D**). The slope of FVC% predicted in the PF-ILD group was −1.42%/6 months (95% CI −1.99 to −0.86), whereas that in the non-PF-ILD group was 2.80%/6 months (95% CI 2.12–3.49) ($p = 0.04$) (**Figure 2E**). The slope of DLCO% predicted also differed between subgroups (−1.84%/6 months, 95% CI −2.43 to −1.25 in the PF-ILD group vs. 1.93%/6 months, 95% CI 1.35 to 2.51 in the non-PF-ILD group, $p = 0.003$) (**Figure 2F**).

Predictive Characteristics Associated With Progressive Fibrosing

Table 3 shows the results of logistic regression analysis for predictors of progressive fibrosing. Multivariable analysis was performed on significant factors obtained from univariate analysis with a *p*-value < 0.2. Although the NLR (OR 0.69, 95% CI 0.55 to 1.08, $p = 0.039$) was significantly associated with PF, the OR included the value 1. Patients with clubbing of fingers (OR 1.52, 95% CI 1.03 to 2.24, $p = 0.035$) and an HRCT-documented UIP-like fibrotic pattern (OR 1.95, 95% CI 1.33 to 2.86, $p = 0.001$) showed a high risk of fibrosis progression.

Predictive Characteristics Associated With Survival

Patients were followed up for a median duration of 3 (2–4) years with 128 (22.1%) deaths during follow-up, and the median overall survival (OS) time for whole patients with fibrosing ILDs was 6 years. In the non-PF group, the median overall survival was not reached, while in the PF-ILD group, 85 of 227 (37.45%) patients died, with a median OS of 5 years (**Supplementary Figure S4**). The median survival time was shorter in patients with hypoxemia (OS: 4 years), baseline DLCO% predicted <50% (OS: 4 years), and UIP-like pattern (OS: 4.5 years). Subgroup analysis based on anti-fibrotic treatment using the log-rank test showed no significant intergroup difference ($p = 0.435$) (**Figure 3**). Within patients in the PF group who received anti-fibrotic treatment, IPF patients showed worse OS (OS: 4.5 years) than non-IPF patients (OS: 6 years) (log-rank test, $p = 0.003$, **Supplementary Figure S5**). **Table 4** shows the results of univariate and multivariate Cox analyses of predictors for all-cause mortality. By multivariate Cox analysis, lower DLCO% predicted (HR 2.25, 95% CI 1.45 to 3.50, $p < 0.001$), hypoxemia (HR 2.08, 95% CI 1.31 to 3.32, $p = 0.002$), and UIP-like fibrosis pattern on HRCT (HR 1.68, 95% CI 1.04 to 2.71, $p = 0.034$) were associated with an increased risk of mortality.

DISCUSSION

We provided a clinical cohort profile of patients with fibrosing ILD in China. A significant percentage of patients with fibrosing ILD tend to develop progressive fibrosing, which is associated with accelerated decline in lung function secondary to progressive fibrosis and symptomatic worsening (Nasser et al., 2021b). Prevalence of non-IPF PF-ILD varied from 28.57% to 39.07% owing to various diagnosis subgroups in our data, consistent with the findings reported by previous studies (approximately 33.0%) (Flaherty et al., 2019; Nasser et al., 2021b). A large-scale survey estimated that 18.0%–32.0% of patients diagnosed with non-IPF ILDs developed progressive fibrosis with overall survival of 61–80 months in the US, France, Germany, Italy, Spain, the

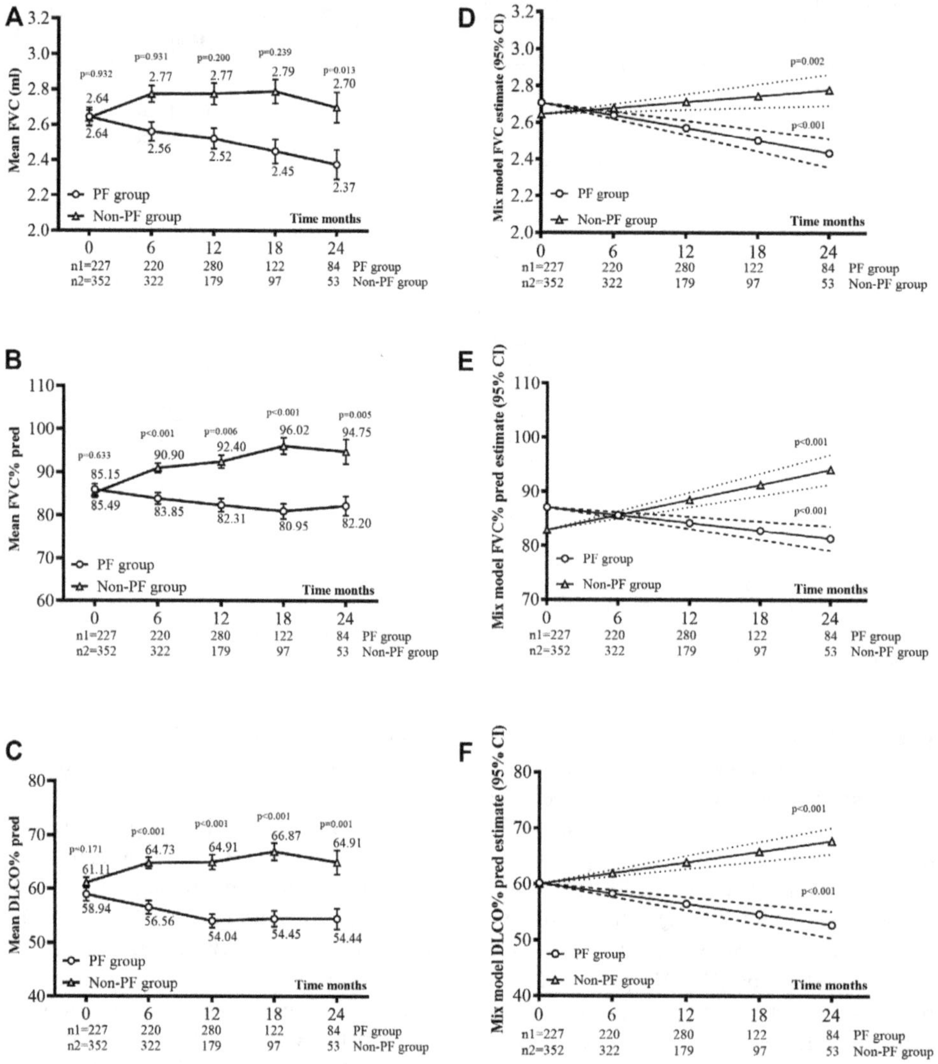

FIGURE 2 | Lung function changes. **(A)**, **(B)**, and **(C)** Mean FVC ml (±SE), mean FVC% predicted (±SE), and mean DLCO% predicted (±SE) during observation. **(D)**, **(E)**, and **(F)** Disease behavior (FVC, FVC% pred, and DLCO% pred) over time was analyzed using a linear mixed model for each group, with a random effect for the intercept and slope. The covariance for the repeated measures was left AR (autoregressive)1: heterogeneous, as this yielded the best fit.

United Kingdom, and Japan (Wijsenbeek et al., 2019). PF-ILD was identified in 135 of 396 (34.1%) patients with non-IPF ILDs in a cohort of Korean patients (Kwon et al., 2021). In another Chinese single-center cohort of 608 patients, 132 patients (21.7%) with ILD met the criteria for PF-ILD (Chen et al., 2021). The difference in findings between previous studies and our study may be attributable to the older age, poorer DLCO% predicted, or various disease classifications used for non-IPF ILDs in our patients. In our study, half of the patients with IPF showed rapid disease progression within 24 months. The clinical course of IPF is variable and difficult to predict, with a median survival time of 2–3 years after diagnosis without anti-fibrotic therapy. However, approximately 25.0% of patients survive over 5 years after the initial diagnosis (Kärkkäinen et al., 2019). Therefore, it is possible that lung function in patients with IPF remained stable or declined only slightly during the first 24 months but eventually led to poor outcomes.

Healthcare utilization is expected to be higher in patients with PF-ILD (Holtze et al., 2018; Wuyts et al., 2020). Hospitalization frequency was higher in the PF-ILD group than in the non-PF-ILD group during follow-up. Patients with PF-ILD received glucocorticoids for primary therapy, which emphasizes the need for alternative treatment. Many clinical trials have confirmed the efficacy of anti-fibrotic drugs to slow disease progression in patients with PF-ILD (Behr et al., 2021; Nambiar et al., 2021). Our data showed a trend of better survival in patients with PF-ILD, though not statistically significant, who received anti-fibrotic treatment; nintedanib and pirfenidone are known to prolong life expectancy in

TABLE 3 | Factors associated with progressive fibrosing.

Covariate	Univariable analysis		Multivariable analysis	
	OR (95% CI)	*p*-value	OR (95% CI)	*p*-value
Age	1.43 (1.02–2.00)	0.039	1.21 (0.85–1.73)	0.294
Male	1.16 (0.83–1.61)	0.400	–	–
BMI	0.85 (0.60–1.20)	0.351	–	–
Smoking	1.22 (0.87–1.71)	0.249	–	–
FVC% pred	0.69 (0.46–1.06)	0.090	0.72 (0.46–1.11)	0.134
DLCO% pred	1.24 (0.87–1.76)	0.237	–	–
Velcro	1.15 (0.82–1.61)	0.406	–	–
Clubbing of fingers	1.71 (1.17–2.48)	0.005	1.52 (1.03–2.24)	0.035
Hypoxemia	1.38 (0.92–2.07)	0.123	1.38 (0.90–2.11)	0.135
Hospitalization at baseline	1.26 (0.87–1.82)	0.219	–	–
UIP-like pattern on HRCT	2.18 (1.51–3.15)	<0.001	1.95 (1.33–2.86)	0.001
WBC	0.82 (0.59–1.15)	0.249	–	–
Neutrophils	0.75 (0.53–1.04)	0.086	0.76 (0.54–1.08)	0.122
Lymphocytes	0.82 (0.59–1.14)	0.237	–	–
Monocyte	0.88 (0.63–1.23)	0.464	–	–
RDW	0.98 (0.70–1.37)	0.913	–	–
LMR	1.08 (0.77–1.51)	0.656	–	–
NLR	0.69 (0.49–0.96)	0.028	0.69 (0.55–1.08)	0.039
PLR	0.94 (0.67–1.32)	0.712	–	–
SIRI	0.85 (0.61–1.19)	0.354	–	–
AISI	1.03 (0.73–1.46)	0.856	–	–

AISI: aggregate index of systemic inflammation; BMI, body mass index; CTD, connective tissue disease; DLCO, diffusion capacity of the lung for carbon monoxide; FVC: forced vital capacity; HRCT, high-resolution computed tomography; MLR, monocyte-to-lymphocyte ratio; NLR, neutrophil-to-lymphocyte ratio; PLR, platelet-to-lymphocyte ratio; RDW: red cell distribution width; SIRI, systemic inflammatory response index; UIP, usual interstitial pneumonia; WBC, white blood cell.

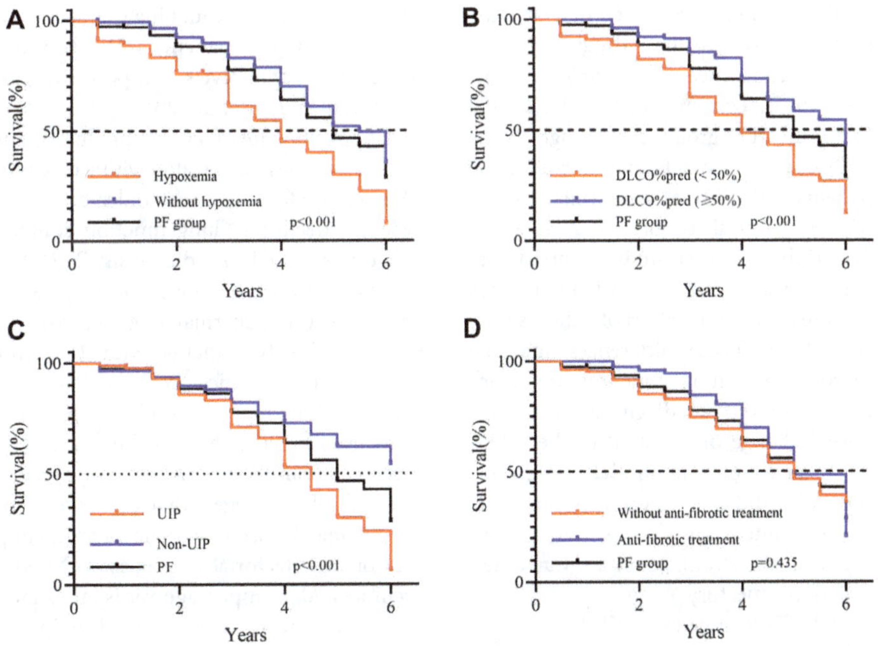

FIGURE 3 | Survival in patients with progressive fibrosing ILD. **(A)** Survival according to with or without hypoxemia at baseline (log-rank test, $p < 0.001$); **(B)** survival according to DLCO% pred at baseline with a 50% threshold (log-rank test, $p < 0.001$); **(C)** survival according to the UIP-like fibrotic pattern on HRCT (log-rank test, $p < 0.001$); **(D)** survival according to with or without anti-fibrotic treatment during observation (log-rank test, $p = 0.435$).

patients with IPF (Costabel et al., 2017; Lancaster et al., 2019). In the INBUILD trial, the annual rate of decline in the FVC in patients with PF-ILD was significantly lower among patients who received nintedanib (−80.8 ml/year) than among those who received a placebo (−187.8 ml/year) (Flaherty et al., 2019). However, only 32.16% of patients receive anti-fibrotic

TABLE 4 | Factors associated with 6-year all-cause mortality in the PF-group.

Covariate	Univariable analysis		Multivariable analysis	
	HR (95% CI)	*p*-value	HR (95% CI)	*p*-value
Age	1.57 (0.99–2.47)	0.054	1.1 (0.67–1.82)	0.698
Male	1.06 (0.69–1.64)	0.777	–	–
BMI	1.02 (0.65–1.58)	0.944	–	–
Smoking	1.23 (0.80–1.88)	0.347	–	–
FVC% pred	1.13 (0.66–1.95)	0.66	–	–
DLCO% pred	2.30 (1.50–3.45)	<0.001	2.25 (1.45–3.50)	<0.001
Velcro	0.97 (0.63–1.49)	0.88	–	–
Clubbing of fingers	0.77 (0.49–1.22)	0.269	–	–
Hypoxemia	2.24 (1.43–3.50)	<0.001	2.08 (1.31–3.32)	0.002
Hospitalization at baseline	0.90 (0.50–1.61)	0.719	–	–
UIP-like pattern on HRCT	0.23 (1.45–3.45)	<0.001	1.68 (1.04–2.71)	0.034
WBC	1.19 (0.78–1.83)	0.419	–	–
Neutrophils	1.09 (0.71–1.67)	0.697	–	–
Lymphocytes	1.24 (0.81–1.89)	0.33	–	–
Monocyte	1.19 (0.76–1.82)	0.429	–	–
RDW	1.15 (0.75–1.77)	0.516	–	–
LMR	0.86 (0.56–1.32)	0.482	–	–
NLR	1.16 (0.76–1.78)	0.495	–	–
PLR	0.78 (0.50–1.21)	0.268	–	–
SIRI	1.39 (0.91–2.13)	0.132	1.17 (0.76–1.82)	0.480
AISI	1.08 (0.69–1.67)	0.746	–	–
Anti-fibrotic treatment	0.84 (0.54–1.32)	0.450		

AISI: aggregate index of systemic inflammation; BMI: body mass index; CTD, connective tissue disease; DLCO, diffusion capacity of the lung for carbon monoxide; FVC, forced vital capacity; HRCT, high-resolution computed tomography; MLR, monocyte-to-lymphocyte ratio; NLR, neutrophil-to-lymphocyte ratio; PLR, platelet-to-lymphocyte ratio; RDW: red cell distribution width; SIRI, systemic inflammatory response index; UIP, usual interstitial pneumonia; WBC, white blood cell.

treatment in our real-world clinical settings, which indicates the possible financial burden associated with these drugs.

Overall, the mean lung function measures remained stable during follow-up in the non-PF-ILD group but showed a decline in the PF-ILD group. In the PF-ILD group, the change in the estimated mean annual FVC was −140 ml. In our study, the decline in the FVC in patients with PF-ILD was similar to that reported by the PROGRESS clinical cohort after 52 weeks (−136 ml) (Nasser et al., 2021b). Another study reported that the mean annual FVC change was −69.9 ml in a United States cohort and −50.0 ml in a United Kingdom cohort of patients with PF-ILD (Oldham et al., 2021). These differences may be attributable to the heterogeneous lung function trajectory across the ILD subgroups. Analysis of diagnosis subgroups showed a mean annual FVC change of −37.2 ml in the CTD-ILD, −92.0 ml in the FHP, and −69.5 ml in the IIP groups (Oldham et al., 2021). We did not perform diagnosis stratification owing to the limited sample size. A greater number of studies that perform the stratification are warranted to investigate the lung function trajectory.

We observed that the HRCT-documented UIP-like fibrotic pattern in patients with fibrosing ILDs was associated with more rapid disease progression, which suggests that morphological patterns may be prognostically significant; our findings are consistent with those reported by previous studies (Nasser et al., 2021b). Moreover, our study showed that clubbing of fingers (enlargement of the ends of the finger accompanied by a downward sloping of the nails) significantly predicted PF-ILD. A previous study reported that the prevalence of clubbing of fingers in cases of fibrosing ILDs ranged from 7.0% to 42.0% (van Manen et al., 2017). Clubbing of fingers is considered an essential clinical finding in patients with fibrosing ILDs and represents decreased oxygen levels and poor prognosis (Kanematsu et al., 1994; van Manen et al., 2017).

Hypoxemia, low DLCO% predicted, and HRCT-documented UIP pattern were associated with worse mortality in patients with PF. Reportedly, male sex, older age, lower FVC or DLCO at baseline, decline in lung function compared with the baseline, subgroups based on diagnosis, HRCT-documented UIP-like fibrotic pattern, or honeycombing were indicators of poor prognosis (Wongkarnjana et al., 2020). Cluster analysis was used to classify patients with ILD into clinical subgroups based on their clinical courses. Patients with the most rapid decline in lung function or fibrosis progression and poor survival were usually clustered together in ILDs or IP with myositis-specific autoantibodies (Adegunsoye et al., 2018; Lia et al., 2022). These findings suggest that evidence of progressive pulmonary fibrosis may be useful to define a group of patients with fibrosing ILD of multifactorial etiologies and poor prognoses. Although accurate and prompt diagnosis is important to enable initiation of optimal management, it is possible to identify patients at high risk of progression through observation of disease behavior despite the specific diagnosis. Validation cohorts are required to confirm mortality predictors.

Given the possible relationship between prognosis and biomarkers obtained by the routinely provided blood cell count test in IPF, we sought to explore the prognostic capacity of the blood cell count and the combined indexes in PF-ILDs. A pooled retrospective analysis of 2,067 IPF patients derived from the clinical trials showed that patients with higher monocyte count had a higher 1-year risk of progression, all-cause mortality, and all-cause hospitalization (Kreuter et al., 2021). On the contrary, we did not observe the relationship between disease progression or mortality and blood cell count and the combined index. According to a multicenter retrospective study, higher baseline NLR and absolute monocyte counts predict worse survival in IPF but not in fHP (Barratt et al., 2021), highlighting the potential divergence in the underlying mechanisms of these diseases. However, our sample size is smaller than the previous reports for the prognostic role of blood cell counts. Second, single peripheral blood cell measures may be influenced by many short-term factors. Further multicenter studies with a larger population would be informative about the applicability of blood cell counts in predicting prognosis.

We provided data on longitudinal clinical outcomes in patients with fibrosing ILD from China. Patients evaluated in a tertiary referral center through a multidisciplinary discussion were routinely followed up every 6–12 months with pulmonary function tests, HRCT, and visits. Unlike previous studies for FP-ILDs (Flaherty et al., 2019; Wijsenbeek et al., 2019; Nasser et al., 2021b) which generally emphasized non-IPF patients, our cohort included both IPF and non-IPF patients as a whole group and also provided separate data for both groups. In this way, the exploration between clinical characteristics and prognosis of patients with PF-ILD is of more clinically utility because it is hard to make specific diagnosis for some ILDs at an early stage, especially for IPF. In addition, we tried to study the relationship between the patient's blood count values and prognosis, which was not explored in PF-ILD patients as a whole group before. The negative results were supported by some previous research studies while opposed by others studying specific diagnosis group of diseases, highlighting cautious use of routine blood test values as prognosis predictors.

Several limitations should be considered: 1) the retrospective and monocentric design of this study may have led to a selection bias. 2) This was a small-scale study in which we observed a reduction in available data on lung function over time, which resulted in an inaccurate estimation of the lung function trajectory. 3) Acute exacerbations, as one of the leading causes of death in patients with IPF (annual incidence of up to 20.0%) (Richeldi, 2015; Kolb et al., 2018; Ruaro et al., 2021; Yoon et al., 2021), were not investigated because some exacerbations were not recorded in the medical system of our hospital. The annual incidence of acute exacerbations in patients with non-IPF PF-ILD was 13.9% (Nasser et al., 2021b; Petnak et al., 2021; Yoon et al., 2021). Further studies are warranted to thoroughly investigate the effects of acute exacerbations. 4) We used all-cause mortality rather than ILD-related mortality as the outcome because all deaths did not occur at the hospital, and some causes of death were not reported reliably.

In summary, we presented a hospital population-based cohort profile of patients with PF-ILDs in China. We reported that 28.57%–53.10% of patients with fibrosing ILD developed a progressive fibrosing feature. Patients with clubbing of fingers or an HRCT-documented UIP pattern showed a high potential risk for PF-ILD. The risk factors associated with mortality in patients with PF-ILD included hypoxemia, low DLCO% predicted, or an HRCT-documented UIP pattern. The relationship between prognosis and blood cell count and the combined index was not observed, highlighting the divergence in the underlying mechanisms of PF-ILDs.

ETHICS STATEMENT

The studies involving human participants were reviewed and approved by the Institutional Review Board of Beijing Chao-Yang Hospital. The patients/participants provided their written informed consent to participate in this study.

AUTHOR CONTRIBUTIONS

The authors were responsible for all content of the manuscript. YW performed data collection, analyzed the data, contributed to interpretation, and wrote the manuscript. ZG, RM, JW, and YF were responsible for recruiting the patients and collecting the data. NW helped in the drafting and revision. QY contributed as primary investigator and was responsible for designing the study, recruiting the patients, analyzing and interpreting the data, and writing the manuscript. All authors read and approved the final manuscript.

ACKNOWLEDGMENTS

We thank all patients who were involved in this study. We express our thanks to Miss Moyang Xu of the University of Michigan and Ann Arbor for polishing the language and grammar of the manuscript.

REFERENCES

1. Abe, M., Tsushima, K., Ishii, D., Shikano, K., Yoshioka, K., Sakayori, M., et al. (2021). Risk Factors for Acute Exacerbation Following Bronchoalveolar Lavage in Patients with Suspected Idiopathic Pulmonary Fibrosis: A Retrospective Cohort Study. *Adv. Respir. Med.* 89 (2), 101–109. doi:10.5603/ARM.a2021.0012
2. Adegunsoye, A., Oldham, J. M., Chung, J. H., Montner, S. M., Lee, C., Witt, L. J., et al. (2018). Phenotypic Clusters Predict Outcomes in a Longitudinal Interstitial Lung Disease Cohort. *Chest* 153 (2), 349–360. doi:10.1016/j.chest.2017.09.026
3. Barratt, S. L., Creamer, A. W., Adamali, H. I., Duckworth, A., Fallon, J., Fidan, S., et al. (2021). Use of Peripheral Neutrophil to Lymphocyte Ratio and Peripheral Monocyte Levels to Predict Survival in Fibrotic Hypersensitivity Pneumonitis (fHP): A Multicentre Retrospective Cohort Study. *BMJ Open Respir. Res.* 8 (1), e001063. doi:10.1136/bmjresp-2021-001063
4. Behr, J., Prasse, A., Kreuter, M., Johow, J., Rabe, K. F., Bonella, F., et al. (2021). Pirfenidone in Patients with Progressive Fibrotic Interstitial Lung Diseases Other Than Idiopathic Pulmonary Fibrosis (RELIEF): a Double-Blind, Randomised, Placebo-Con trolled, Phase 2b Trial. *Lancet Respir. Med.* 9 (5), 476–486. doi:10.1016/s2213-2600(20)30554-3

5. Chen, X., Guo, J., Yu, D., Jie, B., and Zhou, Y. (2021). Predictors of Mortality in Progressive Fibrosing Interstitial Lung Diseases. *Front. Pharmacol.* 12, 754851. doi:10.3389/fphar.2021.754851
6. Churg, A. (2022). Hypersensitivity Pneumonitis: New Concepts and Classifications. *Mod. Pathol.* 35 (Suppl. 1), 15–27. doi:10.1038/s41379-021-00866-y
7. Costabel, U., Albera, C., Lancaster, L. H., Lin, C. Y., Hormel, P., Hulter, H. N., et al. (2017). An Open-Label Study of the Long-Term Safety of Pirfenidone in Patients with Idiopathic Pulmonary Fibrosis (RECAP). *Respiration* 94 (5), 408–415. doi:10.1159/000479976
8. Cottin, V., Hirani, N. A., Hotchkin, D. L., Nambiar, A. M., Ogura, T., Otaola, M., et al. (2018). Presentation, Diagnosis and Clinical Course of the Spectrum of Progressive-Fibrosing Interstitial Lung Diseases. *Eur. Respir. Rev.* 27 (150), 180076. doi:10.1183/16000617.0076-2018
9. Cottin, V., Wollin, L., Fischer, A., Quaresma, M., Stowasser, S., and Harari, S. (2019). Fibrosing Interstitial Lung Diseases: Knowns and Unknowns. *Eur. Respir. Rev.* 28 (151), 180100. doi:10.1183/16000617.0100-2018
10. Flaherty, K. R., Wells, A. U., Cottin, V., Devaraj, A., Walsh, S. L. F., Inoue, Y., et al. (2019). Nintedanib in Progressive Fibrosing Interstitial Lung Diseases. *N. Engl. J. Med.* 381 (18), 1718–1727. doi:10.1056/NEJMoa1908681
11. George, P. M., Spagnolo, P., Kreuter, M., Altinisi k, G., Bonifazi, M., Martinez, F. J., et al. (2020). Progressive Fibrosing Interstitial Lung Disease: Clinical Uncertainties, Consensus Recommendations, and Research Priorities. *Lancet Respir. Med.* 8 (9), 925–934. doi:10.1016/s2213-2600(20)30355-6
12. Gibson, C. D., Kugler, M. C., Deshwal, H., Munger, J. S., and Condos, R. (2020). Advances in Targeted Therapy for Progressive Fibrosing Interstitial Lung Disease. *Lung* 198 (4), 597–608. doi:10.1007/s00408-020-00370-1
13. Hoffmann-Vold, A. M., Allanore, Y., Alves, M., Brunborg, C., Airó, P., Ananieva, L. P., et al. (2021). Progressive Interstitial Lung Disease in Patients with Systemic Sclerosis-Associated Interstitial Lung Disease in the EUSTAR Database. *Ann. Rheum. Dis.* 80 (2), 219–227. doi:10.1136/annrheumdis-2020-217455
14. Holtze, C., Flaherty, K., Kreuter, M., Luppi, F., Moua, T., Vancheri, C., et al. (2018). Healthcare Utilisation and Costs in the Diagnosis and Treatment of Progressive-Fibrosing Interstitial Lung Diseases. *Eur. Respir. Rev.* 27 (150), 180078. doi:10.1183/16000617.0078-2018
15. Johnson, C. (2017). Recent Advances in the Pathogenesis, Prediction, and Management of Rheumatoid Arthritis-Associated Interstitial Lung Disease. *Curr. Opin. Rheumatol.* 29 (3), 254–259. doi:10.1097/bor.0000000000000380
16. Kanematsu, T., Kitaichi, M., Nishimura, K., Nagai, S., and Izumi, T. (1994). Clubbing of the Fingers and Smooth-Muscle Proliferation in Fibrotic Changes in the Lung in Patients with Idiopathic Pulmonary Fibrosis. *Chest* 105 (2), 339–342. doi:10.1378/chest.105.2.339
17. Kärkkäinen, M., Kettunen, H. P., Nurmi, H., Selander, T., Purokivi, M., and Kaarteenaho, R. (2019). Comparison of Disease Progression Subgroups in Idiopathic Pulmonary Fibrosis. *BMC Pulm. Med.* 19 (1), 228. doi:10.1186/s12890-019-0996-2
18. Khanna, D., Tashkin, D. P., Denton, C. P., Renzoni, E. A., Desai, S. R., and Varga, J. (2020). Etiology, Risk Factors, and Biomarkers in Systemic Sclerosis with Interstitial Lung Disease. *Am. J. Respir. Crit. Care Med.* 201 (6), 650–660. doi:10.1164/rccm.201903-0563CI
19. Kolb, M., Bondue, B., Pesci, A., Miyazaki, Y., Song, J. W., Bhatt, N. Y., et al. (2018). Acute Exacerbations of Progressive-Fibrosing Interstitial Lung Diseases. *Eur. Respir. Rev.* 27 (150), 180071. doi:10.1183/16000617.0071-2018
20. Kolb, M., and Vašáková, M. (2019). The Natural History of Progressive Fibrosing Interstitial Lung Diseases. *Respir. Res.* 20 (1), 57. doi:10.1186/s12931-019-1022-1
21. Kreuter, M., Lee, J. S., Tzouvelekis, A., Oldham, J. M., Molyneaux, P. L., Weycker, D., et al. (2021). Monocyte Count as a Prognostic Biomarker in Patients with Idiopathic Pulmonary Fibrosis. *Am. J. Respir. Crit. Care Med.* 204 (1), 74–81. doi:10.1164/rccm.202003-0669OC
22. Kwon, B. S., Choe, J., Chae, E. J., Hwang, H. S., Kim, Y. G., and Song, J. W. (2021). Progressive Fibrosing Interstitial Lung Disease: Prevalence and Clinical Outcome. *Respir. Res.* 22 (1), 282. doi:10.1186/s12931-021-01879-6
23. Lacedonia, D., Correale, M., Tricarico, L., Scioscia, G., Stornelli, S. R., Simone, F., et al. (2022). Survival of Patients with Idiopathic Pulmonary Fibrosis and Pulmonary Hypertension under Therapy with Nintedanib or Pirfenidone. *Intern Emerg. Med.* 17 (3), 815–822. doi:10.1007/s11739-021-02883-w
24. Lancaster, L., Crestani, B., Hernandez, P., Inoue, Y., Wachtlin, D., Loaiza, L., et al. (2019). Safety and Survival Data in Patients with Idiopathic Pulmonary Fibrosis Treated with Nintedanib: Pooled Data from Six Clinical Trials. *BMJ Open Respir. Res.* 6 (1), e000397. doi:10.1136/bmjresp-2018-000397
25. Lee, C. T., Ventura, I. B., Phillips, E. K., Leahy, A., Jablonski, R., Montner, S., et al. (2022). Interstitial Lung Disease in Firefighters: An Emerging Occupational Hazard. *Front. Med. (Lausanne)* 9, 864658. doi:10.3389/fmed.2022.864658
26. Lia, Y., Fana, Y., Wanga, Y., Yanga, S., Dua, X., and Yea, Q. (2022). Phenotypic Clusters and Survival Analyses in Interstitial Pneumonia with Myositis-specific Autoantibodies. *Sarcoidosis Vasc. Diffuse Lung Dis.* 38 (4), e2021047. doi:10. 36141/svdld.v38i4.11368
27. Misharin, A. V., Morales-Nebreda, L., Reyfman, P. A., Cuda, C. M., Walter, J. M., McQuattie-Pimentel, A. C., et al. (2017). Monocyte-derived Alveolar Macrophages Drive Lung Fibrosis and Persist in the Lung over the Life Span. *J. Exp. Med.* 214 (8), 2387–2404. doi:10.1084/jem.20162152
28. Nambiar, A. M., Walker, C. M., and Sparks, J. A. (2021). Monitoring and Management of Fibrosing Interstitial Lung Diseases: a Narrative Review for Practicing Clinicians. *Ther. Adv. Respir. Dis.* 15, 17534666211039771. doi:10.1177/17534666211039771
29. Nasser, M., Larrieu, S., Boussel, L., Si-Mohamed, S., Bazin, F., Marque, S., et al. (2021a). Estimates of Epidemiology, Mortality and Disease Burden Associated with Progressive Fibrosing Interstitial Lung Disease in France (The PROGRESS Study). *Respir. Res.* 22 (1), 162. doi:10.1186/s12931-021-01749-1
30. Nasser, M., Larrieu, S., Si-Mohamed, S., Ahmad, K., Boussel, L., Brevet, M., et al. (2021b). Progressive Fibrosing Interstitial Lung Disease: a Clinical Cohort (The PROGRESS Study). *Eur. Respir. J.* 57 (2), 2002718. doi:10.1183/13993003. 02718-2020
31. Oldham, J. M., Lee, C. T., Wu, Z., Bowman, W. S., Vu Pugashetti, J., Dao, N., et al. (2021). Lung Function Trajectory in Progressive Fibrosing Interstitial Lung Disease. *Eur. Respir. J.* 59 (6), 2101396. doi:10.1183/13993003.01396-2021
32. Olson, A. L., Gifford, A. H., Inase, N., Fernández Pérez, E. R., and Suda, T. (2018). The Epidemiology of Idiopathic Pulmonary Fibrosis and Interstitial Lung Diseases at Risk of a Progressive-Fibrosing Phenotype. *Eur. Respir. Rev.* 27 (150), 180077. doi:10.1183/16000617.0077-2018
33. Orlandi, M., Landini, N., Sambataro, G., Nardi, C., Tofani, L., Bruni, C., et al. (2022). The Role of Chest CT in Deciphering Interstitial Lung Involvement: Systemic Sclerosis versus COVID-19. *Rheumatol. Oxf.* 61 (4), 1600–1609. doi:10.1093/rheumatology/keab615
34. Petnak, T., Lertjitbanjong, P., Thongprayoon, C., and Moua, T. (2021). Impact of Antifibrotic Therapy on Mortality and Acute Exacerbation in Idiopathic Pulmonary Fibrosis: A Systematic Review and Meta-Analysis. *Chest* 160 (5), 1751–1763. doi:10.1016/j.chest.2021.06.049
35. Raghu, G., Collard, H. R., Egan, J. J., Martinez, F. J., Behr, J., Brown, K. K., et al. (2011). An Official ATS/ERS/JRS/ALAT Statement: Idiopathic Pulmonary Fibrosis: Evidence-Based Guidelines for Diagnosis and Management. *Am. J. Respir. Crit. Care Med.* 183 (6), 788–824. doi:10.1164/rccm.2009-040GL
36. Raghu, G., Remy-Jardin, M., Myers, J. L., Richeldi, L., Ryerson, C. J., Lederer, D. J., et al. (2018). Diagnosis of Idiopathic Pulmonary Fibrosis. An Official ATS/ERS/ JRS/ALAT Clinical Practice Guideline. *Am. J. Respir. Crit. Care Med.* 198 (5), e44–e68. doi:10.1164/rccm.201807-1255ST
37. Raghu, G., Remy-Jardin, M., Richeldi, L., Thomson, C. C., Inoue, Y., Johkoh, T., et al. (2022). Idiopathic Pulmonary Fibrosis (An Update) and Progressive Pulmonary Fibrosis in Adults: An Official ATS/ERS/JRS/ALAT Clinical Practice Guideline. *Am. J. Respir. Crit. Care Med.* 205 (9), e18–e47. doi:10.1164/rccm.202202-0399ST
38. Richeldi, L. (2015). Time for Prevention of Idiopathic Pulmonary Fibrosis Exacerbation. *Ann. Am. Thorac. Soc.* 12 Suppl 2, S181–S185. doi:10.1513/AnnalsATS.201504-210AW
39. Ruaro, B., Baratella, E., Confalonieri, P., Wade, B., Marrocchio, C., Geri, P., et al. (2021). High-Resolution Computed Tomography: Lights and Shadows in Improving Care for SSc-ILD Patients. *Diagnostics* 11 (11), 1960. doi:10. 3390/diagnostics11111960

40. Sharma, A., Ferraro, V., Renzoni, E. A., and Morisset, J. (2021). Chronic Hypersensitivity Pneumonitis: Real World Diagnostic Criteria. *Curr. Opin. Pulm. Med.* 27 (5), 414–421. doi:10.1097/mcp.0000000000000799
41. Skibba, M., Drelich, A., Poellmann, M., Hong, S., and Brasier, A. R. (2020). Nanoapproaches to Modifying Epigenetics of Epithelial Mesenchymal Transition for Treatment of Pulmonary Fibrosis. *Front. Pharmacol.* 11, 607689. doi:10.3389/fphar.2020.607689
42. van Manen, M. J. G., Vermeer, L. C., Moor, C. C., Vrijenhoeff, R., Grutters, J. C., Veltkamp, M., et al. (2017). Clubbing in Patients with Fibrotic Interstitial Lung Diseases. *Respir. Med.* 132, 226–231. doi:10.1016/j.rmed.2017.10.021
43. Walsh, S. L. F., Devaraj, A., Enghelmayer, J. I., Kishi, K., Silva, R. S., Patel, N., et al. (2018). Role of Imaging in Progressive-Fibrosing Interstitial Lung Diseases. *Eur. Respir. Rev.* 27 (150), 180073. doi:10.1183/16000617.0073-2018
44. Wang, Y., Hou, Z., Qiu, M., and Ye, Q. (2018). Risk Factors for Primary Sjögren Syndrome-Associated Interstitial Lung Disease. *J. Thorac. Dis.* 10 (4), 2108–2117. doi:10.21037/jtd.2018.03.120
45. Wijsenbeek, M., Kreuter, M., Olson, A., Fischer, A., Bendstrup, E., Wells, C. D., et al. (2019). Progressive Fibrosing Interstitial Lung Diseases: Current Practice in Diagnosis and Management. *Curr. Med. Res. Opin.* 35 (11), 2015–2024. doi:10.1080/03007995.2019.1647040
46. Wongkarnjana, A., Scallan, C., and Kolb, M. R. J. (2020). Progressive Fibrosing Interstitial Lung Disease: Treatable Traits and Therapeutic Strategies. *Curr. Opin. Pulm. Med.* 26 (5), 436–442. doi:10.1097/mcp.0000000000000712
47. Wuyts, W. A., Papiris, S., Manali, E., Kilpeläinen, M., Davidsen, J. R., Miedema, J., et al. (2020). The Burden of Progressive Fibrosing Interstitial Lung Disease: A DELPHI Approach. *Adv. Ther.* 37 (7), 3246–3264. doi:10.1007/s12325-020-01384-0
48. Yang, S., Chai, D., Li, Y., Wang, Y., Zhan, X., Zhang, L., et al. (2022). Patterns of Lung Diseases Predict Survival in Patients with MPO-ANCA-Associated Vasculitis: a Single-Center Retrospective Study. *Clin. Rheumatol.* 41 (3), 783–793. doi:10.1007/s10067-021-05964-5
49. Yoon, H. Y., Lee, S. H., Ha, S., Ryu, J. S., and Song, J. W. (2021). 18F-FDG PET/CT Predicts Acute Exacerbation in Idiopathic Pulmonary Fibrosis after Thoracic Surgery. *BMC Pulm. Med.* 21 (1), 294. doi:10.1186/s12890-021-01659-4

13

Targeting TL1A/DR3 Signaling Offers a Therapeutic Advantage to Neutralizing IL13/IL4Rα in Muco-Secretory Fibrotic Disorders

Hope Steele[1], *Kacey Sachen*[2], *Andrew J. McKnight*[2], *Rachel Soloff*[2] *and Rana Herro*[1,3*]

[1] *Division of Immunobiology, Cincinnati Children's Hospital Medical Center, Cincinnati, OH, United States,* [2] *Kyowa Kirin Pharmaceutical Research, Inc., La Jolla, CA, United States,* [3] *Department of Pediatrics, University of Cincinnati, Cincinnati, OH, United States*

Correspondence:
Rana Herro
rana.herro@cchmc.org

Mucus secretion is an important feature of asthma that highly correlates with morbidity. Current therapies, including administration of mucolytics and anti-inflammatory drugs, show limited effectiveness and durability, underscoring the need for novel effective and longer lasting therapeutic approaches. Here we show that mucus production in the lungs is regulated by the TNF superfamily member 15 (TL1A) acting through the mucus–inducing cytokine IL-13. TL1A induces IL13 expression by innate lymphoid cells leading to mucus production, in addition to promoting airway inflammation and fibrosis. Reciprocally, neutralization of IL13 signaling through its receptor (IL4Rα), completely reverses TL1A-induced mucus secretion, while maintaining airway inflammation and fibrosis. Importance of TL1A is further demonstrated using a preclinical asthma model induced by chronic house dust mite exposure where TL1A neutralization by genetic deletion or antagonistic blockade of its receptor DR3 protected against mucus production and fibrosis. Thus, TL1A presents a promising therapeutic target that out benefits IL13 in reversing mucus production, airway inflammation and fibrosis, cardinal features of severe asthma in humans.

Keywords: mucus, asthma, TL1A, IL13, fibrosis

INTRODUCTION

Many fibro-proliferative disorders of the lung such as asthma and chronic obstructive pulmonary disease (COPD) exhibit increased morbidity associated with mucus hypersecretion (1, 2). Existing therapies are available, but these have varying effectiveness. Bronchodilators do not specifically target mucus hypersecretion (3, 4). Moreover, severe asthmatics become gradually resistant to corticosteroids (5–7). Therefore, there is an absolute necessity to develop novel therapies to limit mucus hypersecretion and improve patient outcomes.

Interleukin-13 (IL13) has recently emerged as a primary target for asthma therapy, with ongoing clinical trials targeting IL13 or approved therapeutics targeting its receptor interleukin-4 receptor α

Abbreviations: IPF, Idiopathic pulmonary fibrosis; TNF, Tumor necrosis factor; TL1A, TNF-like ligand 1A; DR3, Death Receptor 3; ILC, Innate lymphoid cells; COPD, Chronic obstructive pulmonary disease; IL13, Interleukin 13; IL4Rα: Interleukin 4 receptor α; TNFSF15, Tumor necrosis factor superfamily member 15; ClcA1, Chloride channel regulator, Calcium-Activated-1; PAS, Periodic Acid-Schiff; H&E, Hematoxylin and Eosin; i.t., Intratracheal; i.n., Intranasal; i.p., Intraperitoneal.

(IL4Rα) (8, 9). It is thought that IL13 is central for mucus hypersecretion *via* direct effects on bronchial epithelial cells, in addition to promoting smooth muscle contractility, inflammation and fibrosis (10, 11). *In vitro*, lung epithelial cells that were differentiated in an air-liquid interphase and stimulated with IL13, increased their expression of ClcA1, a goblet cell-derived calcium-activated chloride channel tightly linked to mucus production, in addition to the mucin MUC5AC (10). Silencing ClcA1 inhibited IL13-driven mucin production by these cells, indicating that IL13 is dependent on ClcA1 to induce mucus production (10). IL4 another Th2 cytokine that binds to the IL4Rα, is unable to promote MUC5AC production by differentiated goblet cells, as compared to ones treated with IL13 (12). Despite their common receptor, IL4 and IL13 have non redundant activities in asthma. Whereas IL4 acts predominantly in the early phase of asthma development, IL13 is thought to be active in the late phase of allergic reactions. IL4 is involved in regulating T cell proliferation and survival, and IgE synthesis. In contrast, IL-13 is predominantly involved in airway remodeling and mucus hypersecretion (12–14). Several lines of evidence support the contention that IL13, and not IL4, controls mucus production in asthma. In fact, the *in vivo* blockade of IL13 alone, by genetic deletion (15) or antagonistic administration of the IL13Ra2-Ig both prevents and reverses established mucus cell changes (16). Anti-IL4 administration did not reduce the numbers of mucin-secreting cells in the bronchial epithelium of mice induced with ovalbumin (15). Moreover, the *in vivo* administration of recombinant IL13 in the airways enhanced mucus secretion, in IL4-deficient mice (17). Additionally, IL4-deficient Th2 cells adoptively transferred to mice receiving inhaled ovalbumin failed to enhance mucus production by their bronchial epithelium (18). Furthermore, conjugate vaccines against IL4 failed to reduce mucus production in murine model of asthma induced by HDM, as opposed to ones directed against IL13 that abrogated mucus production in the lung bronchial epithelium (14). Collectively this data indicates IL4 is unable to mount a muco-secretory phenotype independently of IL13.

Other soluble molecules could possess similar activities on goblet cells. We have recently discovered that TL1A is able to induce lung fibrosis and tissue remodeling associated with eosinophilic asthma and idiopathic pulmonary fibrosis (IPF) (19). TL1A (aka TNFSF15) is a member of the TNF superfamily that signals through death receptor 3 (DR3) (20, 21). We demonstrated that interrupting TL1A/DR3 signaling, by genetic deletion of the receptor or antagonistic blocking, decreases collagen deposition and smooth muscle accumulation in the lungs in two different models: the allergen-induced eosinophilic asthma model (Th2 asthma) and the bleomycin-induced IPF model (19). Airway resistance in response to methacholine was significantly decreased when active TL1A signaling was lacking (19). Moreover, we showed that the airway administration of recombinant TL1A in isolation is sufficient to promote collagen deposition and smooth muscle hypertrophy. We demonstrated that aside from its pro-inflammatory role, TL1A can exert direct activity on stromal cells (fibroblasts and epithelial cells) to induce fibrosis (19). This was an unprecedented discovery linking TL1A to tissue remodeling and lung fibrosis. Here, we investigated the role of TL1A in mucus production. This is interesting, as mucus plugs and airway obstruction lead to respiratory failure and constitute the main causes of death in asthma and COPD (22, 23).

In this work, we demonstrate that the intra-tracheal administration of TL1A into the airways induces mucus production (aside from fibrosis), and conversely, when blocking TL1A signaling through DR3, mucus production was abrogated in murine eosinophilic asthma. Additionally, we show that TL1A muco-secretory activity is indirect on goblet cells. TL1A induces IL13 production by group 2 innate lymphoid cells (ILC2), which subsequently promotes mucus production. TL1A represents a promising therapeutic target for muco-secretory diseases. This work has tremendous potential significance in human asthma, COPD and cystic fibrosis therapies.

MATERIALS AND METHODS

Mice

Six- to eight-week-old male and female DR3-deficient mice and WT littermates (house on the C57BL/6 x 129 background), derived by Taconic Biosciences (#TF3529; Rensselaer, NY), were bred in-house. Male and female WT C57BL/6 or BALB/c and IL4Rα-deficient mice were purchased from Jackson Laboratories (Bar Harbor, ME). RAG2-deficient mice bred on the BALB/c x 129 background were a generous gift of Dr. Nunzio Bottini (UCSD), and RAG2γc-deficient mice on the BALB/c x 129 background were purchased from Jackson Laboratories (#014593). In all studies, both male and female mice were used. All studies and protocols were approved by and in compliance with the regulations of the Institutional Animal Care and Use Committees of Cincinnati Children's Hospital Medical Center.

Experimental Protocols

Activity of recombinant protein: WT C57BL/6 mice, RAG2-deficient mice, and RAG2γc-deficient mice, were given 10 μg of recombinant mouse TL1A (R&D Systems, Minneapolis, MN) or PBS intratracheally on days 1 and 2 and sacrificed for analyses one day later on day 3. Ocean Ridge Biosciences (Deerfield Beach, FL) performed the RNAseq transcriptomic screen and analysis on the lungs of mice induced with TL1A, *via* Illumina HiSeq 2000 (NCBI SRA database BioProject # PRJNA735223).

Asthma model: WT littermates and DR3-deficient mice on the C57BL/6 x 129 background, from both sexes, were sensitized i.n. on day 0, 7, and 14 with 200 and 100 μg house dust mite extract protein (HDM; GREER Labs Inc, Lenoir, North Carolina; endotoxin levels at 930EU/vial) in PBS, followed by chronic i.n. challenges of 50 μg of HDM protein administered twice a week for the following 4 weeks as previously described (24). Analyses were performed 24 hours after the last challenge. For neutralization of TL1A-DR3 interactions, mouse DR3-Fc (generous gift of Dr. Soloff) or isotype control IgG (BioXCell,

Lebanon, NH) were administered intraperitoneal (i.p.) to WT C57BL/6 mice after the initial sensitization period starting at day 14 and were given every three days until the end of the experiment (100 μg/injection/mouse).

Immunofluorescence Staining of ClcA1, MUC5AC, and α-Smooth Muscle Actin

Paraffin-embedded tissues are sliced 4μm thick each section. Deparaffinization is performed by successive incubation in xylene, followed by 100% ethanol and 75% ethanol for 5 min each time. Sections are washed in PBS before being treated with antigen retrieval solution (Citrate buffer pH 6) for 20 min in the microwave (Power 3) and rested for an additional 20 min at room temperature (RT). The sections are then washed in PBS and incubated in blocking solution containing 10% Donkey Serum and Fc block for 1h at RT. Primary antibodies for ClcA1 (clone EPR12254; Abcam, Cambridge, MA) and MUC5AC (clone 45M1; Abcam) are used at 1:100 dilution according to the manufacturer recommendations and incubation is performed overnight at 4°C. Sections are washed in PBS three times before staining with secondary antibodies Donkey anti-mouse and Donkey anti-rabbit (ImmunoJackson Research, West Grove, PA) at 1:500 dilution for 3h at RT. Sections are then washed in PBS three times and nuclear staining is performed using DAPI at 1:10000 dilution for 5 min at RT. Sections are mounted in ProLong Gold Antifade Mountant (Thermo Fisher Scientific, Waltham, MA) and imaged on Nikon Inverted immunofluorescence microscope.

Immunohistochemistry Staining

PAS, Hematoxylin and Eosin (H&E) and Trichrome stains are performed according to the manufacturers' recommendations (Poly Scientific R&D, Bay Shore, NY and Thermo Fisher Scientific). Sections are scanned using the Zeiss Axioscanner ×20 objective and analyzed using Image-Pro Premier software.

Type 2 Innate Lymphoid Cells Sorting and DR3 Stain

Lung ILC2 are sorted on the following markers CD45.2$^+$Lin$^-$ Thy1.2$^+$ ST2$^+$Sca1$^+$All antibodies are purchased from Biolegend (San Diego, CA) with exception to ST2 (101001PE, MD Biosciences). DR3 stain is performed using the clone 4C12 from Biolegend.

ILC2 Culture and Stimulation With TL1A

ILC2 are cultured for five days in the presence of 50ng/ml IL2, IL7, and IL33 (Peprotech, Rocky Hill, NJ and R&D Systems) followed by two days culture with 10ng/ml IL2, IL7, and IL33 and 100 ng/ml TL1A (R&D Systems# 1896 TL). Measurements of IL13 in the culture supernatants is performed using mouse IL13 DuoSet ELISA (R&D Systems).

Flow Cytometry

BAL and lung cells were treated with RBC lysing buffer (Sigma). Lungs were dissociated using a Lung Dissociation Kit (Miltenyi Biotec) and Gentle MACS (Miltenyi Biotec). LIVE/DEAD cells were stained with Fixable Aqua Dead Cell Staining Kit (Thermo Fisher Scientific), and after Fc block with the 2.4G2 mAb (eBioscience), cells were stained with the following Abs: DR3-PE (4C12; BioLegend), SiglecF (E50-2440; BD Biosciences), CD11b (M1/70; BD Biosciences), CD11c (HL3; BD Biosciences), Ly6G (1A8; BioLegend), ST2-PE (101001PE, MD), CD90.2 (30-H12; BioLegend). For lineage markers for ILC2 staining, the following Abs were used: CD3-FITC (145-2C11; eBioscience), CD4-FITC (GK1.5; eBioscience), CD8- FITC (5H-10-1; BioLegend), CD19-FITC (1D3; BioLegend), NK1.1-FITC (PK136; BioLegend), CD11b-FITC (M1/70; BioLegend), CD11c-FITC (HL3; BD Biosciences), and Gr1-FITC (RB6-8C5; BioLegend). Flow cytometry analysis was performed on a Fortessa (BD Biosciences), and data were analyzed using FlowJo Software (version 10; FlowJo, Ashland, OR). Live CD45+ lung immune cells were separated into T cells (CD3+, CD90.2+), macrophages (CD11b+, CD11c+ SiglecF+), DCs (CD11c+ MHC class II+), neutrophils (GR1+, CD11b+ SigF-), eosinophils (Ly6C+, SigF+, CD11c-) and ILC2 (Lin$^-$ Thy1.2$^+$ ST2$^+$Sca1$^+$).

Statistical Analyses

Statistical analysis was performed using GraphPad Prism software. One way ANOVA or non-parametric Mann-Whitney U test was used where indicated. When One way ANOVA was used, multiple comparison was employed. A *P* value < 0.05 was considered statistically significant. All data are representative of at least three independent experiments with multiple mice as indicated or different donor cell populations.

RESULTS

Intratracheal TL1A Induces a Muco-Secretory Signature in the Lung

We conducted a transcriptomic RNAseq analysis on murine lungs induced with recombinant TL1A, challenged on two successive days and euthanized 24h after the last injection (**Figure 1A**). We discovered that the highest differentially expressed gene in response to TL1A was chloride channel accessory 1 encoding the goblet cell protein ClcA1 (109.700 fold increase), which is involved in mucin synthesis (**Figure 1B**). ClcA1 is thought to signal through TMEM213 to promote MUC5AC production by bronchial epithelial cells stimulated with IL13 (10). In addition to ClcA1, many muco-secretory genes were upregulated in response to TL1A stimulation. These include genes encoding for IL13 (4.166 fold increase), the mucins MUC5AC (5.590 fold increase) and MUC5B (2.268 fold increase), TNFα (4.130 fold increase), TFF2 (3.530 fold increase), TMEM213 (2.776 fold increase) and AREG (2.632 fold increase) (**Figure 1B**). IL4 transcripts were not increased in the lungs of TL1A-induced mice. The intratracheal administration of TL1A in isolation to the airways induces a muco-secretory signature in the lung. Additionally, airway inflammation was increased in TL1A-induced mice compared to PBS (**Supplementary Figures 1A, B**). Flow cytometry analyses of immune cells performed on lung tissue showed a significant increase in T cells, eosinophils, neutrophils, macrophages and

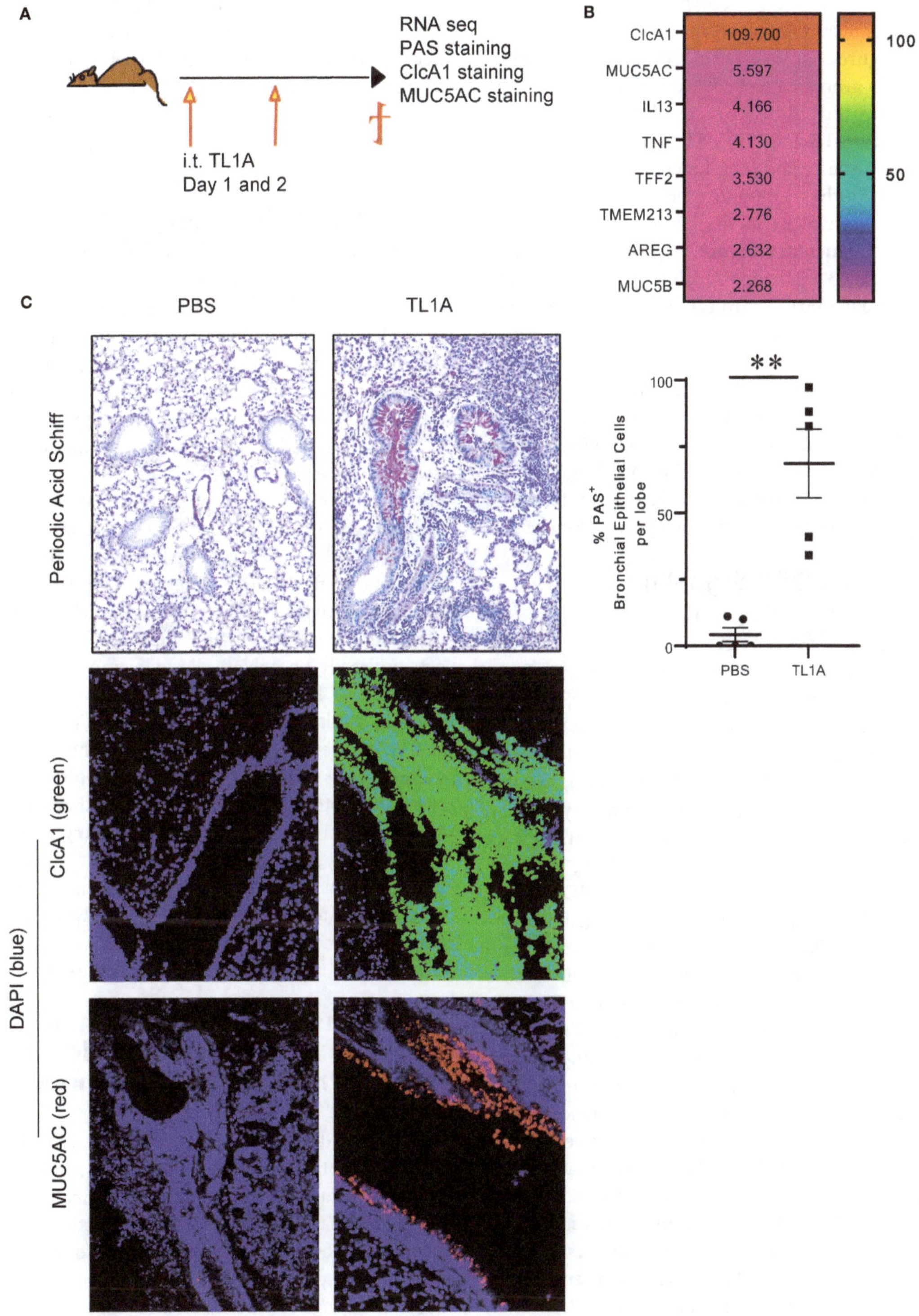

FIGURE 1 | TL1A induces mucus production when administered in isolation into the airways. **(A)** Schematic representation of the protocol used. Briefly, C57BL/6 mice were induced with 10µg of recombinant TL1A i.t. on two successive days. Mice were euthanized 24h after the last i.t. injection, and lungs were harvested for RNAseq analysis, PAS, ClcA1 and MUC5AC stains. **(B)** Heatmap of the top differentially regulated genes involved in mucus production, upregulated in the lungs of TL1A-induced mice. **(C)** Top panel: PAS stain of mucus produced in the lungs and quantified using Image Pro Premier and graphed as %PAS+ bronchial epithelial cells per lobe (right panel). Mid and Lower panels: Immunofluorescence stains of CLcA1 (green), MUC5AC (red) and nuclear DAPI (blue). All results representative of three experiments with four to six mice per group. $^{**}p < 0.005$.

innate lymphoid cells (**Supplementary Figure 1A**). Consistent with the flow analysis, H&E scoring of lung biopsies demonstrated a significant increase in airway inflammation (**Supplementary Figure 1B**). We have additionally monitored fibrosis by scoring trichrome stain of collagen in lung biopsies and showed TL1A-induced mice increased airway fibrosis [**Supplementary Figure 1B** and (19)]. TL1A was able to induce changes in airway resistance and lung function [**Supplementary Figure 1C** and (19)]. Lastly, we monitored levels of IL4, IL5, IL13, TSLP and Periostin transcripts in the lungs of TL1A-induced mice by qPCR (**Supplementary Figure 1D**) and demonstrated mRNA transcripts of IL13 are the most highly increased in TL1A-induced mice (**Supplementary Figure 1D**). IL4 was not enhanced after the intratracheal instillation of TL1A in the airways (**Supplementary Figure 1D**).

After injecting recombinant TL1A directly into the airways, we assessed mucus production by Periodic Acid-Schiff (PAS) stain as well as ClcA1 and MUC5AC expression by immunofluorescence. We observed that the airway administration of 10μg TL1A in isolation into the airways on two successive days, was sufficient to promote mucus production 24h after the last injection (**Figure 1C**).

Interrupting TL1A/DR3 Signaling Decreases Mucus Production in Allergen-Induced Asthma

Chronic challenges with house dust mite in the airways after a sensitization phase, generates an asthma endotype (19, 24) with strong airway eosinophilia (24), Th2 (25) and type 2 innate lymphoid cells infiltrating the lung (26). This model involves type 2 cytokines like IL4, IL5, IL13 and periostin (19), IgE and alarmins like TSLP, IL25 and IL33 (27). We chronically induced wildtype and $DR3^{-/-}$ mice with house dust mite (HDM from Greer Laboratories) for six weeks by first sensitizing the mice using 200μg HDM intranasal (i.n.) at day 0, 100μg HDM i.n. at day 7, and 50μg HDM i.n. at day 14. We then challenged the mice every other day with 50μg i.n. HDM for four weeks and monitored mucus production 24h after the last HDM dose (**Figure 2A**). Strikingly, mucus production assessed by PAS was significantly dampened in mice lacking an active TL1A/DR3 signal. Moreover, we treated wildtype mice induced with chronic HDM, with 100μg DR3-Fc, an antagonist reagent to TL1A, during the challenge phase (starting day 14) twice a week until the end of the experiment. Another group received similar doses of an isotype control to DR3-Fc. We showed that DR3-Fc significantly decreases mucus production, post-disease onset (**Figure 2B**). Additionally, inflammation and fibrosis, assessed by H&E, Trichrome and smooth muscle actin stains respectively, were significantly decreased when TL1A signal was removed by genetic deletion of its receptor DR3 or antagonistic neutralization (DR3-Fc treatment) (**Figure 2C**). Baseline trichrome and H&E scores were comparable between wild type and DR3-deficient mice (**Supplementary Figure 2A**). Flow cytometry analysis on bronchial lavage revealed strong airway eosinophilia compared to neutrophils which were modestly recruited. Additionally, cellular infiltrates were decreased in the bronchial lavage when TL1A signal was interrupted by genetic mutation of its receptor or antagonistic blockade, albeit not significantly (**Supplementary Figure 2B**). Strikingly, Lung ILC2 gated on $CD45.2^{+}Lin^{-}$ $Thy1.2^{+}$ $ST2^{+}Sca1^{+}$ (**Supplementary Figure 2D**), were significantly decreased when TL1A signal was absent (**Supplementary Figure 2C**). Taken together, these data demonstrate that characteristic traits of asthma, including both mucus production and airway inflammation and remodeling, were drastically reversed post-TL1A neutralization.

TL1A Muco-Secretory Activity Is Dependent on IL13/IL4Rα Signaling

IL13 is thought to play a central role in promoting mucus production associated with asthma and COPD, making IL13 neutralizing biologics the focus of both an approved therapeutic, dupilumab, and multiple other ongoing clinical trials (28–31). We questioned whether TL1A muco-secretory activity was dependent on IL13 signaling through its receptor IL4Rα, expressed on goblet cells. To answer this, we injected IL4Rα-deficient mice with recombinant TL1A on two successive days and monitored mucus production at day 3 (**Figure 3A**). Surprisingly, IL4Rα-deficient mice were completely mucus free as compared to wildtype BALB/c mice that induced mucus production after TL1A instillation (**Figure 3B**). TL1A muco-secretory activity is therefore completely dependent on IL13 signaling through its IL4Rα. Thus, we hypothesized that TL1A acts indirectly on goblet cells to promote mucus production by upregulating IL13. Indeed, IL13 transcripts were increased 21.3 folds in wildtype mice induced with TL1A and 17.7 folds in IL4Rα-deficient mice that can't signal through IL13 despite the increase in its transcript expression (**Supplementary Figure 3B**). IL4 transcripts were not increased in neither the wildtype nor the IL4Rα-deficient mice (**Supplementary Figure 3B**). Most importantly, while mucus production was completely abrogated in IL4Rα-deficient mice, inflammation persisted (**Figure 3C**, top). Collagen deposition was lessened in IL4Rα-deficient mice (**Figure 3C**, middle), whereas smooth muscle hypertrophy remained unchanged (**Figure 3C**, bottom).

TL1A Acts on Innate Lymphoid Cells to Promote IL13 Expression Necessary for Mucus Production, Independently of Adaptive Immunity

The two predominant cellular sources of IL13 are T cells and innate lymphoid cells. We first questioned whether TL1A requires adaptive immunity, specifically, whether IL13-expressing T cells drive mucus production. For this purpose, we injected RAG-deficient mice with recombinant TL1A on two successive days and monitored mucus production (**Figure 4A**). Surprisingly, TL1A maintained its capacity to promote mucus production in mice lacking lymphocytes (**Figure 4B**). We therefore concluded that TL1A muco-secretory activity is independent of adaptive immunity.

Alternative to T cells, type 2 innate lymphoid cells (ILC2) are major cellular sources of IL13 and are increased in allergen-induced asthma (32, 33), but not IL4 (13, 34). We therefore questioned whether TL1A induces IL13 production by innate

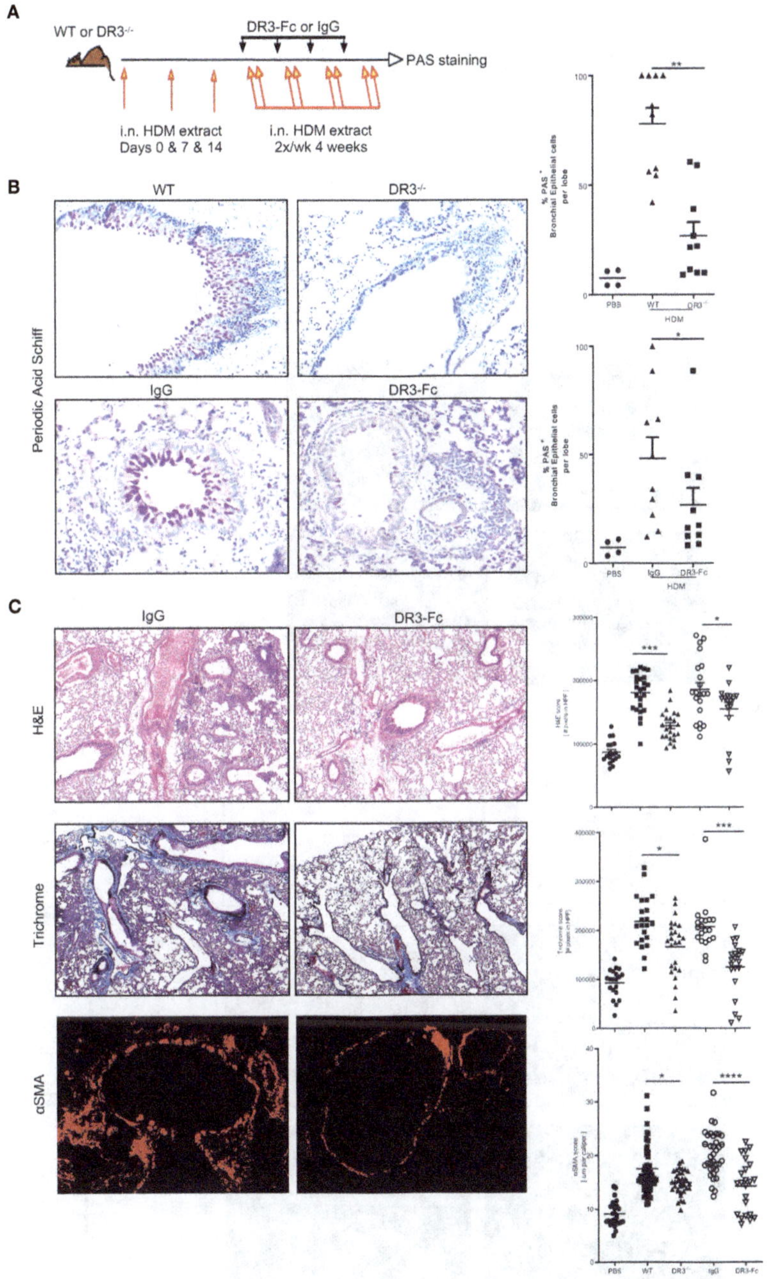

FIGURE 2 | Interrupting TL1A/DR3 signaling decreases mucus production in allergen-induced asthma. **(A)** Schematic representation of protocol used. Briefly, WT littermates and DR3-deficient mice on the C57BL/6 x 129 background were sensitized i.n. on day 0, 7, and 14 with 200 and 100 µg house dust mite extract protein in PBS, followed by chronic i.n. challenges of 50 µg of HDM protein administered twice a week for the following four weeks. Analyses were performed 24 hours after the last challenge. For neutralization of TL1A-DR3 interactions, mouse DR3-Fc or isotype control IgG were administered i.p. to WT C57BL/6 mice after the initial sensitization period starting at day 14 and were given every three days until the end of the experiment (100 µg/injection/mouse). **(B)** PAS stain of mucus produced in the lungs and quantified using Image Pro Premier. **(C)** Inflammation assessed by H&E stain (top panels), collagen deposition assessed by trichrome stain (middle panels), and smooth muscle hypertrophy assessed by αSMA immunofluorescence stain (red) (bottom panels) on lung biopsies of WT C57BL/6 mice after treatment with either IgG or DR3-Fc. Quantifications for each parameter, completed using Image Pro Premier, are shown to the right, including untreated WT C57BL/6 and DR3$^{-/-}$ mice (images not shown). All results representative of three experiments with five mice per group. *$p < 0.05$, ** < 0.005, ***$p < 0.0005$, ****$p < 0.00005$.

lymphoid cells to control mucus production. We injected 10µg of recombinant TL1A on two successive days into RAGγc-deficient mice that lack ILC in addition to lymphocytes (**Figure 4A**). TL1A was unable to induce mucus production in the RAGγc-deficient mice as compared to RAG-deficient mice (**Figure 4B**). Moreover, TL1A increased 14.8 folds IL13 transcripts in the lung

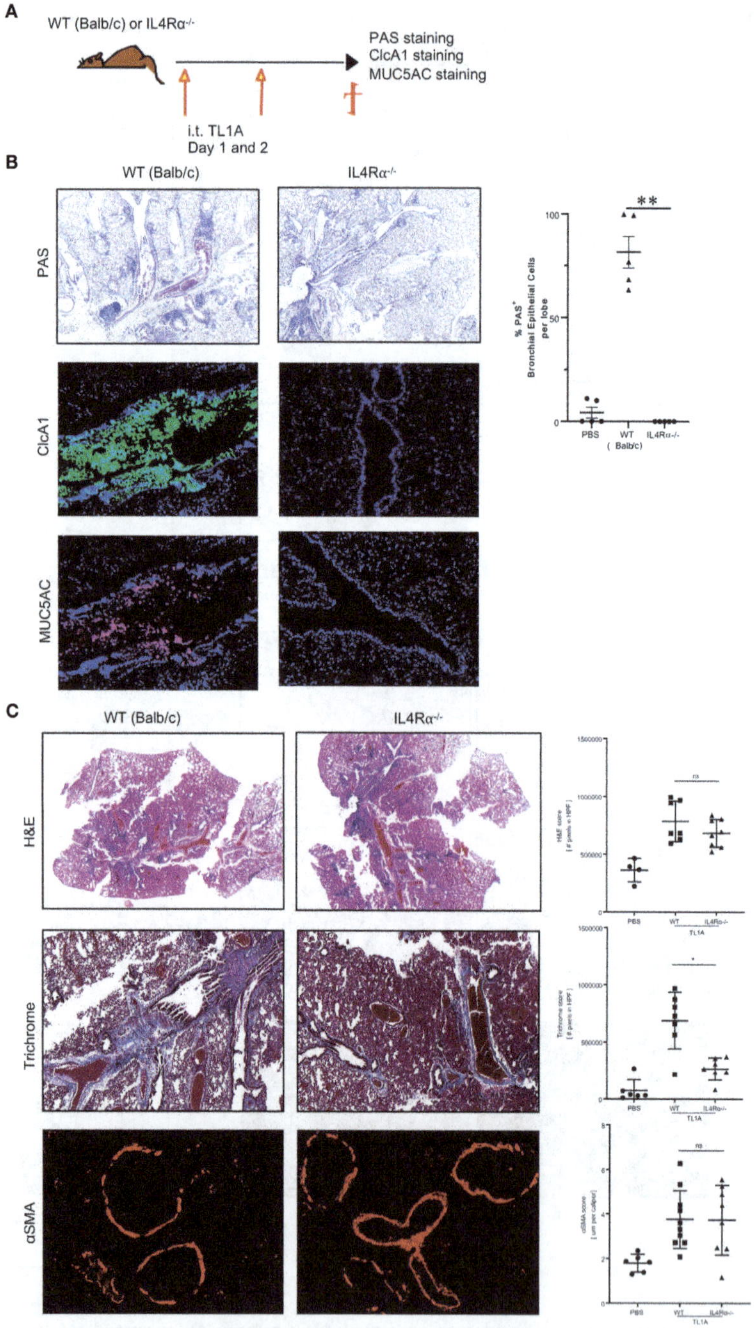

FIGURE 3 | TL1A muco-secretory activity is dependent on IL13/IL4Rα signaling. **(A)** Schematic representation of the protocol used, as previously described in **Figure 1**. **(B)** Top panel: PAS stain of mucus produced in the lungs and quantified using Image Pro Premier (right panel). Mid and Lower panels: Immunofluorescence stains of CLcA1 (green), MUC5AC (red) and nuclear DAPI (blue). **(C)** Inflammation assessed by H&E stain (top panels), collagen deposition assessed by trichrome stain (middle panels), and smooth muscle hypertrophy assessed by αSMA immunofluorescence stain (red) (bottom panels) on lung biopsies of BALB/c and IL4Rα-deficient mice induced with PBS or TL1A. Quantification for each parameter is done using Image Pro Premier. All results representative of three experiments with four to six mice per group. ns, not significant, *p < 0.05, ** < 0.005.

of RAG-deficient mice, whereas TL1A-induced RAGγc-deficient failed to enhance IL13 expression (**Supplementary Figure 3A**). IL4 levels remained unchanged in both RAG and RAGγc-deficient mice, challenged with TL1A (**Supplementary Figure 3A**). This data suggests TL1A acts on ILC to promote IL13 production. To determine whether TL1A exerts a direct effect on ILC, we first verified they express its receptor DR3. We sorted lung ILC2 cells from the lungs of RAG-deficient mice

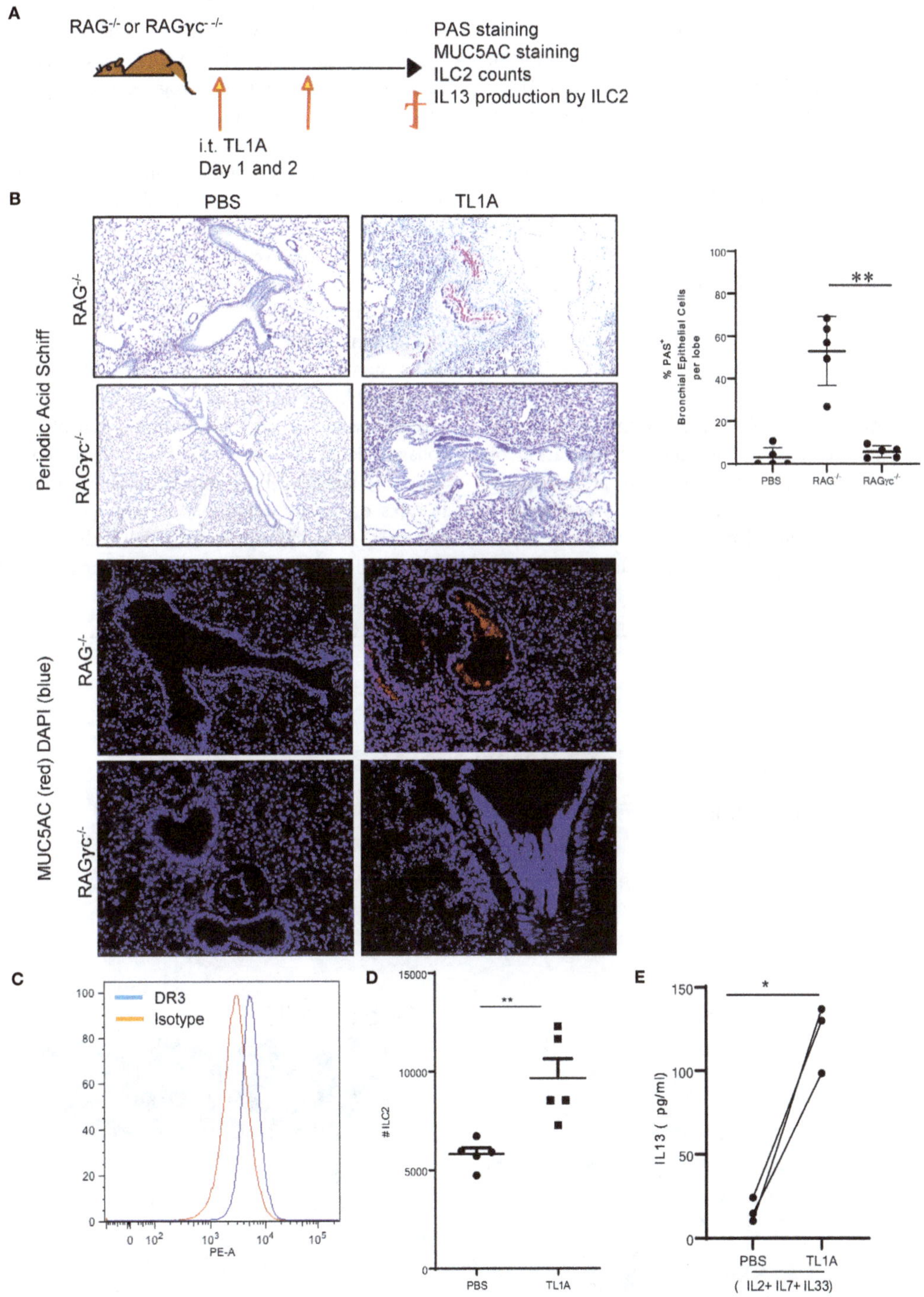

FIGURE 4 | TL1A induces mucus production independently of adaptive immunity, bystander to IL13 production by ILC2. **(A)** Schematic representation of the protocol used, as previously described in **Figure 1**. **(B)** Top panel: PAS stain of mucus produced in the lungs of $RAG^{-/-}$ and $RAG\gamma c^{-/-}$ mice induced with PBS or TL1A and quantified using Image Pro Premier (right graph). Lower panels: Immunofluorescence stains of MUC5AC (red) and nuclear DAPI (blue). **(C)** DR3 staining on ILC2 assessed by flow cytometry (DR3 in blue and Isotype in red). **(D)** Number of lung ILC2 in the left lobe of $RAG^{-/-}$ mice induced with TL1A. **(E)** IL13 levels assessed by ELISA, in the supernatants of ILC2 cultured in the presence of IL2, IL7, and IL33 and stimulated with or without TL1A. All results representative of three experiments with four to six mice per group, or three individual replicate cultures. *$p < 0.05$, **$p < 0.005$.

induced with TL1A and examined DR3 expression. Lung ILC2 sorted on CD45.2$^+$Lin$^-$ Thy1.2$^+$ ST2$^+$Sca1$^+$ expressed DR3 on their surface (**Figure 4C**). *In vivo*, TL1A induced proliferation and activation of lung ILC in RAG-deficient mice (**Figure 4D**). We observed an increase in the numbers of lung ILC2 (**Figure 4D**) as well as upregulation of IL13 production by these cells (**Figure 4E**). ILC2 cultured for five days in the presence of 50ng/ml IL2, IL7, and IL33 followed by two days culture with 10ng/ml IL2, IL7, and/IL33 and 100 ng/ml TL1A, increased IL13 secretion assessed by ELISA in the culture supernatant (**Figure 4E**). We concluded TL1A promotes IL13 production by ILC2, which is necessary for mucus secretion.

DISCUSSION

Mucus plugs are the major cause of death in asthma, COPD and cystic fibrosis. Current therapies involve the administration of mucolytics; however, these aren't always effective at improving patient outcomes and there seems to be an increase in mortality associated with hypersecretory disorders. In this work, we describe, for the first time, a novel activity of TL1A as a driver of mucus production in the lung. To date, the most characterized cytokine involved in mucus production is IL13. It has been shown to drive mucus production by goblet cells differentiated *in vitro*, in Air-Liquid-Interface (ALI) (10). Additionally, silencing IL13 signaling through MAPK inhibition abrogated mucus production in murine models of asthma (35, 36). We have evidence that TL1A drives IL13 production by ILC2, which are increased in asthma. This is consistent with prior findings, showing that TL1A can promote allergic immunopathology through ILC2s (37, 38). Moreover, we show that TL1A can sustain a muco-secretory activity in the absence of T and B cells; however, ILC2 cells were necessary for this activity (**Figure 5**). ILC2 cells stimulated with TL1A, in the presence of the homeostatic cytokines IL2, IL7 and IL33, promoted IL13 production by these innate cells. We demonstrate that blocking TL1A signaling through its receptor DR3, by genetic deletion or antagonist blocking, abrogated mucus and IL13 production. Taken together with our data, which shows that blocking TL1A reduces collagen deposition and smooth muscle hypertrophy [(**Figure 2C** and (19)], targeting TL1A appears to be a novel approach to treat all features of airway inflammation and remodeling associated with asthma. TL1A acts upstream of IL13, driving mucus production through direct activity on ILC2. TL1A can act directly on structural

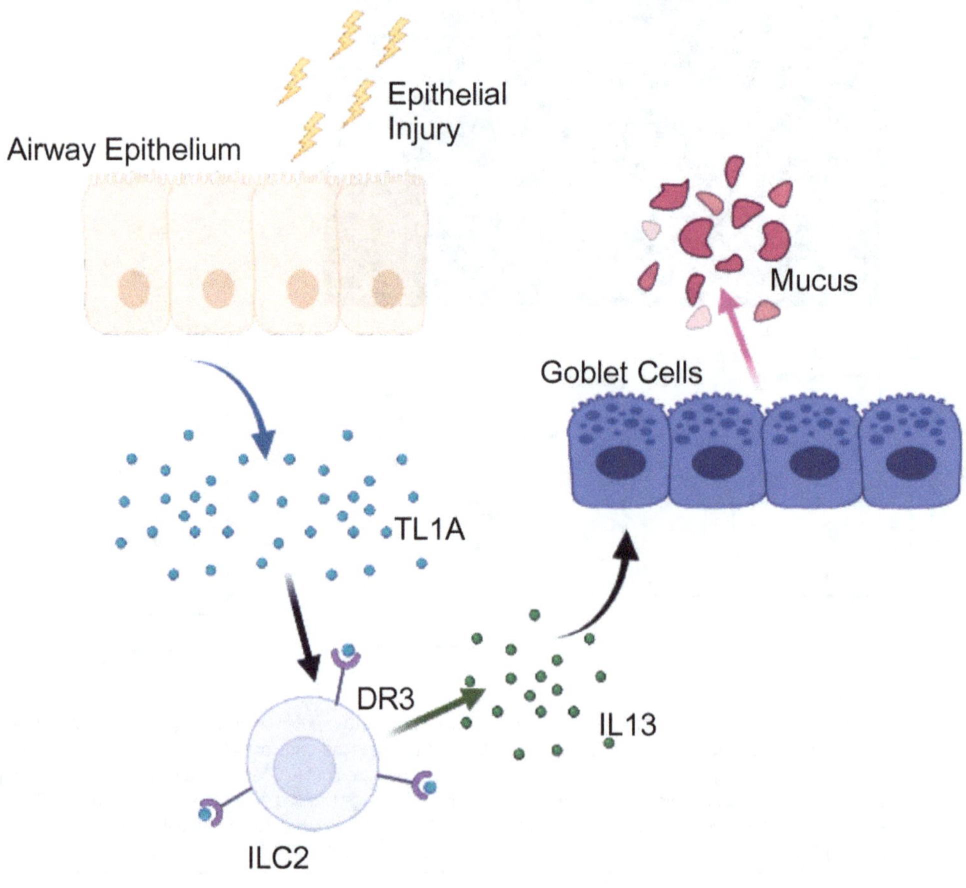

FIGURE 5 | Graphical Abstract. Upon epithelial injury, such as exposure to allergens, TL1A is produced and acts on ILC2 *via* DR3 to promote IL13 secretion, leading to mucus production. Created with BioRender.com.

cells of the lung, namely fibroblasts and epithelial cells, to promote airway remodeling and fibrosis.

Targeting TL1A shows a competitive advantage to neutralizing IL13, as this work shows that IL4Rα-deficient mice sustained an inflammatory response and smooth muscle hypertrophy, despite the absence of mucus and subsequent to the lack of an active IL13 signal. In humans, eight clinical trials failed to demonstrate benefit in neutralizing IL13 in severe asthmatic patients (28, 39). Three monoclonal antibodies directed against IL13 (tralokinumab, lebrikizumab and anrukinzumab) were used to interrogate the role of this cytokine in the pathophysiology of severe asthma and responses to treatment. The primary end points included FEV_1 measurements, Mean ACQ6 scores, and asthma exacerbations recorded by the intake of systemic glucocorticoids and number of hospitalizations (29). All three antibodies showed a pattern of improvement without reaching significant decrease in the endpoints measured. Alternative to anti-IL13 antibodies, IL4Rα antagonists (dupilumab) have been recently FDA approved as add-on-maintenance therapy to treat moderate-to-severe asthma (31). Add-on therapy with dupilumab significantly reduced the oral glucocorticoid dose while simultaneously reducing the rate of severe exacerbations and improving lung function (FEV_1) in patients with glucocorticoid-dependent severe asthma (31). More recently, in the "Liberty Asthma Quest Trial," dupilumab treatment lowered significantly the rates of severe asthma exacerbation and improved lung function as compared to placebo treated controls. Greater benefits were seen in asthmatic patients with higher eosinophilia (31). Nevertheless, the effect of dupilumab on mixed granulocytic or neutrophilic asthma patients that are resistant to steroid treatment remain unanswered. It is becoming evident that neutralizing IL13 is not sufficient to reverse certain features of airway inflammation and fibrosis once established. Consistent with this, our study in the IL4Rα-deficient mice induced with TL1A demonstrated a complete abrogation in mucus production and reduced collagen deposition, while inflammation and fibrosis persisted. IL4 was not increased after TL1A airway challenge whereas IL13 was significantly induced. Additionally, several lines of evidence have refuted the idea that IL4 drives mucus production by bronchial epithelial cells. Interrupting IL13 in isolation by genetic deletion or antagonistic blockade reversed established mucus secretion (15, 16), whereas anti-IL4 blockade did not reduce mucin-secreting goblet cells in a murine model of asthma (15). Vice versa, IL13 administration in IL4-defiicent cells enhanced mucus production (17), supporting a unique role for IL13 in regulating mucus secretion. Collectively, this indicates that IL13, not IL4, controls mucus secretion through IL4Rα signaling.

Recently we showed soluble TL1A can be detected in the bronchial lavage of mice. TL1A is expressed on the surface of alveolar macrophages, dendritic cells, innate lymphoid type 2 cells, and subpopulations of lung structural cells. DR3 was found on CD4 T cells, innate lymphoid type 2 cells, macrophages, fibroblasts, and some epithelial cells and is expressed primarily by alveolar macrophages (19). In asthmatic patients presenting with the eosinophilic endotype, DR3 is upregulated in sputum ILC2 after allergen challenge or by IL2, IL33, and TSLP stimulation *in vitro*. $DR3^+$ILC2 significantly increased IL5 expression upon TL1A stimulation (40). Combined with our data showing TL1A is upstream of IL13, this indicates that targeting TL1A signaling offers an advantage over targeting IL13/IL4Rα or IL5 signaling in isolation to treat mucus secretion associated with asthma.

Taken together, we demonstrate that interrupting TL1A/DR3 signaling abrogates mucus production associated with asthma, post-disease onset. We further show that TL1A acts on ILC2 to promote IL13 secretion leading to mucus production. Aside from its muco-secretory activity, TL1A acts directly on stromal and immune cells, perpetuating fibrosis and airway inflammation. While mucus secretion was dependent on IL13/IL4Rα signaling, in this work, we demonstrate that interrupting IL4Rα was not sufficient to decrease smooth muscle hypertrophy, fibrosis and airway inflammation. Targeting TL1A is therefore, more beneficial than targeting IL13/IL4Rα signaling in asthma and muco-secretory disorders.

ETHICS STATEMENT

The animal study was reviewed and approved by The Institutional Animal Care and Use Committee, Cincinnati Children's Hospital Medical Center.

AUTHOR CONTRIBUTIONS

HS and RH performed experiments and analyzed data. KS, AM, and RS contributed reagents and expertise. RH directed the study and wrote the paper. All authors contributed to the article and approved the submitted version.

ACKNOWLEDGMENTS

We acknowledge Drs. Chandrashekhar Pasare, Sing Sing Way, and Michael Croft for fruitful discussions. We also thank the microscopy core, flow core, and division of veterinary services at Cincinnati Children's Hospital Medical Center for their help.

SUPPLEMENTARY MATERIAL

Supplementary Figure 1 | TL1A induces airway inflammation and remodeling. **(A)** Flow cytometry analyses of cellular infiltration in the lungs of TL1A-induced mice as previously described. Total numbers of leucocytes, T cells, eosinophils, neutrophils, macrophages, and dendritic cells are shown. **(B)** Immunohistochemistry analyses of cellular infiltration assessed by H&E and collagen deposition assessed by Masson Trichrome. Quantifications are shown on the right panel. **(C)** Airway hyperresponsiveness (AHR) to increasing concentrations of methacholine of TL1A versus PBSinduced mice is shown. **(D)** Fold change in mRNA levels of IL4, IL5, IL13, TSLP and periostin in the lungs of TL1A over PBS-induced mice are shown. All results are representative of 5 to 10 mice per group. ****$p < 0.00005$.

Supplementary Figure 2 | TL1A inhibition decreases the infiltration of ILC2 in the lungs and airway fibrosis. **(A)** Quantification of Masson Trichrome and H&E scores in the lungs of HDM-induced mice are shown. **(B)** Flow cytometry analysis of cellular infiltration in the bronchial lavage of mice induced with HDM as previously described. The grey dotted line indicates baseline infiltration. **(C)** Numbers of ILC2 in the left lobe of the lungs of mice induced with HDM. The grey dotted line indicates baseline infiltration. **(D)** Gating strategy of ILC2 cells used during the sorting. All results are representative of 10 mice per group. One-way Anova using a multi-comparison to WT HDM is used to calculate the p values. $^*p < 0.05$, $^{***}p < 0.0005$.

Supplementary Figure 3 | IL13 and IL4 expression in the lungs of TL1A -induced mice. **(A)** Relative expression of IL4 and IL13 in the lungs of RAG and RAGγc-deficient mice induced with TL1A as previously described. **(B)** Relative expression of IL4 and IL13 in the lungs of WT (BALBc) and IL4Rα- deficient mice induced with TL1A as previously described. All results are representative of 4 mice per group. $^*p < 0.05$.

REFERENCES

1. Hauber HP, Foley SC, Hamid Q. Mucin Overproduction in Chronic Inflammatory Lung Disease. *Can Respir J* (2006) 13(6):327–35. doi: 10.1155/2006/901417
2. Fahy JV, Dickey BF. Airway Mucus Function and Dysfunction. *N Engl J Med* (2010) 363(23):2233–47. doi: 10.1056/NEJMra0910061
3. Daviskas E, Anderson SD, Shaw J, Eberl S, Seale JP, Yang IA, et al. Mucociliary Clearance in Patients With Chronic Asthma: Effects of Beta Agonists. *Respirology* (2005) 10(4):426–35. doi: 10.1111/j.1440-1843.2005.00738.x
4. Williams DM, Rubin BK. Clinical Pharmacology of Bronchodilator Medications. *Respir Care* (2018) 63(6):641–54. doi: 10.4187/respcare.06051
5. Chambers ES, Nanzer AM, Pfeffer PE, Richards DF, Timms PM, Martineau AR, et al. Distinct Endotypes of Steroid-Resistant Asthma Characterized by IL-17A(High) and IFN-Gamma(High) Immunophenotypes: Potential Benefits of Calcitriol. *J Allergy Clin Immunol* (2015) 136(3):628–37.e4. doi: 10.1016/j.jaci.2015.01.026
6. Woodruff PG, Boushey HA, Dolganov GM, Barker CS, Yang YH, Donnelly S, et al. Genome-Wide Profiling Identifies Epithelial Cell Genes Associated With Asthma and With Treatment Response to Corticosteroids. *Proc Natl Acad Sci U.S.A.* (2007) 104(40):15858–63. doi: 10.1073/pnas.0707413104
7. Mukherjee M, Svenningsen S, Nair P. Glucocortiosteroid Subsensitivity and Asthma Severity. *Curr Opin Pulm Med* (2017) 23(1):78–88. doi: 10.1097/MCP.0000000000000337
8. Ntontsi P, Papathanassiou E, Loukides S, Bakakos P, Hillas G. Targeted Anti-IL-13 Therapies in Asthma: Current Data and Future Perspectives. *Expert Opin Investig Drugs* (2018) 27(2):179–86. doi: 10.1080/13543784.2018.1427729
9. Bagnasco D, Ferrando M, Varricchi G, Passalacqua G, Canonica GW. A Critical Evaluation of Anti-IL-13 and Anti-IL-4 Strategies in Severe Asthma. *Int Arch Allergy Immunol* (2016) 170(2):122–31. doi: 10.1159/000447692
10. Alevy YG, Patel AC, Romero AG, Patel DA, Tucker J, Roswit WT, et al. IL-13-Induced Airway Mucus Production is Attenuated by MAPK13 Inhibition. *J Clin Invest* (2012) 122(12):4555–68. doi: 10.1172/JCI64896
11. Rael EL, Lockey RF. Interleukin-13 Signaling and its Role in Asthma. *World Allergy Organ J* (2011) 4(3):54–64. doi: 10.1097/WOX.0b013e31821188e0
12. Kondo M, Tamaoki J, Takeyama K, Nakata J, Nagai A. Interleukin-13 Induces Goblet Cell Differentiation in Primary Cell Culture From Guinea Pig Tracheal Epithelium. *Am J Respir Cell Mol Biol* (2002) 27(5):536–41. doi: 10.1165/rcmb.4682
13. Gour N, Wills-Karp M. IL-4 and IL-13 Signaling in Allergic Airway Disease. *Cytokine* (2015) 75(1):68–78. doi: 10.1016/j.cyto.2015.05.014
14. Conde E, Bertrand R, Balbino B, Bonnefoy J, Stackowicz J, Caillot N, et al. Dual Vaccination Against IL-4 and IL-13 Protects Against Chronic Allergic Asthma in Mice. *Nat Commun* (2021) 12(1):2574. doi: 10.1038/s41467-021-22834-5
15. Webb DC, McKenzie AN, Koskinen AM, Yang M, Mattes J, Foster PS. Integrated Signals Between IL-13, IL-4, and IL-5 Regulate Airways Hyperreactivity. *J Immunol* (2000) 165(1):108–13. doi: 10.4049/jimmunol.165.1.108
16. Wills-Karp M, Luyimbazi J, Xu X, Schofield B, Neben TY, Karp CL, et al. Interleukin-13: Central Mediator of Allergic Asthma. *Science* (1998) 282 (5397):2258–61. doi: 10.1126/science.282.5397.2258
17. Grunig G, Warnock M, Wakil AE, Venkayya R, Brombacher F, Rennick DM, et al. Requirement for IL-13 Independently of IL-4 in Experimental Asthma. *Science* (1998) 282(5397):2261–3. doi: 10.1126/science.282.5397.2261
18. Cohn L, Homer RJ, Marinov A, Rankin J, Bottomly K. Induction of Airway Mucus Production By T Helper 2 (Th2) Cells: A Critical Role for Interleukin 4 in Cell Recruitment But Not Mucus Production. *J Exp Med* (1997) 186 (10):1737–47. doi: 10.1084/jem.186.10.1737
19. Herro R, Miki H, Sethi GS, Mills D, Mehta AK, Nguyen XX, et al. TL1A Promotes Lung Tissue Fibrosis and Airway Remodeling. *J Immunol* (2020) 205(9):2414–22. doi: 10.4049/jimmunol.2000665
20. Chinnaiyan AM, O'Rourke K, Yu GL, Lyons RH, Garg M, Duan DR, et al. Signal Transduction by DR3, a Death Domain-Containing Receptor Related to TNFR-1 and CD95. *Science* (1996) 274(5289):990–2. doi: 10.1126/science.274.5289.990
21. Migone TS, Zhang J, Luo X, Zhuang L, Chen C, Hu B, et al. TL1A is a TNF-Like Ligand for DR3 and TR6/DcR3 and Functions as a T Cell Costimulator. *Immunity* (2002) 16(3):479–92. doi: 10.1016/S1074-7613(02)00283-2
22. Dunican EM, Elicker BM, Gierada DS, Nagle SK, Schiebler ML, Newell JD, et al. Mucus Plugs in Patients With Asthma Linked to Eosinophilia and Airflow Obstruction. *J Clin Invest* (2018) 128(3):997–1009. doi: 10.1172/JCI95693
23. Panchabhai TS, Mukhopadhyay S, Sehgal S, Bandyopadhyay D, Erzurum SC, Mehta AC. Plugs of the Air Passages: A Clinicopathologic Review. *Chest* (2016) 150(5):1141–57. doi: 10.1016/j.chest.2016.07.003
24. Doherty TA, Soroosh P, Khorram N, Fukuyama S, Rosenthal P, Cho JY, et al. The Tumor Necrosis Factor Family Member LIGHT is a Target for Asthmatic Airway Remodeling. *Nat Med* (2011) 17(5):596–603. doi: 10.1038/nm.2356
25. Rahimi RA, Nepal K, Cetinbas M, Sadreyev RI, Luster AD. Distinct Functions of Tissue-Resident and Circulating Memory Th2 Cells in Allergic Airway Disease. *J Exp Med* (2020) 217(9):e20190865. doi: 10.1084/jem.20190865
26. Gold MJ, Antignano F, Halim TY, Hirota JA, Blanchet MR, Zaph C, et al. Group 2 Innate Lymphoid Cells Facilitate Sensitization to Local, But Not Systemic, TH2-Inducing Allergen Exposures. *J Allergy Clin Immunol* (2014) 133(4):1142–8. doi: 10.1016/j.jaci.2014.02.033
27. Chen ZG, Zhang TT, Li HT, Chen FH, Zou XL, Ji JZ, et al. Neutralization of TSLP Inhibits Airway Remodeling in a Murine Model of Allergic Asthma Induced by Chronic Exposure to House Dust Mite. *PloS One* (2013) 8(1): e51268. doi: 10.1371/journal.pone.0051268
28. Korenblat P, Kerwin E, Leshchenko I, Yen K, Holweg CTJ, Anzures-Cabrera J, et al. Efficacy and Safety of Lebrikizumab in Adult Patients With Mild-to-Moderate Asthma Not Receiving Inhaled Corticosteroids. *Respir Med* (2018) 134:143–9. doi: 10.1016/j.rmed.2017.12.006
29. Hamann CR, Thyssen JP. Monoclonal Antibodies Against Interleukin 13 and Interleukin 31RA in Development for Atopic Dermatitis. *J Am Acad Dermatol* (2018) 78(3 Suppl 1):S37–42. doi: 10.1016/j.jaad.2017.12.018
30. Rabe KF, Nair P, Brusselle G, Maspero JF, Castro M, Sher L, et al. Efficacy and Safety of Dupilumab in Glucocorticoid-Dependent Severe Asthma. *N Engl J Med* (2018) 378(26):2475–85. doi: 10.1056/NEJMoa1804093
31. Castro M, Corren J, Pavord ID, Maspero J, Wenzel S, Rabe KF, et al. Dupilumab Efficacy and Safety in Moderate-To-Severe Uncontrolled Asthma. *N Engl J Med* (2018) 378(26):2486–96. doi: 10.1056/NEJMoa1804092
32. Spits H, Artis D, Colonna M, Diefenbach A, Di Santo JP, Eberl G, et al. Innate Lymphoid Cells–A Proposal for Uniform Nomenclature. *Nat Rev Immunol* (2013) 13(2):145–9. doi: 10.1038/nri3365
33. Smith SG, Chen R, Kjarsgaard M, Huang C, Oliveria JP, O'Byrne PM, et al. Increased Numbers of Activated Group 2 Innate Lymphoid Cells in the Airways of Patients With Severe Asthma and Persistent Airway Eosinophilia. *J Allergy Clin Immunol* (2016) 137(1):75 86 e8. doi: 10.1016/j.jaci.2015.05.037

34. Price AE, Liang HE, Sullivan BM, Reinhardt RL, Eisley CJ, Erle DJ, et al. Systemically Dispersed Innate IL-13-Expressing Cells in Type 2 Immunity. *Proc Natl Acad Sci USA* (2010) 107(25):11489–94. doi: 10.1073/pnas.1003988107
35. Duan W, Chan JH, McKay K, Crosby JR, Choo HH, Leung BP, et al. Inhaled P38alpha Mitogen-Activated Protein Kinase Antisense Oligonucleotide Attenuates Asthma in Mice. *Am J Respir Crit Care Med* (2005) 171(6):571–8. doi: 10.1164/rccm.200408-1006OC
36. Ma JY, Medicherla S, Kerr I, Mangadu R, Protter AA, Higgins LS. Selective P38alpha Mitogen-Activated Protein Kinase Inhibitor Attenuates Lung Inflammation and Fibrosis in IL-13 Transgenic Mouse Model of Asthma. *J Asthma Allergy* (2008) 1:31–44. doi: 10.2147/JAA.S4199
37. Meylan F, Hawley ET, Barron L, Barlow JL, Penumetcha P, Pelletier M, et al. The TNF-Family Cytokine TL1A Promotes Allergic Immunopathology Through Group 2 Innate Lymphoid Cells. *Mucosal Immunol* (2014) 7(4):958–68. doi: 10.1038/mi.2013.114
38. Yu X, Pappu R, Ramirez-Carrozzi V, Ota N, Caplazi P, Zhang J, et al. TNF Superfamily Member TL1A Elicits Type 2 Innate Lymphoid Cells at Mucosal Barriers. *Mucosal Immunol* (2014) 7(3):730–40. doi: 10.1038/mi.2013.92
39. Lipworth B, Jabbal S, Kuo CR. Anti-Interleukin 13 for Asthma: Stick or Twist? *Lancet Respir Med* (2018) 6(9):e46–e7. doi: 10.1016/S2213-2600(18)30275-3
40. Machida K, Aw M, Salter BMA, Ju X, Mukherjee M, Gauvreau GM, et al. The Role of the TL1A/DR3 Axis in the Activation of Group 2 Innate Lymphoid Cells in Subjects With Eosinophilic Asthma. *Am J Respir Crit Care Med* (2020) 202(8):1105–14. doi: 10.1164/rccm.201909-1722OC

14

Genetics in Idiopathic Pulmonary Fibrosis Pathogenesis, Prognosis and Treatment

Amarpreet Kaur[1], Susan K. Mathai[2] and David A. Schwartz[2]*

[1] Department of Medicine, University of Colorado Denver School of Medicine, Aurora, CO, United States,
[2] Department of Medicine, Division of Pulmonary Sciences and Critical Care Medicine, University of Colorado Denver School of Medicine, Aurora, CO, United States

***Correspondence:**
Susan K. Mathai
susan.mathai@ucdenver.edu

Idiopathic pulmonary fibrosis (IPF), the most common form of idiopathic interstitial pneumonia (IIP), is characterized by irreversible scarring of the lung parenchyma and progressive decline in lung function leading to eventual respiratory failure. The prognosis of IPF is poor with a median survival of 3–5 years after diagnosis and no curative medical therapies. Although the pathogenesis of IPF is not well understood, there is a growing body of evidence that genetic factors contribute to disease risk. Recent studies have identified common and rare genetic variants associated with both sporadic and familial forms of pulmonary fibrosis, with at least one-third of the risk for developing fibrotic IIP explained by common genetic variants. The IPF-associated genetic loci discovered to date are implicated in diverse biological processes, including alveolar stability, host defense, cell–cell barrier function, and cell senescence. In addition, some common variants have also been associated with distinct clinical phenotypes. Better understanding of how genetic variation plays a role in disease risk and phenotype could identify potential therapeutic targets and inform clinical decision-making. In addition, clinical studies should be designed controlling for the genetic backgrounds of subjects, since clinical outcomes and therapeutic responses may differ by genotype. Further understanding of these differences will allow the development of personalized approaches to the IPF management.

Keywords: idiopathic pulmonary fibrosis, MUC5B, pulmonary fibrosis, interstitial lung disease, telomeres

INTRODUCTION

Idiopathic pulmonary fibrosis (IPF) is the most common of the idiopathic interstitial pneumonias (IIPs). IPF is characterized by progressive scarring of the lung parenchyma, which leads to dyspnea and declining pulmonary function and eventually to respiratory failure. The median survival after diagnosis of IPF is 3–5 years (1). In 2011, the American Thoracic Society/European Respiratory Society issued a new classification scheme in which they defined IPF as a specific form of chronic, progressive fibrosing interstitial pneumonia of unknown etiology, occurring mainly in older adults and associated with radiological and/or histopathological pattern of usual interstitial pneumonia (UIP) (2). The prognosis of IPF remains poor despite recently approved medical therapies (3, 4).

Numerous epidemiologic and genetic studies illustrate that genetic and environmental factors contribute to the risk of IPF (5, 6). The most convincing early evidence to support a genetic basis for IPF came from twin studies and studies focusing on familial clustering of the disease, a syndrome termed familial interstitial pneumonia (FIP) (7–9). Recent studies have identified several specific genetic variants that confer risk for development of IPF (10, 11). Discovery of disease-associated genetic variants has improved our understanding of the ways inherited risk factors influence disease risk. However, fundamental questions persist regarding the ways in which complex genetic risk factors interact with environmental exposures to influence disease pathogenesis.

In this review, we briefly discuss the current literature regarding the role of common and rare variants in disease pathogenesis and prognosis and how this may influence clinical management in the future. Genetic variants and loci associated with IPF involve abnormalities in alveolar stability, host defense, cell–cell barrier function, and cell senescence, all of which are all thought to contribute to the pathogenesis of IPF. We conclude by discussing how treatment decisions might be affected by these findings and how better understanding of genetic variation and disease could allow for a more personalized approach to the treatment of IPF.

Rare and Common Variants Associated with IPF

Genetic variants, both rare and common, are associated with sporadic and familial forms of pulmonary fibrosis. Numerous rare variants (those with minor allele frequency of <0.1%) play a role in FIP (≥2 members of the same family with interstitial pneumonia; FIP) (**Table 1**). Familial studies have identified FIP-associated variants related to alveolar stability [*SFTPC* (12, 13), *SFTPA1* (14), *SFTPA2* (15), ATP-binding cassette-type 3 (*ABCA3*) (16), and *NAF1* (17)] as well as five genes linked to telomere biology [*TERT* (18), *TERC* (18), *DKC1* (19), *TINF2* (7, 20), *RTEL1* (21–23), and PARN] (24).

Common variants (defined as minor allele frequency of >5%) also appear to play a role in FIP risk (1). The most widely replicated risk variant (rs35705950), located in the promoter region of *MUC5B*, was initially identified in a combined linkage and association study (41) and has been strongly associated with IPF and FIP. Two large GWAS of IPF subjects (both familial and sporadic) with controls have been conducted in pulmonary fibrosis (10, 11). In addition to confirming the role of *TERT* at 5p15, *MUC5B* at 11p15, and the 3q26 region near *TERC*, the GWAS identified seven newly associated loci, including *FAM13A* (4q22), *DSP* (6q24), *OBFC1* (10q24), *ATP11A* (13q34), *DPP9* (19q13), and chromosomal regions 7q22 and 15q14-15 among others that have been nominally associated (**Table 2**).

Rare variants are thought to be highly penetrant and to have a greater effect size, but given their low frequency, they account for a smaller proportion of overall disease risk in the general population (51). Alternatively, in general, common variants have a smaller effect size but are present at higher frequency and, in aggregate, may contribute to a larger proportion of disease risk (**Figure 1**). However, the *MUC5B* promoter variant rs35705950 is a common variant with a large effect size and therefore accounts for a substantial risk in IPF. In fact, it has been estimated the *MUC5B* promoter variant accounts for 30% of the risk of developing IPF (41, 51).

TABLE 1 | Rare variants in idiopathic pulmonary fibrosis.

Gene	Gene function	Pathological consequence of mutation	Reference
SFTPC	Component of surfactant fluid	Altered trafficking and disrupted proteostasis, increased endoplasmic reticulum (ER) stress	(25–27)
SFTPA2	To modulate innate and adaptive immunity	Increase in ER stress	(15, 25, 28)
ABCA3	Transport of lipids across plasma membrane	Retention of lipids in the ER, ER stress, and apoptotic signaling	(29–31)
TERT	Enzyme in telomerase complex	Telomere shortening	(7, 18, 27, 32–36)
TERC	Template in telomerase complex	Telomere shortening	(7, 18, 27, 32–37)
DKC1	Stabilization of the template in telomerase complex	Telomere shortening	(19, 27, 38)
TINF2	Telomere maintenance	Telomere shortening	(20, 39)
RTELI	DNA helicase	Telomere shortening	(21, 22, 40)
PARN	mRNA stability	Telomere shortening	(21, 24)

Alveolar Stability

Surfactant proteins are synthesized in the endoplasmic reticulum (ER) of alveolar type II cells (AECII) and transported to and stored in the lamellar bodies until secretion into the alveolar space (25, 26). Rare variants identified in the genes encoding surfactant protein C and A (*SFTPC*, *SFTPA1*, and *SFTPA2*) have been associated with pulmonary fibrosis (53). SP-C is a small hydrophobic protein produced by AECIIs that requires the C-terminus for initial folding steps in the ER before secretion into the alveolar space (26). *SFTPC* rare variants are mutations that lie in the BRICHOS domain within the C-terminus of SP-C. The BRICHOS domain is critical for proper folding and trafficking (5, 26). Coding mutations in this region lead to accumulation of misfolded protein resulting in increased ER stress and activation of the unfolded protein response (26, 54). Mutations in the gene that encodes surfactant protein A (*SFTPA2*) have also been linked to FIP (15) and have been associated with increased ER stress as well (28, 55). Rare variants have also been identified in another gene involved with surfactant processing, *ABCA3*, in FIP families (16, 56). *ABCA3* is a transporter protein mainly expressed in AECIIs and is involved in the transport of lipids across plasma membranes (29, 57). In AECIIs, *ABCA3* mutations cause abnormal processing, trafficking, and functionality of the *ABCA* protein, leading to retention of lipids in the ER, ER stress, and apoptotic signaling (30). These mutations are expressed in a recessive manner, where as mutations in *SFTPA2* and *SFTPC* are dominantly expressed (56).

In 2011, Lawson et al. (58) demonstrated that fibrotic remodeling in response to low-dose bleomycin was more severe in mice in which ER stress was induced, either through mutant SFTPC in AECIIs or by administration of tunicamycin, a chemical known to induce ER stress. In addition to effects on apoptosis, ER stress may induce biological pathways involved in cell differentiation (59, 60) through which epithelial cells acquire phenotypic characteristics of mesenchymal cells, a process known as

TABLE 2 | Common variants in idiopathic pulmonary fibrosis (IPF).

Risk allele(s)	Gene	Gene function	Observed effect of risk variant on survival in IPF	Reference
rs408392 rs419598 rs2637988	*IL1RN*	Inhibitor of pro-inflammatory effect of IL-1alpha and IL-1beta		(27, 42)
rs4073 rs2227307	*IL8*	Pro-inflammatory cytokine	Reduced	(43, 44)
rs2609255	*FAM13A*	Signal transduction		(10)
rs3775291	*TLR3*	Pathogen recognition and activation of innate immunity	Reduced	(45)
rs2736100	*TERT*	Enzyme in telomerase complex maintaining telomere length	Reduced	(10, 27, 46, 47)
rs2395655	*HLA-DRB1*	Major histocompatibility complex—immune system		(48)
rs2076295	*DSP*	Tightly links adjacent cells		(10)
rs11191865	*OBFC1*	Stimulates the activity of DNA polymerase-alpha-primase		(10)
rs35705950	*MUC5B*	Influence on rheological properties of airway mucus, mucociliary transport, and airway defense	Improved	(10, 11, 27, 41, 49, 50)
rs7934606	*MUC2*	Mucin production		(10)
rs111521887 rs5743894 rs2743890	*TOLLIP*	Regulator of innate immune responses mediated by toll-like receptor and the transforming growth factor β signaling pathway	Reduced	(11)
rs1278769	*ATP11A*	Phospholipid translocation		(10)
rs7144383	*MDGA2*	Cell–cell interaction		(11)
rs1981997	*MAPT*	Promotes microtubule assembly and stability		(10)
rs17690703	*SPPL2C*	Protein cleavage		(11)
rs12610495	*DPP9*	Cell–cell adhesion		(10)
rs1800470	*TGFB1*	Set of peptides that controls proliferation, differentiation, and other functions in many cell types		(11)

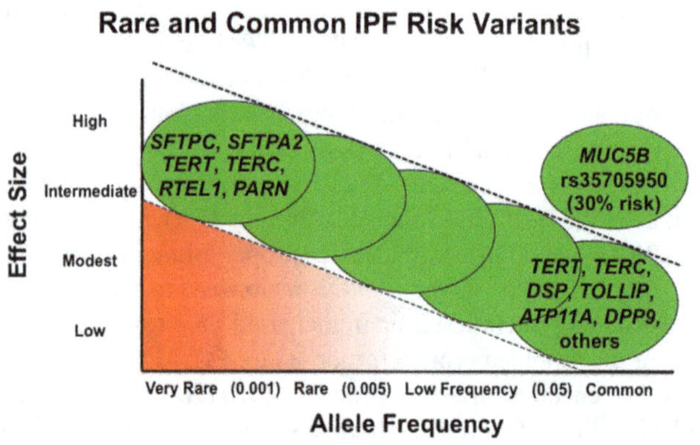

FIGURE 1 | Adapted from figure published previously in BMC Medicine with permission (52).

epithelial-to-mesenchymal transition (EMT), in IPF lungs (61). EMT is hypothesized to increase the number of cells responsible for collagen production and matrix deposition thereby leading to fibrosis (13, 59, 60). To date, published data suggest that ER stress predisposes to AECII apoptosis and subsequent lung fibrosis. Surfactant proteins have been recognized as crucial in maintaining lung alveolar structure and function. However, the precise role of alveolar stability, ER stress, and EMT in IPF pathogenesis remains an area of active investigation.

Cell Senescence

Telomeres are repetitive nucleotide sequences at the ends of chromosomes that protect them from progressive shortening during the normal cell replication process (62). Telomerases restore telomere length and consist of two major components: telomerase reverse transcriptase (encoded by *TERT*) and telomerase RNA (encoded by *TERC*) (18, 37). Mutations in telomerase components were initially identified in the setting of dyskeratosis congenita (DKC), a rare inherited syndrome of telomere shortening characterized by oral leukoplakia, abnormal skin hyperpigmentation, and dystrophic nails, with pulmonary fibrosis present in about 20% of patients; bone marrow failure can also be a complication of DKC (32). More recent studies have found an association between numerous genes in the telomerase maintenance pathway and FIP, including those related to catalytic activity (*TERT* and *TERC*) (7, 32) and telomere stabilization (*DKC1*, *PARN*, and *RTEL1*) (19, 21). These pathogenic variants cause dysfunction of telomerase activity leading to accelerated telomere shortening (32, 63) in peripheral blood and the lung (32–34). Thus far, *TERT* variants are the most frequently identified rare variants associated with pulmonary fibrosis; they are found in ~15% of FIP (7, 32) and in 1–3% of sporadic cases (34). A recent whole-exome sequencing study identified *TERT*, *RTEL1*, and *PARN* variants previously associated with FIP to be associated with sporadic IPF, further supporting the role of telomere dysfunction in IPF pathogenesis and highlighting the genetic commonalities between FIP and sporadic IPF (64).

Telomere dysfunction has further been implicated in IPF as evidence has suggested that short telomeres are not exclusively related to telomerase rare variant mutations. One study found that 25% of sporadic IPF subjects and 24% of familial IPF subjects, without identified mutations for *TERT* or *TERC*, had short telomeres. In addition, all subjects within this specific study who had a mutation in *TERT* or *TERC* and pulmonary fibrosis also had short telomeres (33).

The mechanisms by which telomere defects provoke lung disease are not fully understood. Defects in telomere maintenance have been linked to epithelial cell senescence and an impaired response to epithelial injury (65). During successive cycles of cell division, telomere shortening occurs and eventually leads to activation of the DNA-damage pathways, which result in apoptosis or senescence (32). In certain situations, cellular senescence is appropriate, but premature senescence can impair lung epithelial homeostasis and lead to stimulation of a lung remodeling response (66), resulting in fibrotic lesions (63). One study demonstrated increased epithelial cell senescence in IPF lung tissue by measuring B-galactosidase staining (a marker of senescence) and found that B-galactosidase staining was positive in all IPF cases but was not present in normal lung (67) supporting a role for senescent epithelial cells in IPF pathogenesis. Future studies are necessary to clarify the precise role of cellular senescence in lung injury response and fibrotic remodeling in IPF.

Host Defense

In 2011, genome-wide linkage analysis and targeted genetic sequencing identified a single nucleotide polymorphism (SNP) on chromosome 11 that was associated with both FIP and IPF (41). The SNP, rs35705950, was found to be a gain-of-function variant associated with increased expression of *MUC5B*. Heterozygous (GT) and homozygous (TT) individuals had an odds ratio for developing disease of 6.8 and 20.8 for FIP, and 9.0 and 21.8 for IPF, respectively, supporting the strength of the SNP's association with development of both IPF and FIP (41). *MUC5B* encodes Mucin 5B, which is a major gel-forming mucin in mucus and expressed by airway epithelial cells (68, 69). The association of the *MUC5B* promoter polymorphism with IPF has been replicated and confirmed in nine independent cohorts (10, 11, 49, 50, 70–74), including in a 2013 GWAS (OR for T minor allele = 4.51; 95% CI = 3.91–5.21; $P = 7.21 \times 10^{-95}$) (10). Additional genotyping studies have noted that the *MUC5B* variant is associated with disease in a Mexican cohort of IPF patients, but not in Asian cohorts (75). Most recently, a study of select loci in various European cohorts, including Czech and Greek IPF patients, also confirmed the association between rs35705950 and IPF (76).

MUC5B expression in IPF is localized in the distal airway, respiratory bronchiole, honeycomb cyst (77), and the bronchiolar epithelium (78). Overexpression of *MUC5B* in these areas of the lung and especially in the honeycomb cysts, which are a histopathological finding in IPF (77), further supports the notion that *MUC5B* is important in the pathogenesis of IPF. Evans and colleagues (51) hypothesize that IPF is caused by recurrent injury/repair/regeneration at the bronchoalveolar junction secondary to overexpression of MUC5B, mucociliary dysfunction, retention of particles, ER stress, and disruption of normal reparative and regenerative mechanisms in the distal lung (51).

Interestingly, the *MUC5B* promoter polymorphism may be specific to IIP, since studies have illustrated that rs35705950 is not associated with increased risk of sarcoidosis and scleroderma-related ILD, two other fibrotic lung diseases (10, 50, 70). However, recent data have shown that *MUC5B* rs357057950 variant is associated with radiographic evidence of interstitial lung abnormalities (ILA) studied in the Framingham cohort (79–81). Increasing age and number of copies of *MUC5B* promoter polymorphism were associated with ILA progression, which has been linked to increased mortality (80, 81). In addition, there are some data to suggest that rs357057950 genotype may be associated with higher likelihood of radiographic UIP pattern in the setting of fibrotic IIP (82).

The mechanism by which variants in *MUC5B* confers risk of lung fibrosis is an active area of investigation. Given that mucins play a role in innate immunity (68, 83), immune dysregulation could be a possible mechanism by which increased mucin expression contributes to the pathophysiology of IPF (84). Alternatively, IPF may be a disease of mucociliary clearance in which overexpression of *MUC5B* leads to impaired ciliary function, thereby allowing retention of particles and, subsequently, recurrent lung injury (51).

Several studies have also implicated the human leukocyte antigen (HLA) region in IPF (85–89). The HLA region is located on chromosome 6p21.31 (90), and its main function is regulation of immune response. The DRB1*15:01 allele has been shown to be more prevalent among IPF patients and associated with greater impairment of gas exchange (89). Recently, a genome-wide imputation-based association analysis identified two risk alleles, DRB1*15:01 and DQB1*06:02, found to be associated with fibrotic idiopathic interstitial pneumonias (48). Although not definitive, HLA association with IPF may suggest that autoimmunity may play a role in pulmonary fibrosis; further characterizing the pathophysiologic connection between this genetic variation and disease this remains an area of active investigation.

Epithelial Integrity

The 2013 GWAS by Fingerlin et al. (10) identified multiple susceptibility loci for fibrotic IIP, including two cell–cell adhesion molecules, *DSP* and *DPP9*. *DSP* gene expression was increased in lung tissue of individuals with IIP and varied by genotype for a variant in intron 5 (10, 91). *DSP* encodes for desmoplakin, a critical component of desmosome structure important in cell–cell adhesion. Desmosomes mechanically link cells and stabilize tissue architecture. In addition, they are involved in the regulation of cell proliferation, differentiation, migration, and apoptosis (92). The association between *DSP* variants and IPF, as well as the relationship between *DSP* variants and lung expression of this gene, was confirmed more recently by Mathai et al. (91) IPF lung has higher gene expression of *DSP*. However, IPF subjects with the rs2076295 variant were found to have lower *DSP* expression, suggesting that differential *DSP* expression may play a role in a subset or sub-phenotype of IPF (91). This association further implicates the airway epithelium in the pathogenesis of IPF, as *DSP* appears to be localized primarily to the airway epithelia and not to alveolar epithelial cells. The role of *DSP* in IPF pathogenesis remains an area of active investigation.

PROGNOSIS

Genetic variants, both rare (telomere related) and common (*MUC5B* and *TOLLIP*), may play a role in predicting disease outcomes and have prognostic implications. Short telomeres (<10th percentile adjusted for age) have been identified in a considerable portion of IPF patients, regardless of genetic mutations (33, 34). Patients with shorter telomeres have worse transplant-free survival in multiple independent cohorts (46, 93). Furthermore, a small observational study suggested that increased rates of bone marrow suppression and medication-related complications following lung transplantation are more common in IPF patients with telomerase mutations and/or short telomeres (94). Telomere length testing has been suggested as a component of pretransplant workup in IPF patients, although further prospective study is required before these observations can be utilized routinely in patient care (95).

Common polymorphisms, *MUC5B* and *TOLLIP*, have also shown promise as prognostic indicators (11, 50). A retrospective study of two separate IPF cohorts demonstrated improved survival in patients with the rs35705950 variant (49). In addition, carriers of at least 1 T allele of *MUC5B* polymorphism were found to have at least 50% improved survival and better lung function compared to those with the GG genotype (49). These findings were consistent with previous studies, which demonstrated an association between *MUC5B* variant and less severe pathological changes (96) and slower decline in FVC (50). Similarly, a *TOLLIP* variant was also associated with differential survival. The minor allele at rs5743890 (G) in TOLLIP is protective and associated with reduced susceptibility to IPF. However, those who developed IPF despite having the protective allele had increased mortality (11). At this time, there are no clinical guidelines suggesting genetic testing in the routine care and counseling of IPF patients (95), and further research is needed to identify the clinical implications of these preliminary findings.

TREATMENT

Approaches to therapy in IPF have been limited by the poorly understood pathophysiology of this progressive disease. In addition, the unpredictable clinical course of IPF, lack of validated biomarkers, and low clinical predictive value to animal models (97) have been barriers to identifying therapies. Despite these challenges, recent advances in understanding the pathophysiology of IPF have allowed for identification of novel treatment targets. Currently, two available medications, pirfenidone (4) and ninetedanib (3), have been shown to reduce the rate of lung function decline among IPF patients. However, neither approved drug is curative.

With survival-associated variants (e.g., *MUC5B* and *TOLLIP*) (74), it is possible that genotypes will define subtypes with differential responses to therapy. Identifying distinct sub-phenotypes in IPF may enable the application of targeted therapy on a pathway-specific basis. For example, it may be possible to use telomere length or *TERT* genotype to identify a group of patients who would benefit from telomere-directed therapy (95). Oldham and colleagues (98) found that some carriers with *TOLLIP* polymorphism may benefit from treatment with oral *N*-acetylcysteine (NAC). More specifically, of those that received NAC, subjects with TT genotype for rs3750920 (*TOLLIP*) had decreased risk for the trial's composite end point of death, hospitalization, or 10% decrement in forced vital capacity. In contrast, subjects with the CC genotype for rs3750920 had increased risk for the composite endpoints of the NAC intervention study (98). While NAC has not been shown to be effective in IPF in aggregate (99), it is possible that patients have differential response to this therapy (or other therapies) based on *TOLLIP* genotype (100). More prospectively designed studies are needed before genetic variation can be utilized routinely when choosing therapies for individual patients.

CONCLUSION

This review focuses on the relationship between genetic variants and IPF. In addition to sequence variation, epigenetic changes (such as DNA methylation) (101–104) and gene expression changes are associated with disease risk and phenotype (103, 105, 106). Further studies are necessary to better understand the relationships between genetic variation and epigenetic and gene expression variation in terms of disease risk and phenotype.

Given the growing body of evidence that genetic variants influence disease risk as well as disease progression and clinically meaningful patient outcomes, it will be critical to account for genetic variation in future clinical trials. Such prospective studies and analyses that focus on the relationship between genotype and therapeutic response will be crucial in personalizing and improving IPF therapy.

AUTHOR CONTRIBUTIONS

AK and SM researched and wrote first draft of manuscript; DS edited and revised document. All the authors read and approved final version of manuscript.

REFERENCES

1. Olson AL, Swigris JJ, Lezotte DC, Norris JM, Wilson CG, Brown KK. Mortality from pulmonary fibrosis increased in the United States from 1992 to 2003. *Am J Respir Crit Care Med* (2007) 176(3):277–84. doi:10.1164/rccm.200701-044OC
2. Raghu G, Collard HR, Egan JJ, Martinez FJ, Behr J, Brown KK, et al. An official ATS/ERS/JRS/ALAT statement: idiopathic pulmonary fibrosis: evidence-based guidelines for diagnosis and management. *Am J Respir Crit Care Med* (2011) 183(6):788–824. doi:10.1164/rccm.2009-040GL
3. Richeldi L, du Bois RM, Raghu G, Azuma A, Brown KK, Costabel U, et al. Efficacy and safety of nintedanib in idiopathic pulmonary fibrosis. *N Engl J Med* (2014) 370(22):2071–82. doi:10.1056/NEJMoa1402584
4. King T Jr, Bradford W, Castro-Bernardini S, Fagan E, Glaspole I, Glassberg M, et al. A phase 3 trial of pirfenidone in patients with idiopathic pulmonary fibrosis. *N Engl J Med* (2014) 370(22):2083–92. doi:10.1056/NEJMoa1402582

5. Kropski JA, Lawson WE, Young LR, Blackwell TS. Genetic studies provide clues on the pathogenesis of idiopathic pulmonary fibrosis. *Dis Model Mech* (2013) 6(1):9–17. doi:10.1242/dmm.010736
6. Daccord C, Maher TM. Recent advances in understanding idiopathic pulmonary fibrosis. *F1000Res* (2016) 5:F1000 Faculty Rev–1046. doi:10.12688/f1000research.8209.1
7. Tsakiri KD, Cronkhite JT, Kuan PJ, Xing C, Raghu G, Weissler JC, et al. Adult-onset pulmonary fibrosis caused by mutations in telomerase. *Proc Natl Acad Sci U S A* (2007) 104(18):7552–7. doi:10.1073/pnas.0701009104
8. Bonanni PP, Frymoyer JW, Jacox RF. A family study of idiopathic pulmonary fibrosis: a possible dysproteinemic and genetically determined disease. *Am J Med* (1965) 39(3):411–21. doi:10.1016/0002-9343(65)90208-1
9. Javaheri S, Lederer DH, Pella JA, Mark GJ, Levine BW. Idiopathic pulmonary fibrosis in monozygotic twins. The importance of genetic predisposition. *Chest* (1980) 78(4):591–4. doi:10.1378/chest.78.4.591
10. Fingerlin TE, Murphy E, Zhang W, Peljto AL, Brown KK, Steele MP, et al. Genome-wide association study identifies multiple susceptibility loci for pulmonary fibrosis. *Nat Genet* (2013) 45(6):613–20. doi:10.1038/ng.2609
11. Noth I, Zhang Y, Ma SF, Flores C, Barber M, Huang Y, et al. Genetic variants associated with idiopathic pulmonary fibrosis susceptibility and mortality: a genome-wide association study. *Lancet Respir Med* (2013) 1(4):309–17. doi:10.1016/S2213-2600(13)70045-6
12. Nogee L, Dunbar AE, Wert S, Askin F. A mutation in the surfactant protein C gene associated with familial interstitial lung disease. *N Engl J Med* (2001) 344(8):573–9. doi:10.1056/NEJM200102223440805
13. Tanjore H, Cheng D-S, Degryse AL, Zoz DF, Abdolrasulnia R, Lawson WE, et al. Alveolar epithelial cells undergo epithelial-to-mesenchymal transition in response to endoplasmic reticulum stress. *J Biol Chem* (2011) 286(35):30972–80. doi:10.1074/jbc.M110.181164
14. Nathan N, Giraud V, Picard C, Nunes H, Dastot-Le Moal F, Copin B, et al. Germline SFTPA1 mutation in familial idiopathic interstitial pneumonia and lung cancer. *Hum Mol Genet* (2016) 25(8):1457–67. doi:10.1093/hmg/ddw014
15. Wang Y, Kuan PJ, Xing C, Cronkhite JT, Torres F, Rosenblatt RL, et al. Genetic defects in surfactant protein A2 are associated with pulmonary fibrosis and lung cancer. *Am J Hum Genet* (2009) 84(1):52–9. doi:10.1016/j.ajhg.2008.11.010
16. Crossno PF, Polosukhin VV, Blackwell TS, Johnson JE, Markin C, Moore PE, et al. Identification of early interstitial lung disease in an individual with genetic variations in ABCA3 and SFTPC. *Chest* (2010) 137(4):969–73. doi:10.1378/chest.09-0790
17. Stanley SE, Gable DL, Wagner CL, Carlile TM, Hanumanthu VS, Podlevsky JD, et al. Loss-of-function mutations in the RNA biogenesis factor NAF1 predispose to pulmonary fibrosis-emphysema. *Sci Transl Med* (2016) 8(351):ra107–351. doi:10.1126/scitranslmed.aaf7837
18. Armanios M. Telomerase and idiopathic pulmonary fibrosis. *Mutat Res* (2012) 730(1–2):52–8. doi:10.1016/j.mrfmmm.2011.10.013
19. Kropski JA, Mitchell DB, Markin C, Polosukhin VV, Choi L, Johnson JE, et al. A novel dyskerin (DKC1) mutation is associated with familial interstitial pneumonia. *Chest* (2014) 146(1):e1–7. doi:10.1378/chest.13-2224
20. Alder JK, Stanley SE, Wagner CL, Hamilton M, Hanumanthu VS, Armanios M. Exome sequencing identifies mutant TINF2 in a family with pulmonary fibrosis. *Chest* (2015) 147(5):1361–8. doi:10.1378/chest.14-1947
21. Stuart BD, Choi J, Zaidi S, Xing C, Holohan B, Chen R, et al. Exome sequencing links mutations in PARN and RTEL1 with familial pulmonary fibrosis and telomere shortening. *Nat Genet* (2015) 47(5):512–7. doi:10.1038/ng.3278
22. Cogan JD, Kropski JA, Zhao M, Mitchell DB, Rives L, Markin C, et al. Rare variants in RTEL1 are associated with familial interstitial pneumonia. *Am J Respir Crit Care Med* (2015) 191(6):646–55. doi:10.1164/rccm.201408-1510OC
23. Kannengiesser C, Borie R, Ménard C, Réocreux M, Nitschké P, Gazal S, et al. Heterozygous *RTEL1* mutations are associated with familial pulmonary fibrosis. *Eur Respir J* (2015) 46(2):474–85. doi:10.1183/09031936.00040115
24. Tummala H, Walne A, Collopy L, Cardoso S, de la Fuente J, Lawson S, et al. Poly(A)-specific ribonuclease deficiency impacts telomere biology and causes dyskeratosis congenita. *J Clin Invest* (2015) 125(5):2151–60. doi:10.1172/JCI78963
25. Whitsett JA, Wert SE, Weaver TE. Alveolar surfactant homeostasis and the pathogenesis of pulmonary disease. *Annu Rev Med* (2010) 61(1):105–19. doi:10.1146/annurev.med.60.041807.123500
26. Mulugeta S, Nguyen V, Russo SJ, Muniswamy M, Beers MF. A surfactant protein C precursor protein BRICHOS domain mutation causes endoplasmic reticulum stress, proteasome dysfunction, and caspase 3 activation. *Am J Respir Cell Mol Biol* (2005) 32(6):521–30. doi:10.1165/rcmb.2005-0009OC
27. van Moorsel CHM, Hoffman TW, van Batenburg AA, Klay D, van der Vis JJ, Grutters JC. Understanding idiopathic interstitial pneumonia: a gene-based review of stressed lungs. *Biomed Res Int* (2015) 2015:304186. doi:10.1155/2015/304186
28. Maitra M, Wang Y, Gerard RD, Mendelson CR, Garcia CK. Surfactant protein A2 mutations associated with pulmonary fibrosis lead to protein instability and endoplasmic reticulum stress. *J Biol Chem* (2010) 285(29):22103–13. doi:10.1074/jbc.M110.121467
29. Yamano G, Funahashi H, Kawanami O, Zhao L-X, Ban N, Uchida Y, et al. ABCA3 is a lamellar body membrane protein in human lung alveolar type II cells. *FEBS Lett* (2001) 508(2):221–5. doi:10.1016/S0014-5793(01)03056-3
30. Weichert N, Kaltenborn E, Hector A, Woischnik M, Schams A, Holzinger A, et al. Some ABCA3 mutations elevate ER stress and initiate apoptosis of lung epithelial cells. *Respir Res* (2011) 12:4. doi:10.1186/1465-9921-12-4
31. Cheong N, Madesh M, Gonzales LW, Zhao M, Yu K, Ballard PL, et al. Functional and trafficking defects in ATP binding cassette A3 mutants associated with respiratory distress syndrome. *J Biol Chem* (2006) 281(14):9791–800. doi:10.1074/jbc.M507515200
32. Armanios M, Chen JJ-L, Cogan JD, Alder JK, Ingersoll RG, Markin C, et al. Telomerase mutations in families with idiopathic pulmonary fibrosis. *N Engl J Med* (2007) 356(13):1317–26. doi:10.1056/NEJMoa066157
33. Cronkhite J, Xing C, Raghu G, Chin KM, Torres F, Rosenblatt RL, et al. Telomere shortening in familial and sporadic pulmonary fibrosis. *Am J Respir Crit Care Med* (2008) 178(7):729–37. doi:10.1164/rccm.200804-550OC
34. Alder JK, Chen JJ-L, Lancaster L, Danoff S, Su S, Cogan JD, et al. Short telomeres are a risk factor for idiopathic pulmonary fibrosis. *Proc Natl Acad Sci U S A* (2008) 105(35):13051–6. doi:10.1073/pnas.0804280105
35. Driscoll B, Buckley S, Bui KC, Anderson KD, Warburton D. Telomerase in alveolar epithelial development and repair. *Am J Physiol Lung Cell Mol Physiol* (2000) 279(6):L1191–8.
36. Liu T, Ullenbruch M, Choi YY, Yu H, Ding L, Xaubet A, et al. Telomerase and telomere length in pulmonary fibrosis. *Am J Respir Cell Mol Biol* (2013) 49(2):260–8. doi:10.1165/rcmb.2012-0514OC
37. Chen JL, Greider CW. Telomerase RNA structure and function: implications for dyskeratosis congenita. *Trends Biochem Sci* (2004) 29(4):183–92. doi:10.1016/j.tibs.2004.02.003
38. Heiss NS, Knight SW, Vulliamy TJ, Klauck SM, Wiemann S, Mason PJ, et al. X-linked dyskeratosis congenita is caused by mutations in a highly conserved gene with putative nucleolar functions. *Nat Genet* (1998) 19(1):32–8. doi:10.1038/ng0598-32
39. Kim SH, Kaminker P, Campisi J. TIN2, a new regulator of telomere length in human cells. *Nat Genet* (1999) 23(4):405–12. doi:10.1038/13854
40. Vannier J-B, Sarek G, Boulton SJ. RTEL1: functions of a disease-associated helicase. *Trends Cell Biol* (2014) 24:416–25. doi:10.1016/j.tcb.2014.01.004
41. Seibold MA, Wise AL, Speer MC, Steel MP, Brown KK, Loyd JE, et al. A common MUC5B promoter polymorphism and pulmonary fibrosis. *N Engl J Med* (2012) 364(16):1503–12. doi:10.1056/NEJMoa1013660
42. Korthagen NM, van Moorsel CHM, Kazemier KM, Ruven HJT, Grutters JC. IL1RN genetic variations and risk of IPF: a meta-analysis and mRNA expression study. *Immunogenetics* (2012) 64(5):371–7. doi:10.1007/s00251-012-0604-6
43. Ahn M-H, Park B-L, Lee S-H, Park S-W, Park J-S, Kim D-J, et al. A promoter SNP rs4073T>A in the common allele of the interleukin 8 gene is associated with the development of idiopathic pulmonary fibrosis via the IL-8 protein enhancing mode. *Respir Res* (2011) 12(1):73. doi:10.1186/1465-9921-12-73
44. Richards TJ, Kaminski N, Baribaud F, Flavin S, Brodmerkel C, Horowitz D, et al. Peripheral blood proteins predict mortality in idiopathic

pulmonary fibrosis. *Am J Respir Crit Care Med* (2012) 185(1):67–76. doi:10.1164/rccm.201101-0058OC
45. O'Dwyer DN, Armstrong ME, Trujillo G, Cooke G, Keane MP, Fallon PG, et al. The toll-like receptor 3 L412F polymorphism and disease progression in idiopathic pulmonary fibrosis. *Am J Respir Crit Care Med* (2013) 188(12):1442–50. doi:10.1164/rccm.201304-0760OC
46. Stuart BD, Lee JS, Kozlitina J, Noth I, Devine MS, Glazer CS, et al. Effect of telomere length on survival in patients with idiopathic pulmonary fibrosis: an observational cohort study with independent validation. *Lancet Respir Med* (2014) 2(7):557–65. doi:10.1016/S2213-2600(14)70124-9
47. Kropski JA, Blackwell TS, Loyd JE. The genetic basis of idiopathic pulmonary fibrosis. *Eur Respir J* (2015) 45:1717–27. doi:10.1183/09031936.00163814
48. Fingerlin TE, Zhang W, Yang IV, Ainsworth HC, Russell PH, Blumhagen RZ, et al. Genome-wide imputation study identifies novel HLA locus for pulmonary fibrosis and potential role for auto-immunity in fibrotic idiopathic interstitial pneumonia. *BMC Genet* (2016) 17(1):74. doi:10.1186/s12863-016-0377-2
49. Peljto AL, Zhang Y, Fingerlin TE, Ma SF, Garcia JG, Richards TJ, et al. Association between the MUC5B promoter polymorphism and survival in patients with idiopathic pulmonary fibrosis. *JAMA* (2013) 309(21):2232–9. doi:10.1001/jama.2013.5827
50. Stock CJ, Sato H, Fonseca C, Banya WAS, Molyneaux PL, Adamali H, et al. Mucin 5B promoter polymorphism is associated with idiopathic pulmonary fibrosis but not with development of lung fibrosis in systemic sclerosis or sarcoidosis. *Thorax* (2013) 68(5):436–41. doi:10.1136/thoraxjnl-2012-201786
51. Evans CM, Fingerlin TE, Schwarz MI, Lynch D, Kurche J, Warg L, et al. Idiopathic pulmonary fibrosis: a genetic disease that involves mucociliary dysfunction of the peripheral airways. *Physiol Rev* (2016) 96(4):1567–91. doi:10.1152/physrev.00004.2016
52. Mathai SK, Yang IV, Schwarz MI, Schwartz DA. Incorporating genetics into the identification and treatment of idiopathic pulmonary fibrosis. *BMC Med* (2015) 13:191. doi:10.1186/s12916-015-0434-0
53. Lawson WE, Grant SW, Ambrosini V, Womble KE, Dawson EP, Lane KB, et al. Genetic mutations in surfactant protein C are a rare cause of sporadic cases of IPF. *Thorax* (2004) 59(11):977–80. doi:10.1136/thx.2004.026336
54. Tanjore H, Blackwell TS, Lawson WE. Emerging evidence for endoplasmic reticulum stress in the pathogenesis of idiopathic pulmonary fibrosis. *Am J Physiol Lung Cell Mol Physiol* (2012) 302(8):L721–9. doi:10.1152/ajplung.00410.2011
55. Lawson WE, Crossno PF, Polosukhin VV, Roldan J, Cheng D-S, Lane KB, et al. Endoplasmic reticulum stress in alveolar epithelial cells is prominent in IPF: association with altered surfactant protein processing and herpesvirus infection. *Am J Physiol Lung Cell Mol Physiol* (2008) 294(6):L1119–26. doi:10.1152/ajplung.00382.2007
56. Campo I, Zorzetto M, Mariani F, Kadija Z, Morbini P, Dore R, et al. A large kindred of pulmonary fibrosis associated with a novel ABCA3 gene variant. *Respir Res* (2014) 15(43):15. doi:10.1186/1465-9921-15-43
57. Zhou W, Wang Y. Candidate genes of idiopathic pulmonary fibrosis: current evidence and research. *Appl Clin Genet* (2016) 9:5–13. doi:10.2147/TACG.S61999
58. Lawson WE, Cheng D-S, Degryse AL, Tanjore H, Polosukhin VV, Xu XC, et al. Endoplasmic reticulum stress enhances fibrotic remodeling in the lungs. *Proc Natl Acad Sci U S A* (2011) 108(26):10562–7. doi:10.1073/pnas.1107559108
59. Kim KK, Kugler MC, Wolters PJ, Robillard L, Galvez MG, Brumwell AN, et al. Alveolar epithelial cell mesenchymal transition develops in vivo during pulmonary fibrosis and is regulated by the extracellular matrix. *Proc Natl Acad Sci U S A* (2006) 103(35):13180–5. doi:10.1073/pnas.0605669103
60. Tanjore H, Xu XC, Polosukhin VV, Degryse AL, Li B, Han W, et al. Contribution of epithelial-derived fibroblasts to bleomycin-induced lung fibrosis. *Am J Respir Crit Care Med* (2009) 180(7):657–65. doi:10.1164/rccm.200903-0322OC
61. Marmai C, Sutherland RE, Kim KK, Dolganov GM, Fang X, Kim SS, et al. Alveolar epithelial cells express mesenchymal proteins in patients with idiopathic pulmonary fibrosis. *Am J Physiol Lung Cell Mol Physiol* (2011) 301(1):L71–8. doi:10.1152/ajplung.00212.2010
62. Mathai SK, Schwartz DA, Warg LA. Genetic susceptibility and pulmonary fibrosis. *Curr Opin Pulm Med* (2014) 20(5):429–35. doi:10.1097/MCP.0000000000000074
63. Armanios M, Alder JK, Parry EM, Karim B, Strong MA, Greider CW. Short telomeres are sufficient to cause the degenerative defects associated with aging. *Am J Hum Genet* (2009) 85(6):823–32. doi:10.1016/j.ajhg.2009.10.028
64. Petrovski S, Todd JL, Durheim MT, Wang Q, Chien JW, Kelly FL, et al. An exome sequencing study to assess the role of rare genetic variation in pulmonary fibrosis. *Am J Respir Crit Care Med* (2017) 196(1):82–93. doi:10.1164/rccm.201610-2088OC
65. Armanios M, Blackburn EH. The telomere syndromes. *Nat Rev Genet* (2012) 13(10):693–704. doi:10.1038/nrg3246
66. Alder JK, Guo N, Kembou F, Parry EM, Anderson CJ, Gorgy AI, et al. Telomere length is a determinant of emphysema susceptibility. *Am J Respir Crit Care Med* (2011) 184(8):904–12. doi:10.1164/rccm.201103-0520OC
67. Minagawa S, Araya J, Numata T, Nojiri S, Hara H, Yumino Y, et al. Accelerated epithelial cell senescence in IPF and the inhibitory role of SIRT6 in TGF-beta-induced senescence of human bronchial epithelial cells. *Am J Physiol Lung Cell Mol Physiol* (2011) 300(3):L391–401. doi:10.1152/ajplung.00097.2010
68. Roy MG, Livraghi-Butrico A, Fletcher AA, McElwee MM, Evans SE, Boerner RM, et al. Muc5b is required for airway defence. *Nature* (2014) 505(7483):412–6. doi:10.1038/nature12807
69. Young HWJ, Williams OW, Chandra D, Bellinghausen LK, Pérez G, Suárez A, et al. Central role of Muc5ac expression in mucous metaplasia and its regulation by conserved 5' elements. *Am J Respir Cell Mol Biol* (2007) 37(3):273–90. doi:10.1165/rcmb.2005-0460OC
70. Borie R, Crestani B, Dieude P, Nunes H, Allanore Y, Kannengiesser C, et al. The MUC5B variant is associated with idiopathic pulmonary fibrosis but not with systemic sclerosis interstitial lung disease in the European Caucasian population. *PLoS One* (2013) 8(8):e70621. doi:10.1371/journal.pone.0070621
71. Horimasu Y, Ohshimo S, Bonella F, Tanaka S, Ishikawa N, Hattori N, et al. MUC5B promoter polymorphism in Japanese patients with idiopathic pulmonary fibrosis. *Respirology* (2015) 20(3):439–44. doi:10.1111/resp.12466
72. Wang C, Zhuang Y, Guo W, Cao L, Zhang H, Xu L, et al. Mucin 5B promoter polymorphism is associated with susceptibility to interstitial lung diseases in Chinese males. *PLoS One* (2014) 9(8):e104919. doi:10.1371/journal.pone.0104919
73. van der Vis JJ, Snetselaar R, Kazemier KM, ten Klooster L, Grutters JC, van Moorsel CHM. Effect of Muc5b promoter polymorphism on disease predisposition and survival in idiopathic interstitial pneumonias. *Respirology* (2016) 21(4):712–7. doi:10.1111/resp.12728
74. Wei R, Li C, Zhang M, Jones-Hall YL, Myers JL, Noth I, et al. Association between MUC5B and TERT polymorphisms and different interstitial lung disease phenotypes. *Transl Res* (2014) 163(5):494–502. doi:10.1016/j.trsl.2013.12.006
75. Peljto AL, Selman M, Kim DS, Murphy E, Tucker L, Pardo A, et al. The MUC5B promoter polymorphism is associated with idiopathic pulmonary fibrosis in a Mexican cohort but is rare among Asian ancestries. *Chest* (2015) 147(2):460–4. doi:10.1378/chest.14-0867
76. Kishore A, Žižková V, Kocourková L, Petrkova J, Bouros E, Nunes H, et al. Association study for 26 candidate loci in idiopathic pulmonary fibrosis patients from four European populations. *Front Immunol* (2016) 7:274. doi:10.3389/fimmu.2016.00274
77. Seibold MA, Smith RW, Urbanek C, Groshong SD, Cosgrove GP, Brown KK, et al. The idiopathic pulmonary fibrosis honeycomb cyst contains a mucocilary pseudostratified epithelium. *PLoS One* (2013) 8(3):e58658. doi:10.1371/journal.pone.0058658
78. Nakano Y, Yang IV, Walts AD, Watson AM, Helling BA, Fletcher AA, et al. MUC5B promoter variant rs35705950 affects MUC5B expression in the distal airways in idiopathic pulmonary fibrosis. *Am J Respir Crit Care Med* (2016) 193(4):464–6. doi:10.1164/rccm.201509-1872LE
79. Hunninghake GM, Hatabu H, Okajima Y, Gao W, Dupuis J, Latourelle JC, et al. MUC5B promoter polymorphism and interstitial lung abnormalities. *N Engl J Med* (2013) 368(23):2192–200. doi:10.1056/NEJMoa1216076

80. Araki T, Putman RK, Hatabu H, Gao W, Dupuis J, Latourelle JC, et al. Development and progression of interstitial lung abnormalities in the Framingham heart study. *Am J Respir Crit Care Med* (2016) 194(12):1514–22. doi:10.1164/rccm.201512-2523OC
81. Putman RK, Hatabu H, Araki T, Gudmundsson G, Gao W, Nishino M, et al. Association between interstitial lung abnormalities and all-cause mortality. *JAMA* (2016) 315(7):672–81. doi:10.1001/jama.2016.0518
82. Chung JH, Peljto AL, Chawla A, Talbert JL, McKean DF, Rho B-H, et al. CT imaging phenotypes of pulmonary fibrosis in the MUC5B promoter site polymorphism. *Chest* (2016) 149(5):1215–22. doi:10.1016/j.chest.2015.11.009
83. Parker D, Prince A. Innate immunity in the respiratory epithelium. *Am J Respir Cell Mol Biol* (2011) 45:189–201. doi:10.1165/rcmb.2011-0011RT
84. Zhou Y, Wang X, Liu M, Hu Q, Song L, Ye L, et al. A critical function of toll-like receptor-3 in the induction of anti-human immunodeficiency virus activities in macrophages. *Immunology* (2010) 131(1):40–9. doi:10.1111/j.1365-2567.2010.03270.x
85. Falfán-Valencia R, Camarena A, Juárez A, Becerril C, Montaño M, Cisneros J, et al. Major histocompatibility complex and alveolar epithelial apoptosis in idiopathic pulmonary fibrosis. *Hum Genet* (2005) 118(2):235–44. doi:10.1007/s00439-005-0035-7
86. Aquino-Galvez A, Pérez-Rodríguez M, Camarena Á, Falfan-Valencia R, Ruiz V, Montaño M, et al. MICA polymorphisms and decreased expression of the MICA receptor NKG2D contribute to idiopathic pulmonary fibrosis susceptibility. *Hum Genet* (2009) 125(5–6):639–48. doi:10.1007/s00439-009-0666-1
87. Xue J, Gochuico BR, Alawad AS, Feghali-Bostwick CA, Noth I, Nathan SD, et al. The HLA class II Allele DRB1*1501 is over-represented in patients with idiopathic pulmonary fibrosis. *PLoS One* (2011) 6(2):e14715. doi:10.1371/journal.pone.0014715
88. Zhang J, Xu D, Xu K, Wu B, Zheng M, Chen J, et al. HLA-A and HLA-B gene polymorphism and idiopathic pulmonary fibrosis in a Han Chinese population. *Respir Med* (2012) 106(10):1456–62. doi:10.1016/j.rmed.2012.06.015
89. Zhang H-P, Zou J, Xie P, Gao F, Mu H-J. Association of HLA and cytokine gene polymorphisms with idiopathic pulmonary fibrosis. *Kaohsiung J Med Sci* (2015) 31(12):613–20. doi:10.1016/j.kjms.2015.10.007
90. Erlich HA, Opelz G, Hansen J. HLA DNA typing and transplantation. *Immunity* (2001) 14:347–56. doi:10.1016/S1074-7613(01)00115-7
91. Mathai SK, Pedersen BS, Smith K, Russell P, Schwarz MI, Brown KK, et al. Desmoplakin (DSP) variants are associated with idiopathic pulmonary fibrosis. *Am J Respir Crit Care Med* (2015) 193(10):1151–60. doi:10.1164/rccm.201509-1863OC
92. Huber O, Petersen I. 150th anniversary series: desmosomes and the hallmarks of cancer. *Cell Commun Adhes* (2015) 22(1):15–28. doi:10.3109/15419061.2015.1039642
93. Dai J, Cai H, Li H, Zhuang Y, Min H, Wen Y, et al. Association between telomere length and survival in patients with idiopathic pulmonary fibrosis. *Respirology* (2015) 20(6):947–52. doi:10.1111/resp.12566
94. Silhan LL, Shah PD, Chambers DC, Snyder LD, Riise GC, Wagner CL, et al. Lung transplantation in telomerase mutation carriers with pulmonary fibrosis. *Eur Respir J* (2014) 44(1):178–87. doi:10.1183/09031936.00060014
95. Kropski JA, Young LR, Cogan JD, Mitchell DB, Lancaster LH, Worrell JA, et al. Genetic evaluation and testing of patients and families with idiopathic pulmonary fibrosis. *Am J Respir Crit Care Med* (2016) 195(11):1423–8. doi:10.1164/rccm.201609-1820PP
96. Cosgrove GP, Groshong SD, Peljto AL, Talbert J, McKean D, Markin C, et al. The MUC5B promoter polymorphism is associated with a less severe pathological form of familial interstitial pneumonia (FIP). *Am J Respir Crit Care Med* (2012) 185:A6865. doi:10.1164/ajrccm-conference.2012.185.1_MeetingAbstracts.A6865
97. O'Riordan TG, Smith V, Raghu G. Development of novel agents for idiopathic pulmonary fibrosis. *Chest* (2015) 148(4):1083–92. doi:10.1378/chest.14-3218
98. Oldham JM, Ma S-F, Martinez FJ, Anstrom KJ, Raghu G, Schwartz DA, et al. TOLLIP, MUC5B, and the response to N -acetylcysteine among individuals with idiopathic pulmonary fibrosis. *Am J Respir Crit Care Med* (2015) 192(12):1475–82. doi:10.1164/rccm.201505-1010OC
99. Idiopathic Pulmonary Fibrosis Clinical Research Network, Raghu G, Anstrom KJ, King TE, Lasky JA, Martinez FJ. Prednisone, azathioprine, and N-acetylcysteine for pulmonary fibrosis. *N Engl J Med* (2012) 366(21):1968–77. doi:10.1056/NEJMoa1113354
100. Mathai SK, Newton CA, Schwartz DA, Garcia CK. Pulmonary fibrosis in the era of stratified medicine. *Thorax* (2016) 71(12):1154–60. doi:10.1136/thoraxjnl-2016-209172
101. Helling BA, Yang IV. Epigenetics in lung fibrosis: from pathobiology to treatment perspective. *Curr Opin Pulm Med* (2015) 21(5):454–62. doi:10.1097/MCP.0000000000000191
102. Helling BA, Gerber AN, Kadiyala V, Sasse SK, Pedersen BS, Sparks L, et al. Regulation of MUC5B expression in idiopathic pulmonary fibrosis. *Am J Respir Cell Mol Biol* (2017) 57(1):91–9. doi:10.1165/rcmb.2017-0046OC
103. Yang IV, Pedersen BS, Rabinovich E, Hennessy CE, Davidson EJ, Murphy E, et al. Relationship of DNA methylation and gene expression in idiopathic pulmonary fibrosis. *Am J Respir Crit Care Med* (2014) 190(11):1263–72. doi:10.1164/rccm.201408-1452OC
104. Sanders YY, Ambalavanan N, Halloran B, Zhang X, Liu H, Crossman DK, et al. Altered DNA methylation profile in idiopathic pulmonary fibrosis. *Am J Respir Crit Care Med* (2012) 186(6):525–35. doi:10.1164/rccm.201201-0077OC
105. Yang IV, Burch LH, Steele MP, Savov JD, Hollingsworth JW, McElvania-Tekippe E, et al. Gene expression profiling of familial and sporadic interstitial pneumonia. *Am J Respir Crit Care Med* (2007) 175(1):45–54. doi:10.1164/rccm.200601-062OC
106. Yang IV, Coldren CD, Leach SM, Seibold MA, Murphy E, Lin J, et al. Expression of cilium-associated genes defines novel molecular subtypes of idiopathic pulmonary fibrosis. *Thorax* (2013) 68(12):1114–21. doi:10.1136/thoraxjnl-2012-202943

15

Collagen 1a1 Expression by Airway Macrophages Increases in Fibrotic ILDs and is Associated with FVC Decline and Increased Mortality

Eliza Tsitoura[1], *Athina Trachalaki*[1,2], *Eirini Vasarmidi*[1], *Semeli Mastrodemou*[1], *George A. Margaritopoulos*[2], *Maria Kokosi*[2], *Dionysios Fanidis*[3], *Apostolos Galaris*[3], *Vassilis Aidinis*[3], *Elizabeth Renzoni*[2], *Nikos Tzanakis*[1], *Athol U. Wells*[2†] *and Katerina M. Antoniou*[1*†]

[1] *Laboratory of Molecular and Cellular Pneumonology, Department of Respiratory Medicine, School of Medicine, University of Crete, Heraklion, Greece,* [2] *Interstitial Lung Disease Unit, Royal Brompton and Harefield Hospital National Health Service (NHS) Foundation Trust, Imperial College, London, United Kingdom,* [3] *Division of Immunology, Alexander Fleming Biomedical Sciences Research Centre, Athens, Greece*

Correspondence:
Katerina M. Antoniou
kantoniou@uoc.gr

[†]*These authors have contributed equally to this work*

Within the Interstitial Lung Diseases (ILD), patients with idiopathic pulmonary fibrosis (IPF) and a subset of those with non-IPF fibrotic ILD have a distinct clinical phenotype of progression despite management. This group of patients has been collectively termed the progressive fibrotic phenotype (PFP). Their early recognition may facilitate access to antifibrotic therapies to prevent or slow progression. Macrophages/monocytes within the lung orchestrate the progression and maintenance of fibrosis. A novel role for monocyte-derived macrophages during tissue damage and wound healing is the expression of collagens. We examined Collagen 1a1 expression in airway macrophages from ILD patients at diagnosis. COL1A1 mRNA levels from BAL cells were elevated in IPF and Non-IPF patients. The presence of a UIP pattern and a subsequent progressive phenotype were significantly associated with the higher BAL COL1A1 levels. In Non-IPF patients, higher COL1A1 levels were associated with a more than twofold increase in mortality. The intracellular localisation of COL1A1 in airway macrophages was demonstrated by confocal microscopy in CD45 and CD163 co-staining assays. Additionally, airway macrophages co-expressed COL1A1 with the profibrotic SPP1 gene product osteopontin. The levels of SPP1 mRNA and OPN in the BAL were significantly higher in IPF and Non-IPF patients relative to healthy. Our results suggest that profibrotic airway macrophages are increased in the BAL of patients with IPF and other ILDs and co-express COL1A1 and OPN. Importantly, COL1A1 expression by pro-fibrotic airway macrophages could be a marker of disease progression and poor survival in ILDs.

Keywords: IPF, RA-ILD, NSIP, airway macrophages, SPP1, osteopontin, collagen 1A1, PF-ILD

INTRODUCTION

Interstitial Lung Disease (ILD) is a broad term currently used to include more than 200 different disease entities (1). Connective tissue associated ILD (CTD-ILD) is the most common subtype, whilst idiopathic ILDs lie within the orphan characterization of rare lung diseases. Amongst idiopathic interstitial pneumonias, the most characterized and well-studied is IPF, a lethal chronic disease (1). IPF is distinguished by a clinical phenotype of inexorable progression and a median survival of 3 years, prior to the advent of anti-fibrotic agents (2). Amongst other ILDs, disease behaviour is strikingly diverse, ranging from self-limited, reversible to progressive, IPF-like disease (1–3). A subset of non-IPF ILD patients exhibit a more progressive disease course despite usual management, similar to IPF (PF-ILD) (3–5).

Commonalities in clinical behaviour in IPF and non-IPF ILDs with the PFP suggest common underlying pathogenetic pathways that drive progression, irrespective of the initial trigger (6, 7). Given the strong links between progression and subsequent mortality in non-IPF ILDs, it is vital that algorithms be developed to identify the PFP at presentation. It is known that a pattern of usual interstitial pneumonia (UIP), on biopsy or as judged by CT (UIP or "probable UIP") indicates a higher likelihood of disease progression (8, 9). Molecular biomarkers have also been identified as candidate markers of progression in individual ILDs, including KL-6, PDGF, FGF, VEGF and M-CSF (7, 10).

The role of the innate and adaptive immune systems in the pathogenesis of IPF is not clearly defined (11) and immune cells such as macrophages, monocytes and fibrocytes are subject to intense investigation as novel therapeutic options in IPF effectively alter their activation (12, 13). Macrophages, the most abundant immune cells in the lung, play important roles in tissue remodelling during pulmonary fibrosis (14). Following a fibrotic insult such as bleomycin in murine models, the pool of tissue resident alveolar macrophages is replaced by monocyte-derived macrophages that have distinct phenotypes including the upregulation of pro-fibrotic genes (15). Macrophages produce profibrotic mediators such as transforming growth factor-β (TGF-β) and platelet-derived growth factor (PDGF), directly orchestrating the activation of fibroblast functions and implicated in the aberrant wound-healing cascade during fibrosis (16). Fibrocytes, a minor fraction of circulating leukocytes, portray a dual phenotype of monocytes (CD34, CD45, CD11b) and fibroblasts (collagens I and III, and fibronectin (17) that migrate to the lungs following tissue damage (18). Single-cell RNAseq analyses of the airway cell population from human lungs reveal a plethora of cell entities with monocyte and macrophage markers. This approach is reshaping the field of macrophage/monocyte biology, with the observation that lung macrophage/monocyte populations shift during lung fibrosis towards distinct entities with yet uncharacterised functions (19).

Macrophages were long believed not to produce collagens. However there is cumulative evidence that they express almost all known collagen mRNAs (20, 21). Furthermore, recent evidence from a mouse model of fibrotic scar formation in the heart shows that recruited monocyte-derived macrophages directly contribute to collagen-I fibril formation, suggesting that cell-autonomous production of collagen is a component of the pro-fibrotic monocyte/macrophage response (22). The role of collagen expression by alveolar macrophages in IPF is unknown; however, a recent study showed that Collagen VI is upregulated in macrophages overexpressing Fra-2 in mouse models of pulmonary fibrosis and in IPF tissue macrophages while Col-VI knockout bone marrow chimeras were protected from bleomycin-induced lung fibrosis (23). We have previously observed that mRNA levels of COL1A1 are detectable in BAL cells and are elevated in IPF patients relative to controls (24, 25).

The results of the lung fibrosis cell atlas suggest that macrophage populations in the lungs are distinct in lung fibrosis compared to healthy subjects. Independent studies have identified an increase of alveolar macrophages expressing the *SPP1* gene that encodes for osteopontin (OPN) in fibrotic lungs (15, 19, 26). OPN-expressing macrophages of monocyte origin also accumulate in murine models of hepatosteatosis (27). OPN dramatically increased in the BAL and serum of fibrotic patients and was initially explored as a potential IPF serum biomarker (28, 29). However, results from later studies established a wider pattern of upregulation of OPN in fibrotic disease suggesting a dominant role in the pathogenesis of lung fibrosis (30). OPN may act as a cytokine and a transcription factor and is directly involved in extracellular matrix regulation and collagen expression in fibrotic disorders of the liver, kidneys and heart (31, 32).

In this study, we established that collagen1a1 expression occurs in airway macrophages and increases in pulmonary fibrosis both in mice and humans. We compared the COL1A1 mRNA levels between IPF and non-IPF fibrotic ILDs at diagnosis in order to establish a possible link between disease progression and collagen expression in myeloid cells. In addition, in view of the involvement of OPN in collagen expression, we also examined a possible association of SPP1 and COL1A1 levels in BAL cells.

MATERIALS AND METHODS

Patients

134 patients were prospectively recruited. 69 subjects (ILD, n=50; controls, n=19) were recruited in the Department of Respiratory Medicine, University Hospital of Heraklion, Crete, Greece from May 2012 to December 2018. 65 subjects all with ILD, were recruited in the Royal Brompton Hospital from March 2003 to October 2009.

Patient characteristics are summarised in **Table 1** and **Supplementary Table 1**. Diagnostic sub-groups comprised IPF (n=53) and non-IPF ILDs (n=52). All subjects underwent

Abbreviations: AMs, Airway macrophages; COL1A1, Collagen 1a1; CTD-ILD, Connective tissue associated ILD; GAPDH, glyceraldehyde-3-phosphate dehydrogenase; HP, Hypersensitivity Pneumonitis; ILD, Interstitial Lung Diseases; IPF, Idiopathic Pulmonary Fibrosis; NSIP, Non-Specific Pneumonia; OPN, osteopontin; OP, organising pneumonia; RA-ILD, Rheumatoid Arthritis ILD; SSc-ILD, Scleroderma ILD; SLE, Systemic Lupus erythematosus; SPP1, secreted phosphoprotein 1; UIP, Usual Interstitial Pattern.

TABLE 1 | Patient characteristics.

	Control Group (n = 19)	IPF (n = 53)	Non-IPF (n = 62)	P value
Age	54.1 ± 13.5	68.1 ± 10	59 ± 14	P<0.0001 Control *vs* IPF p=0.001 IPF *vs* Non-IPF p<0.001 Control *vs* Non-IPF ns
gender (female/male)	6/13	8/45	41/21	P<0.0001 *
Smoking History				P<0.0001*
Never	2 (10.5%)	16 (30.8%)	35 (57.4%)	
Ex-smoker	3 (15.8%)	31(59.6%)	6 (32.8%)	
Smoker	14 (73.7%)	5 (9.6%)	20 (9.8%)	
Macrophages	87.3 ± 9	79.1 ± 15.3	79 ± 12.6	P ns
Lymphocytes	9.9 ± 7.6	11 ± 15.2	11 ± 9	P ns
Neutrophils	4.2 ± 1.6	7.3 ± 6.3	6.5 ± 6.2	P=0.006 Control *vs* IPF p<0.001 Control *vs* Non-IPF p<0.001
Eosinophils	0.4 ± 0.5	2 ± 3.3	2.3 ± 2.8	P=0.087 Control *vs* IPF p=0.007 Control *vs* Non-IPF p<0.0001
FVC		78.5 ± 19.7	79.4 ± 25.2	P ns
DLco		52.3 ± 18.5	51 ± 16.5	P ns
CPI		44 ± 15	43 ± 14.7	P ns

**Stands for Chi-square test; "ns" stands for non significant.*

bronchoalveolar lavage (BAL) and chest high resolution computed tomography (HRCT). For the ILD patients BAL and HRCT were part of the initial diagnostic evaluation (33–36).

IPF Group

The diagnosis of IPF was based on ATS/ERS criteria or on multidisciplinary discussion according to the Fleischer criteria (34, 37). Patients were anti-fibrotic naïve.

Non-IPF Group

This category of patients included patients with a known or new diagnosis of Connective tissue disease (CTD-ILD); namely Systemic Sclerosis (SSc), Rheumatoid arthritis (RA), Systemic Lupus erythematous (SLE) or Undifferentiated CTD. Patients with CTD-ILD were enrolled at the initial stages of there ILD diagnosis. Additionally, included patients with Idiopathic Non-Specific Pneumonia (NSIP), Hypersensitivity Pneumonitis (HP) and organizing pneumonia/NSIP overlap (OP/NSIP).

Control Group

Control subjects were undergoing bronchoscopy for the investigation of haemoptysis, without any overt pulmonary comorbidities and with normal bronchoscopy findings and cytology results. Since controls were healthy subjects, no PFTs were performed.

All patients were evaluated with complete pulmonary function tests (PFTs) within one month of bronchoscopy. Lung volumes were measured using body plethysmography and the diffusion capacity (DLco, corrected for haemoglobin) was measured using the single breath technique. The computerized system (Jaeger 2.12; MasterLab, Würzburg, Germany) was used and predicted values were obtained from the standardized lung function testing of the European Coal and Steel Community, Luxembourg (1993).

Patients were classified as non-smokers, current smokers or former smokers (defined as having smoked a minimum of one cigarette a day for a minimum of 1 year, stopping at least 6 months before presentation).

All patients provided written informed consent. The study was approved by the Ethics Committees of the University Hospital of Heraklion (IRB number: 1045 and 17030) and the Royal Brompton Hospital (REC reference 13/LO/0857).

BAL Cell Isolation and Determination of Cellular Composition

BAL fluid was obtained at room temperature. A flexible bronchoscope was wedged into a sub-segmental bronchus of a predetermined region of interest based on radiographical findings. A BAL technique was performed by instilling 180 ml of normal saline in 60-mL aliquots, retrieved by low suction. BAL samples were kept on ice and processed within two hours of collection. Samples were filtered through sterile 70nm cell strainers (BD) and centrifuged at 500g for 5 minutes at 4°C. Cell pellets were re-suspended with cold PBS. Total cell count and cell viability were assessed using Trypan blue (ICN). Differential cell population count was analysed following May-Grunewald-Giemsa staining (25).

Mice

Mice were bred under SPF conditions at the local animal facility at "20–22°C, 55 ± 5% humidity, and a 12-h light/dark cycle; water and food were given ad libitum". All experimentation in mice, in line with the ARRIVE guidelines, was approved by the Veterinary service and Fishery Department of the local governmental prefecture (#2816), following the positive opinion of the Institutional Protocol Evaluation Committee of BSRC Alexander Fleming.

Pulmonary fibrosis was induced through the administration of 0.8U/Kg of bleomycin (Nippon Kayaku) to anesthetized mice (IP ketamine/xylazine/atropine, 100/10/0.05 mg/kg, respectively) *via* the oropharyngeal (OA) route and bronchoalveolar Lavage Fluid (BALF) was collected as previously described (38). In brief, anaesthetized mice were stabilized on a plastic wall. The tongue was carefully pulled out in order to get a clear view of the trachea and at the same time, the nares were blocked to force bleomycin inhalation. The appropriate volume of bleomycin diluted in normal saline (~50μL for each mouse) was directly delivered in the oropharyngeal cavity using a conventional pipette tip. At day 14 after bleomycin administration mice were euthanized and bronchoalveolar fluid was obtained by lavaging the airways with 3mL of normal saline using a cannula through the trachea (three times, 1mL each). Then, BALF cells were collected by a 15 min centrifugation at 1.200rpm/4°C. Cell pellets were resuspended in NucleoZol (Macherey-Nagel, 740404.200) for isolation of total RNA as specified by the manufacturer. SuperScript ™ IV VILO™ (Invitrogen, 11766050) was used following the manufacturers guidelines for reverse transcription.

Quantitative real-time polymerase chain reaction (QRT-PCR) was performed using SoFAst EvaGreen Supermix on a Bio-Rad CFX96 Touch™ Real-Time PCR Detection System (Bio-Rad Laboratories Ltd, CA, USA).Values were normalized to β2-microglobulin (B2M).

RNA Extraction and mRNA Expression

1-1.5 million cells were centrifuged and cell pellets were homogenised in TriReagentTM(MBL) for total RNA, followed by storage at -80°C. Total RNA was isolated as previously described (25). Oligos for RT-PCR amplifications were retrieved from http://www.universalprobelibrary.com. COL1A1: Fwd:5'GGGATTCCCTGGACCTAAAG 3', Rev: 5' GGAACACCTCGCTCTCCA 3', SPP1: Fwd: 5' GGGCT TGGTTGTCAGCAG 3', Rev: 5'TGCAATTCTCATGGTAG TGAGTTT 3', GAPDH: Fwd: 5'AGCCACATCGCTCA GACAC3', Rev: 5'GCCCAATACGACCAAATCC 3'. Primer pairs correspond to gene specific assays #67, 63, and 60 respectively. GAPDH levels were used as an endogenous control for the normalization of mRNA expression levels in BAL samples. Gene expression analysis was performed following incorporation of relative expression values in average (duplicates) normalized by GAPDH. Relative expression values for the patient cohort were calculated by $2^{-\Delta\Delta Ct}$ method, where ΔΔCt =(sample Ct GOI-sample Ct GAPDH)-(Calibrator Ct GOI- Calibrator Ct GAPDH), GOI= gene of interest, calibrator= mean of all Cts. Relative gene expressions were log transformed.

Mouse Q-Real-time PCR was performed on a BioRad CFX96 TouchReal-Time PCR Detection System (Bio-Rad Laboratories Ltd, CA, USA). For the detection of collagen 1α1 transcript we used the following primers: 5'-CTACTACCGGGC CGATGATG-3' (F) & 5'-CGATCCAGTACTCTCCGCTC-3' (R). Values were normalized to the expression of b-2 microglobulin [B2M, primers: 5'-TTCTGGTGCTTGTC TCACTGA-3' (F) & 5'-CAGTATGTTCGGCTTCCCATTC-3' (R)].

Airway Macrophage Cell Culture

0.5 million freshly isolated BAL cells were cultured in DMEM, high glucose, with stable glutamine and sodium pyruvate (Biosera) supplemented with 2% Fetal Calf Serum (FCS) (Biosera) and 1x concentration of penicillin-streptomycin (from 100x concentrated solution, Biosera) in a humidified incubator at 37°C containing 5% CO_2 for 30min, with washes to remove non-adherent cells, such as lymphocytes and eosinophils. In order to avoid changes in gene expression caused by the contact of cells with rigid surfaces that may lead to detectable altered protein levels of COL1A1 or OPN, cells were cultured for a short period of thirty minutes. Cells were fixed with 4% formaldehyde (FA) for 20 min at RT and were stored overnight in 1% FA.

Immunofluorescence

FA fixed cells were washed three time with PBS and permeabilization buffer (0.5%FBS, 0.2%Triton in TBS) was added for 10 minutes followed by antibody blocking buffer (0.5%FCS, 0.1%Triton, 2mg/ml BSA in TBS) for 10 minutes at RT. Primary antibody incubations were carried out for 60 minutes at room temperature in antibody blocking buffer followed by washing with TBS. Secondary antibody incubations were performed for 30 minutes followed by washing with TBS. ToPro-633 or DAPI was added for nuclear staining. Finally, TrueBlack (Biotium) was added for 30 seconds to eliminate autofluorescence signal. COL1A1 was detected with rabbit anti-Col1a1 antibody (TA506380, Boster biologicals) at final concentration 5μg/ml, CD45 with mouse anti-CD45 (M0701, Dako) diluted 1/100 times, CD163 with mouse anti-CD163 (TA506380, Origene) at final concentration 3.5μg/ml, osteopontin was detected with mouse anti-OPN (MAB1433, RnD systems) at final concentration 3μg/ml. Secondary antibodies were: for CD45 and CD163 staining, anti-Mouse Cy3 (M 30010, Thermo Scientific), for OPN staining of fresh BAL cultures Alexa-Anti-mouse 633 (A-21126 Thermo Scientific) or Alexa anti-mouse 488(A11001, Thermo Scientific) and for COL1A1, Alexa-anti-rabbit 488 (A11008, Thermo Scientific). All secondary antibodies were used in 1/500 dilution. Secondary antibody controls were also performed with no background fluorescence. Images were taken by Sp2 Leica confocal microscopy with 63x Plan-Apochromat oil lens. Mean intensity of protein levels/cell were calculated with ImageJ v2.0.0-rc-69/1.52i as follows, photomicrographs, with identical acquisition settings, were adjusted for background, AMs were contoured and mean pixel signal intensity was measured for each cell. 5-8 photomicrographs, depending on cell density and an average of 100 cells per patient sample were measured.

Statistical Analysis

Data were analysed using Prism 8 (Graph Pad) software. Gene expression comparisons between two groups of a normal distribution were performed with Welch's T test, when sample numbers between the populations were unequal or a t-test when population numbers were similar When populations were of a not normal distributions Mann-Whitney test was performed. Gene expression comparisons between more than two groups were performed with one-way Anova and multiple comparisons were performed with Two-stage linear step-up procedure of Benjamini, Krieger and Yekutieli recommended in Prism 8 software. Comparisons of intracellular protein levels/cell obtained by immunofluorescence between the groups were performed with Kruskal-Wallis test and multiple comparisons were performed with Two-stage linear step-up procedure of Benjamini, Krieger and Yekutieli recommended in Prism 8 software.

Survival was analysed using SPSS 25 (IBM) software. Survival analysis was performed using Cox proportional hazard analysis. We used receiver operating characteristics (ROC) curve analysis to select a cut point for COL1A1 that predicted progression and generated hazard ratios (HRs) to compare patients assigned to groups based on the optimal cut-point. A p value less than 0.05 was considered statistically significant (*p<0.05, **p<0.01, ***p<0.001, ****p<0.0001).

RESULTS

COL1A1 mRNA Expression Was Elevated in the BAL Cells From IPF Patients and Experimental Fibrosis in Mice

We have previously observed that mRNA levels of COL1A1 are detectable in BAL cells and are elevated in IPF patients relative to controls (24, 25). Whole BAL cell analyses by RT-PCR in the current cohort confirmed the significant upregulation of COL1A1 mRNA in IPF compared to controls (p=0.0036) (**Figure 1A**). Similar results could be obtained by an alternative approach, using microarray transcriptomic data from BAL cell samples of IPF patients (39). Re-analysis of the above dataset showed that COL1A1 was among the significantly upregulated genes that increased more than 2 fold relative to healthy individuals (0.41 log2FC; 0.0007 p value; 0.008 FDR corrected p value) (**Supplementary Figure 1A**).

We also measured COL1A1 expression by RT-PCR in BAL cells from bleomycin treated mice and found that COL1A1 mRNA was induced by the bleomycin treatment (**Supplementary Figure 1B**). In agreement with our results, re-analysis of RNAseq data from alveolar macrophages isolated from mice fourteen days following bleomycin instillation (40), showed significant upregulation of col1a1 relative to saline treated mice (3.41 log2FC; 1.38e-06 value; 4.4e-05 FDR corrected p value) (**Supplementary Figure 1C**).

COL1A1 mRNA Expression Was Elevated in the BAL Cells From Non-IPF ILD Patients and in Particular Those With UIP Pattern on CT

COL1A1 expression in the BAL was upregulated during fibrosis in both humans and animal models. We therefore sought to examine whether COL1A1 upregulation was specific to IPF or was a characteristic of Non-IPF ILD patients as well. Whole BAL cell mRNA analysis showed that COL1A1 mRNA levels were higher not only in IPF but showed a similar trend in other ILD diagnostic subgroups, collectively compared to controls (one-way Anova test: p=0.03 and Welch's t-test pairwise comparisons, IPF relative to healthy: p=0.036, N-IPF relative to healthy: p=0.051) (**Figure 1A**). Within the non-IPF ILD subgroup, significant differences were observed between the groups, (One-way Anova test: p= 0.04) and in particular RA-ILD and NSIP, showed significantly increased COL1A1 mRNA expression relative to healthy individuals following pairwise comparisons (t-test, p=0.035 and p=0.024 respectively) (**Figure 1B**).

Next, we examined the expression of COL1A1 according to fibrosis pattern on CT, and found that in the whole ILD cohort a UIP pattern was associated with higher COL1A1 levels compared to all other patterns combined (Welch's t-test, p=0.04) (**Figure 1B**). Importantly, within the Non-IPF cohort, patients with a UIP pattern of fibrosis had significantly higher levels of COL1A1 expression (t-test, p=0.04) whilst, in the IPF group, no significant difference was observed between patients with UIP when compared to probable UIP (**Figure 1C**).

Airway Macrophages Express Intracellular COL1A1 in Fibrotic ILDs

The cellular source of COL1A1 in the BAL was examined by immunofluorescence in freshly isolated AMs from BAL of IPF and non IPF f-ILD patients. COL1A1 staining demonstrated a characteristic ER localization, illustrated by a membranous web in the cells (**Figure 2**). Some extent of phagocytosis could not be excluded as COL1A1 positive cytoplasmic vacuoles were also detectable. Furthermore, to confirm that COL1A1 positive cells were of myeloid origin and to exclude the possibility that undetected fibroblasts were responsible for the COL1A1 mRNA measured, cells were co-stained with anti-CD45 a pan-leukocyte marker. As shown in **Figure 2B**, CD45 positive cells showed high COL1A1 expression confirming the expression of COL1A1 by leukocytes. Airway macrophage identity of COL1A1 stained cells was subsequently demonstrated by the co expression of macrophage scavenger receptor CD163 on their surface (**Figure 2C**), which we have previously shown to be elevated in IPF AMs (24).

Intracellular COL1A1 Is Elevated in AMs From f-ILDs

Furthermore, COL1A1 protein levels were semi-quantified by immunofluorescence in formalin fixed whole BAL cell cytospins from samples of IPF, N-IPF and healthy subjects. As shown in **Figure 3A**, COL1A1 expression was heterogeneous among the BAL cells, and was strongly elevated in cells displaying airway macrophage morphology in f-ILD patients. The mean expression of COL1A1/cell calculated from all samples tested per group showed that IPF and N-IPF derived BAL cells had significantly higher COL1A1 expression than healthy subjects (**Figure 3B**). The mean expression of COL1A1/cell for each patient tested, as well as within non-IPF diagnostic subgroups is shown in **Supplementary Figure 2**.

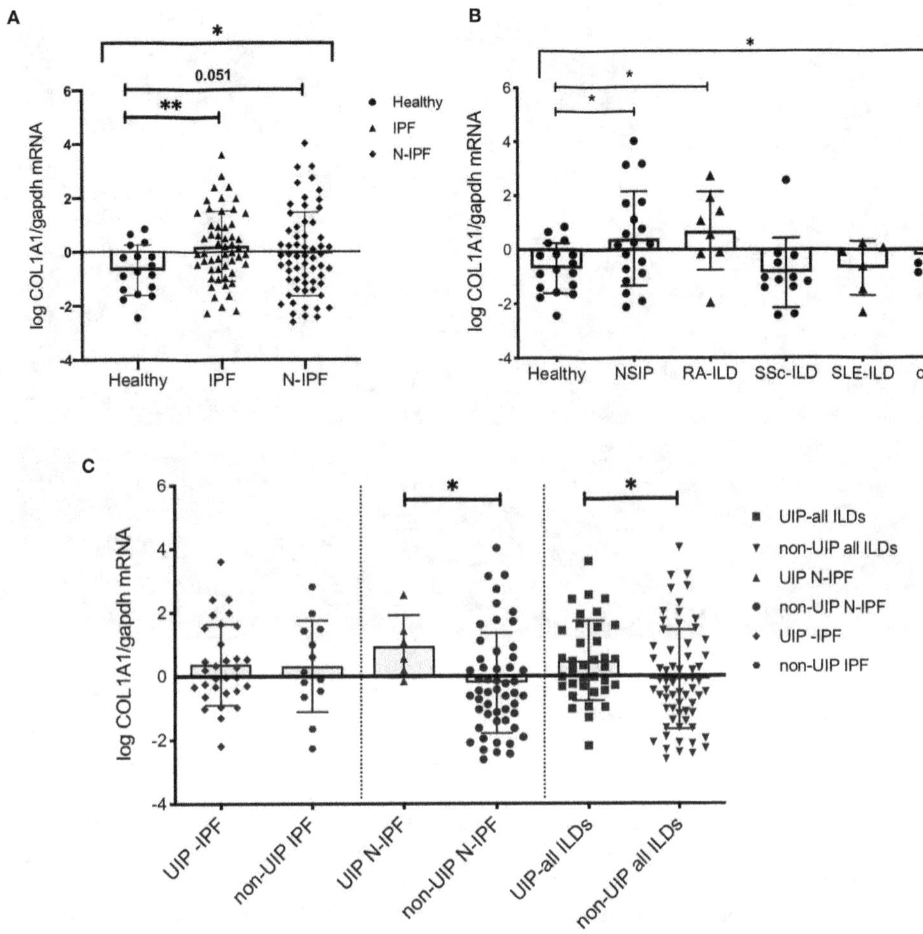

FIGURE 1 | COL1A1 mRNA expression is upregulated in BAL cells from fibrotic ILDs and is higher in ILD patients with UIP *versus* non-UIP patterns of interstitial pneumonia. COL1A1 relative mRNA levels in: **(A)** IPF and N-IPF relative to healthy subjects, (One way Anova test and pairwise t tests), **(B)** COL1A1 expression in whole BAL cells in the ILD diagnostic subgroups relative to heathy. One-way Anova, and pairwise Welch's T tests, p = 0.024), and H *vs* RA p = 0.031 (or Welch's T test p = 0.035). **(C)** Definitive UIP *versus* all other non-UIP patterns in IPF, N-IPF and all ILD patients included in the study. (*p < 0.05, **p < 0.01).

SPP1/OPN Is Elevated in BAL Cells From F-ILDs and Co-Expressed With COL1A1 in AMs

The *SPP1* gene encodes for the cytokine OPN that regulates COL1A1 expression and independent recent studies have shown an increase in a population of pulmonary macrophages expressing SPP1 mRNA in IPF and other ILDs (26). As such, we tested if COL1A1 expression was associated with SPP1 expression in BAL cells. Our results confirmed the increase of SPP1 mRNA in whole BAL cell extracts in IPF relative to healthy subjects however, we found that SPP1 was also significantly elevated in N-IPF relative to both healthy and IPF (Kruskal-Wallis test: p<0.0001, pairwise comparisons IPF relative to healthy: p=0.02, N-IPF relative to healthy: p<0.0001 and N-IPF relative to IPF p: <0.0001) (**Figure 4A**). Within the fibrotic ILDs diagnostic subgroups, NSIP, RA-ILD and SLE-ILD BAL cells had significantly higher SPP1 levels relative to healthy (**Supplementary Figure 3**).

The expression of OPN was evaluated by immunofluorescence in whole BAL cytospins. AMs in N-IPF patients showed particularly high levels of OPN expression when compared to controls (**Figure 4B**), as were NSIP and RA-ILD (**Supplementary Figure 4**). OPN was detected mainly in the outer membrane of AMs, although high levels of cytoplasmic expression were also observed in a fraction of cells in the fibrotic patients (**Figure 4C**). Neutrophils also stained positive for OPN in f-ILDs (**Supplementary Figure 5**).

Finally, we tested if AMs co-expressed OPN and COL1A1. COL1A1 mRNA levels were moderately associated with higher SPP1 mRNA in f-ILDs other than IPF (Pearson's R=0.36, p=0.006). In IPF, SPP1 levels although elevated, did not correlate with COL1A1. However, co-expression of OPN and COL1A1 could be observed in AMs in IPF and N-IPF BAL cultures as shown in **Figure 5**.

Elevated COL1A1 mRNA in BAL Cells Is Associated With Worse Survival and ILD Progression

We subsequently tested possible associations of increased COL1A1 and SPP1 expression with disease severity in IPF and

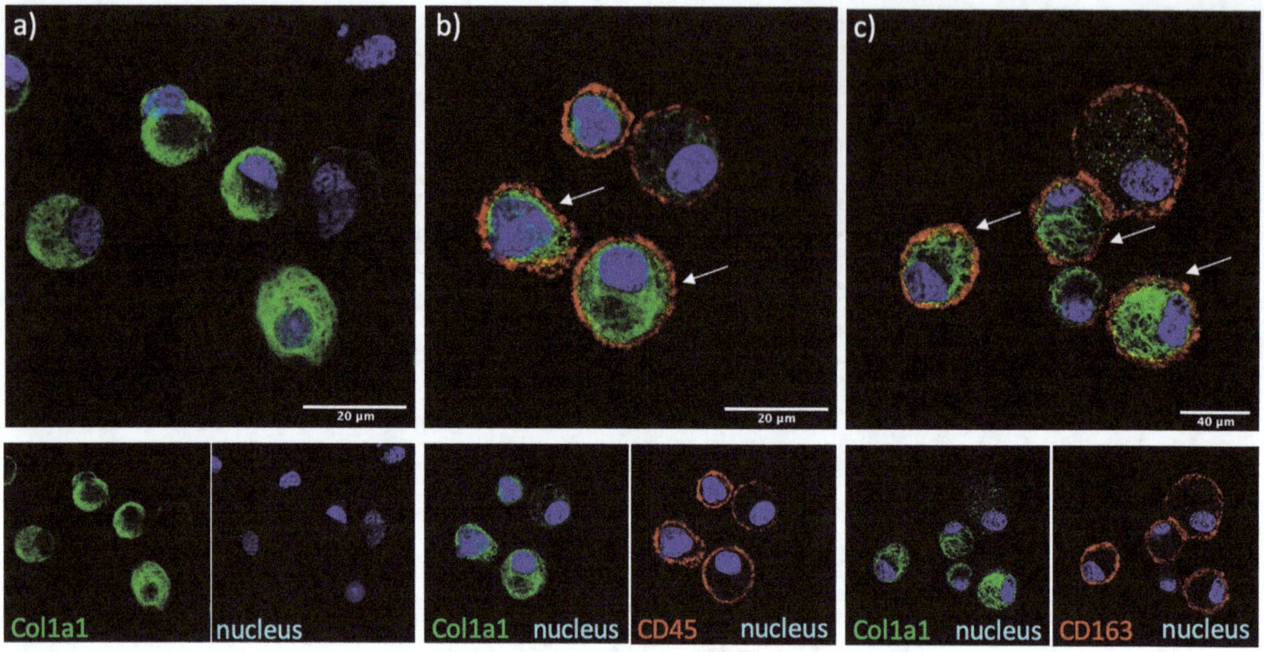

FIGURE 2 | COL1A1 is expressed by cells of myeloid origin and AMs. COL1A1 expression in fresh BAL cultures from a Non-IPF patient with CTD-ILD, stained with rabbit anti-human-COL1A1 and ToPro-633 nuclear stain and **(A)** mouse isotype control, **(B)** mouse anti-CD45 and **(C)** mouse anti-CD163 antibodies. Arrows indicate CD45 and CD163 positive cells expressing COL1A1.

non-IPF patients. In the subgroup of patients with available serial PFTs (n=66), higher COL1A1 relative mRNA expression was associated with 12 month-FVC trends in the whole ILD population (R=-0.38, p=0.001, Pearson correlation). Subgroup analysis revealed that FVC decline was largely associated with higher COL1A1 mRNA in non-IPF patients (n=36) (R=-0.56, p=0.004, Spearman correlation), but not in IPF (n=33) (R=-0.084, p=NS, Spearman correlation) (**Figures 6A–C**).When ILD patients were dichotomized in two categories, stable and progressive ILD, as defined by FVC decline of 10% or more, progressive ILD patients had higher mean COL1A1 mRNA levels compared to stable ILDs (**Figures 6D–F**).

COL1A1 as a continuous variable was linked to higher mortality risk in ILDs (HR 1.3 CI 1.1-1.6, p=0.007), independently of age or disease severity at baseline, CPI (marker of severity) and UIP (independent predictor of worse survival) (HR 1.3; CI 1-1.7, p=0.02). Subgroup analysis of the IPF and N-IPF groups showed that COL1A1 was mostly associated with mortality in the non-IPF cohort with a HR ratio of 1.4 (CI: 1.1-1.8, p=0.01). After adjustment for age, gender, CPI and UIP pattern, COL1A1 remained independently associated with worse survival (HR: 1.6; CI 1.1-2.2 p=0.008) in Non-IPF patients. This was not observed in IPF (HR 1; CI 0.7-1.6, p=NS).

ROC curve-defined cut-off showed that a relative mRNA expression of log 0.5382 was associated with 1.8 times worse risk of mortality in all ILDs (HR 1.8; CI 1.06-3, p=0.03). This remained significant after adjusting for age (HR 1.8; CI 1.2-3.1, p=0.02) or CPI (HR 1.9; 1.1-3.3, p=0.02), but not UIP (HR 1.5 CI 0.8-2.7, p=0.6). Subgroup analysis revealed that the COL1A1 expression above this cut-off was associated with 2.2 times increased risk of death in the non-IPF ILD cohort (HR 2.2; CI 1-4.8, p=0.04) but not in IPF (HR 1.55; CI 0.7-3.2, p=NS). In the Non-IPF group this significant association was independent of age, CPI and UIP (HR 3.8; CI 1.4-10.2 p=0.01). Kaplan Meier curves for the patients with collagen expression above and below the cut-off are shown in **Figures 6G–I**.

SPP1 mRNA expression by airway macrophages in unadjusted analysis was not associated with survival in either group and after adjustment for age, CPI and UIP pattern, SPP1 associate with better outcomes in IPF (HR 0.6; CI 0.4-0.97 p=0.04) but not in the Non-IPF group (HR 0.9, CI 0.7-1.2, p=NS).

DISCUSSION

In this study, we show that alveolar macrophages express collagen 1a1 and this is associated with worse outcomes in ILDs. We examined a cohort of 115 ILD patients and found that the expression of COL1A1 increased in IPF and other progressive ILDs. A UIP pattern of fibrosis was characterised by higher COL1A1 expression in all ILDs and the higher expression was largely associated with worse survival in Non-IPF ILDs. COL1A1 and OPN were abundantly co-expressed in airway macrophages from all ILDs and were significantly higher relative to healthy individuals.

For years, IPF has been considered a distinct disease, of unknown cause, characterised by a UIP pattern of fibrosis and

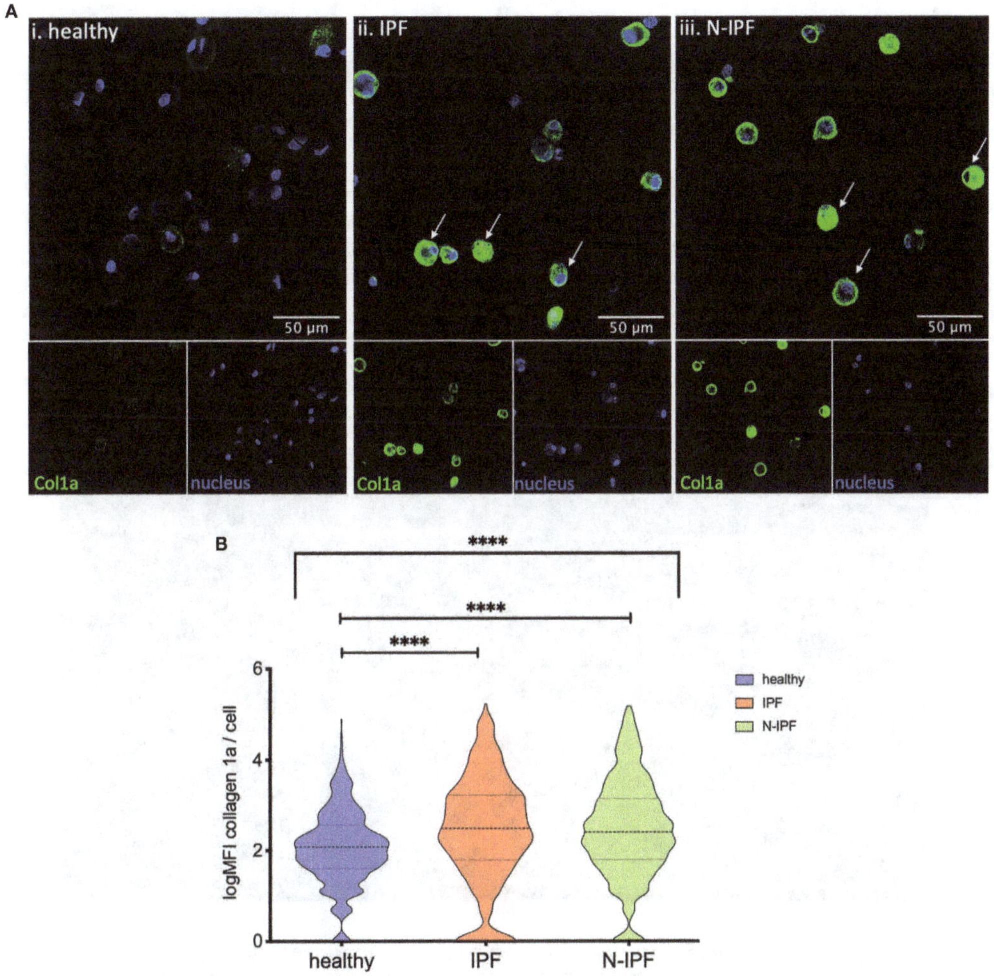

FIGURE 3 | Increased expression of COL1A1 in AMs from fibrotic ILDs. **(A)** Typical images of BAL cytospins stained with anti-human COL1A1 and ToPro-633 nuclear stain from (i) healthy, (ii) IPF, and (iii) a representative N-IPF (RA-ILD) sample. Arrows indicate prominent COL1A1 expression in BAL cells. **(B)** Violin plots of mean log COL1A1 expression/cell per group. (Brown-Forsythe Anova, with pairwise comparisons, ****$p < 0.0001$).

progressive fibrosis leading to dismal prognosis (41). New evidence suggests that some Non-IPF ILD patients may exhibit similar progression despite therapy and it is well known that Non-IPF ILDs can present with a UIP pattern of fibrosis. While the lumping of ILDs is controversial, it has been supported by recent evidence (3). Treatment with Nintedanib, a novel antifibrotic that changed the landscape in IPF treatment (42, 43), has similar efficacy in other PF-ILDs (44, 45), as well as in SSc-ILD (46). Similarly, Pirfenidone, another antifibrotic used in IPF (47), reduces FVC decline in unclassifiable ILDs (48). Based on the commonalities in clinical behaviour of IPF and PF-ILDs with the progressive fibrotic phenotype, it is speculated that common underlying pathogenetic pathways exist and drive fibrosis progression, despite variability of the initial trigger (6, 7).

Biomarkers that could predict progression in fibrotic ILD patients include UIP pattern on CT across different entities such as CTD-ILD (8, 49), hypersensitivity pneumonitis (9) and IPAF (50), severity of the disease at baseline such as DLCO, and/or CPI (51) and genetic or molecular biomarkers including MUC5b polymorphisms (52). Here we show that fibrotic ILD patients with a more progressive phenotype and in particular RA-ILD and NSIP patients, had higher COL1A1 expression than healthy individuals, much similar to IPF. Of particular interest, we showed that within the Non-IPF-ILD cohort higher COL1A1 expression in the BAL at the time of diagnosis was associated with more than two-fold risk of mortality, independently of a UIP pattern, disease severity and age. Similarly, we showed that patients with a UIP pattern of fibrosis, a classic imaging marker of progressive disease, have higher COL1A1 expression. BAL is a largely safe, minimally invasive procedure, used in most ILD centers worldwide for the diagnosis of ILDs (33). The discovery of this novel association between COL1A1 expression and survival could have implications in the management of ILDs, as BAL and COL1A1 measurement could act as a biomarker of progression at the initial stages of the ILD diagnosis. This would be a useful personalised medicine tool to stratify early, patients at

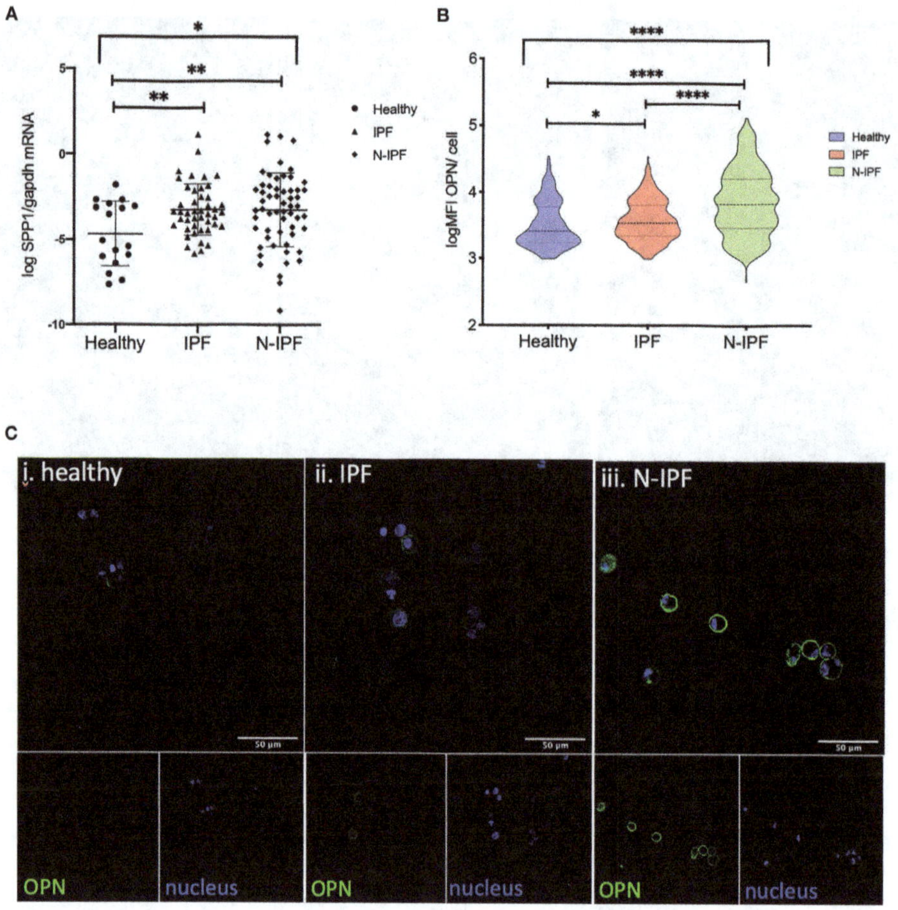

FIGURE 4 | SPP1 and OPN expression in BAL cells. **(A)** SSP1 relative mRNA levels in IPF and N-IPF relative to healthy (Brown-Forsythe Anova, with individual comparisons), **(B)** Violin plots of mean OPN expression/cell per disease group (Kruskal-Wallis test and individual comparisons) and **(C)** Typical Images of BAL cytospins stained with anti-human OPN antibody and ToPro-633 nuclear stain in (i) healthy, (ii) IPF and (iii) N-IPF samples (*$p < 0.05$, **$P < 0.01$, ****$p < 0.0001$).

risk of progression that would benefit from access to antifibrotic therapy before the detrimental progression occurs.

Although the expression of collagens by macrophages may be considered controversial it has been previously demonstrated in animal models. The COL1A1 expression atlas of fibrotic mouse lungs demonstrated that cells with hematopoietic marker CTPRC (encoding for CD45 antigen), CCR2 and CD68 macrophage markers expressed COL1A1 (53). Additionally, our re-analysis of alveolar macrophages isolated from mice fourteen days following bleomycin instillation (40), showed that COL1A1 was significantly upregulated relative to controls. We previously observed that mRNA levels of COL1A1 were detectable in whole BAL cell mRNA and were elevated in IPF patients relative to controls (24, 25). We also performed meta analyses of previously published BAL transcriptomic data from IPF patients (39) showing upregulation of COL1A1 in IPF BAL cells. In that study COL1A1 expression was associated with increased mortality, similarly to our study.

In order to exclude that this higher COL1A1 expression in the BAL might represent the presence of fibroblasts, we showed that COL1A1 was intracellularly expressed in airway macrophages with immunofluorescence and confocal microscopy. Cells with macrophage morphology isolated from BAL and positively stained for CD45 or CD163, were shown to contain high levels of COL1A1. CD163 positive macrophages accumulate in the tissue of fibrotic patients as previously shown (54) and in the BAL of IPF patients (24). According to previous reports that aimed at the identification of markers that would discriminate macrophages and fibrocytes from fibroblasts (21) CD45 was clearly not expressed on fibroblasts. In the same study, similar levels of COL1A1, CD45 and CD163 could be detected on macrophages and fibrocytes. Further characterisation is therefore needed in order to clarify the relative abundance of COL1A1, CD45 and CD163 positive macrophages and fibrocytes in the BAL of ILD patients.

An important finding of our study was that osteopontin and COL1A1 expression were both elevated in airway macrophages. Independent studies of lung macrophages using Single-cell RNAseq analyses have demonstrated the striking upregulation of SPP1 positive macrophages in IPF. Although the molecular

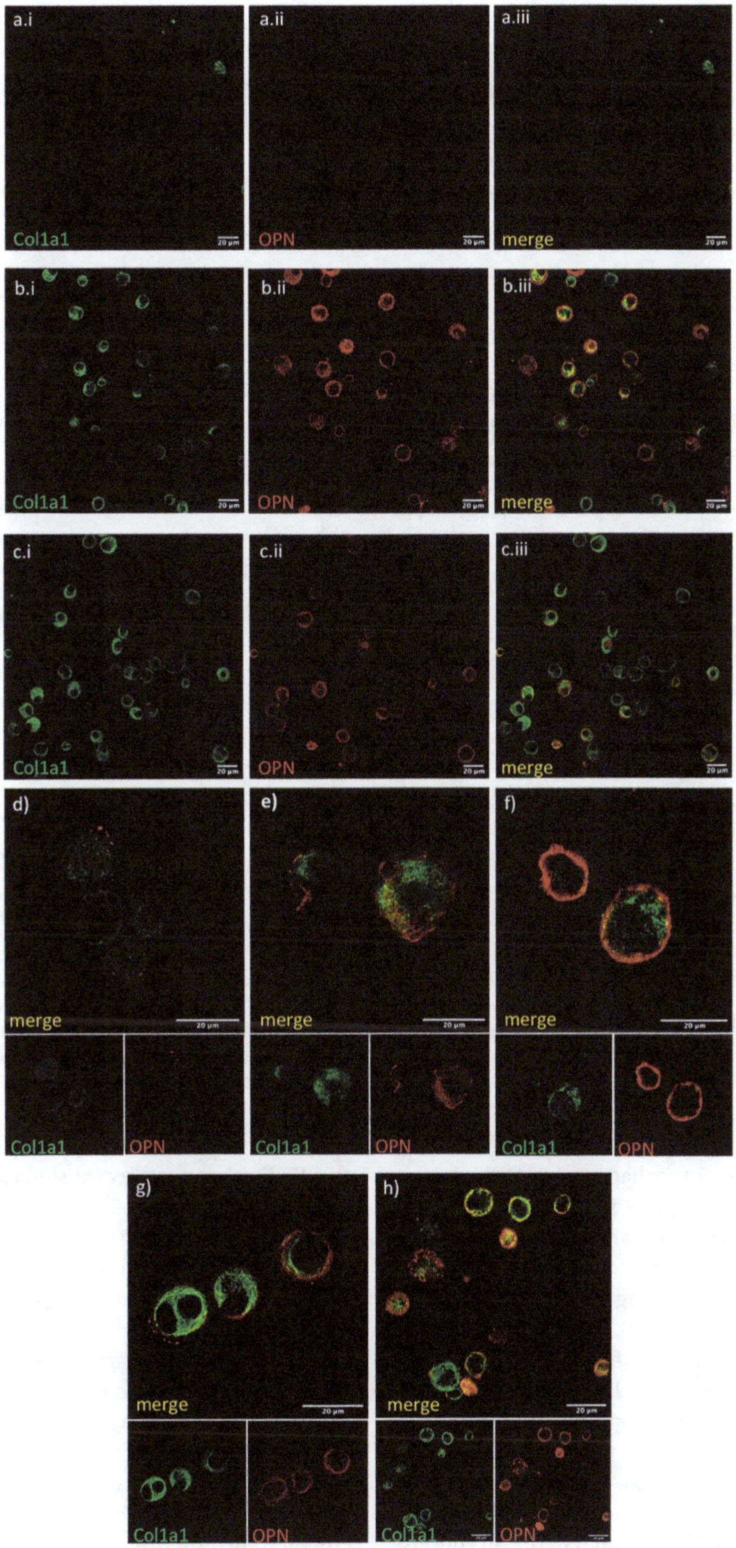

FIGURE 5 | COL1A1 and OPN are coexpressed in AMs from fibrotic ILDs. Fresh BAL cultures were stained with rabbit anti-human-COL1A1and anti-human OPN in healthy **(A, D)**, IPF **(B, E, F)**, and RA-ILD **(C, G, H)**. Panels **(A.i, B.i, C.i)** show COL1A1 stained cells, panels **(A.ii, B.ii, C.ii)** show OPN stained cells and panels **(A.iii, B.iii,C.iii)** are the corresponding merged images. Panels **(D–H)** show merged COL1A1 and OPN images with corresponding single stainings as smaller insets below.

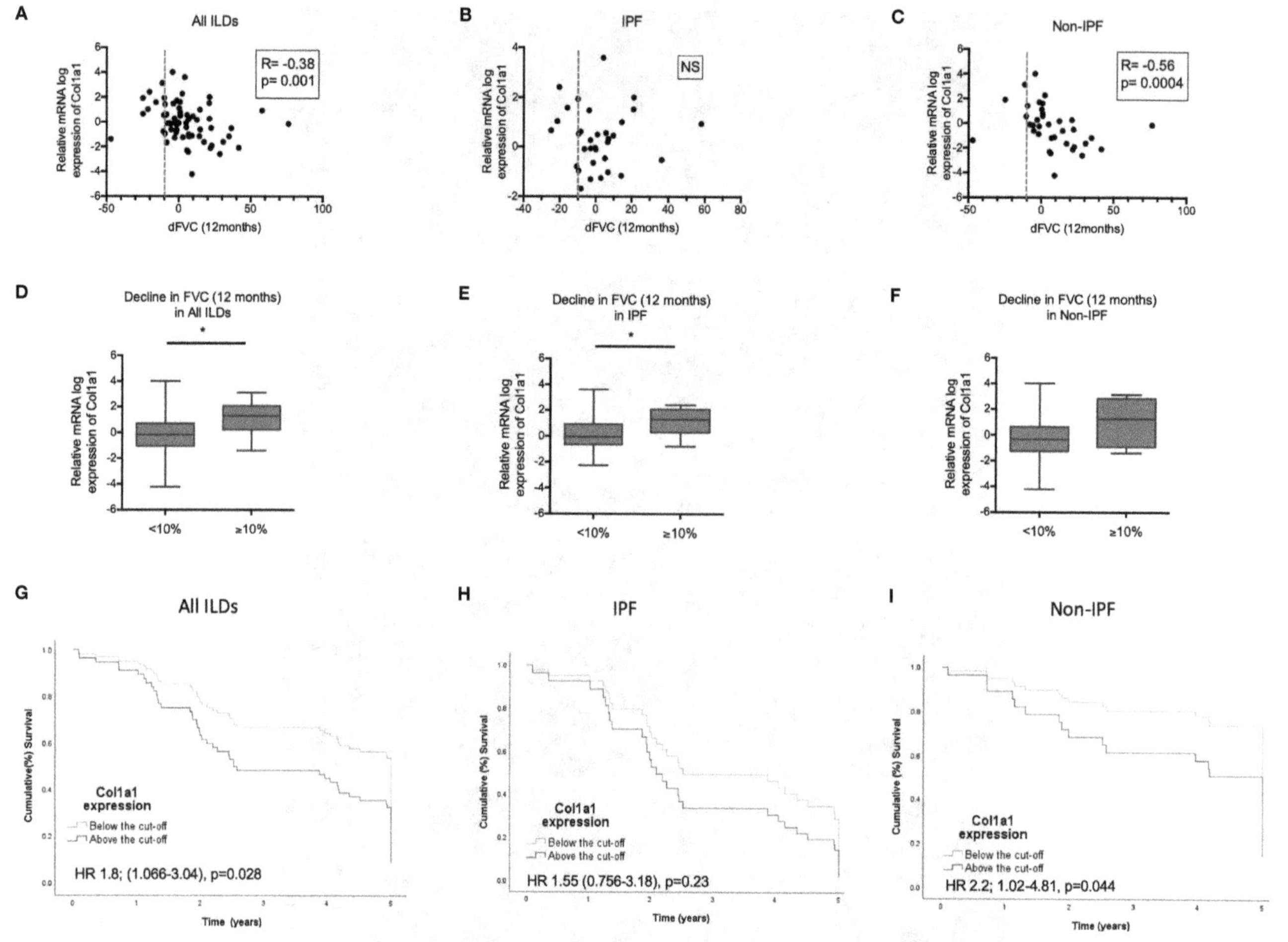

FIGURE 6 | COL1A1 expression in relation to progression and mortality. Spearman correlation coefficient between relative mRNA expression of COL1A1 and FVC decline in 12 months in: **(A)** all ILDs combined (IPF and other ILDs), **(B)** IPF and **(C)** ILDs other than IPF. Comparison of COL1A1 relative mRNA expression in progressors (≥10% FVC decline at 12 months) and non progressors (<10% FVC decline at 12 months in **(D)** all ILDs, **(E)** IPF and **(F)** ILDs other than IPF unpaired T-test or Mann-Whitney tests. Kaplan Mayer Survival curves of patients with high (above the ROC curve-defined cut-off) and low expression of COL1A1 mRNA expression in: **(G)** all ILDs combined, **(H)** IPF and **(I)** ILDs other than IPF. (*$p < 0.05$). HR, Hazard ratio).

mechanism of the induction of collagens by OPN is not thoroughly characterised, recent reports suggest that OPN acts through integrin $\alpha_v\beta_3$ engagement and activation of the phosphoinositide 3-kinase/phosphorylated Akt/nuclear factor kappa B (PI3K/pAkt/NFκB)–signalling pathway at least in hepatic stellate cells (Urtasun et al. Hepatology 2012). Interestingly SPP1 levels correlated with COL1A1 expression in the Non-IPF ILDs but not within the IPF group suggesting a possible uncoupling of collagen expression from OPN in the IPF macrophages. Additionally, we observed that SPP1 mRNA was elevated in the BAL of most ILDs tested, irrespective of disease severity and CT patterns. Intriguingly, increased levels of SPP1 were associated with more favorable outcomes in IPF, in contrast to the rest of the ILDs. Circulating OPN was recently associated with immune complexes-driven profibrotic macrophage activity in SSc-ILD (55) and it could be speculated that OPN plays a more significant role in autoimmune-driven fibrosis as compared to IPF. Furthermore, recent studies with models of tissue repair and scar formation following heart injury showed that osteopontin expressing recruited macrophage populations play both a pro-fibrotic and pro-resolving role (56).

Our work also infers to a less characterised role of airway macrophages in pulmonary fibrosis, as it demonstrates a link between the macrophage derived expression of COL1A1 and fibrotic disease pathogenesis. There are few reports describing a direct role of macrophages in ECM production during fibrosis. A recent mouse model of fibrotic scar formation in the heart shows that recruited monocyte-derived macrophages to the injured site directly contribute to collagen-I fibril formation, suggesting, that collagen production is a component of the pro-fibrotic monocyte/macrophage response (22). Additionally, tumour associated macrophages of monocyte origin were shown to upregulate COL1A1 directly, affecting collagenous matrix organisation in the tumour microenvironment (57). In IPF, monocyte derived macrophages are also believed to play a detrimental role in the disease although the exact mechanism is not understood.

The main limitation of our study is the non-prospective validation of COL1A1 as a biomarker of ILD progression. This was mainly due to the small number of patients with non-IPF ILD and the small number of control patients. Additionally, further work is required for the precise elucidation of the macrophage populations that express COL1A1 as well as, their function. In conclusion our findings suggest that COL1A1 expression by macrophages may be a novel pathogenetic pathway in fibrotic ILDs that is related to worse outcomes. Our observations are exciting as COL1A1 expression could be further evaluated as a biomarker of Progressive ILD and raises hope for the early identification of patients that will develop a Progressive Fibrotic Phenotype.

ETHICS STATEMENT

The studies involving human participants were reviewed and approved by Ethics Committee of the University General Hospital of Heraklion and the Ethics Committee of Royal Brompton Hospital, London, UK.

AUTHOR CONTRIBUTIONS

ET and AT designed study, performed experiments, analyses and wrote the manuscript. EV, GM, and MK collected patient information and critically read the manuscript, SM performed experiments. DF performed meta-analyses from whole transcriptome data. AG performed mouse experiments. VA designed mouse experiments and critically read the manuscript. ER and NT recruited patients and critically read the manuscript. AW and KA designed study, recruited patients, and wrote manuscript. All authors contributed to the article and approved the submitted version.

REFERENCES

1. Travis WD, Costabel U, Hansell DM, King TE Jr, Lynch DA, Nicholson AG, et al. An Official American Thoracic Society/European Respiratory Society Statement: Update of the International Multidisciplinary Classification of the Idiopathic Interstitial Pneumonias. *Am J Respir Crit Care Med* (2013) 188 (6):733–48. doi: 10.1164/rccm.201308-1483ST
2. Antoniou KM, Margaritopoulos GA, Tomassetti S, Bonella F, Costabel U, Poletti V. Interstitial Lung Disease. *Eur Respir Rev* (2014) 23(131):40. doi: 10.1183/09059180.00009113
3. Wells AU, Brown KK, Flaherty KR, Kolb M, Thannickal VJ. What's in a Name? That Which We Call IPF, by Any Other Name Would Act the Same. *Eur Respir J* (2018) 51(5). doi: 10.1183/13993003.00692-2018
4. Cottin V, Wollin L, Fischer A, Quaresma M, Stowasser S, Harari S. Fibrosing Interstitial Lung Diseases: Knowns and Unknowns. *Eur Respir Rev an Off J Eur Respir Soc* (2019) 28(151). doi: 10.1183/16000617.0100-2018
5. Brown KK, Martinez FJ, Walsh SLF, Thannickal VJ, Prasse A, Schlenker-Herceg R, et al. The Natural History of Progressive Fibrosing Interstitial Lung Diseases. *Eur Respir J* (2020) 55(6). doi: 10.1183/13993003.00085-2020
6. Wollin L, Distler JHW, Redente EF, Riches DWH, Stowasser S, Schlenker-Herceg R, et al. Potential of Nintedanib in Treatment of Progressive Fibrosing Interstitial Lung Diseases. *Eur Respir J* (2019) 1900161. doi: 10.1183/13993003.00161-2019
7. Hoffmann-Vold A-M, Weigt SS, Saggar R, Palchevskiy V, Volkmann ER, Liang LL, et al. Endotype–Phenotyping may Predict a Treatment Response in Progressive Fibrosing Interstitial Lung Disease. *EBioMedicine* (2019) 50:379–86. doi: 10.1016/j.ebiom.2019.10.050
8. Jacob J, Hirani N, van Moorsel CHM, Rajagopalan S, Murchison JT, van Es HW, et al. Predicting Outcomes in Rheumatoid Arthritis Related Interstitial Lung Disease. *Eur Respir J* (2019) 53(1). doi: 10.1183/13993003.00869-2018
9. Salisbury ML, Gu T, Murray S, Gross BH, Chughtai A, Sayyouh M, et al. Hypersensitivity Pneumonitis: Radiologic Phenotypes Are Associated With Distinct Survival Time and Pulmonary Function Trajectory. *Chest* (2019) 155 (4):699–711. doi: 10.1016/j.chest.2018.08.1076
10. Kokosi MA, Margaritopoulos GA, Wells AU. Personalised Medicine in Interstitial Lung Diseases. *Eur Respir Rev* (2018) 27(148):170117. doi: 10.1183/16000617.0117-2017
11. Heukels P, Moor CC, von der Thusen JH, Wijsenbeek MS, Kool M. Inflammation and Immunity in IPF Pathogenesis and Treatment. *Respir Med* (2019) 147:79–91. doi: 10.1016/j.rmed.2018.12.015
12. Raghu G, van den Blink B, Hamblin MJ, Brown AW, Golden JA, Ho LA, et al. Long-Term Treatment With Recombinant Human Pentraxin 2 Protein in Patients With Idiopathic Pulmonary Fibrosis: An Open-Label Extension Study. *Lancet Respir Med* (2019) 7(8):657–64. doi: 10.1016/S2213-2600(19) 30172-9
13. Toda M, Mizuguchi S, Minamiyama Y, Yamamoto-Oka H, Aota T, Kubo S, et al. Pirfenidone Suppresses Polarization to M2 Phenotype Macrophages and the Fibrogenic Activity of Rat Lung Fibroblasts. *J Clin Biochem Nutr* (2018) 63 (1):58–65. doi: 10.3164/jcbn.17-111
14. Misharin AV, Morales-Nebreda L, Reyfman PA, Cuda CM, Walter JM, McQuattie-Pimentel AC, et al. Monocyte-Derived Alveolar Macrophages Drive Lung Fibrosis and Persist in the Lung Over the Life Span. *J Exp Med* (2017) 214(8):2387–404. doi: 10.1084/jem.20162152
15. Misharin AV, Morales-Nebreda L, Reyfman PA, Cuda CM, Walter JM, McQuattie-Pimentel AC, et al. Monocyte-Derived Alveolar Macrophages Drive Lung Fibrosis and Persist in the Lung Over the Life Span. *J Exp Med* (2017) 214(8):2387–404. doi: 10.1084/jem.20162152
16. Zhang L, Wang Y, Wu G, Xiong W, Gu W, Wang CY. Macrophages: Friend or Foe in Idiopathic Pulmonary Fibrosis? *Respir Res* (2018) 19(1):170. doi: 10.1186/s12931-018-0864-2
17. Reilkoff RA, Bucala R, Herzog EL. Fibrocytes: Emerging Effector Cells in Chronic Inflammation. *Nat Rev Immunol* (2011) 11(6):427–35. doi: 10.1038/nri2990
18. Moore BB, Kolodsick JE, Thannickal VJ, Cooke K, Moore TA, Hogaboam C, et al. CCR2-Mediated Recruitment of Fibrocytes to the Alveolar Space After Fibrotic Injury. *Am J Pathol* (2005) 166(3):675–84. doi: 10.1016/S0002-9440 (10)62289-4
19. Reyfman PA, Walter JM, Joshi N, Anekalla KR, McQuattie-Pimentel AC, Chiu S, et al. Single-Cell Transcriptomic Analysis of Human Lung Provides Insights Into the Pathobiology of Pulmonary Fibrosis. *Am J Respir Crit Care Med* (2019) 199(12):1517–36. doi: 10.1164/rccm.201712-2410OC
20. Schnoor M, Cullen P, Lorkowski J, Stolle K, Robenek H, Troyer D, et al. Production of Type VI Collagen by Human Macrophages: A New Dimension

in Macrophage Functional Heterogeneity. *J Immunol (Baltimore Md 1950)* (2008) 180(8):5707–19. doi: 10.4049/jimmunol.180.8.5707
21. Pilling D, Fan T, Huang D, Kaul B, Gomer RH. Identification of Markers That Distinguish Monocyte-Derived Fibrocytes From Monocytes, Macrophages, and Fibroblasts. *PloS One* (2009) 4(10):e7475. doi: 10.1371/journal.pone.0007475
22. Simoes FC, Cahill TJ, Kenyon A, Gavriouchkina D, Vieira JM, Sun X, et al. Macrophages Directly Contribute Collagen to Scar Formation During Zebrafish Heart Regeneration and Mouse Heart Repair. *Nat Commun* (2020) 11(1):600. doi: 10.1038/s41467-019-14263-2
23. Ucero AC, Bakiri L, Roediger B, Suzuki M, Jimenez M, Mandal P, et al. Fra-2-Expressing Macrophages Promote Lung Fibrosis in Mice. *J Clin Invest* (2019) 129(8):3293–309. doi: 10.1172/JCI125366
24. Tsitoura E, Vasarmidi E, Bibaki E, Trachalaki A, Koutoulaki C, Papastratigakis G, et al. Accumulation of Damaged Mitochondria in Alveolar Macrophages With Reduced OXPHOS Related Gene Expression in IPF. *Respir Res* (2019) 20(1):264. doi: 10.1186/s12931-019-1196-6
25. Tsitoura E, Wells AU, Karagiannis K, Lasithiotaki I, Vasarmidi E, Bibaki E, et al. MiR-185/AKT and miR-29a/Collagen 1a Pathways Are Activated in IPF BAL Cells. *Oncotarget* (2016) 7(46):74569–81. doi: 10.18632/oncotarget.12740
26. Morse C, Tabib T, Sembrat J, Buschur KL, Bittar HT, Valenzi E, et al. Proliferating SPP1/MERTK-Expressing Macrophages in Idiopathic Pulmonary Fibrosis. *Eur Respir J* (2019) 54(2). doi: 10.1183/13993003.02441-2018
27. Remmerie A, Martens L, Thoné T, Castoldi A, Seurinck R, Pavie B, et al. Osteopontin Expression Identifies a Subset of Recruited Macrophages Distinct From Kupffer Cells in the Fatty Liver. *Immunity* (2020) 53(3):641–57.e14. doi: 10.1016/j.immuni.2020.08.004
28. Pardo A, Gibson K, Cisneros J, Richards TJ, Yang Y, Becerril C, et al. Up-Regulation and Profibrotic Role of Osteopontin in Human Idiopathic Pulmonary Fibrosis. *PloS Med* (2005) 2(9):e251. doi: 10.1371/journal.pmed.0020251
29. White ES, Xia M, Murray S, Dyal R, Flaherty CM, Flaherty KR, et al. Plasma Surfactant Protein-D, Matrix Metalloproteinase-7, and Osteopontin Index Distinguishes Idiopathic Pulmonary Fibrosis From Other Idiopathic Interstitial Pneumonias. *Am J Respir Crit Care Med* (2016) 194(10):1242–51. doi: 10.1164/rccm.201505-0862OC
30. Neighbors M, Cabanski CR, Ramalingam TR, Sheng XR, Tew GW, Gu C, et al. Prognostic and Predictive Biomarkers for Patients With Idiopathic Pulmonary Fibrosis Treated With Pirfenidone: *Post-Hoc* Assessment of the CAPACITY and ASCEND Trials. *Lancet Respir Med* (2018) 6(8):615–26. doi: 10.1016/S2213-2600(18)30185-1
31. Song Z, Chen W, Athavale D, Ge X, Desert R, Das S, et al. Osteopontin Takes Center Stage in Chronic Liver Disease. *Hepatol (Baltimore Md)* (2020) 73 (4):1594–1608. doi: 10.1002/hep.31582
32. Vianello E, Kalousová M, Dozio E, Tacchini L, Zima T, Corsi Romanelli MM. Osteopontin: The Molecular Bridge Between Fat and Cardiac-Renal Disorders. *Int J Mol Sci* (2020) 21(15). doi: 10.3390/ijms21155568
33. Molyneaux PL, Smith JJ, Saunders P, Chua F, Wells AU, Renzoni EA, et al. Bronchoalveolar Lavage Is Safe and Well Tolerated in Individuals With Idiopathic Pulmonary Fibrosis: An Analysis of the PROFILE Study. *Am J Respir And Crit Care Med* (2020) 3(1):136–9. doi: 10.1164/rccm.202004-1138LE
34. Raghu G, Remy-Jardin M, Myers JL, Richeldi L, Ryerson CJ, Lederer DJ, et al. Diagnosis of Idiopathic Pulmonary Fibrosis. An Official ATS/ERS/JRS/ALAT Clinical Practice Guideline. *Am J Respir Crit Care Med* (2018) 198(5):e44–68. doi: 10.1164/rccm.201807-1255ST
35. Torres P, Rabahi MF, Moreira M, Escuissato DL, Meirelles GSP, Marchiori E. Importance of Chest HRCT in the Diagnostic Evaluation of Fibrosing Interstitial Lung Diseases. *Jornal Brasileiro Pneumologia Publicacao Oficial da Sociedade Bras Pneumologia e Tisilogia* (2021) 47(3):e20200096. doi: 10.36416/1806-3756/e20200096
36. Lynch DA, Sverzellati N, Travis WD, Brown KK, Colby TV, Galvin JR, et al. Diagnostic Criteria for Idiopathic Pulmonary Fibrosis: A Fleischner Society White Paper. *Lancet Respir Med* (2018) 6(2):138–53. doi: 10.1016/S2213-2600 (17)30433-2
37. Lynch DA, Sverzellati N, Travis WD, Brown KK, Colby TV, Galvin JR, et al. Diagnostic Criteria for Idiopathic Pulmonary Fibrosis: A Fleischner Society White Paper. *Lancet Respir Med* (2018) 6(2):138–53. doi: 10.1016/S2213-2600 (17)30433-2
38. Barbayianni I, Ninou I, Tzouvelekis A, Aidinis V. Bleomycin Revisited: A Direct Comparison of the Intratracheal Micro-Spraying and the Oropharyngeal Aspiration Routes of Bleomycin Administration in Mice. *Front Med* (2018) 5:269. doi: 10.3389/fmed.2018.00269
39. Prasse A, Binder H, Schupp JC, Kayser G, Bargagli E, Jaeger B, et al. BAL Cell Gene Expression Is Indicative of Outcome and Airway Basal Cell Involvement in Idiopathic Pulmonary Fibrosis. *Am J Respir Crit Care Med* (2019) 199 (5):622–30. doi: 10.1164/rccm.201712-2551OC
40. Xie N, Cui H, Ge J, Banerjee S, Guo S, Dubey S, et al. Metabolic Characterization and RNA Profiling Reveal Glycolytic Dependence of Profibrotic Phenotype of Alveolar Macrophages in Lung Fibrosis. *Am J Physiol Lung Cell Mol Physiol* (2017) 313(5):L834–l44. doi: 10.1152/ajplung.00235.2017
41. Ley B, Collard HR, King TE. Clinical Course and Prediction of Survival in Idiopathic Pulmonary Fibrosis. *Am J Respir Crit Care Med* (2011) 183(4):431–40. doi: 10.1164/rccm.201006-0894CI
42. Richeldi L, du Bois RM, Raghu G, Azuma A, Brown KK, Costabel U, et al. Efficacy and Safety of Nintedanib in Idiopathic Pulmonary Fibrosis. *New Engl J Med* (2014) 370(22):2071–82. doi: 10.1056/NEJMoa1402584
43. Antoniou K, Markopoulou K, Tzouvelekis A, Trachalaki A, Vasarmidi E, Organtzis J, et al. Efficacy and Safety of Nintedanib in a Greek Multicentre Idiopathic Pulmonary Fibrosis Registry: A Retrospective, Observational, Cohort Study. *ERJ Open Res* (2020) 6(1):00172–2019. doi: 10.1183/23120541.00172-2019
44. Flaherty KR, Wells AU, Cottin V, Devaraj A, Walsh SLF, Inoue Y, et al. Nintedanib in Progressive Fibrosing Interstitial Lung Diseases. *New Engl J Med* (2019) 381(18):1718–27. doi: 10.1056/NEJMoa1908681
45. Wells AU, Flaherty KR, Brown KK, Inoue Y, Devaraj A, Richeldi L, et al. Nintedanib in Patients With Progressive Fibrosing Interstitial Lung Diseases-Subgroup Analyses by Interstitial Lung Disease Diagnosis in the INBUILD Trial: A Randomised, Double-Blind, Placebo-Controlled, Parallel-Group Trial. *Lancet Respir Med* (2020) 8(5):453–60. doi: 10.1016/S2213-2600(20)30036-9
46. Distler O, Highland KB, Gahlemann M, Azuma A, Fischer A, Mayes MD, et al. Nintedanib for Systemic Sclerosis–Associated Interstitial Lung Disease. *New Engl J Med* (2019) 380(26):2518–28. doi: 10.1056/NEJMoa1903076
47. Margaritopoulos GA, Trachalaki A, Wells AU, Vasarmidi E, Bibaki E, Papastratigakis G, et al. Pirfenidone Improves Survival in IPF: Results From a Real-Life Study. *BMC Pulm Med* (2018) 18(1):177. doi: 10.1186/s12890-018-0736-z
48. Maher TM, Corte TJ, Fischer A, Kreuter M, Lederer DJ, Molina-Molina M, et al. Pirfenidone in Patients With Unclassifiable Progressive Fibrosing Interstitial Lung Disease: A Double-Blind, Randomised, Placebo-Controlled, Phase 2 Trial. *Lancet Respir Med* (2020) 8(2):147–57. doi: 10.1016/S2213-2600 (19)30341-8
49. Chan C, Ryerson CJ, Dunne JV, Wilcox PG. Demographic and Clinical Predictors of Progression and Mortality in Connective Tissue Disease-Associated Interstitial Lung Disease: A Retrospective Cohort Study. *BMC Pulm Med* (2019) 19(1):192. doi: 10.1186/s12890-019-0943-2
50. Oldham JM, Adegunsoye A, Valenzi E, Lee C, Witt L, Chen L, et al. Characterisation of Patients With Interstitial Pneumonia With Autoimmune Features. *Eur Respir J* (2016) 47(6):1767–75. doi: 10.1183/13993003.01565-2015
51. Jacob J, Bartholmai BJ, Rajagopalan S, Egashira R, Brun AL, Kokosi M, et al. Unclassifiable-Interstitial Lung Disease: Outcome Prediction Using CT and Functional Indices. *Respir Med* (2017) 130:43–51. doi: 10.1016/j.rmed.2017.07.007
52. Juge PA, Lee JS, Ebstein E, Furukawa H, Dobrinskikh E, Gazal S, et al. MUC5B Promoter Variant and Rheumatoid Arthritis With Interstitial Lung Disease. *N Engl J Med* (2018) 379(23):2209–19. doi: 10.1056/NEJMoa1801562
53. Tsukui T, Sun KH, Wetter JB, Wilson-Kanamori JR, Hazelwood LA, Henderson NC, et al. Collagen-Producing Lung Cell Atlas Identifies Multiple Subsets With Distinct Localization and Relevance to Fibrosis. *Nat Commun* (2020) 11(1):1920. doi: 10.1038/s41467-020-15647-5
54. Nouno T, Okamoto M, Ohnishi K, Kaieda S, Tominaga M, Zaizen Y, et al. Elevation of Pulmonary CD163(+) and CD204(+) Macrophages Is Associated With the Clinical Course of Idiopathic Pulmonary Fibrosis Patients. *J Thorac Dis* (2019) 11(9):4005–17. doi: 10.21037/jtd.2019.09.03

55. Gao X, Jia G, Guttman A, DePianto DJ, Morshead KB, Sun KH, et al. Osteopontin Links Myeloid Activation and Disease Progression in Systemic Sclerosis. *Cell Rep Med* (2020) 1(8):100140. doi: 10.1016/j.xcrm.2020.100140
56. Bevan L, Lim ZW, Venkatesh B, Riley PR, Martin P, Richardson RJ. Specific Macrophage Populations Promote Both Cardiac Scar Deposition and Subsequent Resolution in Adult Zebrafish. *Cardiovasc Res* (2020) 116 (7):1357–71. doi: 10.1093/cvr/cvz221
57. Afik R, Zigmond E, Vugman M, Klepfish M, Shimshoni E, Pasmanik-Chor M, et al. Tumor Macrophages Are Pivotal Constructors of Tumor Collagenous Matrix. *J Exp Med* (2016) 213(11):2315–31. doi: 10.1084/jem.20151193

16

The Role of Immune and Inflammatory Cells in Idiopathic Pulmonary Fibrosis

*Omkar Desai, Julia Winkler, Maksym Minasyan and Erica L. Herzog**

Section of Pulmonary, Critical Care and Sleep Medicine, Department of Internal Medicine, Yale School of Medicine, New Haven, CT, United States

***Correspondence:**
Erica L. Herzog
erica.herzog@yale.edu*

The contribution of the immune system to idiopathic pulmonary fibrosis (IPF) remains poorly understood. While most sources agree that IPF does not result from a primary immunopathogenic mechanism, evidence gleaned from animal modeling and human studies suggests that innate and adaptive immune processes can orchestrate existing fibrotic responses. This review will synthesize the available data regarding the complex role of professional immune cells in IPF. The role of innate immune populations such as monocytes, macrophages, myeloid suppressor cells, and innate lymphoid cells will be discussed, as will the activation of these cells *via* pathogen-associated molecular patterns derived from invading or commensural microbes, and danger-associated molecular patterns derived from injured cells and tissues. The contribution of adaptive immune responses driven by T-helper cells and B cells will be reviewed as well. Each form of immune activation will be discussed in the context of its relationship to environmental and genetic factors, disease outcomes, and potential therapies. We conclude with discussion of unanswered questions and opportunities for future study in this area.

Keywords: innate immunity, adaptive immunity, macrophage, lymphocyte, fibroproliferation

INTRODUCTION

Idiopathic pulmonary fibrosis (IPF) is a chronic, progressive, fibrotic disease of unknown etiology characterized by the radiographic and histopathologic pattern of usual interstitial pneumonia (UIP) (1, 2). It is known to have outcomes similar to some cancers, with mortality approaching 50% within 3–5 years after diagnosis (1). Although the origin of this disease is not known, several risk factors have been identified, including cigarette smoking (3), chronic viral infections (4), gastroesophageal reflux (5), and genetic predisposition (6), which will be discussed throughout this article as appropriate. The mechanistic relationship of these risk factors to disease development and progression has yet to be determined.

The pathogenic cascade of lung fibrosis is thought to be initiated by perpetuated microinjuries to the alveolar epithelium that engenders a dysregulated wound healing response (7). Through poorly understood processes involving the recruitment and activation of myofibroblasts, normal lung tissue is obliterated by the accumulation of extracellular matrix (ECM) components (8). The basic science and translational research conducted throughout the last few decades has allowed substantial insight into the mechanisms driving IPF (9). In addition, the tireless efforts of investigators conducting clinical trials have resulted in the development of anti-fibrotic therapies with the potential to delay the rate of lung function decline in some patients (10, 11). A central concept of these developments has been the emerging consensus that IPF does not appear to be a direct result of immune cell dysfunction but rather that immune and inflammatory cells can permit, promote, or suppress fibro-proliferation driven by native lung fibroblasts (**Figure 1**). This article reviews the evidence in support of this hypothesis.

HISTORICAL PERSPECTIVE

In order to understand the controversy surrounding the role of the immune system in IPF a brief overview of the disease state is required. IPF is defined as the presence of UIP in the absence of an identifiable underlying cause. Examination of lung tissue from patients with IPF reveals a paucity, but not absence, of inflammatory cells, when compared to pathologies, such as non-specific interstitial pneumonia, acute respiratory distress syndrome, organizing pneumonia (OP), and granulomatous processes such as hypersensitivity pneumonitis (HP) (12). Similarly, CT scan criteria specify that large areas of ground glass opacities—typically reflective of inflammatory process—are inconsistent with UIP (1). Classical signs of autoimmunity are absent on physical examination and laboratory testing, as is clinical evidence of an identifiable antigen-driven immune response (1). In addition, the long history of failed immunotherapies, such as administration of interferon gamma (13), neutralization of TNFα (14), and suppression of acute inflammatory responses with low dose Prednisone and Azathioprine (15), suggests that IPF does not result from a primary immunopathogenic process. These clinical observations have been interpreted by some sources as indicating the pathogenesis of IPF lacks an immune component (9). However, this array of findings is unlikely to suggest that the immune system is not involved. On the contrary, the worsening of clinical outcomes by classical immunosuppression suggests, if anything, that certain immune responses might be protective and others might be harmful. Thus, better understanding of all forms of immunity has the potential to advance the understanding of IPF.

INNATE VS ADAPTIVE IMMUNITY

The immune response is stratified into innate processes, which respond immediately to chemical or physical patterns of the stimulus, and adaptive immunity, which involves a highly specific antigen-driven response. Both arms of the immune system appear to be activated in IPF. The data supporting this concept are presented below.

INNATE IMMUNE CELLS

The innate immune system forms the first line of defense against pathogens. Its recognition of antigens is mainly dependent on pattern recognition by innate immune receptors. These cell populations are central to both host defense and tissue homeostasis. Macrophages and neutrophils are among the best studied innate immune cells in regard to IPF, though a contribution of monocyte-derived cells, such as fibrocytes and myeloid-derived suppressor cells (MDSCs), and of innate lymphoid cells (ILCs), has also been proposed. It should also be noted that parenchymal cells, such as epithelial cells and fibroblasts, also show abnormalities in innate

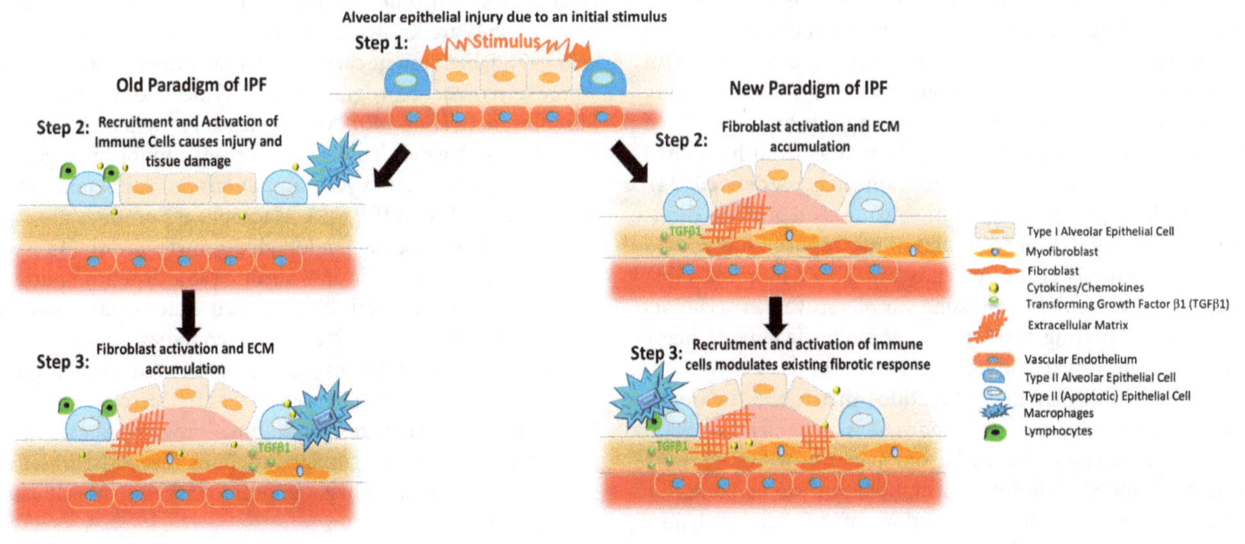

FIGURE 1 | Changing paradigms regarding the proposed pathogenesis of idiopathic pulmonary fibrosis (IPF). The left column presents previous concepts of IPF. In this setting, an initial stimulus affects the alveolar epithelium (blue and pale pink shapes). As shown in the middle panel on the left, this process results in the generation of apoptotic epithelial cells (light blue) and the recruitment and activation of various immune cells including various populations of macrophages (blue) and lymphocytes (green) that produce cytokines and chemokines (yellow). As shown in the third panel on the left, these inflammatory cells and substances induce the activation of fibroblasts (red) and myofibroblasts (orange) to result in TGFβ1 activation (small light green circles) and the deposition of excessively stiff and biochemically abnormal extracellular matrix (ECM, red crosshatched lines). Observations gleaned from clinical trials and experimental modeling have refined this paradigm, however, to result in the scheme shown on the right. In this newer model, the stimuli affecting the lung epithelium leads to fibroblast activation and ECM accumulation that can occur without a primary immunopathogenic component (second panel on left). Once the fibrotic response is established, resident and recruited immune cells, such as macrophages and lymphocytes, modulate existing responses through a variety of mechanisms.

immune activation (16). However, because these stromal populations are not considered to be classical or professional immune cells, their potential and largely speculative contribution to the immunopathogenesis of IPF will not be discussed in this review.

Macrophages

Macrophages are innate immune cells that not only act as antimicrobial phagocytes in the lungs but also play a key role in the pathogenesis of fibrotic lung disease (17). Of the immunopathogenic mechanisms discussed in this review, macrophage-driven processes are among the most extensively studied with reports of fibrosis-promoting properties dating back nearly 50 years (18). Macrophages can regulate both injury and repair in various models of fibrosis and macrophage heterogeneity has emerged as an important area of study in IPF (9). Prior classification schemes proposed the existing of two phenotypes, namely classically activated M1 macrophages that arise in response to INFγ and TNFα, and alternatively activated M2 macrophages that arise in response to stimulation with IL-4, IL-10, IL-13, and TGFβ1 (19). The central concept has been that M1 macrophages suppress, and M2 macrophages promote, fibroproliferation and uncontrolled repair (17). While recent evidence suggests that a dichotomous stratification oversimplifies the functional heterogeneity of these highly plastic cells (20), the M1/M2 distinction is useful when considering functional distinction in broad terms. In this context, a relative excess of M1 macrophages leads to epithelial cell death and failure of repair such as that seen in acute exacerbation of IPF (AE-IPF), while an excess of M2 macrophages leads to the aberrant and dysregulated repair responses that characterize progressive fibrosis (21). At least one endogenous macrophage-driven pathomechanism identified in AE-IPF is characterized by M2 macrophage activation and upregulation of M2 cytokines (22). Detailed studies performed in several mouse models of IPF demonstrate the heterogeneous and highly plastic nature of lung macrophages, with a contribution from both long-lived resident alveolar macrophages (23), as well as from interstitial macrophages that are at least partially bone marrow derived (24). While the difference in surface marker expression prevents direct translation of highly detailed studies of macrophage subtypes in the mouse, synthesis of the currently available data reveals that the accumulation of cells expressing various scavenger receptors and fibrosis-promoting markers is a common feature of many forms of lung fibrosis including IPF (21, 25, 26).

Macrophages display many functions that frame them as a central contributor to fibrotic responses. As early as the 1980s, alveolar macrophages obtained from patients with IPF were shown to stimulate fibroblast accumulation *via* a paracrine mechanism involving the production of soluble mediators typically associated with alternative activation (18). More recent work using lung-derived macrophages confirms the fibroblast-stimulating properties of macrophages (21), and also reveals that circulating monocytes in patients with IPF appear to be programmed with this property prior to actually entering the lung (21). Further studies using animal modeling reveal that removal (27, 28) or repolarizing (27) of interstitial macrophages is both preventative and therapeutic in several mouse models of IPF. This latter mechanism is the conceptual basis for administration of the large pentraxin protein serum amyloid P to patients with IPF (27, 29), which is currently under investigation for multiple forms of fibrosis including IPF. While several studies indicate that macrophages might also participate in other forms of lung fibrosis *via* the regulation of epithelial cell activation (30), this area remains largely unexplored in the context of IPF.

A large body of evidence supports the concept that macrophages produce soluble mediators that regulate fibrotic responses (17) but the mechanism(s) through which they adopt this activation state remains incompletely determined. As increasing body of evidence, however, indicates that interactions with dead or dying cells may be involved (31). In this process, called "efferocytosis," macrophages (either lung resident or recruited) participate in the engulfment of apoptotic cells causes the transcriptional activation of TGFβ (32). In fact, alveolar macrophages produce TGFβ1 in both humans (33) and mice (30) and Cre-mediated removal of TGFβ1 expression in LysM-expressing cells prevents collagen accumulation and histologic evidence of remodeling in several commonly used animal models (30). These results suggest one potential mechanism through which macrophages contribute to fibrosing lung disease. However, in addition to their role in apoptotic cell clearance and TGFβ production, macrophages produce cytokines, such as TNFα, IL-1, IL-6, IL-8, IL-10, and IL-12, and chemokines, such CXCL1, CXCL2, CXCL9, CXCL10, CXCL12, CCL5, CCL17, and CCL18 (34). Their production of lipid mediators such as eicosanoids might contribute to fibrosis (35), though this function has not been specifically studied in either IPF samples or currently used mouse models (36). Macrophages also participate in ECM remodeling through the secretion of matrix metalloproteinases (37) and by direct ingestion and recycling of collagen (38). In other clinical contexts and modeling systems, macrophages are known to direct the metabolic fate of adjacent cells (39), which might carry substantial implications for fibrosis where glycolytic reprogramming has been observed to drive fibroblast activation (40). Macrophages participate in surfactant recycling (41) which could be of critical importance given the known association between mutations in surfactant proteins and susceptibility to IPF (42). Macrophages produce angiogenic factors such as vascular endothelial growth factor (43), which can be both pro- (44) or anti-fibrotic (45), depending upon the timing of expression and the target cell. Macrophages have been shown to rescue intestinal stem cell phenotypes *via* the delivery of WNT-containing exosomes (46) and while a similar effect has yet to be seen in IPF, given the recently reported association between innate immune activation and lung progenitor cell survival (47), it is possible that similar functions may exist in IPF. The potential role of macrophages in pulmonary fibrosis is illustrated in **Figure 2**.

These data reveal a robust and important relationship between macrophages and fibroproliferation in the IPF lung and lead to the critical question of whether therapies targeting macrophage activation might stabilize or restore lung function in patients with IPF. The few clinical trials conducted in this area have yielded disappointing results. For example, as direct suppression of M1 responses with TNFα neutralization with Etanercept failed to improve clinical outcomes (14). Similar results were seen in a study that sought to inhibit macrophage recruitment *via* treatment

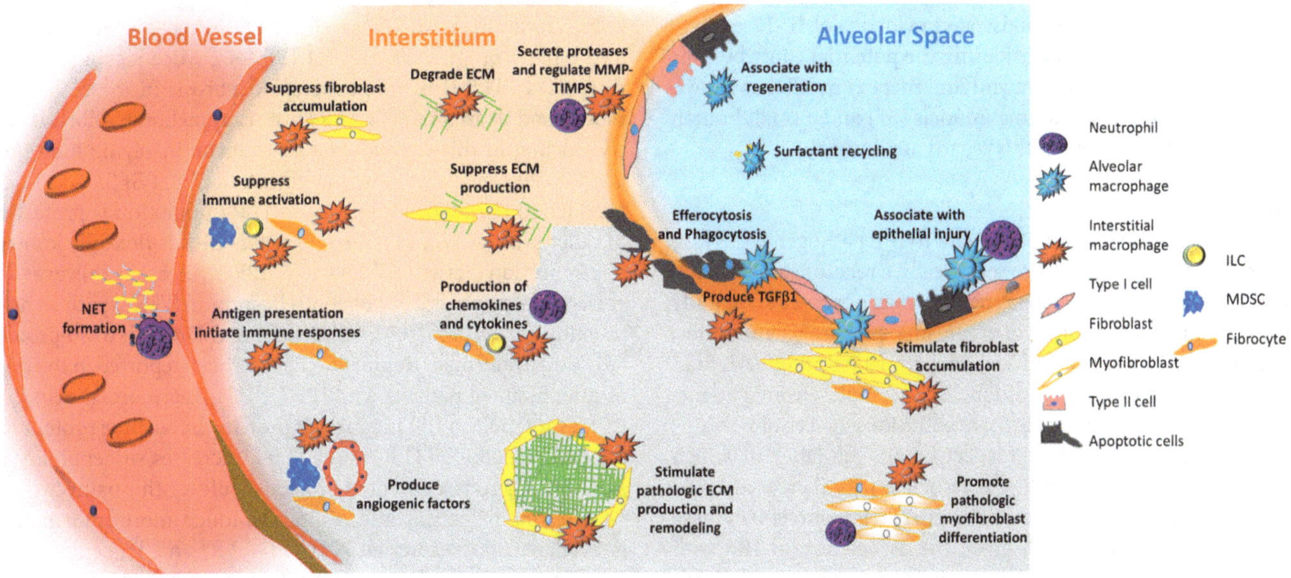

FIGURE 2 | Potential role of innate immunity in pulmonary fibrosis. In response to interactions with pathogen-associated molecular patterns or danger-associated molecular patterns, or to stimulation with various mediators, macrophages—both alveolar (aqua irregular shape) and interstitial (red irregular shape)—can adopt fibrosis modifying properties. These functions include production of TGFβ1, production of soluble mediators that cause fibroblast accumulation and activation, production of TIMPS and MMPS that participate in extracellular matrix (ECM) remodeling, production of angiogenic factors, secretion of lipid mediators, regulation of structural cell injury and stem cell renewal, and surfactant recycling. Neutrophils (purple polymorphonuclear circle) produce neutrophil elastase (NE), TIMPS, and MMPs that dictate whether ECM accumulates or is degraded. Neutrophils also participate in the formation of neutrophil extracellular traps, which may promote fibrosis *via* the production of TGFβ1 and subsequent myofibroblast activation. Circulating fibrocytes (orange spindle shaped cells) are bone marrow-derived mesenchymal cells that enter the lung *via* the vasculature. Once in the lung they adopt multiple functions that would be expected to modulate fibrogenesis including the ability to differentiate into fibroblasts and myofibroblasts, production of ECM, contraction of wounds, participate in antigen presentation, production of chemokines and cytokines, and regulation of angiogenesis *via* production of soluble mediators. Myeloid-derived suppressor cells (MDSC, blue) are immunosuppressive cells that show an association with ECM remodeling and pulmonary hypertension. Innate lymphoid cells (ILCs) produce cytokines that may regulate fibroblast accumulation and ECM production. In the above figure, the functions of each cell are depicted in font matching the cell's color. Note that cells are not drawn to scale.

with Carlumab, a monoclonal antibody targeting chemokine C-C chemokine ligand 2 (48). While these data could be viewed as negative, they are in fact incredibly helpful as they reveal that targeting the alternative activation state or specific function of macrophages, rather than the M1 phenotype or broadly active aspect such as recruitment, is more likely to be of benefit in a complex disease such as IPF. This concept is the conceptual basis for the ongoing Phase II trial of Pentraxin 5, an acute phase reactant that interferes with innate immune activation by binding to debris and inhibiting Fcγ receptor driven inflammatory process in phagocytic cells (49). The mechanism(s) though which the extrinsic features of the lung microenvironment might result in sterile inflammation and fibrosis are presented below.

ACTIVATION OF PROFESSIONAL IMMUNE CELLS IN IPF: PATHOGEN-ASSOCIATED MOLECULAR PATTERNS (PAMPs) VS DANGER-ASSOCIATED MOLECULAR PATTERNS (DAMPs)

Pathogen-Associated Molecular Patterns

A dominant mechanism through which innate immune cells adopt fibrosis-promoting properties likely involves the recognition of innate immune agonists by pattern recognition receptors (PRRs). Ligands for PRRs fall into two classes. Those derived from invading microorganisms are called "PAMPs" and those derived from injured cells and tissues are called "DAMPs" (50). While both inflammatory and parenchymal cells contain PRRs, we will, for the sake of clarity, restrict this particular review to the professional immune cells that have been classically accepted as the first line of host defense (51). Because IPF is not believed to result from a primary infectious process, until recently, the concept of PAMPs has been little studied (31). However, over the last two decades, data gleaned from human and animal studies have linked certain viruses and bacteria with IPF.

Viruses

Several viruses are proposed as playing a role in the development of IPF. For example, Epstein–Barr virus (EBV, a member of the Herpes family) is enriched in bronchoalveolar lavage (BAL) fluid and lung biopsy tissue of IPF patients when compared with healthy controls (52, 53), and is thought to act *via* upregulating TGFβ1 expression and inducing mesenchymal properties in lung epithelial cells (54). In addition, Cytomegalovirus is thought to accelerate existing fibrosis in bleomycin-treated mice by enhancing TGFβ1 activation and increasing detection of both phospho-SMAD2 and Vimentin (55). A strong association with

Herpesvirus saimiri was seen in a human study, wherein the infected epithelial cells demonstrated evidence of IL-17 expression of viral origin (56). Considering the potential contributions of viruses, the use of adjuvant antiviral therapy in IPF has shown potential benefit both in animal models (57) and a small human study (58) although data in this regard are limited.

Bacteria

The potential contribution of bacteria to IPF pathogenesis is also an area of active investigation. Specifically, a relationship between total bacterial load and poor prognosis was observed in a study in which enriched detection of organisms, such as Haemophilus, Streptococcus, Neisseria and Veillonella, was found in BAL fluid of IPF patients (59). In addition, BAL samples from patients with IPF contain augmented concentrations of certain strains of Staphylococcus and Streptococcus (60), the latter of which was shown in profiling studies to associate with increased NOD receptor signaling and poor outcomes (61). The source(s) of these bacteria is not clear though given the association of IPF with GERD (62), one possibility is that ongoing microaspiration leads to repeated inoculation with oral and gastric organisms. Thus, the concept of the microbiome is gaining traction in IPF and forms the basis for studies examining antibiotics as a novel treatment approach (63).

Danger-Associated Molecular Patterns

Immune responses are also initiated in the absence of pathogen recognition. Here, damage to previously intact cells and tissue results in the accumulation of substances with the potential to function as "DAMPs." In uninjured tissues, DAMP-mediated inflammatory processes contribute to homeostasis by allowing the regulated removal of debris, thereby facilitating the resolution of injury and the achievement of repair (31). Abnormal responses to DAMP recognition has been described as one form of immunosenescence (64) and it is intriguing to consider this concept in relationship to the telomerase mutations that are associated with the IPF disease state. Excessive accumulation of DAMPs, however, activates PRRs to engender a microenvironment rich in sterile inflammation (65). These responses may differ from PAMP-driven inflammatory responses (66). Another form of innate immune ligands derived from homeostatic mechanism (HAMPs) has recently been described (67), but because these moieties have not been studied in the context of IPF, they will not be discussed further in our review.

A number of substances are classified as DAMPs. The easiest to conceptualize may be intracellular components such as nucleic acids and organelles that are passively released from necrotic cells. DAMPs might also be actively released by cells *via* the exocytosis of membrane bound vesicles or endosomes. Still another class of DAMPs is generated by the transformation of inert proteins such as collagens into signaling molecules such as collagen fragments. These entities are recognized by innate immune receptors that for the most part have the ability to be activated *via* pathogens as well (31). The activation of these receptors can be protective or harmful depending on the nature of the ligand and the specific receptor. For example, animal modeling reveals that mice lacking toll-like receptor 3 (TLR3) suffer increased fibrosis in the bleomycin model, and the Leu412 Phe polymorphism in the gene encoding TLR3 (which recognizes dsRNA as well as free RNA) has been implicated in a rapidly progressive form of IPF (68). Mice lacking toll-like receptor 4 (TLR4) manifest increased fibrosis in the bleomycin model, and treatment with TLR4 agonists ameliorates fibrosis and remodeling in this setting *via* a mechanism involving lung progenitor cell renewal (47) and augmentation of TGFβ1 and IL-17 production (69). However, because TLR4 inhibition is protective in other settings (70, 71), the role of this PRR is not fully known. A connection between TLR4 and IPF may exist, however, as enrichment of several endogenous ligands for TLR4, such as high mobility group box 1 (72, 73), tenascin-C (74–76), S100 protein (73), and hyaluronan fragments (77), has been reported in the BAL or lung tissue of patients with IPF (78). Furthermore, the finding that a mutation in toll interacting protein, an adaptor protein for toll-like receptor 2 (TLR2) and TLR4, increases susceptibility to IPF (79), suggests a potential protective role for this pathway.

In terms of pathogenic responses, much more information is available. For example, NACHT, LLR, and PYD domains-containing protein 3 (NALP3) inflammasome activation leads to IL-1β production and fibrosis in bleomycin treated animals (80, 81). While the relevance of these results to the human disease state is not directly established, lung tissue from patients with IPF show increased concentrations of uric acid (82), and BAL from these patients contained an increase in free ATP (83), both of which are known inflammasome activators (81, 84). Inflammasome activation in IPF may also occur *via* toll-like receptor 9 (TLR9) as detection of this PRR (85) and its endogenous ligand mitochondrial DNA are both increased in IPF (86). In fact, direct exposure of previously normal fibroblasts to either endogenous TLR9 agonists such as unmethylated CpG-rich DNA derived from mitochondria (mtDNA) (86) or synthetic TLR9 agonists enacts a transition to an αSMA expressing, myofibroblastic phenotype (87). However, because mice with ubiquitous deletion of TLR9 develop worsened fibrosis in several experimental settings (88), likely due to inflammatory nature of these models, the role of TLR9 in IPF has been difficult to understand. Thus, this is an area that would benefit from additional studies and improved models that more accurately represent the microenvironment of the diseased human lung.

Neutrophils

Neutrophils are innate immune cells that possess several functions through which they might participate in fibrosis. Neutrophilia in BAL fluid has been associated with early mortality in IPF (89) and concentrations of the neutrophil chemoattractant, CXCL8, are increased in IPF (90). Furthermore, levels of alveolar epithelial marker, cytokeratin 19, in BAL fluid correlated to neutrophil concentrations, suggesting an association between neutrophils and epithelial injury in this context (91).

Neutrophils might also contribute to fibrosis *via* their regulation of ECM turnover. Neutrophil elastase (NE), the main proteolytic product of alveolar neutrophils, is increased in BAL fluid of IPF patients (92). NE generates DAMPs by degrading various ECM components, such as collagens I, II, III, IV, fibronectin, laminin, and elastin (93, 94), and *ex vivo* work demonstrates that NE can induce fibroblast proliferation and myofibroblast differentiation (95). NE deficient mice are protected from the fibrosis seen in both the bleomycin and asbestos models (93, 95), and the NE inhibitor, Sivelestat, is protective in the bleomycin model (96). Neutrophils also control ECM homeostasis through their regulation of the net balance between MMPs and TIMPs (97, 98), particularly the pro-fibrotic MMP-2, MMP-8, and MMP-9 (99). Batimastat, a synthetic inhibitor of MMP, when used in bleomycin-induced mice, resulted in reduced MMP-2, MMP-9, and TIMP-1 level in BAL fluid and was, therefore, useful in preventing pulmonary fibrosis (100), though the relevance of these findings to human IPF remains unclear.

One newly described fibrosis-promoting function of neutrophils is the generation of extracellular neutrophil traps. These pro-inflammatory collections of chromatin and neutrophils regulate both immune cell function (101) and fibroblast activation (102). While enhanced detection of intrapulmonary neutrophil extracellular traps (NETs) has been reported in both the bleomycin model and in some forms of fibrotic ILD (102), a specific association with IPF has yet to be fully described. Further studies are warranted to understand whether NETS play a role in IPF pathogenesis.

To summarize, neutrophils are innate immune cells that are associated with the production of cytokines and chemokines, presence of injury, regulation of ECM turnover, and generation of NETs. All of these functions would be expected to result in fibroblast activation and ECM accumulation (**Figure 2**). However, because the pathology of UIP is not characterized by neutrophil accumulation—and, in fact, the presence of neutrophils would lead to a pathologic diagnosis other than UIP—the role of neutrophils remains unclear.

Fibrocytes

Fibrocytes are circulating, bone marrow-derived mesenchymal progenitor cells that can migrate into lung tissue and further differentiate into fibroblasts and myofibroblasts (103). These cells are believed to derive from monocyte-based progenitors. They comprise only a small fraction of circulating leukocytes in normal humans, but are found abundantly in pathologic conditions characterized by macrophage-driven inflammation and persistent fibroblast activation such as IPF (104). These cells express hematopoietic and progenitor cell markers, CD45 and CD34, and also produce ECM proteins such as collagens I and III, vimentin and fibronectin (105). Similarly, they can be induced to express αSMA (106) and participate in the contraction of artificial wounds (107, 108). However, despite their documented ability to both produce ECM and display functions of myofibroblasts in a variety of modeling systems, consistent evidence of these properties in human lung tissue remains scarce. Thus, in recent years, attention has focused on alternate functions of these highly plastic cells. Fibrocytes not only express receptors for chemokines, such as CCR3, CCR5, CCR7, and CXCR4, but also produce inflammatory cytokines, TNF-α, IL-6, IL-8, and IL-10, and chemokines, MIP-1α, MIP-1β, MCP-1, and GRO-α (109, 110). They participate in antigen presentation (111, 112) and angiogenesis (113), and in some settings are able to control the activation of adjacent fibroblasts *via* paracrine means (114). Thus, fibrocytes display an array of functions that would be expected to influence the development and progression of lung fibrosis (**Figure 2**), though their specific contribution to IPF is currently not defined and requires further investigation.

Myeloid-Derived Suppressor Cells (MDSCs)

Myeloid-derived suppressor cells are a heterogeneous group of immature myeloid immune cells, which appear to be related to poor prognosis in certain forms of cancers (115). MDSCs play a role in the immune system through their suppressive action on T cells (116). They promote regulatory T cell (Treg) expansion and restrain T-cell activation (117) and are associated with a number of diseases characterized by fibrosis and pathologic remodeling. Thus, it is perhaps not surprising that one recent study found that elevated concentrations of peripheral blood MDSCs, defined by the surface markers HLA-DR, CD33, CD11b, CD14, and CD66b, reflect poor lung function in patients with IPF (118). Another experiment with bleomycin-induced mice showed that MDSCs triggered vascular remodeling and pulmonary hypertension, and that preventing their recruitment *via* neutralization of CXCR2 normalized the pulmonary pressure (119). While the relationship between vascular abnormalities and parenchymal fibrosis remains poorly understood, accumulating evidence suggests that these events might significantly impact parenchymal homeostasis during injury and repair (45). Thus, therapeutic strategies targeting the activity of MDSCs or restricting their accumulation and expansion in peripheral blood may be a novel approach to disease modification, though more work is needed to understand their relevance to human disease (118).

Innate Lymphoid Cells

Innate lymphoid cells are newly identified lymphoid cell populations that do not express the recombination activating gene and are classified into three subgroups: ILC1, which include natural killer cells that produce IFN-γ as well as CD127lo and CD127hi ILCs (120); ILC2, which produce type 2 cytokines, such as IL-5 and IL-13; and lastly, ILC3 that produce IL-17 and IL-22 (121). ILCs in the lung interact with epithelial cells, natural killer T cells, and myeloid cells to form an immune system network (122). ILC2 are activated quickly by environmental antigens and pathogens to release large quantities of IL-13, thereby suggesting a potential role in pulmonary fibrosis (123). ILCs have been identified in the IPF lung (124) though studies of their role in this disease remain in the nascent stages. Thus, this is an area that would benefit from additional study.

ADAPTIVE IMMUNE RESPONSES: T CELLS AND B CELLS

As noted above, the role of lymphocytes in fibrosis is poorly understood and controversial. The failure of IPF to improve in response to lymphocyte-modulating therapies, and the observation that lymphocytes are not required for the development of experimentally induced fibrosis in mice (125), has contributed to this situation. However, substantial and outcome predictive abnormalities in lymphocyte subsets and activation have been described in the lungs and blood of IPF patients, and animal modeling shows that certain lymphocyte populations are sufficient to induce or modify mammalian lung fibrosis. Thus, lymphocytes might participate in fibrosis *via* as yet undefined mechanisms. The evidence supporting this concept is reviewed below.

T Lymphocytes

Relative to samples obtained from normal individuals, lung tissue and BAL fluid from patients with IPF are enriched for several population of T lymphocytes (126). In the tissue, these lymphoid aggregates contain CD3+ T lymphocytes (127) and evaluation of the peripheral blood supports these findings to some extent. Specifically, transcriptional profiling of PBMCs found that a signature characterized by reduced expression of T cell regulatory genes related to the immune checkpoint CTLA-4 was associated with reduced event free survival (128) and these findings were recently recapitulated in a landmark study involving six independent IPF cohorts from centers across the US and Europe (129). These findings recapitulate an earlier study in which reduced expression of the costimulatory molecule CD28 on circulating T cells was seen to be a predictor of poor outcomes (130). Because treatment with the lymphocyte-modulating agent Azathioprine results in impaired function of molecules that function as immune checkpoints (131), it is intriguing to speculate that the worsened outcomes seen in the Azathioprine-treated subjects in the PANTHER trial (15) relates to aberrant activation of CD4+ T lymphocytes. In this light, it is also interesting that the checkpoint inhibitors used as cancer immunotherapy can cause inflammatory ILD (132) though to date a specific relationship with IPF has not been shown. CD4+ T lymphocytes are divided into several subpopulations, among which the best studied in IPF are T-helper cells, as shown in **Figure 3**. T-helper cells comprise several classically defined subpopulations based on their pattern of cytokine expression. In the below paragraphs, the data regarding specific T-helper populations in the context of IPF will be presented.

Th1/Th2 Cells

Perhaps the most studied concept in T-helper biology as it relates to pulmonary fibrosis is the contributions of Th1 and Th2 cells. Animal modeling, and some human data, suggests that the relative proportions of these populations might enact the balance between injury and repair. Here, Th1 cells and their secretory products are thought of as being anti-fibrotic and Th2 cells and their mediators are considered pro-fibrotic (133). For example, Th1 cells release IL-12, which is a potent inducer of IFNγ, and several studies have reported a relative reduction in IFNγ levels in the BAL or circulation of patients with IPF (134). In addition, a bleomycin study in mice found that IL-12-attenuated pulmonary fibrosis *via* modulation of IFNγ production, thus presenting a protective role of Th1 associated mediators in fibrosis (135). These findings are supported by other work showing that attenuation of Th1 differentiation *via* targeting of the transcription factor T-bet increased bleomycin-induced lung injury (136). Conversely, studies that focused on the Th2 cytokines IL-4 and IL-13 showed them to stimulate fibroblast proliferation, collagen production, and fibroblast to myofibroblast differentiation—thereby rendering Th2 cells fibrogenic (137). In addition, detection of Th2 cells and their secretory mediators appears to be enhanced in the lungs and blood of patients with IPF (137–140). However, systemic administration of recombinant

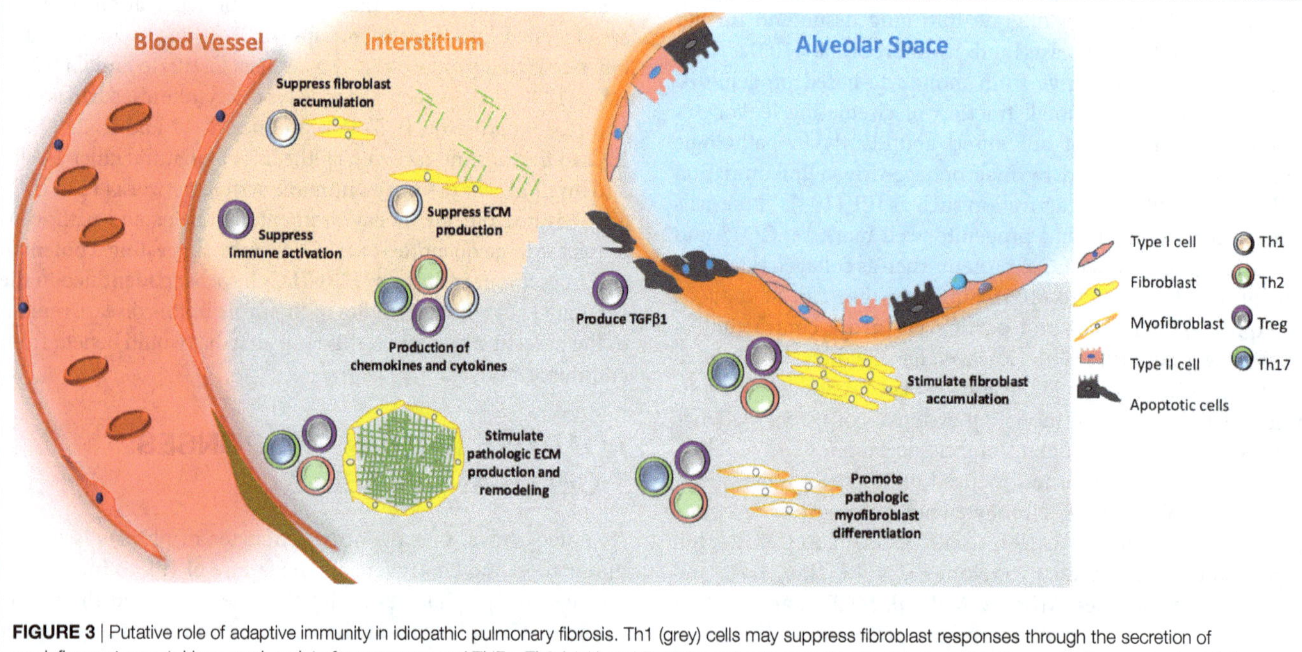

FIGURE 3 | Putative role of adaptive immunity in idiopathic pulmonary fibrosis. Th1 (grey) cells may suppress fibroblast responses through the secretion of pro-inflammatory cytokines, such as interferon gamma and TNFα. Th2 (pink) and Th17 (green) cells stimulate fibroblast proliferation, activation, and extracellular matrix (ECM) production through their secretion of IL-4 and IL-13 (Th2) and IL-17 (Th17). Tregs (purple) may either promote fibrosis through production of PDGFβ and TGFβ1, or suppress fibrosis *via* poorly understood effects on fibrocyte accumulation. Note that image is not drawn to scale.

IFNγ (which would simulate the presence of Th1 biology) and monoclonal antibody-mediated neutralization of IL-13 (which would specifically target Th2 responses) failed to demonstrate efficacy in randomized, placebo-controlled trials of patients with IPF (141, 142). Therefore, the concept of the Th1/Th2 balance as a central mediator of IPF may require re-evaluation and the development of strategies to better and more efficaciously target their secretory products. The potential role of Th1 and Th2 cells is shown in **Figure 3**.

Th17 Cells

The role of Th17 cells in IPF is also incompletely defined. Th17 cells produce cytokines, such as IL-17 and IL-22, which are host-defensive cytokine in many infectious conditions but also promote inflammatory pathology in various diseases such as autoimmune conditions (143). As shown in **Figure 3,** the functions of IL-17 include stimulation of ECM production, collagen disposition, and mediation of TGF-β signaling (144). Increased detection of IL-17 in the lung tissue, BAL, and serum of IPF patients suggests a potential relationship with disease. These human findings are supported by murine studies in which administration of IL-17A is sufficient to induce collagen accumulation and fibrotic lesions (144, 145), and that neutralization of IL-17 can reduce fibrosis in several animal models (146, 147). Furthermore, in silica-induced lung fibrosis, neutralization of IL-17A delayed T-cell-driven immune responses and consequently slowed the progression of lung inflammation and fibrosis (148). Interestingly, recent work has expanded the concept of IL-17 in fibrosis beyond lymphocytes, as one recent studying in an experimental model of HP found neutrophils and monocytes/macrophages to be a dominant source of IL-17A (149). Similar findings have not been described in IPF. While IL-22, another product of Th17 cells, appears to be protective in the bleomycin model (150) BAL concentrations do not differ between IPF and control (151). Because anti-IL-17 treatment has not been tested in IPF, the efficacy of neutralizing Th17 cells and their secretory products as a therapeutic approach in IPF is currently not known.

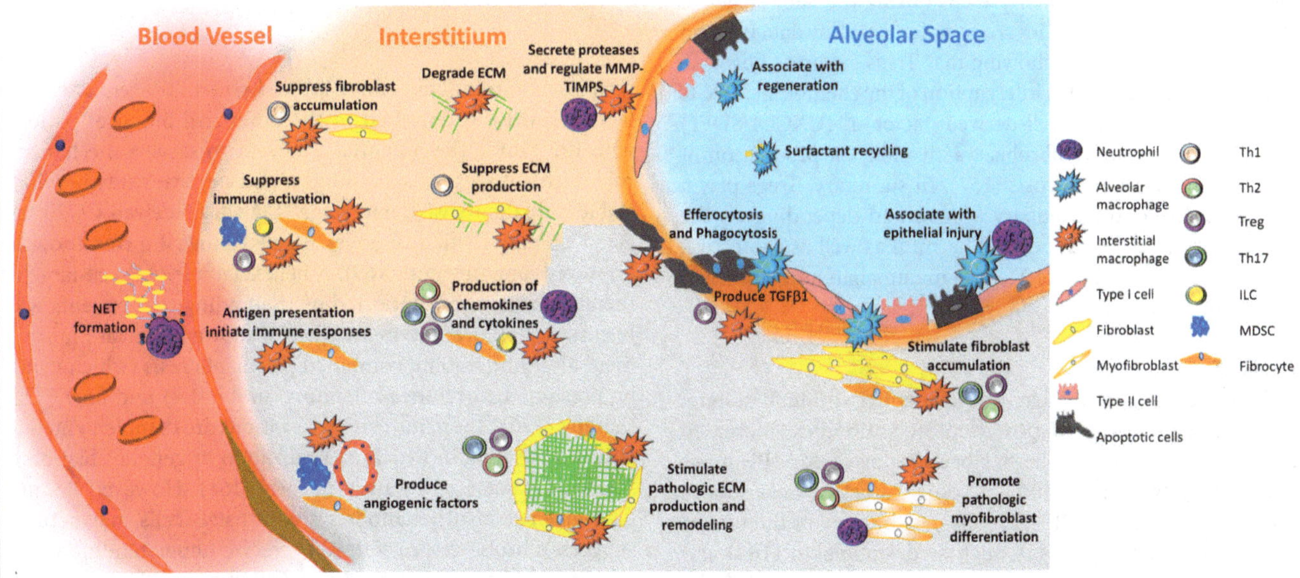

FIGURE 4 | Unifying schematic of immunopathogenic mechanisms of idiopathic pulmonary fibrosis (IPF) reveals that many important fibrosis-promoting processes may be regulated by input from both the innate and adaptive immune systems. Currently available data suggest that innate mechanisms may dominate. For example, both alveolar and interstitial macrophages respond to innate immune ligands present in pathogen-associated molecular patterns or danger-associated molecular patterns to assume adopt fibrosis modifying properties, including production of TGFβ1, paracrine regulation of fibroblast accumulation and activation, production of TIMPS and MMPS that participate in extracellular matrix (ECM) remodeling, production of angiogenic factors, secretion of lipid mediators, regulation of structural cell injury and stem cell renewal, and surfactant recycling. Macrophages might also suppress fibrosis by stimulating a regenerative program in epithelial stem cells, by regulating MMPs and TIMPS, and by directly degrading collagen and ECM. Neutrophils may promote fibrosis *via* the formation of neutrophil extracellular traps (NETs), which may promote fibrosis *via* the production of TGFβ1 and subsequent myofibroblast activation. However, neutrophils may also suppress fibrosis by regulating the MMP:TIMP balance and producing neutrophil elastase (NE) which degrades ECM. Circulating fibrocytes possess several fibromodulatory, including the ability to differentiate into fibroblasts and myofibroblasts, production of ECM, contraction of wounds, participate in antigen presentation, production of chemokines and cytokines, and regulation of angiogenesis *via* production of soluble mediators. Myeloid-derived suppressor cells (blue) display show an association with ECM remodeling and pulmonary hypertension. Innate lymphoid cells (ILCs) produce cytokines that may regulate fibroblast accumulation and ECM production. In terms of the adaptive immune response, Th1 cells may suppress fibroblast responses through the secretion of pro-inflammatory cytokines while Th2 and Th17 cells stimulate fibroblast proliferation, activation, and ECM production. Tregs either promote fibrosis through production of PDGFβ and TGFβ1, or suppress fibrosis *via* poorly understood effects on fibrocyte accumulation. B cells are not shown in this figure given the largely speculative nature of their role in IPF. The redundancy and opposing effects of these functions likely accounts for the failure of IPF to respond to classical forms of immunosuppression. Given the pronounced contribution of the innate immune system, interventions targeting the recognition of, or response to, innate immune ligands might be of benefit.

Regulatory T Cells

The role of Tregs in pulmonary fibrosis has been gaining acceptance in the recent years. Due to their ability to produce both IL-10 and TGFβ1, Tregs have the potential to both promote or suppress fibrosis depending on the context. For example, a now seminal 2009 study reported marked suppression of functional CD4+, CD25high, FoxP3+ cells in the BAL and peripheral blood of IPF patients (152), thereby showing, for the first time, a relationship between impaired Tregs and IPF. However, more recent studies in this area have actually shown an increase in Tregs, and an imbalance of the Treg/Th17 axis in IPF patients (153). In addition, a population of aberrantly activated Tregs identified by expression of the neuroimmune molecule Semaphorin 7a+ was sufficient to engender TGF-β1 induced fibrosis in the adult mouse lung (154) *via* undefined mechanisms. A synthesis of this information suggests that recruited or lung resident Tregs might be fibrosis-suppressive or fibrosis-stimulatory depending on their interaction with the local milieu (155). This concept is supported by experimental data from a bleomycin model showing that Tregs may stimulate TGFβ1 production and collagen accumulation when present during the injury phase, but might reduce these endpoints when present during the later stages of the model (155). These studies are complemented by data from an LPS model of lung injury showing that Tregs suppress fibrocyte recruitment and fibrosis *via* interruption of the chemokine C-X-C motif ligand 4/stromal cell-derived factor 1 (CXCL4/SDF1) axis (156), but promote fibroblast activation *via* production of PDGFβ in a model of silicosis (157). In summary, Tregs play a controversial role in pulmonary fibrosis and depending on the stage of fibrosis, they can be both harmful as well as protective. The putative contribution of Tregs to mammalian lung fibrosis is depicted in **Figure 3**.

BOX 1 | Unanswered questions regarding the immune and inflammatory cells in idiopathic pulmonary fibrosis (IPF).

- To what extent do data obtained from mouse models reflect the situation in the fibrotic human lung? Can mimetics be developed that more accurately simulate the IPF disease state?
- Do events in the peripheral blood truly reflect events occurring in the diseased lung?
- Do the innate immune abnormalities seen in IPF represent a unique form of immunosenescence?
- Can therapies targeting macrophage activation stabilize or restore lung function in patients with IPF?
- Does the altered microbiome cause pathogen-associated molecular pattern-driven innate immune activation in IPF and are antimicrobial therapies efficacious in IPF?
- Does perpetuated microinjury cause danger-associated molecular pattern (DAMP)-driven innate immune activation in IPF and are therapies targeting DAMPs and their receptors efficacious in IPF?
- Are neutrophil extracellular traps an important part of IPF pathogenesis?
- What is the role of fibrocytes and myeloid-derived suppressor cells in IPF?
- Do innate lymphoid cells participate in IPF?
- How does the relative balance of T-helper cells participate in IPF and can this contribution be targeted in a safe and efficacious manner?
- Are B cells involved in the development of IPF?
- Can immune events detected in the circulation be used to guide personalized therapies in IPF?

B Cells

B cells represent another arm of the adaptive immune system. Functioning primarily as producers of antibodies, increased detection of CD20+ B cells has been reported for IPF lungs (158). A variety of novel autoantibodies targeting neoepitopes have been reported in IPF (159–163), with many of the targets being structural cell proteins, such as desmoplakin (164) and periplakin (159). In addition, while the presence of clinically relevant positive serology effectively rules out IPF as a diagnosis, recent work demonstrates that patients with low level titers of autoantibodies might have worsened clinical outcomes than those patients lacking these findings (160). Presence of autoantibodies can be linked to poor survival as seen in a recent study wherein high levels of anti-vimentin were associated with worsened pulmonary function and prognosis (165). Similar findings were observed with the presence of anti-HSP70 autoantibodies in patients with IPF (166). Further evidence of a potential role for humoral responses in the pathogenesis of IPF is provided by the detection of antibodies targeting BPI fold containing family B, member 1 (167) though to date the mechanistic impact of these observations remain elusive. While B cell subtypes and function have not been specifically phenotyped in large-scale clinical studies, evidence does exist supporting a role for B cells in some forms of this disease. For example, detection of B lymphocyte stimulator, which is also known as B-cell-activating factor (BAFF), is enriched in the lungs and blood of patients with IPF (168). The potential of B cells to serve a mechanistic role in this disease is shown by a retrospective study in which stable outpatients with end stage ILD who received CD20 targeted therapy (which removes B cells) showed a trend toward improved lung function (169). A beneficial role of B-cell-targeted therapies is further supported by the finding that patients with respiratory failure due to an AE-IPF showed clinical improvement after undergoing combined plasmapheresis (which would be presumed to remove offending antibodies) and anti-CD20 therapy (170). These human observations are complemented by animal modeling in which neutralization or genetic ablation of BAFF attenuates pulmonary fibrosis (168). However, because data gleaned in other models show that B cells may actually suppress fibrotic response (171), precise understanding of the relationship between B cells and IPF remains elusive and the potential contribution these cells to IPF pathogenesis remains a query in need of further study. Due to the largely speculative nature of their relationship with fibrosis, B cells are not included in **Figure 3**.

CONCLUSION

As can be seen, the cells of the immune system show a rich and multifaceted contribution to IPF. When viewed in contrast with the epithelial cells that are believed to be the primary site of injury, and with fibroblasts, which are viewed as the driver of matrix deposition and remodeling, the more heterogeneous contribution of the innate and adaptive immune systems shown in **Figure 4** is nuanced and unlikely to respond to a single intervention. This aspect, combined with the relative ease of isolating immune cells and substances from the BAL and circulation renders the immune system an attractive area for the development of immunopathogenesis-based personalized therapies based on easily accessible biomarkers. Areas of particular interest and important questions in this context, which are shown in **Box 1**, would benefit from concerted efforts performed in large-scale multicenter recruitment efforts, leveraging of existing datasets and registries, and the generation of improved modeling systems that more faithfully recapitulate the complex microenvironment of the fibrotic human lung and improve the understanding and treatment of IPF on a global scale.

AUTHOR CONTRIBUTIONS

OD wrote manuscript, JW made figures and wrote manuscript, MM wrote manuscript, and EH wrote manuscript. All authors approved final version.

REFERENCES

1. Raghu G, Collard HR, Egan JJ, Martinez FJ, Behr J, Brown KK, et al. An official ATS/ERS/JRS/ALAT statement: idiopathic pulmonary fibrosis: evidence-based guidelines for diagnosis and management. *Am J Respir Crit Care Med* (2011) 183(6):788–824. doi:10.1164/rccm.2009-040GL
2. American Thoracic Society. Idiopathic pulmonary fibrosis: diagnosis and treatment. International consensus statement. American Thoracic Society (ATS), and the European Respiratory Society (ERS). *Am J Respir Crit Care Med* (2000) 161(2 Pt 1):646–64. doi:10.1164/ajrccm.161.2.ats3-00
3. Baumgartner KB, Samet JM, Stidley CA, Colby TV, Waldron JA. Cigarette smoking: a risk factor for idiopathic pulmonary fibrosis. *Am J Respir Crit Care Med* (1997) 155(1):242–8. doi:10.1164/ajrccm.155.1.9001319
4. Enomoto T, Usuki J, Azuma A, Nakagawa T, Kudoh S. Diabetes mellitus may increase risk for idiopathic pulmonary fibrosis. *Chest* (2003) 123(6):2007–11. doi:10.1378/chest.123.6.2007
5. Raghu G, Freudenberger TD, Yang S, Curtis JR, Spada C, Hayes J, et al. High prevalence of abnormal acid gastro-oesophageal reflux in idiopathic pulmonary fibrosis. *Eur Respir J* (2006) 27(1):136–42. doi:10.1183/09031936.06.00037005
6. Hodgson U, Laitinen T, Tukiainen P. Nationwide prevalence of sporadic and familial idiopathic pulmonary fibrosis: evidence of founder effect among multiplex families in Finland. *Thorax* (2002) 57(4):338–42. doi:10.1136/thorax.57.4.338
7. Fernandez IE, Eickelberg O. New cellular and molecular mechanisms of lung injury and fibrosis in idiopathic pulmonary fibrosis. *Lancet* (2012) 380(9842):680–8. doi:10.1016/S0140-6736(12)61144-1
8. Wynn TA. Integrating mechanisms of pulmonary fibrosis. *J Exp Med* (2011) 208(7):1339–50. doi:10.1084/jem.20110551
9. Blackwell TS, Tager AM, Borok Z, Moore BB, Schwartz DA, Anstrom KJ, et al. Future directions in idiopathic pulmonary fibrosis research. An NHLBI workshop report. *Am J Respir Crit Care Med* (2014) 189(2):214–22. doi:10.1164/rccm.201306-1141WS
10. Richeldi L, du Bois RM, Raghu G, Azuma A, Brown KK, Costabel U, et al. Efficacy and safety of nintedanib in idiopathic pulmonary fibrosis. *N Engl J Med* (2014) 370(22):2071–82. doi:10.1056/NEJMoa1402584
11. King TE Jr, Bradford WZ, Castro-Bernardini S, Fagan EA, Glaspole I, Glassberg MK, et al. A phase 3 trial of pirfenidone in patients with idiopathic pulmonary fibrosis. *N Engl J Med* (2014) 370(22):2083–92. doi:10.1056/NEJMoa1402582
12. Travis WD, Costabel U, Hansell DM, King TE Jr, Lynch DA, Nicholson AG, et al. An official American Thoracic Society/European Respiratory Society statement: update of the international multidisciplinary classification of the idiopathic interstitial pneumonias. *Am J Respir Crit Care Med* (2013) 188(6):733–48. doi:10.1164/rccm.201308-1483ST
13. King TE Jr, Albera C, Bradford WZ, Costabel U, Hormel P, Lancaster L, et al. Effect of interferon gamma-1b on survival in patients with idiopathic pulmonary fibrosis (INSPIRE): a multicentre, randomised, placebo-controlled trial. *Lancet* (2009) 374(9685):222–8. doi:10.1016/S0140-6736(09)60551-1
14. Raghu G, Brown KK, Costabel U, Cottin V, du Bois RM, Lasky JA, et al. Treatment of idiopathic pulmonary fibrosis with etanercept: an exploratory, placebo-controlled trial. *Am J Respir Crit Care Med* (2008) 178(9):948–55. doi:10.1164/rccm.200709-1446OC
15. Idiopathic Pulmonary Fibrosis Clinical Research Network, Raghu G, Anstrom KJ, King TE Jr, Lasky JA, Martinez FJ. Prednisone, azathioprine, and N-acetylcysteine for pulmonary fibrosis. *N Engl J Med* (2012) 366(21):1968–77. doi:10.1056/NEJMoa1113354
16. Selman M, Pardo A. Role of epithelial cells in idiopathic pulmonary fibrosis: from innocent targets to serial killers. *Proc Am Thorac Soc* (2006) 3(4):364–72. doi:10.1513/pats.200601-003TK
17. Wynn TA, Vannella KM. Macrophages in tissue repair, regeneration, and fibrosis. *Immunity* (2016) 44(3):450–62. doi:10.1016/j.immuni.2016.02.015
18. Bitterman PB, Wewers MD, Rennard SI, Adelberg S, Crystal RG. Modulation of alveolar macrophage-driven fibroblast proliferation by alternative macrophage mediators. *J Clin Invest* (1986) 77(3):700–8. doi:10.1172/JCI112364
19. Pechkovsky DV, Prasse A, Kollert F, Engel KM, Dentler J, Luttmann W, et al. Alternatively activated alveolar macrophages in pulmonary fibrosis-mediator production and intracellular signal transduction. *Clin Immunol* (2010) 137(1):89–101. doi:10.1016/j.clim.2010.06.017
20. Gordon S, Pluddemann A, Martinez Estrada F. Macrophage heterogeneity in tissues: phenotypic diversity and functions. *Immunol Rev* (2014) 262(1):36–55. doi:10.1111/imr.12223
21. Zhou Y, Peng H, Sun H, Peng X, Tang C, Gan Y, et al. Chitinase 3-like 1 suppresses injury and promotes fibroproliferative responses in Mammalian lung fibrosis. *Sci Transl Med* (2014) 6(240):240ra76. doi:10.1126/scitranslmed.3007096
22. Schupp JC, Binder H, Jager B, Cillis G, Zissel G, Muller-Quernheim J, et al. Macrophage activation in acute exacerbation of idiopathic pulmonary fibrosis. *PLoS One* (2015) 10(1):e0116775. doi:10.1371/journal.pone.0116775
23. Larson-Casey JL, Deshane JS, Ryan AJ, Thannickal VJ, Carter AB. Macrophage Akt1 kinase-mediated mitophagy modulates apoptosis resistance and pulmonary fibrosis. *Immunity* (2016) 44(3):582–96. doi:10.1016/j.immuni.2016.01.001
24. Peng X, Moore M, Mathur A, Zhou Y, Sun H, Gan Y, et al. Plexin C1 deficiency permits synaptotagmin 7-mediated macrophage migration and enhances mammalian lung fibrosis. *FASEB J* (2016) 30:4056–70. doi:10.1096/fj.201600373R
25. Christmann RB, Sampaio-Barros P, Stifano G, Borges CL, de Carvalho CR, Kairalla R, et al. Association of interferon- and transforming growth factor beta-regulated genes and macrophage activation with systemic sclerosis-related progressive lung fibrosis. *Arthritis Rheumatol* (2014) 66(3):714–25. doi:10.1002/art.38288
26. Zhou Y, He CH, Herzog EL, Peng X, Lee CM, Nguyen TH, et al. Chitinase 3-like-1 and its receptors in Hermansky-Pudlak syndrome-associated lung disease. *J Clin Invest* (2015) 125(8):3178–92. doi:10.1172/JCI79792
27. Murray LA, Chen Q, Kramer MS, Hesson DP, Argentieri RL, Peng X, et al. TGF-beta driven lung fibrosis is macrophage dependent and blocked by Serum amyloid P. *Int J Biochem Cell Biol* (2011) 43(1):154–62. doi:10.1016/j.biocel.2010.10.013
28. Gibbons MA, MacKinnon AC, Ramachandran P, Dhaliwal K, Duffin R, Phythian-Adams AT, et al. Ly6Chi monocytes direct alternatively activated profibrotic macrophage regulation of lung fibrosis. *Am J Respir Crit Care Med* (2011) 184(5):569–81. doi:10.1164/rccm.201010-1719OC
29. Murray LA, Rosada R, Moreira AP, Joshi A, Kramer MS, Hesson DP, et al. Serum amyloid P therapeutically attenuates murine bleomycin-induced pulmonary fibrosis via its effects on macrophages. *PLoS One* (2010) 5(3):e9683. doi:10.1371/journal.pone.0009683
30. Young LR, Gulleman PM, Short CW, Tanjore H, Sherrill T, Qi A, et al. Epithelial-macrophage interactions determine pulmonary fibrosis susceptibility in Hermansky-Pudlak syndrome. *JCI Insight* (2016) 1(17):e88947. doi:10.1172/jci.insight.88947

31. Ellson CD, Dunmore R, Hogaboam CM, Sleeman MA, Murray LA. Danger-associated molecular patterns and danger signals in idiopathic pulmonary fibrosis. *Am J Respir Cell Mol Biol* (2014) 51(2):163–8. doi:10.1165/rcmb.2013-0366TR
32. Freire-de-Lima CG, Xiao YQ, Gardai SJ, Bratton DL, Schiemann WP, Henson PM. Apoptotic cells, through transforming growth factor-beta, coordinately induce anti-inflammatory and suppress pro-inflammatory eicosanoid and NO synthesis in murine macrophages. *J Biol Chem* (2006) 281(50):38376–84. doi:10.1074/jbc.M605146200
33. Toossi Z, Hirsch CS, Hamilton BD, Knuth CK, Friedlander MA, Rich EA. Decreased production of TGF-beta 1 by human alveolar macrophages compared with blood monocytes. *J Immunol* (1996) 156(9):3461–8.
34. Arango Duque G, Descoteaux A. Macrophage cytokines: involvement in immunity and infectious diseases. *Front Immunol* (2014) 5:491. doi:10.3389/fimmu.2014.00491
35. Huang SK, Peters-Golden M. Eicosanoid lipid mediators in fibrotic lung diseases: ready for prime time? *Chest* (2008) 133(6):1442–50. doi:10.1378/chest.08-0306
36. Castelino FV. Lipids and eicosanoids in fibrosis: emerging targets for therapy. *Curr Opin Rheumatol* (2012) 24(6):649–55. doi:10.1097/BOR.0b013e328356d9f6
37. Rohani MG, McMahan RS, Razumova MV, Hertz AL, Cieslewicz M, Pun SH, et al. MMP-10 regulates collagenolytic activity of alternatively activated resident macrophages. *J Invest Dermatol* (2015) 135(10):2377–84. doi:10.1038/jid.2015.167
38. Madsen DH, Leonard D, Masedunskas A, Moyer A, Jurgensen HJ, Peters DE, et al. M2-like macrophages are responsible for collagen degradation through a mannose receptor-mediated pathway. *J Cell Biol* (2013) 202(6):951–66. doi:10.1083/jcb.201301081
39. Biswas SK, Mantovani A. Orchestration of metabolism by macrophages. *Cell Metab* (2012) 15(4):432–7. doi:10.1016/j.cmet.2011.11.013
40. Xie N, Tan Z, Banerjee S, Cui H, Ge J, Liu RM, et al. Glycolytic reprogramming in myofibroblast differentiation and lung fibrosis. *Am J Respir Crit Care Med* (2015) 192(12):1462–74. doi:10.1164/rccm.201504-0780OC
41. Wright JR. Clearance and recycling of pulmonary surfactant. *Am J Physiol* (1990) 259(2 Pt 1):L1–12.
42. Lawson WE, Grant SW, Ambrosini V, Womble KE, Dawson EP, Lane KB, et al. Genetic mutations in surfactant protein C are a rare cause of sporadic cases of IPF. *Thorax* (2004) 59(11):977–80. doi:10.1136/thx.2004.026336
43. Stockmann C, Kerdiles Y, Nomaksteinsky M, Weidemann A, Takeda N, Doedens A, et al. Loss of myeloid cell-derived vascular endothelial growth factor accelerates fibrosis. *Proc Natl Acad Sci U S A* (2010) 107(9):4329–34. doi:10.1073/pnas.0912766107
44. Barratt SL, Blythe T, Jarrett C, Ourradi K, Shelley-Fraser G, Day MJ, et al. Differential expression of VEGF-Axxx isoforms is critical for development of pulmonary fibrosis. *Am J Respir Crit Care Med* (2017) 196(4):479–93. doi:10.1164/rccm.201603-0568OC
45. Murray LA, Habiel DM, Hohmann M, Camelo A, Shang H, Zhou Y, et al. Antifibrotic role of vascular endothelial growth factor in pulmonary fibrosis. *JCI Insight* (2017) 2(16):e92192. doi:10.1172/jci.insight.92192
46. Saha S, Aranda E, Hayakawa Y, Bhanja P, Atay S, Brodin NP, et al. Macrophage-derived extracellular vesicle-packaged WNTs rescue intestinal stem cells and enhance survival after radiation injury. *Nat Commun* (2016) 7:13096. doi:10.1038/ncomms13096
47. Liang J, Zhang Y, Xie T, Liu N, Chen H, Geng Y, et al. Hyaluronan and TLR4 promote surfactant-protein-C-positive alveolar progenitor cell renewal and prevent severe pulmonary fibrosis in mice. *Nat Med* (2016) 22(11):1285–93. doi:10.1038/nm.4192
48. Raghu G, Martinez FJ, Brown KK, Costabel U, Cottin V, Wells AU, et al. CC-chemokine ligand 2 inhibition in idiopathic pulmonary fibrosis: a phase 2 trial of carlumab. *Eur Respir J* (2015) 46(6):1740–50. doi:10.1183/13993003.01558-2014
49. Castano AP, Lin SL, Surowy T, Nowlin BT, Turlapati SA, Patel T, et al. Serum amyloid P inhibits fibrosis through Fc gamma R-dependent monocyte-macrophage regulation in vivo. *Sci Transl Med* (2009) 1(5):5ra13. doi:10.1126/scitranslmed.3000111
50. Tang D, Kang R, Coyne CB, Zeh HJ, Lotze MT. PAMPs and DAMPs: signal 0s that spur autophagy and immunity. *Immunol Rev* (2012) 249(1):158–75. doi:10.1111/j.1600-065X.2012.01146.x
51. Mogensen TH. Pathogen recognition and inflammatory signaling in innate immune defenses. *Clin Microbiol Rev* (2009) 22(2):240–73, Table of Contents. doi:10.1128/CMR.00046-08
52. Tang YW, Johnson J, Cruz-Gervis R, Graham B, Brigham K, Oates J, et al. Increased detection of herpesvirus DNA in idiopathic pulmonary fibrosis. *Chest* (2001) 120(1 Suppl):74S–5S. doi:10.1378/chest.120.1_suppl.S74-a
53. Manika K, Alexiou-Daniel S, Papakosta D, Papa A, Kontakiotis T, Patakas D, et al. Epstein-Barr virus DNA in bronchoalveolar lavage fluid from patients with idiopathic pulmonary fibrosis. *Sarcoidosis Vasc Diffuse Lung Dis* (2007) 24(2):134–40.
54. Sides MD, Klingsberg RC, Shan B, Gordon KA, Nguyen HT, Lin Z, et al. The Epstein-Barr virus latent membrane protein 1 and transforming growth factor – beta1 synergistically induce epithelial – mesenchymal transition in lung epithelial cells. *Am J Respir Cell Mol Biol* (2011) 44(6):852–62. doi:10.1165/rcmb.2009-0232OC
55. Li Y, Gao J, Wang G, Fei G. Latent cytomegalovirus infection exacerbates experimental pulmonary fibrosis by activating TGF-beta1. *Mol Med Rep* (2016) 14(2):1297–301. doi:10.3892/mmr.2016.5366
56. Folcik VA, Garofalo M, Coleman J, Donegan JJ, Rabbani E, Suster S, et al. Idiopathic pulmonary fibrosis is strongly associated with productive infection by herpesvirus saimiri. *Mod Pathol* (2014) 27(6):851–62. doi:10.1038/modpathol.2013.198
57. Mora AL, Torres-Gonzalez E, Rojas M, Xu J, Ritzenthaler J, Speck SH, et al. Control of virus reactivation arrests pulmonary herpesvirus-induced fibrosis in IFN-gamma receptor-deficient mice. *Am J Respir Crit Care Med* (2007) 175(11):1139–50. doi:10.1164/rccm.200610-1426OC
58. Egan JJ, Adamali HI, Lok SS, Stewart JP, Woodcock AA. Ganciclovir antiviral therapy in advanced idiopathic pulmonary fibrosis: an open pilot study. *Pulm Med* (2011) 2011:240805. doi:10.1155/2011/240805
59. Molyneaux PL, Cox MJ, Willis-Owen SA, Mallia P, Russell KE, Russell AM, et al. The role of bacteria in the pathogenesis and progression of idiopathic pulmonary fibrosis. *Am J Respir Crit Care Med* (2014) 190(8):906–13. doi:10.1164/rccm.201403-0541OC
60. Han MK, Zhou Y, Murray S, Tayob N, Noth I, Lama VN, et al. Lung microbiome and disease progression in idiopathic pulmonary fibrosis: an analysis of the COMET study. *Lancet Respir Med* (2014) 2(7):548–56. doi:10.1016/S2213-2600(14)70069-4
61. Huang Y, Ma SF, Espindola MS, Vij R, Oldham JM, Huffnagle GB, et al. Microbes are associated with host innate immune response in idiopathic pulmonary fibrosis. *Am J Respir Crit Care Med* (2017) 196(2):208–19. doi:10.1164/rccm.201607-1525OC
62. Lee JS, Collard HR, Raghu G, Sweet MP, Hays SR, Campos GM, et al. Does chronic microaspiration cause idiopathic pulmonary fibrosis? *Am J Med* (2010) 123(4):304–11. doi:10.1016/j.amjmed.2009.07.033
63. Kawamura K, Ichikado K, Yasuda Y, Anan K, Suga M. Azithromycin for idiopathic acute exacerbation of idiopathic pulmonary fibrosis: a retrospective single-center study. *BMC Pulm Med* (2017) 17(1):94. doi:10.1186/s12890-017-0437-z
64. Huang J, Xie Y, Sun X, Zeh HJ III, Kang R, Lotze MT, et al. DAMPs, ageing, and cancer: the 'DAMP Hypothesis'. *Ageing Res Rev* (2015) 24(Pt A):3–16. doi:10.1016/j.arr.2014.10.004
65. Land WG. The role of damage-associated molecular patterns in human diseases: part I – promoting inflammation and immunity. *Sultan Qaboos Univ Med J* (2015) 15(1):e9–21.
66. Piccinini AM, Zuliani-Alvarez L, Lim JM, Midwood KS. Distinct microenvironmental cues stimulate divergent TLR4-mediated signaling pathways in macrophages. *Sci Signal* (2016) 9(443):ra86. doi:10.1126/scisignal.aaf3596
67. Liston A, Masters SL. Homeostasis-altering molecular processes as mechanisms of inflammasome activation. *Nat Rev Immunol* (2017) 17(3):208–14. doi:10.1038/nri.2016.151
68. O'Dwyer DN, Armstrong ME, Trujillo G, Cooke G, Keane MP, Fallon PG, et al. The toll-like receptor 3 L412F polymorphism and disease progression in idiopathic pulmonary fibrosis. *Am J Respir Crit Care Med* (2013) 188(12):1442–50. doi:10.1164/rccm.201304-0760OC
69. Liu HZ, Yang HZ, Mi S, Cui B, Hua F, Hu ZW. Toll like receptor 2 mediates bleomycin-induced acute lung injury, inflammation and fibrosis in mice. *Yao Xue Xue Bao* (2010) 45(8):976–86.
70. He Z, Zhu Y, Jiang H. Inhibiting toll-like receptor 4 signaling ameliorates pulmonary fibrosis during acute lung injury induced by lipopolysaccharide:

an experimental study. *Respir Res* (2009) 10:126. doi:10.1186/1465-9921-10-126

71. Li XX, Jiang DY, Huang XX, Guo SL, Yuan W, Dai HP. Toll-like receptor 4 promotes fibrosis in bleomycin-induced lung injury in mice. *Genet Mol Res* (2015) 14(4):17391–8. doi:10.4238/2015.December.21.8
72. Li LC, Gao J, Li J. Emerging role of HMGB1 in fibrotic diseases. *J Cell Mol Med* (2014) 18(12):2331–9. doi:10.1111/jcmm.12419
73. Park JS, Svetkauskaite D, He Q, Kim JY, Strassheim D, Ishizaka A, et al. Involvement of toll-like receptors 2 and 4 in cellular activation by high mobility group box 1 protein. *J Biol Chem* (2004) 279(9):7370–7. doi:10.1074/jbc.M306793200
74. Bhattacharyya S, Wang W, Morales-Nebreda L, Feng G, Wu M, Zhou X, et al. Tenascin-C drives persistence of organ fibrosis. *Nat Commun* (2016) 7:11703. doi:10.1038/ncomms11703
75. Midwood K, Sacre S, Piccinini AM, Inglis J, Trebaul A, Chan E, et al. Tenascin-C is an endogenous activator of toll-like receptor 4 that is essential for maintaining inflammation in arthritic joint disease. *Nat Med* (2009) 15(7):774–80. doi:10.1038/nm.1987
76. Carey WA, Taylor GD, Dean WB, Bristow JD. Tenascin-C deficiency attenuates TGF-ss-mediated fibrosis following murine lung injury. *Am J Physiol Lung Cell Mol Physiol* (2010) 299(6):L785–93. doi:10.1152/ajplung.00385.2009
77. Jiang D, Liang J, Fan J, Yu S, Chen S, Luo Y, et al. Regulation of lung injury and repair by toll-like receptors and hyaluronan. *Nat Med* (2005) 11(11):1173–9. doi:10.1038/nm1315
78. Huebener P, Schwabe RF. Regulation of wound healing and organ fibrosis by toll-like receptors. *Biochim Biophys Acta* (2013) 1832(7):1005–17. doi:10.1016/j.bbadis.2012.11.017
79. Noth I, Zhang Y, Ma SF, Flores C, Barber M, Huang Y, et al. Genetic variants associated with idiopathic pulmonary fibrosis susceptibility and mortality: a genome-wide association study. *Lancet Respir Med* (2013) 1(4):309–17. doi:10.1016/S2213-2600(13)70045-6
80. Tian R, Zhu Y, Yao J, Meng X, Wang J, Xie H, et al. NLRP3 participates in the regulation of EMT in bleomycin-induced pulmonary fibrosis. *Exp Cell Res* (2017) 357(2):328–34. doi:10.1016/j.yexcr.2017.05.028
81. Gasse P, Riteau N, Charron S, Girre S, Fick L, Petrilli V, et al. Uric acid is a danger signal activating NALP3 inflammasome in lung injury inflammation and fibrosis. *Am J Respir Crit Care Med* (2009) 179(10):903–13. doi:10.1164/rccm.200808-1274OC
82. Markart P, Luboeinski T, Korfei M, Schmidt R, Wygrecka M, Mahavadi P, et al. Alveolar oxidative stress is associated with elevated levels of nonenzymatic low-molecular-weight antioxidants in patients with different forms of chronic fibrosing interstitial lung diseases. *Antioxid Redox Signal* (2009) 11(2):227–40. doi:10.1089/ARS.2008.2105
83. Riteau N, Gasse P, Fauconnier L, Gombault A, Couegnat M, Fick L, et al. Extracellular ATP is a danger signal activating P2X7 receptor in lung inflammation and fibrosis. *Am J Respir Crit Care Med* (2010) 182(6):774–83. doi:10.1164/rccm.201003-0359OC
84. Braga TT, Forni MF, Correa-Costa M, Ramos RN, Barbuto JA, Branco P, et al. Soluble uric acid activates the NLRP3 inflammasome. *Sci Rep* (2017) 7:39884. doi:10.1038/srep39884
85. Trujillo G, Meneghin A, Flaherty KR, Sholl LM, Myers JL, Kazerooni EA, et al. TLR9 differentiates rapidly from slowly progressing forms of idiopathic pulmonary fibrosis. *Sci Transl Med* (2010) 2(57):57ra82. doi:10.1126/scitranslmed.3001510
86. Ryu C, Sun H, Gulati M, Herazo-Maya JD, Chen Y, Osafo-Addo A, et al. Extracellular mitochondrial DNA is generated by fibroblasts and predicts death in idiopathic pulmonary fibrosis. *Am J Respir Crit Care Med* (2017) 196:1571–81. doi:10.1164/rccm.201612-2480OC
87. Kirillov V, Siler JT, Ramadass M, Ge L, Davis J, Grant G, et al. Sustained activation of toll-like receptor 9 induces an invasive phenotype in lung fibroblasts: possible implications in idiopathic pulmonary fibrosis. *Am J Pathol* (2015) 185(4):943–57. doi:10.1016/j.ajpath.2014.12.011
88. Luckhardt TR, Coomes SM, Trujillo G, Stoolman JS, Vannella KM, Bhan U, et al. TLR9-induced interferon beta is associated with protection from gammaherpesvirus-induced exacerbation of lung fibrosis. *Fibrogenesis Tissue Repair* (2011) 4:18. doi:10.1186/1755-1536-4-18
89. Kinder BW, Brown KK, Schwarz MI, Ix JH, Kervitsky A, King TE Jr. Baseline BAL neutrophilia predicts early mortality in idiopathic pulmonary fibrosis. *Chest* (2008) 133(1):226–32. doi:10.1378/chest.07-1948
90. Xaubet A, Agusti C, Luburich P, Barbera JA, Carrion M, Ayuso MC, et al. Interleukin-8 expression in bronchoalveolar lavage cells in the evaluation of alveolitis in idiopathic pulmonary fibrosis. *Respir Med* (1998) 92(2):338–44. doi:10.1016/S0954-6111(98)90118-4
91. Inage M, Nakamura H, Kato S, Saito H, Abe S, Hino T, et al. Levels of cytokeratin 19 fragments in bronchoalveolar lavage fluid correlate to the intensity of neutrophil and eosinophil-alveolitis in patients with idiopathic pulmonary fibrosis. *Respir Med* (2000) 94(2):155–60. doi:10.1053/rmed.1999.0712
92. Obayashi Y, Yamadori I, Fujita J, Yoshinouchi T, Ueda N, Takahara J. The role of neutrophils in the pathogenesis of idiopathic pulmonary fibrosis. *Chest* (1997) 112(5):1338–43. doi:10.1378/chest.112.5.1338
93. Chua F, Dunsmore SE, Clingen PH, Mutsaers SE, Shapiro SD, Segal AW, et al. Mice lacking neutrophil elastase are resistant to bleomycin-induced pulmonary fibrosis. *Am J Pathol* (2007) 170(1):65–74. doi:10.2353/ajpath.2007.060352
94. Hedstrom L. Serine protease mechanism and specificity. *Chem Rev* (2002) 102(12):4501–24. doi:10.1021/cr000033x
95. Gregory AD, Kliment CR, Metz HE, Kim KH, Kargl J, Agostini BA, et al. Neutrophil elastase promotes myofibroblast differentiation in lung fibrosis. *J Leukoc Biol* (2015) 98(2):143–52. doi:10.1189/jlb.3HI1014-493R
96. Takemasa A, Ishii Y, Fukuda T. A neutrophil elastase inhibitor prevents bleomycin-induced pulmonary fibrosis in mice. *Eur Respir J* (2012) 40(6):1475–82. doi:10.1183/09031936.00127011
97. Kruger P, Saffarzadeh M, Weber AN, Rieber N, Radsak M, von Bernuth H, et al. Neutrophils: between host defence, immune modulation, and tissue injury. *PLoS Pathog* (2015) 11(3):e1004651. doi:10.1371/journal.ppat.1004651
98. Beeh KM, Beier J, Kornmann O, Buhl R. Sputum matrix metalloproteinase-9, tissue inhibitor of metalloprotinease-1, and their molar ratio in patients with chronic obstructive pulmonary disease, idiopathic pulmonary fibrosis and healthy subjects. *Respir Med* (2003) 97(6):634–9. doi:10.1053/rmed.2003.1493
99. Henry MT, McMahon K, Mackarel AJ, Prikk K, Sorsa T, Maisi P, et al. Matrix metalloproteinases and tissue inhibitor of metalloproteinase-1 in sarcoidosis and IPF. *Eur Respir J* (2002) 20(5):1220–7. doi:10.1183/09031936.02.00022302
100. Corbel M, Caulet-Maugendre S, Germain N, Molet S, Lagente V, Boichot E. Inhibition of bleomycin-induced pulmonary fibrosis in mice by the matrix metalloproteinase inhibitor batimastat. *J Pathol* (2001) 193(4):538–45. doi:10.1002/path.826
101. Kaplan MJ, Radic M. Neutrophil extracellular traps: double-edged swords of innate immunity. *J Immunol* (2012) 189(6):2689–95. doi:10.4049/jimmunol.1201719
102. Chrysanthopoulou A, Mitroulis I, Apostolidou E, Arelaki S, Mikroulis D, Konstantinidis T, et al. Neutrophil extracellular traps promote differentiation and function of fibroblasts. *J Pathol* (2014) 233(3):294–307. doi:10.1002/path.4359
103. Strieter RM, Keeley EC, Burdick MD, Mehrad B. The role of circulating mesenchymal progenitor cells, fibrocytes, in promoting pulmonary fibrosis. *Trans Am Clin Climatol Assoc* (2009) 120:49–59.
104. Reilkoff RA, Bucala R, Herzog EL. Fibrocytes: emerging effector cells in chronic inflammation. *Nat Rev Immunol* (2011) 11(6):427–35. doi:10.1038/nri2990
105. Gomperts BN, Strieter RM. Fibrocytes in lung disease. *J Leukoc Biol* (2007) 82(3):449–56. doi:10.1189/jlb.0906587
106. Hong KM, Belperio JA, Keane MP, Burdick MD, Strieter RM. Differentiation of human circulating fibrocytes as mediated by transforming growth factor-beta and peroxisome proliferator-activated receptor gamma. *J Biol Chem* (2007) 282(31):22910–20. doi:10.1074/jbc.M703597200
107. Kao HK, Chen B, Murphy GF, Li Q, Orgill DP, Guo L. Peripheral blood fibrocytes: enhancement of wound healing by cell proliferation, re-epithelialization, contraction, and angiogenesis. *Ann Surg* (2011) 254(6):1066–74. doi:10.1097/SLA.0b013e3182251559
108. Herzog EL, Bucala R. Fibrocytes in health and disease. *Exp Hematol* (2010) 38(7):548–56. doi:10.1016/j.exphem.2010.03.004
109. Quan TE, Cowper SE, Bucala R. The role of circulating fibrocytes in fibrosis. *Curr Rheumatol Rep* (2006) 8(2):145–50. doi:10.1007/s11926-006-0055-x
110. Chesney J, Metz C, Stavitsky AB, Bacher M, Bucala R. Regulated production of type I collagen and inflammatory cytokines by peripheral blood fibrocytes. *J Immunol* (1998) 160(1):419–25.

111. Chesney J, Bacher M, Bender A, Bucala R. The peripheral blood fibrocyte is a potent antigen-presenting cell capable of priming naive T cells in situ. *Proc Natl Acad Sci U S A* (1997) 94(12):6307–12. doi:10.1073/pnas.94.12.6307
112. Fan X, Liang HP. Circulating fibrocytes: a potent cell population in antigen-presenting and wound healing. *Chin J Traumatol* (2010) 13(2):111–6.
113. Brunet I, Gordon E, Han J, Cristofaro B, Broqueres-You D, Liu C, et al. Netrin-1 controls sympathetic arterial innervation. *J Clin Invest* (2014) 124(7):3230–40. doi:10.1172/JCI75181
114. Madala SK, Edukulla R, Schmidt S, Davidson C, Ikegami M, Hardie WD. Bone marrow-derived stromal cells are invasive and hyperproliferative and alter transforming growth factor-alpha-induced pulmonary fibrosis. *Am J Respir Cell Mol Biol* (2014) 50(4):777–86. doi:10.1165/rcmb.2013-0042OC
115. Lindau D, Gielen P, Kroesen M, Wesseling P, Adema GJ. The immunosuppressive tumour network: myeloid-derived suppressor cells, regulatory T cells and natural killer T cells. *Immunology* (2013) 138(2):105–15. doi:10.1111/imm.12036
116. Gabrilovich DI, Nagaraj S. Myeloid-derived suppressor cells as regulators of the immune system. *Nat Rev Immunol* (2009) 9(3):162–74. doi:10.1038/nri2506
117. Zoso A, Mazza EM, Bicciato S, Mandruzzato S, Bronte V, Serafini P, et al. Human fibrocytic myeloid-derived suppressor cells express IDO and promote tolerance via Treg-cell expansion. *Eur J Immunol* (2014) 44(11):3307–19. doi:10.1002/eji.201444522
118. Fernandez IE, Greiffo FR, Frankenberger M, Bandres J, Heinzelmann K, Neurohr C, et al. Peripheral blood myeloid-derived suppressor cells reflect disease status in idiopathic pulmonary fibrosis. *Eur Respir J* (2016) 48(4):1171–83. doi:10.1183/13993003.01826-2015
119. Bryant AJ, Shenoy V, Fu C, Marek G, Lorentsen KJ, Herzog EL, et al. Myeloid-derived suppressor cells are necessary for development of pulmonary hypertension. *Am J Respir Cell Mol Biol* (2017) 58(2):170–180. doi:10.1165/rcmb.2017-0214OC
120. Kiessling R, Klein E, Pross H, Wigzell H. "Natural" killer cells in the mouse. II. Cytotoxic cells with specificity for mouse Moloney leukemia cells. Characteristics of the killer cell. *Eur J Immunol* (1975) 5(2):117–21. doi:10.1002/eji.1830050209
121. Sonnenberg GF, Artis D. Innate lymphoid cells in the initiation, regulation and resolution of inflammation. *Nat Med* (2015) 21(7):698–708. doi:10.1038/nm.3892
122. Lai DM, Shu Q, Fan J. The origin and role of innate lymphoid cells in the lung. *Mil Med Res* (2016) 3:25. doi:10.1186/s40779-016-0093-2
123. Peebles RS Jr. At the bedside: the emergence of group 2 innate lymphoid cells in human disease. *J Leukoc Biol* (2015) 97(3):469–75. doi:10.1189/jlb.3BT0814-383R
124. Monticelli LA, Sonnenberg GF, Abt MC, Alenghat T, Ziegler CG, Doering TA, et al. Innate lymphoid cells promote lung-tissue homeostasis after infection with influenza virus. *Nat Immunol* (2011) 12(11):1045–54. doi:10.1031/ni.2131
125. Helene M, Lake-Bullock V, Zhu J, Hao H, Cohen DA, Kaplan AM. T cell independence of bleomycin-induced pulmonary fibrosis. *J Leukoc Biol* (1999) 65(2):187–95. doi:10.1002/jlb.65.2.187
126. Fireman E, Vardinon N, Burke M, Spizer S, Levin S, Endler A, et al. Predictive value of response to treatment of T-lymphocyte subpopulations in idiopathic pulmonary fibrosis. *Eur Respir J* (1998) 11(3):706–11.
127. Nuovo GJ, Hagood JS, Magro CM, Chin N, Kapil R, Davis L, et al. The distribution of immunomodulatory cells in the lungs of patients with idiopathic pulmonary fibrosis. *Mod Pathol* (2012) 25(3):416–33. doi:10.1038/modpathol.2011.166
128. Herazo-Maya JD, Noth I, Duncan SR, Kim S, Ma SF, Tseng GC, et al. Peripheral blood mononuclear cell gene expression profiles predict poor outcome in idiopathic pulmonary fibrosis. *Sci Transl Med* (2013) 5(205):205ra136. doi:10.1126/scitranslmed.3005964
129. Herazo-Maya JD, Sun J, Molyneaux PL, Li Q, Villalba JA, Tzouvelekis A, et al. Validation of a 52-gene risk profile for outcome prediction in patients with idiopathic pulmonary fibrosis: an international, multicentre, cohort study. *Lancet Respir Med* (2017) 5(11):857–68. doi:10.1016/S2213-2600(17)30349-1
130. Gilani SR, Vuga LJ, Lindell KO, Gibson KF, Xue J, Kaminski N, et al. CD28 down-regulation on circulating CD4 T-cells is associated with poor prognoses of patients with idiopathic pulmonary fibrosis. *PLoS One* (2010) 5(1):e8959. doi:10.1371/journal.pone.0008959
131. Tiede I, Fritz G, Strand S, Poppe D, Dvorsky R, Strand D, et al. CD28-dependent Rac1 activation is the molecular target of azathioprine in primary human CD4+ T lymphocytes. *J Clin Invest* (2003) 111(8):1133–45. doi:10.1172/JCI16432
132. Delaunay M, Cadranel J, Lusque A, Meyer N, Gounant V, Moro-Sibilot D, et al. Immune-checkpoint inhibitors associated with interstitial lung disease in cancer patients. *Eur Respir J* (2017) 50(2):1700050. doi:10.1183/13993003.00050-2017
133. Luzina IG, Todd NW, Iacono AT, Atamas SP. Roles of T lymphocytes in pulmonary fibrosis. *J Leukoc Biol* (2008) 83(2):237–44. doi:10.1189/jlb.0707504
134. Prior C, Haslam PL. In vivo levels and in vitro production of interferon-gamma in fibrosing interstitial lung diseases. *Clin Exp Immunol* (1992) 88(2):280–7. doi:10.1111/j.1365-2249.1992.tb03074.x
135. Keane MP, Belperio JA, Burdick MD, Strieter RM. IL-12 attenuates bleomycin-induced pulmonary fibrosis. *Am J Physiol Lung Cell Mol Physiol* (2001) 281(1):L92–7. doi:10.1152/ajplung.2001.281.1.L92
136. Xu J, Mora AL, LaVoy J, Brigham KL, Rojas M. Increased bleomycin-induced lung injury in mice deficient in the transcription factor T-bet. *Am J Physiol Lung Cell Mol Physiol* (2006) 291(4):L658–67. doi:10.1152/ajplung.00006.2006
137. Saito A, Okazaki H, Sugawara I, Yamamoto K, Takizawa H. Potential action of IL-4 and IL-13 as fibrogenic factors on lung fibroblasts in vitro. *Int Arch Allergy Immunol* (2003) 132(2):168–76. doi:10.1159/000073718
138. Postlethwaite AE, Holness MA, Katai H, Raghow R. Human fibroblasts synthesize elevated levels of extracellular matrix proteins in response to interleukin 4. *J Clin Invest* (1992) 90(4):1479–85. doi:10.1172/JCI116015
139. Liu X, Kohyama T, Wang H, Zhu YK, Wen FQ, Kim HJ, et al. Th2 cytokine regulation of type I collagen gel contraction mediated by human lung mesenchymal cells. *Am J Physiol Lung Cell Mol Physiol* (2002) 282(5):L1049–56. doi:10.1152/ajplung.00321.2001
140. Kimura T, Ishii Y, Yoh K, Morishima Y, Iizuka T, Kiwamoto T, et al. Overexpression of the transcription factor GATA-3 enhances the development of pulmonary fibrosis. *Am J Pathol* (2006) 169(1):96–104. doi:10.2353/ajpath.2006.051160
141. Raghu G, Brown KK, Bradford WZ, Starko K, Noble PW, Schwartz DA, et al. A placebo-controlled trial of interferon gamma-1b in patients with idiopathic pulmonary fibrosis. *N Engl J Med* (2004) 350(2):125–33. doi:10.1056/NEJMoa030511
142. Parker JM, Glaspole IN, Lancaster LH, Haddad TJ, She D, Roseti SL, et al. A phase 2 randomized controlled study of tralokinumab in subjects with idiopathic pulmonary fibrosis. *Am J Respir Crit Care Med* (2017) 197(1):94–103. doi:10.1164/rccm.201704-0784OC
143. Onishi RM, Gaffen SL. Interleukin-17 and its target genes: mechanisms of interleukin-17 function in disease. *Immunology* (2010) 129(3):311–21. doi:10.1111/j.1365-2567.2009.03240.x
144. Wilson MS, Madala SK, Ramalingam TR, Gochuico BR, Rosas IO, Cheever AW, et al. Bleomycin and IL-1beta-mediated pulmonary fibrosis is IL-17A dependent. *J Exp Med* (2010) 207(3):535–52. doi:10.1084/jem.20092121
145. Lei L, Zhao C, Qin F, He ZY, Wang X, Zhong XN. Th17 cells and IL-17 promote the skin and lung inflammation and fibrosis process in a bleomycin-induced murine model of systemic sclerosis. *Clin Exp Rheumatol* (2016) 34 Suppl 100(5):14–22.
146. Mi S, Li Z, Yang HZ, Liu H, Wang JP, Ma YG, et al. Blocking IL-17A promotes the resolution of pulmonary inflammation and fibrosis via TGF-beta1-dependent and -independent mechanisms. *J Immunol* (2011) 187(6):3003–14. doi:10.4049/jimmunol.1004081
147. Dong Z, Lu X, Yang Y, Zhang T, Li Y, Chai Y, et al. IL-27 alleviates the bleomycin-induced pulmonary fibrosis by regulating the Th17 cell differentiation. *BMC Pulm Med* (2015) 15:13. doi:10.1186/s12890-015-0012-4
148. Chen Y, Li C, Weng D, Song L, Tang W, Dai W, et al. Neutralization of interleukin-17A delays progression of silica-induced lung inflammation and fibrosis in C57BL/6 mice. *Toxicol Appl Pharmacol* (2014) 275(1):62–72. doi:10.1016/j.taap.2013.11.012
149. Hasan SA, Eksteen B, Reid D, Paine HV, Alansary A, Johannson K, et al. Role of IL-17A and neutrophils in fibrosis in experimental hypersensitivity pneumonitis. *J Allergy Clin Immunol* (2013) 131(6):1663–73. doi:10.1016/j.jaci.2013.01.015

150. Liang SC, Tan XY, Luxenberg DP, Karim R, Dunussi-Joannopoulos K, Collins M, et al. Interleukin (IL)-22 and IL-17 are coexpressed by Th17 cells and cooperatively enhance expression of antimicrobial peptides. *J Exp Med* (2006) 203(10):2271–9. doi:10.1084/jem.20061308
151. Whittington HA, Armstrong L, Uppington KM, Millar AB. Interleukin-22: a potential immunomodulatory molecule in the lung. *Am J Respir Cell Mol Biol* (2004) 31(2):220–6. doi:10.1165/rcmb.2003-0285OC
152. Kotsianidis I, Nakou E, Bouchliou I, Tzouvelekis A, Spanoudakis E, Steiropoulos P, et al. Global impairment of CD4+CD25+FOXP3+ regulatory T cells in idiopathic pulmonary fibrosis. *Am J Respir Crit Care Med* (2009) 179(12):1121–30. doi:10.1164/rccm.200812-1936OC
153. Galati D, De Martino M, Trotta A, Rea G, Bruzzese D, Cicchitto G, et al. Peripheral depletion of NK cells and imbalance of the Treg/Th17 axis in idiopathic pulmonary fibrosis patients. *Cytokine* (2014) 66(2):119–26. doi:10.1016/j.cyto.2013.12.003
154. Reilkoff RA, Peng H, Murray LA, Peng X, Russell T, Montgomery R, et al. Semaphorin 7a+ regulatory T cells are associated with progressive idiopathic pulmonary fibrosis and are implicated in transforming growth factor-beta1-induced pulmonary fibrosis. *Am J Respir Crit Care Med* (2013) 187(2):180–8. doi:10.1164/rccm.201206-1109OC
155. Boveda-Ruiz D, D'Alessandro-Gabazza CN, Toda M, Takagi T, Naito M, Matsushima Y, et al. Differential role of regulatory T cells in early and late stages of pulmonary fibrosis. *Immunobiology* (2013) 218(2):245–54. doi:10.1016/j.imbio.2012.05.020
156. Garibaldi BT, D'Alessio FR, Mock JR, Files DC, Chau E, Eto Y, et al. Regulatory T cells reduce acute lung injury fibroproliferation by decreasing fibrocyte recruitment. *Am J Respir Cell Mol Biol* (2013) 48(1):35–43. doi:10.1165/rcmb.2012-0198OC
157. Lo Re S, Lecocq M, Uwambayinema F, Yakoub Y, Delos M, Demoulin JB, et al. Platelet-derived growth factor-producing CD4+ Foxp3+ regulatory T lymphocytes promote lung fibrosis. *Am J Respir Crit Care Med* (2011) 184(11):1270–81. doi:10.1164/rccm.201103-0516OC
158. Todd NW, Scheraga RG, Galvin JR, Iacono AT, Britt EJ, Luzina IG, et al. Lymphocyte aggregates persist and accumulate in the lungs of patients with idiopathic pulmonary fibrosis. *J Inflamm Res* (2013) 6:63–70. doi:10.2147/JIR.S40673
159. Taille C, Grootenboer-Mignot S, Boursier C, Michel L, Debray MP, Fagart J, et al. Identification of periplakin as a new target for autoreactivity in idiopathic pulmonary fibrosis. *Am J Respir Crit Care Med* (2011) 183(6):759–66. doi:10.1164/rccm.201001-0076OC
160. Lee JS, Kim EJ, Lynch KL, Elicker B, Ryerson CJ, Katsumoto TR, et al. Prevalence and clinical significance of circulating autoantibodies in idiopathic pulmonary fibrosis. *Respir Med* (2013) 107(2):249–55. doi:10.1016/j.rmed.2012.10.018
161. Wallace WA, Roberts SN, Caldwell H, Thornton E, Greening AP, Lamb D, et al. Circulating antibodies to lung protein(s) in patients with cryptogenic fibrosing alveolitis. *Thorax* (1994) 49(3):218–24. doi:10.1136/thx.49.3.218
162. Yang Y, Fujita J, Bandoh S, Ohtsuki Y, Yamadori I, Yoshinouchi T, et al. Detection of antivimentin antibody in sera of patients with idiopathic pulmonary fibrosis and non-specific interstitial pneumonia. *Clin Exp Immunol* (2002) 128(1):169–74. doi:10.1046/j.1365-2249.2002.01811.x
163. Fujita J, Dobashi N, Ohtsuki Y, Yamadori I, Yoshinouchi T, Kamei T, et al. Elevation of anti-cytokeratin 19 antibody in sera of the patients with idiopathic pulmonary fibrosis and pulmonary fibrosis associated with collagen vascular disorders. *Lung* (1999) 177(5):311–9. doi:10.1007/PL00007649
164. Mathai SK, Pedersen BS, Smith K, Russell P, Schwarz MI, Brown KK, et al. Desmoplakin variants are associated with idiopathic pulmonary fibrosis. *Am J Respir Crit Care Med* (2016) 193(10):1151–60. doi:10.1164/rccm.201509-1863OC
165. Li FJ, Surolia R, Li H, Wang Z, Kulkarni T, Liu G, et al. Autoimmunity to vimentin is associated with outcomes of patients with idiopathic pulmonary fibrosis. *J Immunol* (2017) 199(5):1596–605. doi:10.4049/jimmunol.1700473
166. Kahloon RA, Xue J, Bhargava A, Csizmadia E, Otterbein L, Kass DJ, et al. Patients with idiopathic pulmonary fibrosis with antibodies to heat shock protein 70 have poor prognoses. *Am J Respir Crit Care Med* (2013) 187(7):768–75. doi:10.1164/rccm.201203-0506OC
167. Shum AK, Alimohammadi M, Tan CL, Cheng MH, Metzger TC, Law CS, et al. BPIFB1 is a lung-specific autoantigen associated with interstitial lung disease. *Sci Transl Med* (2013) 5(206):206ra139. doi:10.1126/scitranslmed.3006998
168. Francois A, Gombault A, Villeret B, Alsaleh G, Fanny M, Gasse P, et al. B cell activating factor is central to bleomycin- and IL-17-mediated experimental pulmonary fibrosis. *J Autoimmun* (2015) 56:1–11. doi:10.1016/j.jaut.2014.08.003
169. Keir GJ, Maher TM, Ming D, Abdullah R, de Lauretis A, Wickremasinghe M, et al. Rituximab in severe, treatment-refractory interstitial lung disease. *Respirology* (2014) 19(3):353–9. doi:10.1111/resp.12214
170. Donahoe M, Valentine VG, Chien N, Gibson KF, Raval JS, Saul M, et al. Autoantibody-targeted treatments for acute exacerbations of idiopathic pulmonary fibrosis. *PLoS One* (2015) 10(6):e0127771. doi:10.1371/journal.pone.0127771
171. Arras M, Louahed J, Simoen V, Barbarin V, Misson P, van den Brule S, et al. B lymphocytes are critical for lung fibrosis control and prostaglandin E2 regulation in IL-9 transgenic mice. *Am J Respir Cell Mol Biol* (2006) 34(5):573–80. doi:10.1165/rcmb.2004-0383OC

17

Dendritic Cells are the Intriguing Players in the Puzzle of Idiopathic Pulmonary Fibrosis Pathogenesis

Marialuisa Bocchino[1*], *Serena Zanotta*[2], *Ludovica Capitelli*[1] *and Domenico Galati*[2]

[1] Respiratory Medicine Division, Department of Clinical Medicine and Surgery, Federico II University, Naples, Italy,
[2] Hematology–Oncology and Stem Cell Transplantation Unit, Department of Hematology and Developmental Therapeutics, Istituto Nazionale Tumori-IRCCS-Fondazione G. Pascale, Naples, Italy

***Correspondence:**
Marialuisa Bocchino
marialuisa.bocchino@unina.it

Idiopathic pulmonary fibrosis (IPF) is the most devastating progressive interstitial lung disease that remains refractory to treatment. Pathogenesis of IPF relies on the aberrant cross-talk between injured alveolar cells and myofibroblasts, which ultimately leads to an aberrant fibrous reaction. The contribution of the immune system to IPF remains not fully explored. Recent evidence suggests that both innate and adaptive immune responses may participate in the fibrotic process. Dendritic cells (DCs) are the most potent professional antigen-presenting cells that bridge innate and adaptive immunity. Also, they exert a crucial role in the immune surveillance of the lung, where they are strategically placed in the airway epithelium and interstitium. Immature DCs accumulate in the IPF lung close to areas of epithelial hyperplasia and fibrosis. Conversely, mature DCs are concentrated in well-organized lymphoid follicles along with T and B cells and bronchoalveolar lavage of IPF patients. We have recently shown that all sub-types of peripheral blood DCs (including conventional and plasmacytoid DCs) are severely depleted in therapy naïve IPF patients. Also, the low frequency of conventional CD1c^{+} DCs is predictive of a worse prognosis. The purpose of this mini-review is to focus on the main evidence on DC involvement in IPF pathogenesis. Unanswered questions and opportunities for future research ranging from a better understanding of their contribution to diagnosis and prognosis to personalized DC-based therapies will be explored.

Keywords: idiopathic pulmonary fibrosis, dendritic cells, immunity, cancer, immunotherapy

INTRODUCTION

Idiopathic pulmonary fibrosis (IPF) is a progressive and devastating fatal lung disease that usually remains refractory to treatment (1–3), with an estimated median survival of 2 to 5 years from the first diagnosis. In the last two decades, disease incidence has steadily increased, varying from 2.8 to 19 cases per 100.000 people per year in Europe and North America, respectively (1). Disease behavior is also highly variable, with associated comorbidities potentially exerting a detrimental impact on prognosis (4, 5). The current availability of anti-fibrotic drugs (i.e., nintedanib and pirfenidone) has improved patients' short-term life expectancy through the slowdown of the lung function decline and the reduction of hospitalization rate and episodes of acute exacerbation (6).

Despite many efforts, the pathogenesis of IPF has not yet been elucidated. No longer considered just an inflammatory disorder (7), IPF pathogenesis likely relies on the aberrant cross-talk between injured alveolar cells and myofibroblasts. This interaction ultimately promotes a pro-fibrotic microenvironment through the engagement of a vicious circle supported, among others, by oxidative stress (8–10). The immune system's contribution to IPF remains poorly understood, with several pieces of emerging evidence suggesting that both innate and adaptive responses can orchestrate the fibrotic process (11–13). In this scenario, dendritic cells (DCs) may play a significant role because of their involvement in the lungs' immune surveillance, where they are strategically placed within the airway epithelium and interstitium (14).

Notably, DCs encompass a heterogeneous family of bone marrow-derived cells recognized as the most specialized and potent antigen-presenting cells (APCs) of the immune system (15, 16). DCs are located in almost all tissues, where they detect and process Ags for presentation to T lymphocytes, thus establishing a tailored link between innate and adaptive immune responses. Besides, DCs are pivotal in regulating the delicate interplay between immunity and tolerance (17–19) as they promote the deletion of clonal autoreactive immature T cells in the thymus. Conversely, DCs interact in the periphery with T cells to achieve immune tolerance by inducing T-cell anergy, T cell deletion, and amplification and stimulation of regulatory T cell (Treg) subsets (18, 19). Due to their pleiotropic functions and properties within the immune system, DCs have been broadly studied in different experimental and internal medicine areas, including transplantation, allergy, autoimmunity, infectious diseases, cancer (20), and, more recently, fibrosis. Significant efforts have explored the fibrogenesis of different organs, including the liver, the kidney, and the heart (21–24).

The present review aims to offer an overview including the most relevant contributions in the field of IPF to focus on the emerging evidence addressing the role of DCs in disease pathogenesis and clinical behavior and potentially in immune-targeted therapy development.

DEVELOPMENT OF DENDRITIC CELLS

DCs originate from bone marrow progenitors through hematopoiesis, a finely regulated development process that involves several cellular and molecular events. Recent studies have identified a common DC precursor, the human granulocyte-monocyte-DC progenitor (GMDP), which supports the development of all the three major human DC subtypes (25). The GMDPs, through an intermediate maturation state into monocyte-dendritic progenitors (MDPs), differentiate into the common DC progenitors (CDPs). CDPs are restricted to the bone marrow, where they give rise to plasmacytoid DCs (pDCs) and conventional DC precursors (pre-cDCs). Frequencies of pre-cDCs increase in response to circulating FMS-like tyrosine kinase-3 Ligand (Flt3L) and then terminally differentiate into conventional DC (cDC) subsets in the periphery (25, 26). Accordingly, colony-stimulating factor-1 (CSF-1) and granulocyte-macrophage colony-stimulating factor (GM-CSF) are major cytokines required for human DC differentiation. In particular, Flt3L is a crucial regulator of DC commitment to both cDCs and pDCs (27–29). Additional transcription factors such as Ikaros, PU.1, growth factor independent 1 transcriptional repressor (GFi1), interferon regulatory factor 8 (IRF8), basic leucine zipper ATF-like transcription factor 3 (BATF3), and inhibitor of DNA binding 2 (ID2) synergistically regulate DC development and subset specification through the engagement of different signaling pathways (30–35), as illustrated in **Figure 1**.

CLASSIFICATION AND FUNCTION OF DENDRITIC CELL SUBTYPES

In humans, blood DC subtypes include $CD11c^+$cDCs, that are $CD1c^+$ or $CD141^+$ cells, and $CD11c^-$ pDCs, including $CD123^+$ or $CD303^+$ cells. Conventional DCs, previously termed type-1 ($CD1c^+$) and type-2 ($CD141^+$) myeloid DCs (mDCs), have recently reclassified as cDC2 and cDC1, respectively (36–38) (**Figure 1**). Conventional DCs exert a key function ranging from pathogen detection to cancer immunity as they are critical, through antigen presentation, to initiate specific T-cell responses. On the other, pDCs display high anti-viral activities due to their ability to produce type I interferon and are thought to be involved in immune tolerance (39, 40).

Finally, a new DC subtype is represented by the so-called monocyte-derived DCs (mo-DCs). Evidence shows that mo-DCs arise from monocytes recruited to the inflammatory site and express CD11c, CD1c, CD1a, FcεR1, IRF4, and ZBTB46. It is thought that mo-DCs promote $CD4^+$ T cell polarization within inflammatory contexts (41). A synoptical view of the previous and actual classification of DCs is reported in **Table 1**.

DENDRITIC CELL ACTIVATION AND FUNCTIONAL MATURATION

Mature DCs display phenotypic and functional profiles distinct from their naïve (immature) counterparts. Immature DCs express low levels of major histocompatibility complex (MHC) and co-stimulatory molecules and are usually found in peripheral tissues where they play as sentinels for immune monitoring. These cells can endocytose and process antigens but are poorly effective in generating peptide-MHC complexes to ensure optimal antigen presentation and efficient T-cell activation (42–45). Tissue damage, inflammatory processes, microorganisms, and tumor-derived products may promote the maturation of DCs. After that, these cells lose endocytic activity, increase MHC-peptide complexes, up-regulate co-stimulatory molecules, and secrete inflammatory cytokines essential for the activation of T-cell responses (46, 47). Lastly, following maturation, DCs acquire an increased migratory potential that allows them to move into different compartments, such as non-lymphoid and lymphoid tissues and blood (48, 49).

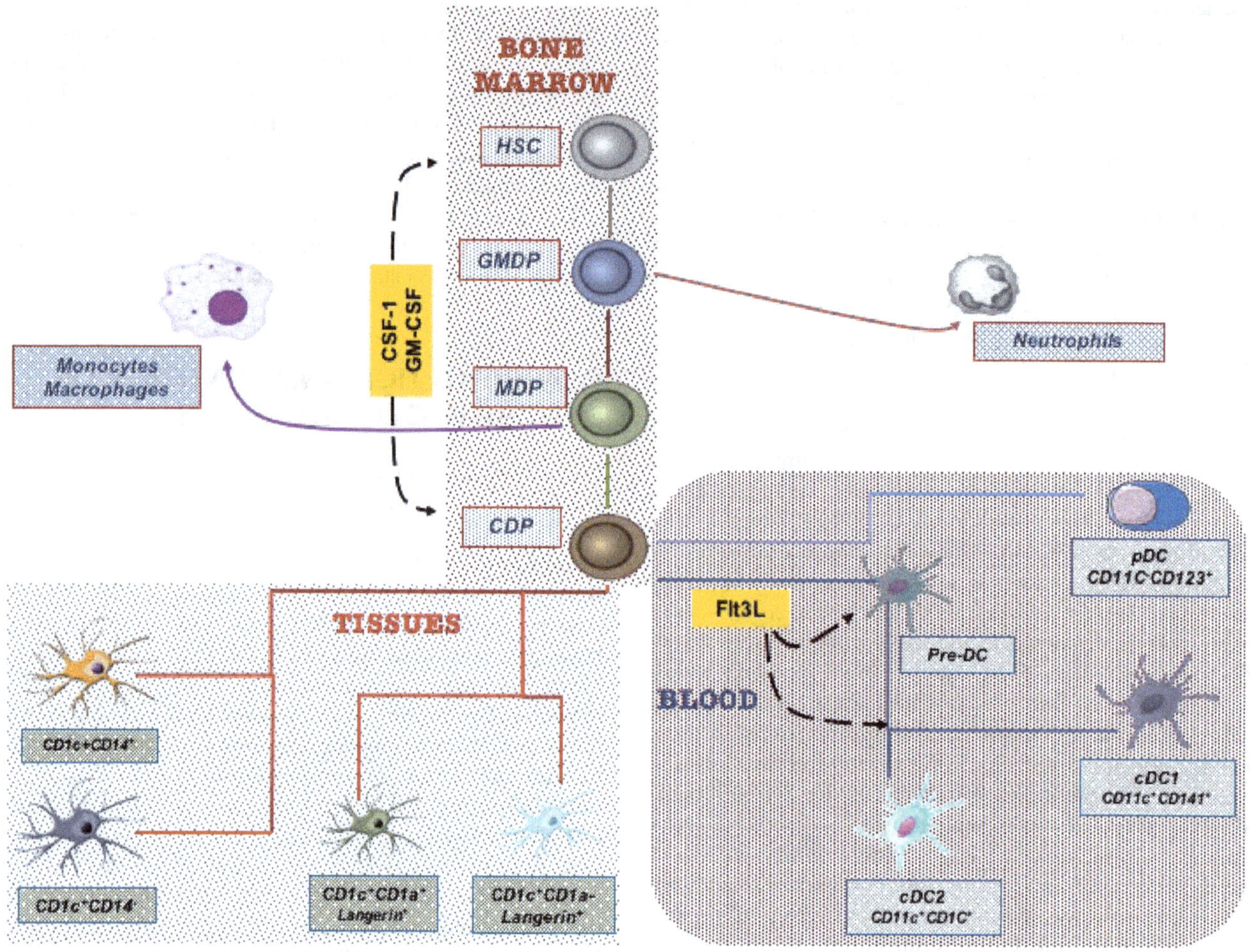

FIGURE 1 | Dendritic cells (DCs) derive from hematopoietic stem cells in the bone marrow. Progenitor cells give rise in the final step to Common Derived Progenitors (CDPs) that differentiate in the blood circulating DC subtypes and in lung tissue DC subsets.

DENDRITIC CELL SUBSETS IN THE HUMAN LUNG MICROENVIRONMENT

Due to their anatomy and function, the lungs are vital organs constantly exposed to the external environment. Consequently, inhaled particles of different nature and origin and potential pathogens need to be efficiently counteracted by a finely adjusted immune response to preserve lung health (50). The activity of lung DCs mainly depends on their organ distribution. For instance, DCs located in the alveolar septa have many dendritic projections able to continuously sample, while those located in the conducting airways seem to do so most rarely (51). Usually, DCs exist in an immature state in the lung periphery, skilled to take up inhaled particulate and soluble antigens. Upon activation, lung DCs, as previously described, become qualified to (52) induce a tailor-made immune response by T-cells (T-helper cell (Th) type 1, Th2, or Th17, depending on the type of pathogen) and B-cells (53, 54).

The lack of validated markers and technical difficulties ìn obtaining human lung tissues for investigation has significantly limited human lung DC subsets' characterization and functional studies. Since the first observations by Demetds et al., who initially identified human lung DC subsets through the BDCA markers previously applied to characterize blood DCs (55), understanding pulmonary DC subtypes has improved chiefly only in the last few years. In particular, both genomic and functional studies have shown that human epithelial-associated DCs can be divided into four major subpopulations: pDCs, cDC2 CD1c$^+$, cDC1 CD141$^{+,}$ and mo-DCs (36–38, 41). More recently, lung DCs have been reclassified into five subtypes based on the differential expression of Langerin, CD1c, and CD14 (56). Interestingly, transcriptome analysis performed in bronchoalveolar lavage (BAL) samples has revealed in the human lower respiratory tract the existence of Langerin$^+$, CD14$^{+,}$ and CD14$^-$ subsets of CD1c DCs functionally related with alveolar macrophages. Noteworthy, the higher mRNA expression levels of several dendritic cell-associated genes,

TABLE 1 | Synoptical classification of dendritic cell subsets.

Dendritic cell (DC) subtypes based on CD11c expression		Specific DC markers	Old classification	New classification
Myeloid / Conventional	$CD11c^+$ DC	**CD1c / BDCA-1**	Type-1 Myeloid DC (mDC1)	**Conventional DC2 (cDC2)**
Myeloid / Conventional	$CD11c^+$ DC	**CD141 / BDCA-3**	Type-2 Myeloid DC (mDC2)	**Conventional DC1 (cDC1)**
Plasmacytoid	$CD11c^-$ DC	**CD123** **CD303 / BDCA-2**	Plasmacytoid DC (pDC)	**Plasmacytoid DC (pDC)**
Monocyte-derived DC	$CD11c^+$ DC	**CD1c** **CD1a** **FcεR1** **CD206**	–	**Monocyte-derived DC (mo-DC)**

DC, dendritic cell; mDC, myeloid DC; cDC, conventional DC; Mo-DC, monocyte-derived DC; pDC, plasmacytoid DC; BDCA, Blood Dendritic Cell Antigen; FcεR1, Fc Fragment of IgE Receptor 1.

including CD1, FLT3, CX3CR1, and CCR6, have disclosed a specific gene signature of DCs distinct from that of monocytes/macrophages (56). **Figure 1** synthetically depicts the DC subtype differentiation in the lung.

THE ROLE OF DCs IN IPF PATHOGENESIS

The involvement of DCs in the pathogenesis of IPF is a challenging field of relatively recent interest, with only a few reports available in humans.

In 2006 it was first reported that fully mature DCs expressing CD40, CD83, CD86, and DC-lysosome-associated membrane protein, along with non-proliferating B and T lymphocytes, contribute to the creation of ectopic organized lymphoid structures in the lung of IPF patients (57). Conversely, immature DC subsets seem to heavily infiltrate the IPF lungs, specifically in areas of epithelial hyperplasia and fibrosis, and to be present in the BAL fluid (58–60). It is thought that fibroblastic foci of IPF patients can orchestrate blood immature DC recruitment through chemokines' expression (CCL19, CXCL12, and CCL21) (58, 61). This effect may maintain a condition of chronic inflammation by maturing DCs *in situ* within ectopic lymphoid follicles. Two physiologically relevant models showed that both human and mouse lung fibroblasts are critically involved in DC trafficking by secreting chemokines that play a crucial role in fibrosis and inflammation (62). Accordingly, co-cultures of DCs with lung fibroblasts from control subjects and IPF patients further confirmed the *in vitro* ability of lung fibroblasts to modulate the activation and maturation of DCs. These findings suggest that IPF fibroblasts might sustain chronic inflammation and immune responses by locally maintaining a pool of immature DCs (63). In a clinical trial published in 2015, the DC-specific growth factor Flt3L was found to increase cDC1 and cDC2 cell populations' precursors in bone marrow biopsies and peripheral blood samples from healthy volunteers (64). Following this finding, Flt3L has further been shown to be up-regulated in the serum and lung tissue of IPF patients, likely contributing to the accumulation of lung DCs during pulmonary fibrogenesis (65).

We previously showed that quantitative reduction of blood DCs was a feature shared by other respiratory diseases, including chronic obstructive pulmonary disease (COPD) and obstructive sleep apnea (66–68). We have recently also investigated the distribution of peripheral DCs subtypes in a prospective cohort of therapy naïve IPF patients. All blood DC subsets were severely depleted in the context of a pro-inflammatory milieu characterized by high expression levels of reactive oxygen species (ROS) and interleukin (IL)-6. In agreement with data previously reported, we likely attributed such a depletion, at least in part, to an increased cell turnover and recruitment at the lung level. Noteworthy, IL-6 levels and perturbations of the cDC2 subset were not influenced by anti-fibrotic therapies but were associated with reduced survival. Of note, low frequencies of cDC2 were an independent predictive biomarker of worse prognosis (69). **Figure 2** shows the role of DC subtypes undergoing the maturation process in the fibrotic lung tissue. Certainly, as mentioned, DCs involvement is not exclusive to IPF as it may also affect other respiratory diseases. In this context, it is worthy of note the report by Naessens T et al. The Authors have shown that cDC2 are potent inducers of T follicular helper cells and contribute to tertiary lymphoid tissue formation in the lung of COPD patients (70).

THE WAY FORWARD: SIMILARITIES WITH CANCER BIOLOGY AND RATIONALE FOR IMMUNE-TARGETED THERAPIES

In the light of the above evidence, DCs appear to play a role in the fibrotic process and, more specifically, in IPF pathogenesis. IPF notably shares many similarities with lung cancer, ranging from genetics to clinical behavior (71). It is also estimated that the overall cancer incidence in IPF patients is 29 cases per 1000 persons-years, with lung neoplasms being the most frequent ones (72). DC alterations have been widely studied and characterized in solid and blood malignancies (73). Like the liver fibrosis model leading to tumorigenesis (22), DC imbalance and functional impairment may represent a pathogenic bridge between IPF and cancer. This aspect merits further investigation for its prevention and therapeutic repercussions (13, 69). In this regard, DC-based treatments represent emerging alternatives to conventional chemotherapy in cancer patients (74), while such an approach is conceptually missing in fibrosis-related diseases. The lack of animal models that faithfully reproduce IPF pathogenesis is undoubtedly a significant limit in this setting. Despite this, the bleomycin model of inflammation-driven pulmonary fibrosis has still helped explore different purposes over time. In this regard, it has been shown that the immune-mediator VAG539 was able to attenuate the hallmarks of bleomycin-induced lung injury

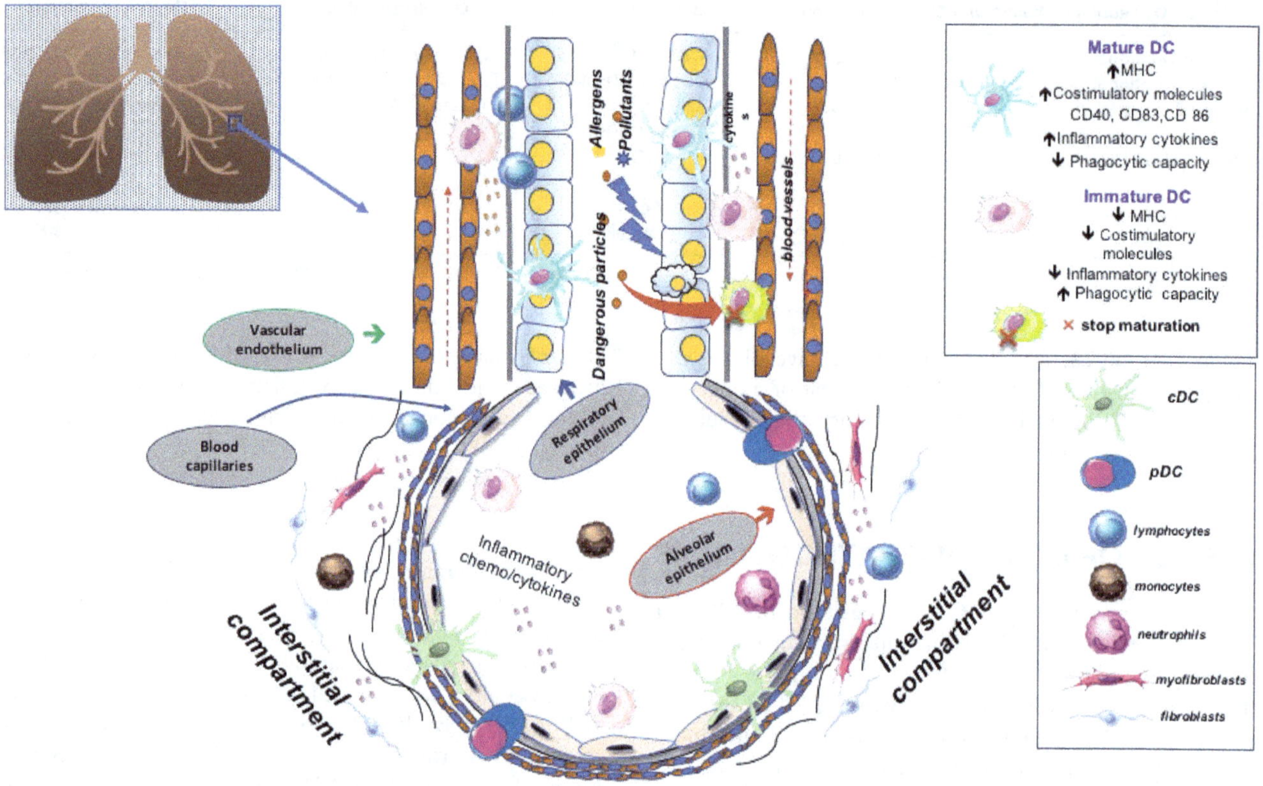

FIGURE 2 | Dendritic cells (DC) are located in the lung interstitium and alveoli, where they act as sentinel cells. Any imbalance of their frequency distribution and functional status may have significant consequences in disease pathogenesis. Emerging evidence suggests that plenty of local factors along with different arrays of chemo-cytokines can modulate DCs maturation in the lung of patients affected by idiopathic pulmonary fibrosis, thus affecting their tolerogenic or immunogenic properties.

through the inactivation of DCs, suggesting a crucial role of these cells across the modulation of both inflammation and fibrosis (75). Likewise, infusion of CD11c-diphtheria toxin (DT) receptor (DTR) in bleomycin-treated mice prompted DCs depletion, thus mitigating lung fibrosis (76). Indeed, both studies have some limitations. First, the expression of aryl hydrocarbon receptor as the key molecular target of VAG539 is not restricted to DCs (77), and, second, the infusion of DT to CD11c-DTR mice depletes not only DCs but also pulmonary macrophages as CD11c is highly expressed on both cell types (78). Even with the awareness of these limitations, we believe that this area of interest deserves wider attention. Accordingly, recent clinical trials have explored the safety and efficacy of recombinant human Flt3L in healthy volunteers and cancer therapy to trigger DC expansion in humans (79–81). Interestingly, recombinant Flt3L increased the numbers of $CD11b^{+}$ DCs, reducing lung fibrosis in wild-type (WT) mice exposed to AdTGF-beta1 (65).

IPF remains, for the most part, an unexplored field due to the non-recognition of the trigger cause. Perturbations of the lung microbiome and viral infections have been hypothesized to have a potential link with the development of IPF (82–86). Therefore, it is not negligible that any dysregulation of DCs, as major APCs and anti-viral effectors, may actively contribute to the puzzle of IPF pathogenesis through a wider involvement at different levels. Overall, accumulated evidence and related considerations further strengthen the concept that participation of DCs in the fibrotic process could be a driving force for future deepening.

CONCLUSION

Interpreting the involvement of the immune response in the pathogenesis of IPF has become a prosperous field of investigation only in recent years. New reports reveal expanding potential pathogenic roles for DCs in lung fibrosis. These findings promise to open new scenarios to understand better the cause and the biological mechanisms underlying the disease. Further efforts and challenges will be to evaluate their potential in terms of easy to perform biomarkers predictive of clinical behavior and targets of immune-based treatments. In analogy with cancer, combination therapy strategies with anti-fibrotic drugs could optimistically represent a milestone shortly.

AUTHOR CONTRIBUTIONS

All authors contributed to the article and approved the submitted version.

REFERENCES

1. Hutchinson J, Fogarty A, Hubbard R, McKeever T. Global Incidence and Mortality of Idiopathic Pulmonary Fibrosis: A Systematic Review. *Eur Respir J* (2015) 46(3):795–806. doi: 10.1183/09031936.00185114
2. Raghu G, Remy-Jardin M, Myers JL, Richeldi L, Ryerson CJ, Lederer DJ, et al. Diagnosis of Idiopathic Pulmonary Fibrosis. An Official ATS/ERS/JRS/ALAT Clinical Practice Guideline. *Am J Respir Crit Care Med* (2018) 198(5):e44–68. doi: 10.1164/rccm.201807-1255ST
3. Raghu G, Collard HR, Egan JJ, Martinez FJ, Behr J, Brown KK, et al. An Official ATS/ERS/JRS/ALAT Statement: Idiopathic Pulmonary Fibrosis: Evidence-Based Guidelines for Diagnosis and Management. *Am J Respir Crit Care Med* (2011) 183(6):788–824. doi: 10.1164/rccm.2009-040GL
4. Kreuter M, Ehlers-Tenenbaum S, Palmowski K, Bruhwyler J, Oltmanns U, Muley T, et al. Impact of Comorbidities on Mortality in Patients With Idiopathic Pulmonary Fibrosis. *PloS One* (2016) 11(3):e0151425. doi: 10.1371/journal.pone.0151425
5. Torrisi SE, Ley B, Kreuter M, Wijsenbeek M, Vittinghoff E, Collard HR, et al. The Added Value of Comorbidities in Predicting Survival in Idiopathic Pulmonary Fibrosis: A Multicentre Observational Study. *Eur Respir J* (2019) 53(3):1–10. doi: 10.1183/13993003.01587-2018
6. Maher TM, Strek ME. Anti-Fibrotic Therapy for Idiopathic Pulmonary Fibrosis: Time to Treat. *Respir Res* (2019) 20(1):205. doi: 10.1186/s12931-019-1161-4
7. Selman M, Pardo A. Idiopathic Pulmonary Fibrosis: Misunderstandings Between Epithelial Cells and Fibroblasts? *Sarcoidosis Vasc Diffuse Lung Dis* (2004) 21(3):165–72. doi: 10.1164/rccm.201312-2221PP
8. Selman M, Pardo A. Revealing the Pathogenic and Aging-Related Mechanisms of the Enigmatic Idiopathic Pulmonary Fibrosis. An Integral Model. *Am J Respir Crit Care Med* (2014) 189(10):1161–72. doi: 10.1164/rccm.201312-2221PP
9. Hill C, Jones MG, Davies DE, Wang Y. Epithelial-Mesenchymal Transition Contributes to Pulmonary Fibrosis Via Aberrant Epithelial/Fibroblastic Cross-Talk. *J Lung Health Dis* (2019) 3(2):31–5. doi: 10.29245/2689-999X/2019/2.1149
10. Bocchino M, Agnese S, Fagone E, Svegliati S, Grieco D, Vancheri C, et al. Reactive Oxygen Species are Required for Maintenance and Differentiation of Primary Lung Fibroblasts in Idiopathic Pulmonary Fibrosis. *PloS One* (2010) 5 (11):e14003. doi: 10.1371/journal.pone.0014003
11. Galati D, De Martino M, Trotta A, Rea G, Bruzzese D, Cicchitto G, et al. Peripheral Depletion of NK Cells and Imbalance of the Treg/Th17 Axis in Idiopathic Pulmonary Fibrosis Patients. *Cytokine* (2014) 66(2):119–26. doi: 10.1016/j.cyto.2013.12.003
12. Desai O, Winkler J, Minasyan M, Herzog EL. The Role of Immune and Inflammatory Cells in Idiopathic Pulmonary Fibrosis. *Front Med (Lausanne)* (2018) 5:43. doi: 10.3389/fmed.2018.00043
13. Shenderov K, Collins SL, Powell JD, Horton MR. Immune Dysregulation as a Driver of Idiopathic Pulmonary Fibrosis. *J Clin Invest* (2021) 131(2):1–12. doi: 10.1172/JCI143226
14. Worbs T, Hammerschmidt SI, Forster R. Dendritic Cell Migration in Health and Disease. *Nat Rev Immunol* (2017) 17(1):30–48. doi: 10.1038/nri.2016.116
15. Banchereau J, Briere F, Caux C, Davoust J, Lebecque S, Liu YJ, et al. Immunobiology of Dendritic Cells. *Annu Rev Immunol* (2000) 18:767–811. doi: 10.1146/annurev.immunol.18.1.767
16. Steinman RM. Decisions About Dendritic Cells: Past, Present, and Future. *Annu Rev Immunol* (2012) 30:1–22. doi: 10.1146/annurev-immunol-100311-102839
17. Banchereau J, Steinman RM. Dendritic Cells and the Control of Immunity. *Nature* (1998) 392(6673):245–52. doi: 10.1038/32588
18. Cools N, Ponsaerts P, Van Tendeloo VF, Berneman ZN. Balancing Between Immunity and Tolerance: An Interplay Between Dendritic Cells, Regulatory T Cells, and Effector T Cells. *J Leukoc Biol* (2007) 82(6):1365–74. doi: 10.1189/jlb.0307166
19. Steinman RM, Banchereau J. Taking Dendritic Cells Into Medicine. *Nature* (2007) 449(7161):419–26. doi: 10.1038/nature06175
20. Lipscomb MF, Masten BJ. Dendritic Cells: Immune Regulators in Health and Disease. *Physiol Rev* (2002) 82(1):97–130. doi: 10.1152/physrev.00023.2001
21. Baskic D, Vukovic V, Popovic S, Jovanovic D, Mitrovic S, Djurdjevic P, et al. Chronic Hepatitis C: Conspectus of Immunological Events in the Course of Fibrosis Evolution. *PloS One* (2019) 14(7):e0219508. doi: 10.1371/journal.pone.0219508
22. Lurje I, Hammerich L, Tacke F. Dendritic Cell and T Cell Cross-Talk in Liver Fibrogenesis and Hepatocarcinogenesis: Implications for Prevention and Therapy of Liver Cancer. *Int J Mol Sci* (2020) 21(19):1–25. doi: 10.3390/ijms21197378
23. Rogers NM, Ferenbach DA, Isenberg JS, Thomson AW, Hughes J. Dendritic Cells and Macrophages in the Kidney: A Spectrum of Good and Evil. *Nat Rev Nephrol* (2014) 10(11):625–43. doi: 10.1038/nrneph.2014.170
24. Wang H, Kwak D, Fassett J, Liu X, Yao W, Weng X, et al. Role of Bone Marrow-Derived CD11c(+) Dendritic Cells in Systolic Overload-Induced Left Ventricular Inflammation, Fibrosis and Hypertrophy. *Basic Res Cardiol* (2017) 112(3):25. doi: 10.1007/s00395-017-0615-4
25. Lee J, Breton G, Oliveira TY, Zhou YJ, Aljoufi A, Puhr S, et al. Restricted Dendritic Cell and Monocyte Progenitors in Human Cord Blood and Bone Marrow. *J Exp Med* (2015) 212(3):385–99. doi: 10.1084/jem.20141442
26. Breton G, Zheng S, Valieris R, Tojal da Silva I, Satija R, Nussenzweig MC. Human Dendritic Cells (Dcs) are Derived From Distinct Circulating Precursors That are Precommitted to Become CD1c+ or CD141+ Dcs. *J Exp Med* (2016) 213(13):2861–70. doi: 10.1084/jem.20161135
27. Maraskovsky E, Daro E, Roux E, Teepe M, Maliszewski CR, Hoek J, et al. In Vivo Generation of Human Dendritic Cell Subsets by Flt3 Ligand. *Blood* (2000) 96(3):878–84. doi: 10.1182/blood.V96.3.878.015k15_878_884
28. Marroquin CE, Westwood JA, Lapointe R, Mixon A, Wunderlich JR, Caron D, et al. Mobilization of Dendritic Cell Precursors in Patients With Cancer by Flt3 Ligand Allows the Generation of Higher Yields of Cultured Dendritic Cells. *J Immunother* (2002) 25(3):278–88. doi: 10.1097/00002371-200205000-00011
29. Anandasabapathy N, Feder R, Mollah S, Tse SW, Longhi MP, Mehandru S, et al. Classical Flt3L-Dependent Dendritic Cells Control Immunity to Protein Vaccine. *J Exp Med* (2014) 211(9):1875–91. doi: 10.1084/jem.20131397
30. Hambleton S, Salem S, Bustamante J, Bigley V, Boisson-Dupuis S, Azevedo J, et al. IRF8 Mutations and Human Dendritic-Cell Immunodeficiency. *N Engl J Med* (2011) 365(2):127–38. doi: 10.1056/NEJMoa1100066
31. Anderson KL, Perkin H, Surh CD, Venturini S, Maki RA, Torbett BE. Transcription Factor PU.1 is Necessary for Development of Thymic and Myeloid Progenitor-Derived Dendritic Cells. *J Immunol* (2000) 164(4):1855–61. doi: 10.4049/jimmunol.164.4.1855
32. Wu L, Nichogiannopoulou A, Shortman K, Georgopoulos K. Cell-Autonomous Defects in Dendritic Cell Populations of Ikaros Mutant Mice Point to a Developmental Relationship With the Lymphoid Lineage. *Immunity* (1997) 7(4):483–92. doi: 10.1016/s1074-7613(00)80370-2
33. Rathinam C, Geffers R, Yucel R, Buer J, Welte K, Moroy T, et al. The Transcriptional Repressor Gfi1 Controls STAT3-Dependent Dendritic Cell Development and Function. *Immunity* (2005) 22(6):717–28. doi: 10.1016/j.immuni.2005.04.007
34. Poulin LF, Reyal Y, Uronen-Hansson H, Schraml BU, Sancho D, Murphy KM, et al. DNGR-1 is a Specific and Universal Marker of Mouse and Human Batf3-Dependent Dendritic Cells in Lymphoid and non-Lymphoid Tissues. *Blood* (2012) 119(25):6052–62. doi: 10.1182/blood-2012-01-406967
35. Spits H, Couwenberg F, Bakker AQ, Weijer K, Uittenbogaart CH. Id2 and Id3 Inhibit Development of CD34(+) Stem Cells Into Predendritic Cell (Pre-DC)2 But Not Into Pre-DC1. Evidence for a Lymphoid Origin of Pre-DC2. *J Exp Med* (2000) 192(12):1775–84. doi: 10.1084/jem.192.12.1775
36. Villani AC, Satija R, Reynolds G, Sarkizova S, Shekhar K, Fletcher J, et al. Single-Cell RNA-Seq Reveals New Types of Human Blood Dendritic Cells, Monocytes, and Progenitors. *Science* (2017) 356(6335):1–12. doi: 10.1126/science.aah4573
37. Ziegler-Heitbrock L, Ancuta P, Crowe S, Dalod M, Grau V, Hart DN, et al. Nomenclature of Monocytes and Dendritic Cells in Blood. *Blood* (2010) 116 (16):e74–80. doi: 10.1182/blood-2010-02-258558
38. Mildner A, Jung S. Development and Function of Dendritic Cell Subsets. *Immunity* (2014) 40(5):642–56. doi: 10.1016/j.immuni.2014.04.016
39. Dai H, Thomson AW, Rogers NM. Dendritic Cells as Sensors, Mediators, and Regulators of Ischemic Injury. *Front Immunol* (2019) 10:2418. doi: 10.3389/fimmu.2019.02418

40. Haniffa M, Collin M, Ginhoux F. Ontogeny and Functional Specialization of Dendritic Cells in Human and Mouse. *Adv Immunol* (2013) 120:1–49. doi: 10.1016/B978-0-12-417028-5.00001-6
41. Collin M, Bigley V. Human Dendritic Cell Subsets: An Update. *Immunology* (2018) 154(1):3–20. doi: 10.1111/imm.12888
42. Lutz MB, Schuler G. Immature, Semi-Mature and Fully Mature Dendritic Cells: Which Signals Induce Tolerance or Immunity? *Trends Immunol* (2002) 23(9):445–9. doi: 10.1016/s1471-4906(02)02281-0
43. Dudek AM, Martin S, Garg AD, Agostinis P. Immature, Semi-Mature, and Fully Mature Dendritic Cells: Toward a DC-Cancer Cells Interface That Augments Anticancer Immunity. *Front Immunol* (2013) 4:438. doi: 10.3389/fimmu.2013.00438
44. Mahnke K, Schmitt E, Bonifaz L, Enk AH, Jonuleit H. Immature, But Not Inactive: The Tolerogenic Function of Immature Dendritic Cells. *Immunol Cell Biol* (2002) 80(5):477–83. doi: 10.1046/j.1440-1711.2002.01115.x
45. Manicassamy S, Pulendran B. Dendritic Cell Control of Tolerogenic Responses. *Immunol Rev* (2011) 241(1):206–27. doi: 10.1111/j.1600-065X.2011.01015.x
46. Mellman I. Dendritic Cells: Master Regulators of the Immune Response. *Cancer Immunol Res* (2013) 1(3):145–9. doi: 10.1158/2326-6066.CIR-13-0102
47. Reis e Sousa C. Dendritic Cells in a Mature Age. *Nat Rev Immunol* (2006) 6 (6):476–83. doi: 10.1038/nri1845
48. Bertho N, Adamski H, Toujas L, Debove M, Davoust J, Quillien V. Efficient Migration of Dendritic Cells Toward Lymph Node Chemokines and Induction of T(H)1 Responses Require Maturation Stimulus and Apoptotic Cell Interaction. *Blood* (2005) 106(5):1734–41. doi: 10.1182/blood-2004-10-3991
49. Ohl L, Mohaupt M, Czeloth N, Hintzen G, Kiafard Z, Zwirner J, et al. CCR7 Governs Skin Dendritic Cell Migration Under Inflammatory and Steady-State Conditions. *Immunity* (2004) 21(2):279–88. doi: 10.1016/j.immuni.2004.06.014
50. Schlitzer A, McGovern N, Ginhoux F. Dendritic Cells and Monocyte-Derived Cells: Two Complementary and Integrated Functional Systems. *Semin Cell Dev Biol* (2015) 41:9–22. doi: 10.1016/j.semcdb.2015.03.011
51. Kopf M, Schneider C, Nobs SP. The Development and Function of Lung-Resident Macrophages and Dendritic Cells. *Nat Immunol* (2015) 16(1):36–44. doi: 10.1038/ni.3052
52. Condon TV, Sawyer RT, Fenton MJ, Riches DW. Lung Dendritic Cells At the Innate-Adaptive Immune Interface. *J Leukoc Biol* (2011) 90(5):883–95. doi: 10.1189/jlb.0311134
53. Lambrecht BN, Prins JB, Hoogsteden HC. Lung Dendritic Cells and Host Immunity to Infection. *Eur Respir J* (2001) 18(4):692–704.
54. Lambrecht BN, Hammad H. Lung Dendritic Cells: Targets for Therapy in Allergic Disease. *Handb Exp Pharmacol* (2009) 188):99–114. doi: 10.1007/978-3-540-71029-5_5
55. Demedts IK, Brusselle GG, Vermaelen KY, Pauwels RA. Identification and Characterization of Human Pulmonary Dendritic Cells. *Am J Respir Cell Mol Biol* (2005) 32(3):177–84. doi: 10.1165/rcmb.2004-0279OC
56. Patel VI, Booth JL, Duggan ES, Cate S, White VL, Hutchings D, et al. Transcriptional Classification and Functional Characterization of Human Airway Macrophage and Dendritic Cell Subsets. *J Immunol* (2017) 198 (3):1183–201. doi: 10.4049/jimmunol.1600777
57. Marchal-Somme J, Uzunhan Y, Marchand-Adam S, Valeyre D, Soumelis V, Crestani B, et al. Cutting Edge: non-Proliferating Mature Immune Cells Form a Novel Type of Organized Lymphoid Structure in Idiopathic Pulmonary Fibrosis. *J Immunol* (2006) 176(10):5735–9. doi: 10.4049/jimmunol.176.10.5735
58. Marchal-Somme J, Uzunhan Y, Marchand-Adam S, Kambouchner M, Valeyre D, Crestani B, et al. Dendritic Cells Accumulate in Human Fibrotic Interstitial Lung Disease. *Am J Respir Crit Care Med* (2007) 176(10):1007–14. doi: 10.1164/rccm.200609-1347OC
59. Greer AM, Matthay MA, Kukreja J, Bhakta NR, Nguyen CP, Wolters PJ, et al. Accumulation of BDCA1(+) Dendritic Cells in Interstitial Fibrotic Lung Diseases and Th2-High Asthma. *PloS One* (2014) 9(6):e99084. doi: 10.1371/journal.pone.0099084
60. Tsoumakidou M, Karagiannis KP, Bouloukaki I, Zakynthinos S, Tzanakis N, Siafakas NM. Increased Bronchoalveolar Lavage Fluid CD1c Expressing Dendritic Cells in Idiopathic Pulmonary Fibrosis. *Respiration* (2009) 78 (4):446–52. doi: 10.1159/000226244
61. Luther SA, Bidgol A, Hargreaves DC, Schmidt A, Xu Y, Paniyadi J, et al. Differing Activities of Homeostatic Chemokines CCL19, CCL21, and CXCL12 in Lymphocyte and Dendritic Cell Recruitment and Lymphoid Neogenesis. *J Immunol* (2002) 169(1):424–33. doi: 10.4049/jimmunol.169.1.424
62. Kitamura H, Cambier S, Somanath S, Barker T, Minagawa S, Markovics J, et al. Mouse and Human Lung Fibroblasts Regulate Dendritic Cell Trafficking, Airway Inflammation, and Fibrosis Through Integrin Alphavbeta8-Mediated Activation of TGF-Beta. *J Clin Invest* (2011) 121(7):2863–75. doi: 10.1172/JCI45589
63. Freynet O, Marchal-Somme J, Jean-Louis F, Mailleux A, Crestani B, Soler P, et al. Human Lung Fibroblasts may Modulate Dendritic Cell Phenotype and Function: Results From a Pilot in Vitro Study. *Respir Res* (2016) 17:36. doi: 10.1186/s12931-016-0345-4
64. Breton G, Lee J, Zhou YJ, Schreiber JJ, Keler T, Puhr S, et al. Circulating Precursors of Human CD1c+ and CD141+ Dendritic Cells. *J Exp Med* (2015) 212(3):401–13. doi: 10.1084/jem.20141441
65. Tort Tarres M, Aschenbrenner F, Maus R, Stolper J, Schuette L, Knudsen L, et al. The FMS-Like Tyrosine Kinase-3 Ligand/Lung Dendritic Cell Axis Contributes to Regulation of Pulmonary Fibrosis. *Thorax* (2019) 74:947–57. doi: 10.1136/thoraxjnl-2018-212603
66. Galati D, Zanotta S, Corazzelli G, Bruzzese D, Capobianco G, Morelli E, et al. Circulating Dendritic Cells Deficiencies as a New Biomarker in Classical Hodgkin Lymphoma. *Br J Haematol* (2019) 184(4):594–604. doi: 10.1111/bjh.15676
67. Galgani M, Fabozzi I, Perna F, Bruzzese D, Bellofiore B, Calabrese C, et al. Imbalance of Circulating Dendritic Cell Subsets in Chronic Obstructive Pulmonary Disease. *Clin Immunol* (2010) 137(1):102–10. doi: 10.1016/j.clim.2010.06.010
68. Galati D, Zanotta S, Canora A, Polistina GE, Nicoletta C, Ghinassi G, et al. Severe Depletion of Peripheral Blood Dendritic Cell Subsets in Obstructive Sleep Apnea Patients: A New Link With Cancer? *Cytokine* (2020) 125:154831. doi: 10.1016/j.cyto.2019.154831
69. Galati D, Zanotta S, Polistina GE, Coppola A, Capitelli L, Bocchino M. Circulating Dendritic Cells are Severely Decreased in Idiopathic Pulmonary Fibrosis With a Potential Value for Prognosis Prediction. *Clin Immunol* (2020) 215:108454. doi: 10.1016/j.clim.2020.108454
70. Naessens T, Morias Y, Hamrud E, Gehrmann U, Budida R, Mattsson J, et al. Human Lung Conventional Dendritic Cells Orchestrate Lymphoid Neogenesis During Chronic Obstructive Pulmonary Disease. *Am J Respir Crit Care Med* (2020) 202(4):535–48. doi: 10.1164/rccm.201906-1123OC
71. Tzouvelekis A, Gomatou G, Bouros E, Trigidou R, Tzilas V, Bouros D. Common Pathogenic Mechanisms Between Idiopathic Pulmonary Fibrosis and Lung Cancer. *Chest* (2019) 156(2):383–91. doi: 10.1016/j.chest.2019.04.114
72. Lee HY, Lee J, Lee CH, Han K, Choi SM. Risk of Cancer Incidence in Patients With Idiopathic Pulmonary Fibrosis: A Nationwide Cohort Study. *Respirology* (2021) 26(2):180–7. doi: 10.1111/resp.13911
73. Galati D, Corazzelli G, De Filippi R, Pinto A. Dendritic Cells in Hematological Malignancies. *Crit Rev Oncol Hematol* (2016) 108:86–96. doi: 10.1016/j.critrevonc.2016.10.006
74. Galati D, Zanotta S, Bocchino M, De Filippi R, Pinto A. The Subtle Interplay Between Gamma Delta T Lymphocytes and Dendritic Cells: Is There a Role for a Therapeutic Cancer Vaccine in the Era of Combinatorial Strategies? *Cancer Immunol Immunother* (2021). doi: 10.1007/s00262-020-02805-3
75. Bantsimba-Malanda C, Marchal-Somme J, Goven D, Freynet O, Michel L, Crestani B, et al. A Role for Dendritic Cells in Bleomycin-Induced Pulmonary Fibrosis in Mice? *Am J Respir Crit Care Med* (2010) 182(3):385–95. doi: 10.1164/rccm.200907-1164OC
76. Ding L, Liu T, Wu Z, Hu B, Nakashima T, Ullenbruch M, et al. Bone Marrow Cd11c+ Cell-Derived Amphiregulin Promotes Pulmonary Fibrosis. *J Immunol* (2016) 197(1):303–12. doi: 10.4049/jimmunol.1502479
77. Mulero-Navarro S, Fernandez-Salguero PM. New Trends in Aryl Hydrocarbon Receptor Biology. *Front Cell Dev Biol* (2016) 4:45. doi: 10.3389/fcell.2016.00045
78. van Rijt LS, Jung S, Kleinjan A, Vos N, Willart M, Duez C, et al. In Vivo Depletion of Lung CD11c+ Dendritic Cells During Allergen Challenge Abrogates the Characteristic Features of Asthma. *J Exp Med* (2005) 201 (6):981–91. doi: 10.1084/jem.20042311

79. Galati D, Zanotta S. Empowering Dendritic Cell Cancer Vaccination: The Role of Combinatorial Strategies. *Cytotherapy* (2018) 20(11):1309–23. doi: 10.1016/j.jcyt.2018.09.007
80. Anandasabapathy N, Breton G, Hurley A, Caskey M, Trumpfheller C, Sarma P, et al. Efficacy and Safety of CDX-301, Recombinant Human Flt3L, At Expanding Dendritic Cells and Hematopoietic Stem Cells in Healthy Human Volunteers. *Bone Marrow Transplant* (2015) 50(7):924–30. doi: 10.1038/bmt.2015.74
81. Galati D, Zanotta S. Hematologic Neoplasms: Dendritic Cells Vaccines in Motion. *Clin Immunol* (2017) 183:181–90. doi: 10.1016/j.clim.2017.08.016
82. Lipinski JH, Moore BB, O'Dwyer DN. The Evolving Role of the Lung Microbiome in Pulmonary Fibrosis. *Am J Physiol Lung Cell Mol Physiol* (2020) 319(4):L675–L82. doi: 10.1152/ajplung.00258.2020
83. Invernizzi R, Molyneaux PL. The Contribution of Infection and the Respiratory Microbiome in Acute Exacerbations of Idiopathic Pulmonary Fibrosis. *Eur Respir Rev* (2019) 28(152):1–6. doi: 10.1183/16000617.0045-2019
84. Tong X, Su F, Xu X, Xu H, Yang T, Xu Q, et al. Alterations to the Lung Microbiome in Idiopathic Pulmonary Fibrosis Patients. *Front Cell Infect Microbiol* (2019) 9:149. doi: 10.3389/fcimb.2019.00149
85. Sheng G, Chen P, Wei Y, Yue H, Chu J, Zhao J, et al. Viral Infection Increases the Risk of Idiopathic Pulmonary Fibrosis: A Meta-Analysis. *Chest* (2020) 157 (5):1175–87. doi: 10.1016/j.chest.2019.10.032
86. Moore BB, Moore TA. Viruses in Idiopathic Pulmonary Fibrosis. Etiology and Exacerbation. *Ann Am Thorac Soc* (2015) 12 Suppl 2:S186–92. doi: 10.1513/AnnalsATS.201502-088AW

18

Integrating Patient Perspectives into Personalized Medicine in Idiopathic Pulmonary Fibrosis

*Catharina C. Moor, Peter Heukels, Mirjam Kool and Marlies S. Wijsenbeek**

Department of Respiratory Medicine, Erasmus Medical Center, University Hospital Rotterdam, Rotterdam, Netherlands

Correspondence:
Marlies S. Wijsenbeek
m.wijsenbeek-lourens@erasmusmc.nl

Idiopathic pulmonary fibrosis (IPF) is a progressive and ultimately fatal disease which has a major impact on patients' quality of life (QOL). Except for lung transplantation, there is no curative treatment option. Fortunately, two disease-modifying drugs that slow down disease decline were recently approved. Though this is a major step forward, these drugs do not halt or reverse the disease, nor convincingly improve health-related QOL. In daily practice, disease behavior and response to therapy greatly vary among patients. It is assumed that this is related to the multiple biological pathways and complex interactions between genetic, molecular, and environmental factors that are involved in the pathogenesis of IPF. Recently, research in IPF has therefore started to focus on developing targeted therapy through identifying genetic risk factors and biomarkers. In this rapidly evolving field of personalized medicine, patient factors such as lifestyle, comorbidities, preferences, and experiences with medication should not be overlooked. This review describes recent insights and methods on how to integrate patient perspectives into personalized medicine. Furthermore, it provides an overview of the most used patient-reported outcome measures in IPF, to facilitate choices for both researchers and clinicians when incorporating the patient voice in their research and care. To enhance truly personalized treatment in IPF, biology should be combined with patient perspectives.

Keywords: idiopathic pulmonary fibrosis, health-related quality of life, personalized medicine, patient-reported outcomes, personomics, patient experiences

INTRODUCTION

> *Give different ones [therapeutic drinks] to different patients, for the sweet ones do not benefit everyone, nor do the astringent ones, nor are all patients able to drink the same things*
> ***Hippocrates*** (1)

Idiopathic pulmonary fibrosis (IPF) is the most common idiopathic interstitial pneumonia (2). IPF is characterized by progressive decline of lung function, with a median survival of only 3–5 years (3). Common symptoms as breathlessness, cough, and fatigue have a major impact on the quality of life (QOL) of patients (4). IPF occurs more often in men than women and usually affects elderly patients, aged 50 years and above (3). There are two approved anti-fibrotic drugs that slow down disease decline, but these drugs do not halt or reverse the disease, and ultimately IPF remains a fatal disease (5, 6). The heterogeneity in disease behavior and response to therapy in IPF has (further) stimulated research to identify possible distinct underlying genetic, molecular, and environmental factors associated with IPF (7, 8).

The potential to enhance personalized treatment has prompted excitement also in the IPF field (7). Until now, the focus of personalized medicine has been on physiology and the use of this biological information to predict response to treatment and to develop targeted therapy (9). In this process, patient factors should not be overlooked. For real personalized treatment patient perceptions and preferences should also be taken into account. In this article, we focus on recent insights and methods on how to integrate patient perspectives into personalized medicine.

Impact of Disease

Idiopathic pulmonary fibrosis is a heterogeneous disease, with a highly variable disease course (10, 11). Additionally, different phenotypes of IPF exist. Most patients have a slow disease progression, while some patients display relative stable periods followed by acute exacerbations and a small group of patients experiences a rapid decline in lung function (12). Uncertainty about the disease course and prognosis can cause emotional distress and anxiety, and, as a result, IPF has a major impact on most patients' health-related quality of life (HRQOL). HRQOL can be defined as a patient's perceived well-being affected by disease and treatment of the disease (13). IPF affects patients in almost every domain of life; hence, the burden of the disease is high, not just for patients but also for their partners and families. Patients often struggle with loss of independence because of functional limitations and deteriorating symptoms. Not only can breathlessness, cough, and fatigue diminish QOL, but also other symptoms such as sleep disorders, loss of appetite, and psychological problems can (14–18).

Most clinical trials in IPF that have been performed so far, have shown no convincing improvement of patient HRQOL (5, 6, 19). To date, the main focus in research has been to stabilize or improve physiological outcomes rather than HRQOL. Physiological parameters, such as lung function, do not correlate well with HRQOL measurements (20, 21). To our knowledge for parameters as imaging and biomarkers, relationships with HRQOL have not yet been established. Thus, decline in lung function does not adequately reflect the perceived impact of the disease on patients' lives.

Every person has a different lifestyle, personal circumstances, and coping strategies. These factors can play an important role in how a disease manifests itself; hence, the same disease affects each person in a different way (16, 22, 23). Medication may show promising results at group level in randomized controlled trials, but still in some individual patients, treatment may fail (22). For example, the side effects of medication may outweigh the positive effects of medication in daily practice, or the burden of treatment might be too high for patients. To improve and personalize treatment of IPF, we should also include patient perspectives and QOL.

Personomics

Personalized, stratified, or precision medicine is a broad term which can be referred to as "delivering the right treatment to the right patient at the right time" (24). Personalized medicine has gained increasing attention during the past decade (22, 25). However, the concept is not new; Hippocrates already mentioned the importance of a personalized approach to diagnosis and treatment in the fifth century BC, stating that "individuality of human beings affects predisposition to disease and response to treatment," and also noting that "not all patients are able to drink the same therapeutic drinks" (1, 26). His concepts already include the notion that experiences with treatment differ among patients. This idea is also acknowledged by Britten et al., who suggest that because individuals are more than their genetic profile, the main concept of stratified medicine is too limited at the moment (22). Personalized treatment comprises not only "biology," but should also focus on patient perspectives, needs, experiences, personality, environment, lifestyle, and other personal circumstances (**Figure 1**) (9, 22). Accordingly, the term "personomics" has been introduced to capture a patient's life circumstances that may alter disease behavior and response to treatment (23). Below we will briefly touch on the role of biology and other aspects of personalized medicine as shown in **Figure 1**, but the focus will be on patient perspectives.

Current View of Personalized Medicine in IPF

In other fields, especially oncology, personalized medicine has dramatically changed clinical practice during the last few years. Biomarkers have been used to develop targeted therapy and allocate patients to individual treatment plans (27–29).

Currently, the diagnosis of IPF is based on clinical, radiological, and pathological findings (3). The exact etiology of IPF is, however, incompletely understood. One of the proposed hypotheses is the concept of dysfunctional wound healing: repeated epithelial injury and dysfunctional regeneration possibly in combination with a dysregulated immune system normally facilitating wound healing leads to fibrogenesis and, as a consequence, excessive scarring of the lung tissue (11, 30). Epithelial injury might be caused by risk factors such as cigarette smoking, micro-aspiration of gastric content, and lead to development of IPF in susceptible individuals (11). At present, it is assumed that multiple biological pathways and complex interactions between genetic, molecular, and environmental factors are involved in the pathogenesis of IPF. Improved understanding of the pathogenesis of IPF has led to the identification of potential molecular biomarkers (7, 11, 31–33). Genome-wide association studies found genetic mutations that correlate with disease risk and possibly also disease progression (34–37); subsequently, the first examples of drug–gene interactions in IPF were found (38). To date, the value of biomarkers in IPF has not been fully clarified, and, therefore biomarkers or genetic endotyping are not yet used in clinical practice (7, 33).

Novel studies in IPF suggest that the "respiratory microbiome" is also involved in IPF pathogenesis, disease progression, and mortality (39–41). Patients with IPF have a higher bacterial burden and abundance of specific pathogens in the lung microbiome than the normal population. Furthermore, interactions have been found between specific gene expression and an altered lung microbiome in IPF, which is the first evidence for host-environmental interactions in IPF (42, 43). The lung microbiome may serve as a prognostic factor in the future, and clinical trials aimed at altering the microbiome of patients with IPF have already started (44).

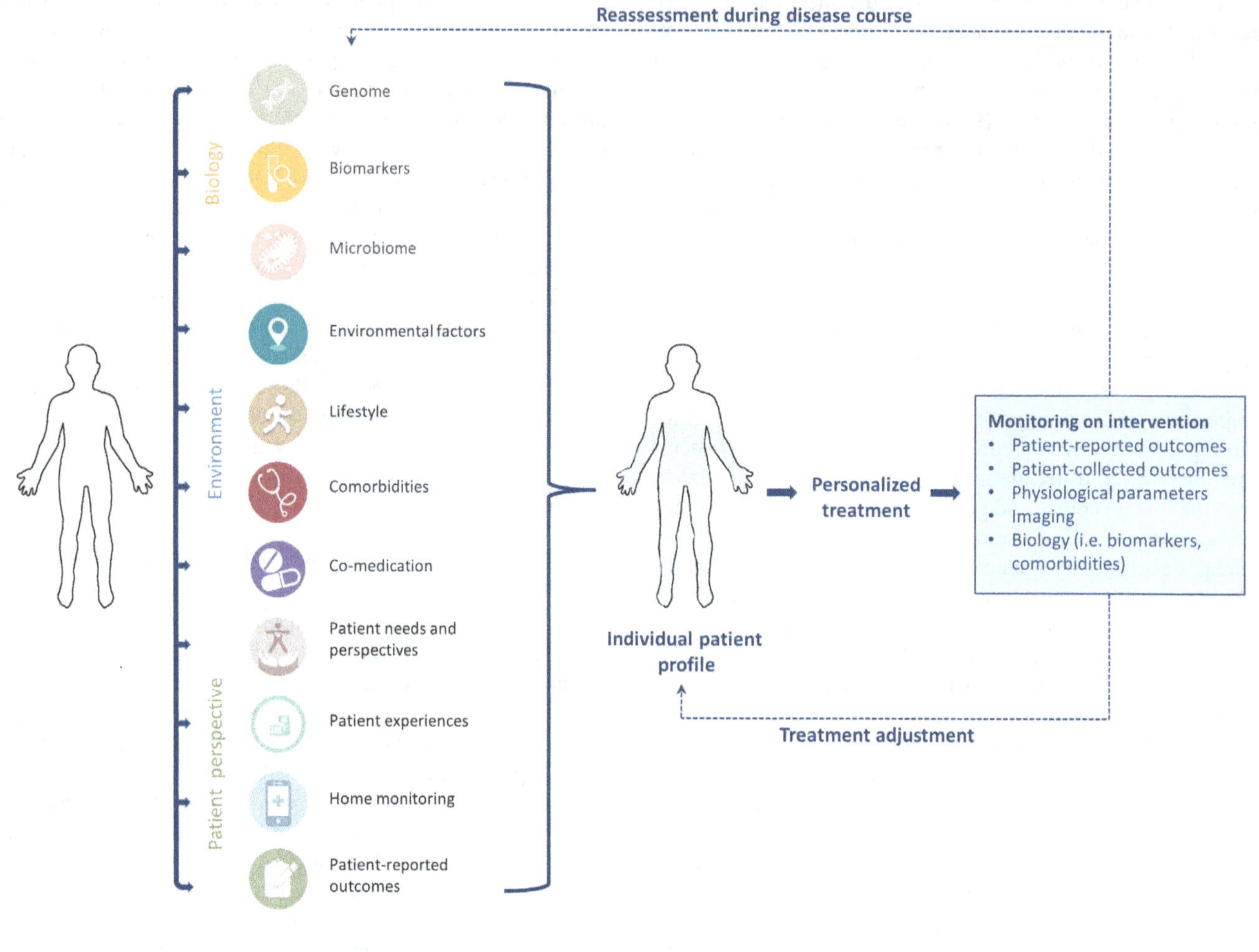

FIGURE 1 | To enhance tailored treatment in idiopathic pulmonary fibrosis, "biology" should be combined with patient factors to generate an individual patient profile. Close monitoring, timely reassessment, and treatment adjustment during the disease course are required to optimize personalized care.

A detailed description of (molecular) biology and its current role and potential in the IPF field is beyond the scope of this review.

HOW TO INTEGRATE PERSONOMICS INTO PERSONALIZED MEDICINE

Patient Needs and Perspectives in IPF Care

The importance of engaging patients in IPF care has gained increasing attention during the last several years (45). Recent qualitative studies have reported a need for better education about IPF, information about specific treatment options and palliative care, and access to specialist centers and specialist nurses. Additionally, more support for caregivers is warranted (16, 17, 46–48). These recommendations underscore the idea that not only pharmacological treatment but also non-pharmacological treatment options such as oxygen therapy, pulmonary rehabilitation, psychological support, and palliative care, are an important part of personalized management. With regard to pharmacological treatment, it is important to assess the needs and perspectives of patients before starting treatment, thereby enhancing shared decision-making. For instance, some side effects of disease-modifying drugs might have a devastating impact on one patient, but be far less bothersome to other patients (22). At the moment, over-use and under-use of medication, compliance problems, and waste of medication are not unusual in IPF (22, 49, 50). Non-adherence to medication could therefore be prevented when patients' preferences and lifestyle are taken into account (9). Since patient preferences and needs may change because of disease progression or personal circumstances, an important aspect of disease management is iterative evaluation of the situation of individual patients (16, 46, 51). Only in this way can "holistic" personalized care be given in IPF.

Comorbidities and Co-Medication

Holistic care also means looking further than the lungs. IPF is associated with a number of pulmonary and extra-pulmonary comorbidities, such as pulmonary hypertension, respiratory infection, cardiovascular disease, emphysema, lung cancer, diabetes mellitus, venous thromboembolism, and gastroesophageal reflux (52–56). Comorbidities are more prevalent in patients with IPF than in the normal population and have a negative influence on QOL and survival (54, 56–58). Hence, early identification and treatment of comorbid conditions have the potential to improve QOL, functional outcomes, and survival for patients with IPF (53). Kreuter et al. (54) proposed the "IPF comorbidome," which visually displays prevalence of comorbidities and their strength of association with mortality in patients with IPF. This comorbidome could be used to predict prognosis for individual patients with IPF, and thus enhance personalized treatment.

Moreover, extra attention should be paid to the frail, elderly patients who have multiple comorbidities and functional impairment (55). As a consequence, these patients might have a higher risk of harmful side effects of disease-modifying medication and should be closely monitored during treatment. Besides, polypharmacy may play an important role in this group of patients. It is generally known that polypharmacy decreases medication compliance, increases risk of adverse drug events, and might lead to impaired functional status and cognitive impairment in elderly patients (59). Furthermore, co-medication can also interfere with disease-modifying medication, and subsequently increase side effects or reduce treatment efficacy (60). Accordingly, co-medication could play an important role in the choice of pharmacological treatment in IPF. Expected risk–benefit ratio, comorbidities, and co-medication should be taken into account before pharmacological treatment is started in individual patients.

MEASURING QOL AND MONITORING TREATMENT RESPONSE

It remains challenging how to measure patients' disease burden, experiences, and response to treatment in IPF. For this purpose, it is important to receive structured patient input throughout the whole disease course, starting already when the diagnosis is established. At present, digital solutions can facilitate more collaboration with patients in monitoring disease behavior, their experiences, and response to therapy (**Figure 2**).

Patient-Reported Outcome Measures (PROMs) in IPF

A PRO is defined as "any report of the status of a patient's health condition that comes directly from the patient, without interpretation of the patient's response by a clinician or anyone else" (61). Patient-reported outcome measures (PROMs) can be used to measure (HR)QOL, assess symptoms, and evaluate disease progression. There is a difference between generic and disease-specific PROMs. Disease-specific PROMs are developed to assess symptoms and (HR)QOL in a specific disease, whereas generic PROMs address more general questions and can be used in the whole population (62). One of the most commonly used generic PROMs in IPF trials are the short-form 36 and the Euroqol-5D, which is also a widely accepted instrument for economic evaluation in healthcare (63, 64). An overview of the most widely used PROMs in IPF is given in **Table 1**.

Disease-Specific PROMs

Although PROMs can play an important role to improve care for IPF, only a few well-validated, disease-specific questionnaires have been developed (19). Until a few years ago, most questionnaires used in clinical trials in IPF were originally intended for other chronic diseases (64, 65, 68). The validity of these questionnaires, such as the Saint George Respiratory Questionnaire (SGRQ) and COPD Assessment Test, has been confirmed in patients with IPF (66, 68). For the SGRQ, even an adapted version, the SGRQ-I, has been developed (67). This revised PROM consists of questions from the original SGRQ that were most relevant for patients with IPF. The reliability and validity of the SGRQ-I are comparable with the SGRQ. However, PROMs which are developed in a target population from the start, are thought to be more precise in capturing changes in HRQOL for this group of patients

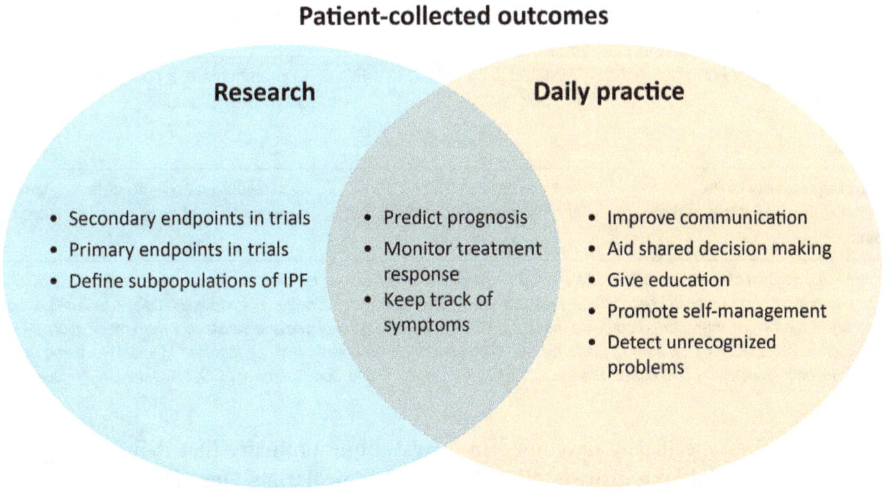

FIGURE 2 | Patient-reported and recorded outcomes can be used to enhance personalized treatment.

TABLE 1 | Overview of most used patient-reported outcomes in IPF.

Patient-reported outcome measure	Description	Validation studies and MCID	Advantages	Disadvantages
Disease-specific				
SGRQ (65)	Fifty-item questionnaire with three domains assessing HRQOL in chronic respiratory diseases	Validated in IPF; MCID in IPF: five to eight points (66)	Used in many clinical trials in IPF	Originally developed for COPD and asthma; lengthy, difficult questionnaire
SGRQ-I (67)	IPF-specific version of original SGRQ; contains 34 items	Validity comparable with SGRQ	Questions more relevant for IPF than SGRQ	Responsiveness and MCID not known yet; limited experience
CAT (68)	Composed of eight symptom items on a 0–5 response scale	Validated in IPF	Simple and quick instrument	Originally developed for COPD; limited experience in IPF
K-BILD (21)	Fifteen-item health status questionnaire in ILD with three domains	Validated in IPF MCID in IPF: five points (69)	Brief developed in ILD including IPF patients	Limited experience in clinical trials, though increasingly used
L-IPF (70) (revised version ATAQ-IPF)	Contains two modules with different domains	Currently in validation process	Adapted with feedback from patients	Not available yet
IPF-PROM (71)	Concise questionnaire to asses QOL in IPF	Study is ongoing	Developed with patients and caregivers	Not available yet
PESaM (72)	Generic and disease-specific module; evaluates patients' expectations, experiences, and satisfaction with disease-modifying drugs	Currently in validation process	Developed together with IPF patients	Not validated yet; responsiveness unknown
IPF-PREM (73)	Questionnaire to assess experiences with care delivery	Study is ongoing	Measures experiences of patients	Not available yet
Domain-specific				
UCSD (74)	Contains 24 items on a 0–5 response scale assessing dyspnea in the last week	Validated in IPF; MCID in IPF: eight points	Already used in different IPF trials; valid to assess change in dyspnea in IPF	Takes considerably more time compared with other dyspnea measures; not originally developed in IPF
mMRC (75)	Consists of one question with five grades for the level of dyspnea	Not validated in IPF	Quick, easy tool for use in daily practice; relates to disease progression	Responsiveness in IPF unclear; not originally developed in IPF
BDI-TDI (76)	BDI scores three components of dyspnea on baseline; TDI measures changes compared with baseline	Not validated in IPF; MCID in COPD: one point (76)	Measures both baseline and change over time	Only interview-administered or computerized version; not originally developed in IPF
Borg Scale (77)	Level of dyspnea scored on a scale from 0 to 10	Not validated in IPF; MCID in COPD: one point (78)	Useful during 6-min walk test in daily practice	Only measures dyspnea during exertion, does not measure dyspnea over time; not originally developed in IPF
HADS (79)	Consist of 14 items in the subscales anxiety and depression	Not validated in IPF; MCID in COPD: 1.5 points (79)	Reliable screening tool for anxiety and depression	Should not be used as diagnostic test; not originally developed in IPF
CQLQ (80)	Consists of 28 cough-specific questions in six domains	Validated in IPF; MCID in IPF: five points	Comprehensive; responsive outcome measure	Good validity for total score in IPF, but not for all domains; limited experience in IPF; not originally developed in IPF
LCQ (81)	Chronic cough quality of life questionnaire with 19 items in three domains	Not validated in IPF; MCID in chronic cough: 1.3 points (82)	High reliability; ability to detect a response to change	Limited experience in IPF; not originally developed in IPF

IPF, idiopathic pulmonary fibrosis; MCID, minimal clinically important difference; ILD, interstitial lung disease; HRQOL, health-related quality of life; SGRQ, Saint George Respiratory Questionnaire; K-BILD, Kings' Brief Interstitial Lung Disease health status questionnaire; L-IPF, living with idiopathic pulmonary fibrosis; ATAQ-IPF, a tool to assess quality of life in IPF; IPF-PROM, idiopathic pulmonary fibrosis—patient-reported outcome measure; PESaM, patient experiences and satisfaction with medication; IPF-PREM, idiopathic pulmonary fibrosis—patient-reported experience measure; UCSD, University of California San Diego shortness of breath; mMRC, modified Medical Research Council; BDI-TDI, baseline and transition dyspnea indexes; HADS, Hospital Anxiety and Depression Scale; CQLQ, Cough Quality of Life Questionnaire; LCQ, Leicester Cough Questionnaire.

(58). One of the first questionnaires specifically developed in a population of patients with interstitial lung diseases (ILDs), among whom patients with IPF, is the Kings' Brief Interstitial Lung Disease health status questionnaire (21). This is a brief, valid questionnaire that is increasingly used in IPF and other ILD clinical trials. One of the emerging PROMs in IPF is the "living with idiopathic pulmonary fibrosis" (L-IPF) questionnaire, which is a revised, electronic version of the ATAQ-IPF (a tool to assess quality of life in IPF). The L-IPF was adapted from the ATAQ-IPF following feedback from patients, and a validation study is underway at the moment (70). Another questionnaire which is currently being developed with the help of a multidisciplinary group of patients and carers is the IPF-PROM (71).

Domain-Specific PROMs

Additionally, domain-specific PROMs, which are questionnaires related to a specific symptom or organ, can be used to capture and objectify different aspects of disease. A few measures to evaluate breathlessness, such as the University of California San Diego Shortness of Breath Questionnaire, the modified Medical Research Council scale, the baseline and transition dyspnea indexes, and the Borg scale, are commonly used in IPF, although none were originally developed for IPF (74–77). Even though cough is a major problem in IPF, no specific cough questionnaires for IPF exist. However, the Leicester Cough Questionnaire and the Cough Quality of Life Questionnaire are currently used instead (80, 83). A widely known PROM to assess anxiety and depression is the Hospital Anxiety and Depression Scale, which is increasingly used in IPF (79). No specific fatigue questionnaires for IPF exist; however, the Fatigue Assessment Scale, originally developed for sarcoidosis, is used and might be adapted for IPF in the future (84).

PROs in Research and Daily Practice

PROs could be very helpful to enhance personalized treatment in IPF (**Figure 2**). Until now, PROMs have been mainly used for research purposes, as a secondary endpoint in clinical trials. The most used primary endpoint in IPF trials is forced vital capacity, which is accepted as a surrogate measure for mortality (85). One study showed that HRQOL, assessed with the SGRQ, is also an independent prognostic factor for mortality in IPF (86). PROMs probably reflect another dimension of disease compared with traditional physiological parameters (86). In the future, PROMs could possibly be used to predict treatment success in IPF.

PROM uses in daily practice can allow healthcare providers and patients to gain more insight into the individual disease and patient behavior. In a study of Sampson et al. (46), most patients were uncertain about their own disease course and progression and had difficulties interpreting objective hospital-based parameters. PROMs could allow both patients and healthcare providers to keep track of symptoms and disease progression easily. PRO results can even be used as a simple tool to communicate with patients, educate them, promote self-management, and aid shared decision making during the course of the disease (19, 87). A systematic review in oncology has shown strong evidence that routine collecting of PROs improved patient-centered care, patient satisfaction, and detection of unrecognized problems (88).

Patient-Reported Experience Measures in IPF

Optimal treatment requires close monitoring of the balance between the effects and side effects of disease-modifying drugs. Nonetheless, to our knowledge, a reliable measure to assess patient experiences with medication in IPF is not yet available in clinical practice. For this reason, a consortium of doctors, scientists, and patient representatives has joined forces to develop the patient experiences and satisfaction with medications (PESaM) questionnaire, which has a generic module and a disease-specific part for IPF (84). The PESaM questionnaire focuses on perceived effectiveness, side effects, and ease of use of medication and its impact on patients' lives. This patient-reported experience measure (PREM) could not only be used in future clinical trials, but also in clinical practice to help with better detection of side effects and adjustment of medication. Moreover, Russell and colleagues, together with patients, are currently developing the "IPF-PREM." This is a measure to assess patient experiences with healthcare and can possibly be used to improve the quality of care for patients (69).

Home Monitoring

Ideally, for a better tailored treatment, frequent monitoring with a low burden for the patient is needed. In the last decade, the use of e-health in chronic diseases has been growing, and shows mostly promising results (89–91). E-health involves the exchange of data between a patient and a healthcare provider using information and communication technologies (92). By using e-health tools, patients may better understand their health condition and become actively involved in the management of their own disease. It allows frequent monitoring in between regular visits and collection of PROs at home (93). Recently, a study showed that daily home spirometry in a population of patients with IPF was highly feasible and informative (94). Home-based spirometry predicts disease decline and mortality better than hospital-based measurements. Routine home spirometry could be very helpful to identify patients with rapid decline in lung function and to evaluate response to treatment. The authors suggest that daily home spirometry will allow for more individualized patient care. The feasibility of home-based spirometry in IPF was confirmed by Johannson et al. (95), who additionally showed that home spirometry might reduce sample size as well as the length of future clinical trials. Another promising example of home monitoring in IPF is the longitudinal follow-up of physical activity with activity trackers worn by patients at home (96). Decline in physical activity can provide reliable, objective data on disease progression and could be integrated into a home monitoring program. A comprehensive home monitoring program, consisting of an e-health tool combined with home spirometry and online collecting of PROs, has the potential to enhance trial design, stimulate self-management, allow for early treatment adaption to minimize side effects, prevent hospital admissions, and subsequently improve personalized management and QOL for patients with IPF.

CONCLUSION

The potential to enhance personalized treatment has prompted excitement also in the IPF field. In the future, patients' genetic, biomarker, and microbiome profiles may guide clinical trial design and treatment decisions. In this process, patient perspectives should not be overlooked. Only by integrating biological information with patient-reported and patient-collected information, will we be able to realize truly personalized treatment.

AUTHOR CONTRIBUTIONS

All authors conceptualized and designed the review, CM and MW wrote the paper, PH and MK provided critical feedback and input. All authors agree to be accountable for the content of the work and approved the manuscript.

REFERENCES

1. Potter P. *Hippocrates Vol VI. Diseases, Internal Affections*. Cambridge, MA, London: Harvard University Press, William Heinemann LTD (1988).
2. American Thoracic Society, European Respiratory Society. American Thoracic Society/European Respiratory Society international multidisciplinary consensus classification of the idiopathic interstitial pneumonias. This joint statement of the American Thoracic Society (ATS), and the European Respiratory Society (ERS) was adopted by the ATS board of directors, June 2001 and by the ERS Executive Committee, June 2001. *Am J Respir Crit Care Med* (2002) 165(2):277–304. doi:10.1164/ajrccm.165.2.ats01
3. Raghu G, Collard HR, Egan JJ, Martinez FJ, Behr J, Brown KK, et al. An official ATS/ERS/JRS/ALAT statement: idiopathic pulmonary fibrosis: evidence-based guidelines for diagnosis and management. *Am J Respir Crit Care Med* (2011) 183(6):788–824. doi:10.1164/rccm.2009-040GL
4. *The Voice of the Patient: A Series of Reports from the U.S. Food and Drug Administration's (FDA's) Patient-Focused Drug Development Initiative*. Center for Drug Evaluation and Research (CDER) US Food and Drug Administration (FDA) (2015).
5. Richeldi L, du Bois RM, Raghu G, Azuma A, Brown KK, Costabel U, et al. Efficacy and safety of nintedanib in idiopathic pulmonary fibrosis. *N Engl J Med* (2014) 370(22):2071–82. doi:10.1056/NEJMoa1402584
6. King TE Jr, Bradford WZ, Castro-Bernardini S, Fagan EA, Glaspole I, Glassberg MK, et al. A phase 3 trial of pirfenidone in patients with idiopathic pulmonary fibrosis. *N Engl J Med* (2014) 370(22):2083–92. doi:10.1056/NEJMoa1402582
7. Spagnolo P, Tzouvelekis A, Maher TM. Personalized medicine in idiopathic pulmonary fibrosis: facts and promises. *Curr Opin Pulm Med* (2015) 21(5):470–8. doi:10.1097/MCP.0000000000000187
8. Macagno F, Varone F, Leone PM, Mari PV, Panico L, Berardini L, et al. New treatment directions for IPF: current status of ongoing and upcoming clinical trials. *Expert Rev Respir Med* (2017) 11(7):533–48. doi:10.1080/17476348.2017.1335601
9. Di Paolo A, Sarkozy F, Ryll B, Siebert U. Personalized medicine in Europe: not yet personal enough? *BMC Health Serv Res* (2017) 17(1):289. doi:10.1186/s12913-017-2205-4
10. Clarke DL, Murray LA, Crestani B, Sleeman MA. Is personalised medicine the key to heterogeneity in idiopathic pulmonary fibrosis? *Pharmacol Ther* (2017) 169:35–46. doi:10.1016/j.pharmthera.2016.09.010
11. Spagnolo P, Cottin V. Genetics of idiopathic pulmonary fibrosis: from mechanistic pathways to personalised medicine. *J Med Genet* (2017) 54(2):93–9. doi:10.1136/jmedgenet-2016-103973
12. Ley B, Collard HR, King TE Jr. Clinical course and prediction of survival in idiopathic pulmonary fibrosis. *Am J Respir Crit Care Med* (2011) 183(4):431–40. doi:10.1164/rccm.201006-0894CI
13. Ebrahim S. Clinical and public health perspectives and applications of health-related quality of life measurement. *Soc Sci Med* (1995) 41(10):1383–94. doi:10.1016/0277-9536(95)00116-O
14. Swigris JJ, Stewart AL, Gould MK, Wilson SR. Patients' perspectives on how idiopathic pulmonary fibrosis affects the quality of their lives. *Health Qual Life Outcomes* (2005) 3:61. doi:10.1186/1477-7525-3-61
15. Duck A, Spencer LG, Bailey S, Leonard C, Ormes J, Caress AL. Perceptions, experiences and needs of patients with idiopathic pulmonary fibrosis. *J Adv Nurs* (2015) 71(5):1055–65. doi:10.1111/jan.12587
16. Overgaard D, Kaldan G, Marsaa K, Nielsen TL, Shaker SB, Egerod I. The lived experience with idiopathic pulmonary fibrosis: a qualitative study. *Eur Respir J* (2016) 47(5):1472–80. doi:10.1183/13993003.01566-2015
17. Russell AM, Ripamonti E, Vancheri C. Qualitative European survey of patients with idiopathic pulmonary fibrosis: patients' perspectives of the disease and treatment. *BMC Pulm Med* (2016) 16:10. doi:10.1186/s12890-016-0171-y
18. Yount SE, Beaumont JL, Chen SY, Kaiser K, Wortman K, Van Brunt DL, et al. Health-related quality of life in patients with idiopathic pulmonary fibrosis. *Lung* (2016) 194(2):227–34. doi:10.1007/s00408-016-9850-y
19. Wijsenbeek M, van Manen M, Bonella F. New insights on patient-reported outcome measures in idiopathic pulmonary fibrosis: only PROMises? *Curr Opin Pulm Med* (2016) 22(5):434–41. doi:10.1097/MCP.0000000000000294
20. Swigris JJ, Esser D, Conoscenti CS, Brown KK. The psychometric properties of the St George's Respiratory Questionnaire (SGRQ) in patients with idiopathic pulmonary fibrosis: a literature review. *Health Qual Life Outcomes* (2014) 12:124. doi:10.1186/s12955-014-0124-1
21. Patel AS, Siegert RJ, Brignall K, Gordon P, Steer S, Desai SR, et al. The development and validation of the King's Brief Interstitial Lung Disease (K-BILD) health status questionnaire. *Thorax* (2012) 67(9):804–10. doi:10.1136/thoraxjnl-2012-201581
22. Britten N, Pope C, Halford S, Richeldi L. What if we made stratified medicine work for patients? *Lancet Respir Med* (2016) 4(1):8–10. doi:10.1016/S2213-2600(15)00499-3
23. Ziegelstein RC. Personomics. *JAMA Intern Med* (2015) 175(6):888–9. doi:10.1001/jamainternmed.2015.0861
24. MRC. (2017). Available from: https://www.mrc.ac.uk/research/initiatives/stratified-medicine/
25. Brownell R, Kaminski N, Woodruff PG, Bradford WZ, Richeldi L, Martinez FJ, et al. Precision medicine: the new frontier in idiopathic pulmonary fibrosis. *Am J Respir Crit Care Med* (2016) 193(11):1213–8. doi:10.1164/rccm.201601-0169CI
26. Sykiotis GP, Kalliolias GD, Papavassiliou AG. Pharmacogenetic principles in the Hippocratic writings. *J Clin Pharmacol* (2005) 45(11):1218–20. doi:10.1177/0091270005281091
27. Daccord C, Maher TM. Recent advances in understanding idiopathic pulmonary fibrosis. *F1000Res* (2016) 5:F1000 Faculty Rev–1046. doi:10.12688/f1000research.8209.1
28. Dietel M. Molecular pathology: a requirement for precision medicine in cancer. *Oncol Res Treat* (2016) 39(12):804–10. doi:10.1159/000453085
29. Vargas AJ, Harris CC. Biomarker development in the precision medicine era: lung cancer as a case study. *Nat Rev Cancer* (2016) 16(8):525–37. doi:10.1038/nrc.2016.56
30. Hoyne GF, Elliott H, Mutsaers SE, Prele CM. Idiopathic pulmonary fibrosis and a role for autoimmunity. *Immunol Cell Biol* (2017) 95(7):577–83. doi:10.1038/icb.2017.22
31. Maher TM. Beyond the diagnosis of idiopathic pulmonary fibrosis; the growing role of systems biology and stratified medicine. *Curr Opin Pulm Med* (2013) 19(5):460–5. doi:10.1097/MCP.0b013e328363f4b7
32. Hambly N, Shimbori C, Kolb M. Molecular classification of idiopathic pulmonary fibrosis: personalized medicine, genetics and biomarkers. *Respirology* (2015) 20(7):1010–22. doi:10.1111/resp.12569
33. Ley B, Brown KK, Collard HR. Molecular biomarkers in idiopathic pulmonary fibrosis. *Am J Physiol Lung Cell Mol Physiol* (2014) 307(9):L681–91. doi:10.1152/ajplung.00014.2014
34. Fingerlin TE, Murphy E, Zhang W, Peljto AL, Brown KK, Steele MP, et al. Genome-wide association study identifies multiple susceptibility loci for pulmonary fibrosis. *Nat Genet* (2013) 45(6):613–20. doi:10.1038/ng.2609
35. Seibold MA, Wise AL, Speer MC, Steele MP, Brown KK, Loyd JE, et al. A common MUC5B promoter polymorphism and pulmonary fibrosis. *N Engl J Med* (2011) 364(16):1503–12. doi:10.1056/NEJMoa1013660
36. Peljto AL, Zhang Y, Fingerlin TE, Ma SF, Garcia JG, Richards TJ, et al. Association between the MUC5B promoter polymorphism and survival in patients with idiopathic pulmonary fibrosis. *JAMA* (2013) 309(21):2232–9. doi:10.1001/jama.2013.5827
37. Noth I, Zhang Y, Ma SF, Flores C, Barber M, Huang Y, et al. Genetic variants associated with idiopathic pulmonary fibrosis susceptibility and mortality:

a genome-wide association study. *Lancet Respir Med* (2013) 1(4):309–17. doi:10.1016/S2213-2600(13)70045-6
38. Oldham JM, Ma SF, Martinez FJ, Anstrom KJ, Raghu G, Schwartz DA, et al. TOLLIP, MUC5B, and the response to N-acetylcysteine among individuals with idiopathic pulmonary fibrosis. *Am J Respir Crit Care Med* (2015) 192(12):1475–82. doi:10.1164/rccm.201505-1010OC
39. Molyneaux PL, Cox MJ, Willis-Owen SA, Mallia P, Russell KE, Russell AM, et al. The role of bacteria in the pathogenesis and progression of idiopathic pulmonary fibrosis. *Am J Respir Crit Care Med* (2014) 190(8):906–13. doi:10.1164/rccm.201403-0541OC
40. Han MK, Zhou Y, Murray S, Tayob N, Noth I, Lama VN, et al. Lung microbiome and disease progression in idiopathic pulmonary fibrosis: an analysis of the COMET study. *Lancet Respir Med* (2014) 2(7):548–56. doi:10.1016/S2213-2600(14)70069-4
41. Molyneaux PL, Cox MJ, Wells AU, Kim HC, Ji W, Cookson WO, et al. Changes in the respiratory microbiome during acute exacerbations of idiopathic pulmonary fibrosis. *Respir Res* (2017) 18(1):29. doi:10.1186/s12931-017-0511-3
42. Molyneaux PL, Willis-Owen SAG, Cox MJ, James P, Cowman S, Loebinger M, et al. Host-microbial interactions in idiopathic pulmonary fibrosis. *Am J Respir Crit Care Med* (2017) 195(12):1640–50. doi:10.1164/rccm.201607-1408OC
43. Huang Y, Ma SF, Espindola MS, Vij R, Oldham JM, Huffnagle GB, et al. Microbes are associated with host innate immune response in idiopathic pulmonary fibrosis. *Am J Respir Crit Care Med* (2017) 196(2):208–19. doi:10.1164/rccm.201607-1525OC
44. ClinicalTrials.gov. *CleanUP IPF for the Pulmonary Trials Cooperative (CleanUp-IPF), NCT02759120*. (2017). Available from: https://clinicaltrials.gov/ct2/show/NCT02759120
45. Russell AM, Swigris JJ. What's it like to live with idiopathic pulmonary fibrosis? Ask the experts. *Eur Respir J* (2016) 47(5):1324–6. doi:10.1183/13993003.00109-2016
46. Sampson C, Gill BH, Harrison NK, Nelson A, Byrne A. The care needs of patients with idiopathic pulmonary fibrosis and their carers (CaNoPy): results of a qualitative study. *BMC Pulm Med* (2015) 15:155. doi:10.1186/s12890-015-0145-5
47. van Manen MJG, Kreuter M, van den Blink B, Oltmanns U, Palmowski K, Brunnemer E, et al. What patients with pulmonary fibrosis and their partners think: a live, educative survey in the Netherlands and Germany. *ERJ Open Res* (2017) 3(1):00065-2016. doi:10.1183/23120541.00065-2016
48. Bonella F, Wijsenbeek M, Molina-Molina M, Duck A, Mele R, Geissler K, et al. European IPF patient charter: unmet needs and a call to action for healthcare policymakers. *Eur Respir J* (2016) 47(2):597–606. doi:10.1183/13993003.01204-2015
49. Cottin V, Maher T. Long-term clinical and real-world experience with pirfenidone in the treatment of idiopathic pulmonary fibrosis. *Eur Respir Rev* (2015) 24(135):58–64. doi:10.1183/09059180.00011514
50. Koschel DCV, Skold M, Tomassetti S, Azuma A, Giot C, Yocum D, et al. Pirfenidone post-authorization safety registry (PASSPORT) – interim analysis of IPF treatment. *Eur Respir J* (2014) 44:1904.
51. van Manen MJ, Geelhoed JJ, Tak NC, Wijsenbeek MS. Optimizing quality of life in patients with idiopathic pulmonary fibrosis. *Ther Adv Respir Dis* (2017) 11(3):157–69. doi:10.1177/1753465816686743
52. Raghu G, Amatto VC, Behr J, Stowasser S. Comorbidities in idiopathic pulmonary fibrosis patients: a systematic literature review. *Eur Respir J* (2015) 46(4):1113–30. doi:10.1183/13993003.02316-2014
53. Suzuki A, Kondoh Y. The clinical impact of major comorbidities on idiopathic pulmonary fibrosis. *Respir Investig* (2017) 55(2):94–103. doi:10.1016/j.resinv.2016.11.004
54. Kreuter M, Ehlers-Tenenbaum S, Palmowski K, Bruhwyler J, Oltmanns U, Muley T, et al. Impact of comorbidities on mortality in patients with idiopathic pulmonary fibrosis. *PLoS One* (2016) 11(3):e0151425. doi:10.1371/journal.pone.0151425
55. Fulton BG, Ryerson CJ. Managing comorbidities in idiopathic pulmonary fibrosis. *Int J Gen Med* (2015) 8:309–18. doi:10.2147/IJGM.S74880
56. Hyldgaard C, Hilberg O, Bendstrup E. How does comorbidity influence survival in idiopathic pulmonary fibrosis? *Respir Med* (2014) 108(4):647–53. doi:10.1016/j.rmed.2014.01.008
57. Collard HR, Ward AJ, Lanes S, Cortney Hayflinger D, Rosenberg DM, Hunsche E. Burden of illness in idiopathic pulmonary fibrosis. *J Med Econ* (2012) 15(5):829–35. doi:10.3111/13696998.2012.680553
58. Kreuter M, Swigris J, Pittrow D, Geier S, Klotsche J, Prasse A, et al. Health related quality of life in patients with idiopathic pulmonary fibrosis in clinical practice: insights-IPF registry. *Respir Res* (2017) 18(1):139. doi:10.1186/s12931-017-0621-y
59. Maher RL, Hanlon J, Hajjar ER. Clinical consequences of polypharmacy in elderly. *Expert Opin Drug Saf* (2014) 13(1):57–65. doi:10.1517/14740338.2013.827660
60. Jo HE, Randhawa S, Corte TJ, Moodley Y. Idiopathic pulmonary fibrosis and the elderly: diagnosis and management considerations. *Drugs Aging* (2016) 33(5):321–34. doi:10.1007/s40266-016-0366-1
61. *Guidance for Industry. Patient-Reported Outocome Measures: Use in Medical Product Development to Support Labeling Claims*. US Department of Health and Human Services, Food and Drug Administration (2009). Available from: https://www.fda.gov/downloads/drugs/guidances/ucm193282.pdf
62. Black N. Patient reported outcome measures could help transform healthcare. *BMJ* (2013) 346:f167. doi:10.1136/bmj.f167
63. Brooks R. EuroQol: the current state of play. *Health Policy* (1996) 37(1):53–72. doi:10.1016/0168-8510(96)00822-6
64. Ware JE Jr, Sherbourne CD. The MOS 36-item short-form health survey (SF-36). I. Conceptual framework and item selection. *Med Care* (1992) 30(6):473–83. doi:10.1097/00005650-199206000-00002
65. Jones PW, Quirk FH, Baveystock CM. The St George's respiratory questionnaire. *Respir Med* (1991) 85(Suppl B):25–31; discussion 33–7. doi:10.1016/S0954-6111(06)80166-6
66. Swigris JJ, Brown KK, Behr J, du Bois RM, King TE, Raghu G, et al. The SF-36 and SGRQ: validity and first look at minimum important differences in IPF. *Respir Med* (2010) 104(2):296–304. doi:10.1016/j.rmed.2009.09.006
67. Yorke J, Jones PW, Swigris JJ. Development and validity testing of an IPF-specific version of the St George's respiratory questionnaire. *Thorax* (2010) 65(10):921–6. doi:10.1136/thx.2010.139121
68. Matsuda T, Taniguchi H, Ando M, Kondoh Y, Kimura T, Kataoka K, et al. COPD assessment test for measurement of health status in patients with idiopathic pulmonary fibrosis: a cross-sectional study. *Respirology* (2017) 22(4):721–7. doi:10.1111/resp.12936
69. Sinha APAS, Birring SS. The King's Brief Interstitial Lung Disease (K-BILD) questionnaire; an updated minimal important difference. *Eur Respir J* (2016) 48(Suppl 60):PA808. doi:10.1183/13993003.congress-2016.PA808
70. Graney B, Johnson N, Evans CJ, Ryan A, Matsui A, Raimundo K, et al. Living with idiopathic pulmonary fibrosis (L-IPF): developing a patient-reported symptom and impact questionnaire to assess health-related quality of life in IPF. *Am J Respir Crit Care Med* (2017) 195:A5353.
71. Russell AM, Doyle AM, Fleming S, Burdett C, Ross D, Aden Z, et al. Development of a patient reported outcome measure (PROM) in idiopathic pulmonary fibrosis (IPF): incorporating a research partnership with patients. *Am J Respir Crit Care Med* (2015) 191:A5190.
72. Kimman ML, Rotteveel AH, Wijsenbeek M, Mostard R, Tak NC, van Jaarsveld X, et al. Development and pretesting of a questionnaire to assess patient experiences and satisfaction with medications (PESaM questionnaire). *Patient* (2017) 10(5):629–42. doi:10.1007/s40271-017-0234-z
73. Russell AM, Sonecha S, Datta A, Hewitt R, Howell I, Elliott A, Wickremasinghe M. Development of patient reported experience measure (PREM) for idiopathic pulmonary fibrosis (IPF). *Thorax* (2016) 71:A238. doi:10.1136/thoraxjnl-2016-209333.419
74. Swigris JJ, Han M, Vij R, Noth I, Eisenstein EL, Anstrom KJ, et al. The UCSD shortness of breath questionnaire has longitudinal construct validity in idiopathic pulmonary fibrosis. *Respir Med* (2012) 106(10):1447–55. doi:10.1016/j.rmed.2012.06.018
75. Nishiyama O, Taniguchi H, Kondoh Y, Kimura T, Kato K, Kataoka K, et al. A simple assessment of dyspnoea as a prognostic indicator in idiopathic pulmonary fibrosis. *Eur Respir J* (2010) 36(5):1067–72. doi:10.1183/09031936.00152609
76. Mahler DA, Witek TJ Jr. The MCID of the transition dyspnea index is a total score of one unit. *COPD* (2005) 2(1):99–103. doi:10.1081/COPD-200050666
77. Borg GA. Psychophysical bases of perceived exertion. *Med Sci Sports Exerc* (1982) 14(5):377–81. doi:10.1249/00005768-198205000-00012
78. Jones PW, Beeh KM, Chapman KR, Decramer M, Mahler DA, Wedzicha JA. Minimal clinically important differences in pharmacological trials. *Am J Respir Crit Care Med* (2014) 189(3):250–5. doi:10.1164/rccm.201310-1863PP

79. Matsuda T, Taniguchi H, Ando M, Kondoh Y, Kimura T, Kataoka K, et al. Depression is significantly associated with the health status in patients with idiopathic pulmonary fibrosis. *Intern Med* (2017) 56(13):1637–44. doi:10.2169/internalmedicine.56.7019
80. Lechtzin N, Hilliard ME, Horton MR. Validation of the cough quality-of-life questionnaire in patients with idiopathic pulmonary fibrosis. *Chest* (2013) 143(6):1745–9. doi:10.1378/chest.12-2870
81. Birring SS, Prudon B, Carr AJ, Singh SJ, Morgan MD, Pavord ID. Development of a symptom specific health status measure for patients with chronic cough: Leicester Cough Questionnaire (LCQ). *Thorax* (2003) 58(4):339–43. doi:10.1136/thorax.58.4.339
82. Raj AA, Pavord DI, Birring SS. Clinical cough IV: what is the minimal important difference for the Leicester Cough Questionnaire? *Handb Exp Pharmacol* (2009) 187:311–20. doi:10.1007/978-3-540-79842-2_16
83. Key AL, Holt K, Hamilton A, Smith JA, Earis JE. Objective cough frequency in idiopathic pulmonary fibrosis. *Cough* (2010) 6:4. doi:10.1186/1745-9974-6-4
84. Kotecha J, Atkins C, Wilson A. Patient confidence and quality of life in idiopathic pulmonary fibrosis and sarcoidosis. *Sarcoidosis Vasc Diffuse Lung Dis* (2016) 33(4):341–8.
85. Collard HR, Bradford WZ, Cottin V, Flaherty KR, King TE Jr, Koch GG, et al. A new era in idiopathic pulmonary fibrosis: considerations for future clinical trials. *Eur Respir J* (2015) 46(1):243–9. doi:10.1183/09031936.00200614
86. Furukawa T, Taniguchi H, Ando M, Kondoh Y, Kataoka K, Nishiyama O, et al. The St. George's Respiratory Questionnaire as a prognostic factor in IPF. *Respir Res* (2017) 18(1):18. doi:10.1186/s12931-017-0503-3
87. Santana MJ, Feeny D. Framework to assess the effects of using patient-reported outcome measures in chronic care management. *Qual Life Res* (2014) 23(5):1505–13. doi:10.1007/s11136-013-0596-1
88. Chen J, Ou L, Hollis SJ. A systematic review of the impact of routine collection of patient reported outcome measures on patients, providers and health organisations in an oncologic setting. *BMC Health Serv Res* (2013) 13:211. doi:10.1186/1472-6963-13-211
89. Koff PB, Jones RH, Cashman JM, Voelkel NF, Vandivier RW. Proactive integrated care improves quality of life in patients with COPD. *Eur Respir J* (2009) 33(5):1031–8. doi:10.1183/09031936.00063108
90. Rasmussen LM, Phanareth K, Nolte H, Backer V. Internet-based monitoring of asthma: a long-term, randomized clinical study of 300 asthmatic subjects. *J Allergy Clin Immunol* (2005) 115(6):1137–42. doi:10.1016/j.jaci.2005.03.030
91. Denis F, Lethrosne C, Pourel N, Molinier O, Pointreau Y, Domont J, et al. Randomized trial comparing a web-mediated follow-up with routine surveillance in lung cancer patients. *J Natl Cancer Inst* (2017) 109:9. doi:10.1093/jnci/djx029
92. World Health Organization. *eHealth*. (2017). Available from: http://www.who.int/ehealth/en/
93. Wicks P, Stamford J, Grootenhuis MA, Haverman L, Ahmed S. Innovations in e-health. *Qual Life Res* (2014) 23(1):195–203. doi:10.1007/s11136-013-0458-x
94. Russell AM, Adamali H, Molyneaux PL, Lukey PT, Marshall RP, Renzoni EA, et al. Daily home spirometry: an effective tool for detecting progression in idiopathic pulmonary fibrosis. *Am J Respir Crit Care Med* (2016) 194(8):989–97. doi:10.1164/rccm.201511-2152OC
95. Johannson KA, Vittinghoff E, Morisset J, Lee JS, Balmes JR, Collard HR. Home monitoring improves endpoint efficiency in idiopathic pulmonary fibrosis. *Eur Respir J* (2017) 50(1):1602406. doi:10.1183/13993003.02406-2016
96. Bahmer T, Kirsten AM, Waschki B, Rabe KF, Magnussen H, Kirsten D, et al. Prognosis and longitudinal changes of physical activity in idiopathic pulmonary fibrosis. *BMC Pulm Med* (2017) 17(1):104. doi:10.1186/s12890-017-0444-0

19

Protective Role of the Nucleic Acid Sensor STING in Pulmonary Fibrosis

Florence Savigny, Corinne Schricke, Norinne Lacerda-Queiroz, Mélanie Meda, Mégane Nascimento, Sarah Huot-Marchand, Felipe Da Gama Monteiro, Bernhard Ryffel, Aurélie Gombault, Marc Le Bert, Isabelle Couillin and Nicolas Riteau**

Experimental and Molecular Immunology and Neurogenetics Laboratory (INEM), CNRS Orleans (UMR7355) and University of Orleans, Orleans, France

***Correspondence:**
Isabelle Couillin
couillin@cnrs-orleans.fr
Nicolas Riteau
nicolas.riteau@cnrs-orleans.fr

Idiopathic pulmonary fibrosis (IPF) is the most common and severe type of interstitial lung disease for which current treatments display limited efficacy. IPF is largely driven by host-derived danger signals released upon recurrent local tissue damage. Here we explored the roles of self-DNA and stimulator of interferon genes (STING), a protein belonging to an intracellular DNA sensing pathway that leads to type I and/or type III interferon (IFN) production upon activation. Using a mouse model of IPF, we report that STING deficiency leads to exacerbated pulmonary fibrosis with increased collagen deposition in the lungs and excessive remodeling factors expression. We further show that STING-mediated protection does not rely on type I IFN signaling nor on IL-17A or TGF-β modulation but is associated with dysregulated neutrophils. Together, our data support an unprecedented immunoregulatory function of STING in lung fibrosis.

Keywords: idiopathic pulmonary fibrosis, STING, self-DNA recognition, mice, IL-28

INTRODUCTION

Idiopathic pulmonary fibrosis (IPF) is the most common type of idiopathic interstitial pneumonia (1, 2), characterized by progressive lung scarring causing shorter life expectancy and high mortality rate (2, 3). While the etiology is still unclear, it is believed that the physiopathology relies on repeated local micro-injuries triggering DNA damage, unbalanced cell death and aberrant tissue remodeling with extracellular matrix components and ultimately fibrosis (1–4). Immune cells such as macrophages, neutrophils and T helper 17 (Th17) cells recruited to the lung tissue are known to display important proinflammatory and profibrotic functions (5). Self-derived danger-associated molecular patterns (DAMPS) are considered as important contributors (6), such as ATP (7) and uric acid (8) to the pathology. In this study, we hypothesize that self-nucleic acid sensing might also contribute to IPF. Pathogen-derived nucleic acid sensing through pathogen recognition receptors (PRRs) is an effective strategy to detect invading microorganisms and trigger innate and adaptive immune responses (9). However, recent literature clearly established that PRRs such as STING are also involved in self-nucleic acid sensing (10, 11). STING is an endoplasmic reticulum (ER)-associated membrane protein activated by cyclic dinucleotides (CDNs) produced as second messengers by microorganisms or synthesized by enzymes such as cyclic GMP-AMP synthase (cGAS) in response to binding either host- or pathogen-derived cytosolic dsDNA (12, 13). Of note, in addition to cGAS other cytosolic receptors such as DDX41 and IFI16 sense DNA or CDNs to activate STING (12, 13). Activated STING translocates from the ER membrane to the Golgi apparatus, induces nuclear factor κB (NF-κB) and interferon regulatory factor 3 (IRF3) transcription factors activation leading to the production of type I IFNs and other cytokines involved in host immune responses (14). Recent studies showed that STING stimulation can also lead to type III interferon production (15–17). The type III IFN family comprises IFN-λ1 (IL-29), IFN-λ2 (IL-28A), IFN-λ3 (IL-28B), and the newly identified IFN-λ4 in human and IFN-λ2 (IL-28A) and IFN-λ3 (IL-28B) in mice (18). Type III IFN are less well characterized and are thought to function similarly as type I IFN, although in a more restricted manner as their effects are most evident on epithelial cells and neutrophils (18, 19).

Detection of aberrant self-nucleic acids in the cytosol, either mitochondrial DNA (mtDNA) or nuclear DNA (14, 20), is implicated in the development of autoimmune diseases and sterile inflammation (21). Since IPF physiopathology involves unbalanced cell death processes, we investigated whether self-nucleic acid release and its sensing by the STING pathway are participating in the response (1–4). We employed the classical murine model of human IPF using airway exposure to bleomycin (BLM), a potent cytotoxic drug used as chemotherapy but causing pulmonary fibrosis in a fraction of treated patients (22). We show that intranasal BLM administration leads to increased levels of self-DNA in the airways and upregulated cGAS and STING expressions. We report that STING deficiency leads to an exacerbated lung fibrosis independently of type I IFN signaling and characterized by a prolonged neutrophilic inflammation. As a whole, our data show that STING is protective against BLM-induced pulmonary fibrosis in a mechanism that may rely on neutrophilic inflammation resolution.

MATERIAL AND METHODS

Mice

Wild-type C57BL/6J (WT) mice were purchased from Janvier laboratory (Janvier Laboratory, France). Mice deficient for STING (*Sting*$^{-/-}$) were provided by Glen Barber (23), *Cgas*$^{-/-}$ by Zhijian Chen (24) and *Ifnar1*$^{-/-}$ by Michel Aguet (25) and bred in our specific pathogen-free animal facility at CNRS (TAAM UPS44, Orleans, France). For experiments, adult (8–14-week-old) males were transferred to experimental animal facility and monitored daily.

Ethics

All animal experiments complied with the French Government animal experiment regulations and were submitted to the "Ethics Committee for Animal Experimentation of CNRS Campus Orleans" (CCO) under number CLE CCO 2015-1087 and approved under APAFIS#19361. Clinical score was determined daily based on mice appearance and behavior. Appearance was determined based on standard parameters including eye, fur and ear monitoring (https://www.nc3rs.org.uk/grimacescales) and behavior monitoring included mobility, posture and social interaction.

Treatments

Bleomycin sulfate (7.5 and 3 mg/kg for day 1 and day 14 experiments, respectively; Bellon Laboratories) in saline or saline alone were administered through the airways by nasal instillation in a volume of 40-µl under light isoflurane anesthesia.

Bronchoalveolar Lavage and Cell Counts

Mice were euthanized by CO_2 overdose using Prodigy Lab Control Unit (Smartbox) and bronchoalveolar lavage fluid (BALF) was performed as previously described (7). Differential cell counts were routinely performed on cytospin preparation (Cytospin 3, Thermo Shandon) after May-Grünwald Giemsa staining (Sigma-Aldrich, St Louis, MO) according to the manufacturer's instructions and at least 200 cells were counted using standard morphological criteria.

Lung Homogenization

After BALF collection, lungs were perfused with isoton to flush the vascular content and homogenized by a rotor-stator (Ultra-turrax®) in 1 ml of PBS. The extracts were centrifuged for 10 min at 9,000 g and the supernatants stored at -80°C.

Lung Histology

Lung left lobes were fixed in 4% buffered formaldehyde, processed and paraffin-embedded under standard conditions. Lung sections (3 µm) were stained with hematoxylin and eosin (H&E) or Sirius red/Fast green. The slides were scanned using NanoZoomer (Hamamatsu Photonics France) and lung fibrosis scored using the Ashcroft modified scale (26).

Mediator Measurement

BALF supernatants and lung homogenates were analyzed using ELISA assay kits for murine CXCL1/KC, MMP-9, and TIMP-1 according to manufacturer's instructions (R&D system, Minneapolis, MN). TGF-β1–3 contents in the lungs were assessed by multiplex assay according to manufacturer's instructions (Merck, Darmstadt, Germany).

Collagen Assay

BALF collagen content was measured using the Sircol collagen dye binding assay (Biocolor Ltd., Northern Ireland) according to the manufacturer's instructions.

Double-Stranded DNA Quantification

Cell-free double-stranded DNA (dsDNA) was measured in the BALF fluid using Quant-iTPicoGreen dsDNA reagent (Invitrogen, Carlsbad, CA), according to the manufacturer's protocol.

Quantitative PCR

RNA was purified from lung homogenates using Tri-Reagent (Sigma-Aldrich, Saint-Louis, MO) extraction protocol. RNA reverse transcription into cDNA was carried out with GoTaq qPCR-Master Mix (Promega, Madison, WI). RT-qPCR was performed with Fast SYBR Green Master mix (Promega) on an ARIA MX (Agilent Technologies, Santa Clara, CA). Primers *Tmem173* (#QT00261590) encoding for STING, *Mb21d1* (#QT00131929) encoding for cGAS, and *Fn1* (#QT00135758) encoding for fibronectin were purchased from Qiagen (Qiagen, Hilden, Germany). RNA expression was normalized to *Gapdh* (#QT00166768, Qiagen, Hilden, Germany) expression and analyzed using the ΔΔCt method.

Flow Cytometry

Lungs were cut in small pieces and digested using a 1mg/ml DNase (DN25, Sigma-Aldrich, St Louis, MO)/125 µg/ml collagenase (Liberase™, Sigma-Aldrich, St Louis, MO) solution for 45 min at 37°C and filtered on 40 µm cell strainer. BALF and lung single cell suspensions were incubated for 20 min at RT with Fc block (Thermo Fisher Scientific, Waltham, MA), washed and stained with surface markers including a Fixable Viability Dye eFluor 780 (Thermo Fisher Scientific, Waltham, MA). Cells were fixed and permeabilized using Fixation/Permeabilization kit (Thermo Fisher Scientific, Waltham, MA) and stained with intracellular markers. For IL-17 staining (clone eBio17B7), lung cell suspensions were incubated for 5 h at 37°C in presence of brefeldin A (BFA; Thermo Fisher Scientific, Waltham, MA) to prevent protein secretion. Antibody clones and dilutions used are detailed in **Supplementary Table 1**. All samples were acquired on an LSR Fortessa flow cytometer (BD Biosciences, San Jose, CA) and analyzed using FlowJo software (TreeStar).

Immunoblot

20µg of proteins (Pierce BCA protein assay, Thermo Fisher Scientific, Waltham, MA) were denatured by boiling (95°C, 5 min) in reducing SDS sample buffer, separated by SDS-PAGE and transferred to nitrocellulose membranes (GE Healthcare Life Sciences, Amersham, UK). After blocking in 5% Blotting-Grade Blocker (BioRad, France) and washing in Tris-Buffered saline (TBS)- 0,1% Tween® 20, membranes were incubated with primary mouse anti-STING (Abcam, ref ab92605), anti-cGAS (Cell Signaling Technology, ref 3165) or anti-IL-28 (Santa Cruz Biotechnology, ref sc-137151) antibodies in TBS-BSA (Bovine Serum Albumine) 1%- azide 0,5 mM overnight at 4°C. Membranes were washed and incubated with relevant secondary antibody conjugated to horseradish peroxidase (HRP) 2 h at RT. Anti-actin antibody was already HRP-conjugated (Sigma-Aldrich, ref A3854). Detection was performed with ECL Western-blotting Detection Reagent (GE Healthcare Life Sciences, Amersham, UK) and luminescence acquired using Multi-application gel imaging system PXi software (Syngene). Bands intensity were quantified using ImageJ (NIH, USA).

Immunofluorescence

Lung tissues were fixed in 4% paraformaldehyde (PFA) (Sigma-Aldrich, St Louis, MO) and then dehydrated in 30% sucrose solution for 2 weeks at 4°C. Lungs were embedded in tissue-teck (OCT®) and stored at -80°C. 10-µm lung sections were cut on cryostat (Leica, Solms, Germany) and heated at 80°C for 30 min in 10 mM citrate pH = 6. Lung cells were permeabilized with 0.5% Triton X-100, blocked in 1% BSA 10% SVF 0.1% Triton X-100 in PBS for 1 h, washed three times in TBS, and incubated overnight with rabbit anti-STING (ab92605 1/50, Abcam) in PBS containing 2% BSA, 10% FCS, and 0.5% Triton X-100 at 4°C. Lung sections were TBS washed and incubated with anti-rabbit IgG Alexa 532 secondary antibody (1/100) for 1 h at RT. After washing, cells were counterstained with DAPI for 10 min at RT, PBS washed, and mounted onto microscope slides (mowiol). Slides were observed using a Zeiss Axiovert 200M microscope coupled with a Zeiss LSM 510 Meta scanning device (Carl Zeiss Co. Ltd., Jena, Germany). The inverted microscope was equipped with a Plan-Apochromat 63X objective (NA = 1.4). Images were acquired using Zeiss LSM Image Browser (Carl Zeiss Co. Ltd., Jena, Germany).

Statistical Analyses

Statistical tests of selected populations were performed using Mann-Whitney non-parametric test. Weight variation plots were analyzed using two-way ANOVA corrected for multiple comparisons employing Tuckey's test. Results were considered significant at $p < 0.05$.

RESULTS

BLM Administration Induces Airway Self-DNA Release and Lung cGAS and STING Expressions

To address a potential role for self-DNA recognition by the cGAS/STING pathway in the establishment of pulmonary fibrosis, we measured double stranded (ds) DNA content in the bronchoalveolar lavage fluid (BALF) as well as cGAS and STING expressions in the lungs at the fibrotic phase (14 days after BLM instillation). As compared to saline (NaCl) control wild-type (WT) mice, we noted that dsDNA content is significantly increased in the BALF of BLM-treated WT mice (**Figure 1A**) and BLM treatment leads to a strong increase of cGAS (*Mb21d1*) (**Figure 1B**) and STING (*Tmem173*) (**Figure 1C**) gene expressions in the lungs. Of note, *Mb21d1* and *Tmem173* expressions are reduced in absence of STING and cGAS, respectively, suggesting retroactive loops at the gene expression level. We next assessed cGAS and STING protein expressions in saline- or BLM-treated WT mice, cGAS (*Cgas*$^{-/-}$) or STING (*Sting*$^{-/-}$) deficient mice. Both cGAS and STING protein expressions are increased in the lungs of BLM-treated WT mice and cGAS or STING levels are not impaired by the absence of STING or cGAS, respectively (**Figures 1D, E**). We also assessed STING expression in pulmonary tissue by immunofluorescence and show that it is expressed in both bronchial epithelial cells and infiltrating cells (**Figures 1F, G**).

Regarding the acute inflammatory phase (1 day after BLM instillation), we observed that despite a strong increase of BALF dsDNA content (**Supplementary Figure 1A**), cGAS or STING deficiency had no major impact on total BALF cell numbers (**Supplementary Figure 1B**) or neutrophil frequencies (**Supplementary Figure 1C**). Lung levels of the neutrophil attractant chemokine CXCL1 as well as the remodeling factors MMP-9 and TIMP-1 (**Supplementary Figures 1D–F**) were also unchanged among BLM-treated groups suggesting minor cGAS/STING contribution in early inflammation. Nevertheless, persistent enhanced airway dsDNA in the BALF associated with a strong increase of lung cGAS and STING expressions at

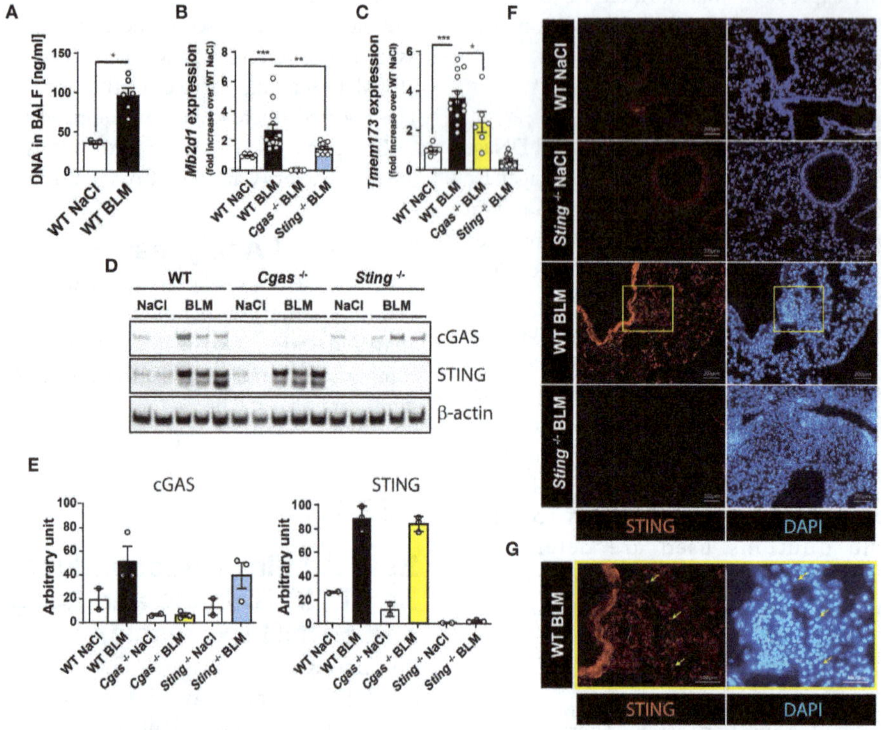

FIGURE 1 | Increased BALF dsDNA content as well as cGAS and STING expressions. C57BL/6 WT, *Cgas*$^{-/-}$ and *Sting*$^{-/-}$ mice were treated with NaCl or BLM (3 mg/kg intranasally) and BALF and lungs were collected after 14 days. **(A)** BALF cell-free dsDNA content. **(B)** *Mb21d1* (cGAS) and **(C)** *Tmem173* (STING) gene expressions. STING protein expression by **(D)** Western-Blotting and **(E)** semi-quantitative band analysis. **(F)** STING expression in the lungs assessed by immunofluorescence. The yellow box is magnified in **(G)** and yellow arrows illustrate STING positive infiltrating cells. Data are representative of 2-3 independent experiments, showed as mean ± SEM, *p < 0.05; ***p < 0.001.

the fibrotic stage led us to investigate a role for this pathway in the establishment of pulmonary fibrosis.

STING Deficiency Leads to Increased Pulmonary Fibrosis

As compared to BLM-treated WT or *Cgas*$^{-/-}$ mice, *Sting*$^{-/-}$ mice exhibit higher body weight loss (**Figure 2A**) with occasional succumbing animals. The remodeling factors MMP-9 (**Figure 2B**) and TIMP-1 (**Figure 2C**) were also increased in the lungs of STING deficient animals as compared to their WT relatives 14 days post BLM administration. This was accompanied by higher lung cell accumulation as shown by H&E staining of lung micrographs (**Figure 2D**) and CD4^{+} T lymphocyte numbers assessed by flow cytometry (**Figure 2E**). Sirius Red/Fast Green collagen staining also shows extended areas of fibrosis and increased collagen deposition (**Figure 2F**), further confirmed by fibrosis score using Ashcroft modified scale (26) (**Figure 2G**). BALF collagen content was also increased in *Sting*$^{-/-}$ mice as compared to their WT relatives (**Figure 2H**). Interestingly, BLM-treated *Cgas*$^{-/-}$ mice display intermediate bodyweight loss (**Figure 2A**), MMP-9 production (**Figure 2B**) and fibrosis (**Figures 2F, G**), suggesting that other DNA sensors might be involved. Of note, BLM-induced increased levels of the important pro-fibrotic factor TGF-β were not significantly altered in cGAS or STING deficient mice (**Figure 2I**), arguing for a role of another pro-fibrotic pathway in absence of STING.

STING-Mediated Protection Is Type I IFN Signaling Independent

STING signaling pathway is a well-characterized type I IFN inducer (14). We thus utilized mouse deficient for type I IFN receptor (*Ifnar1*$^{-/-}$) to test the hypothesis of a type I IFN-dependent role of STING. In contrast to BLM-treated *Sting*$^{-/-}$ mice, *Ifnar1*$^{-/-}$ displayed comparable body weight loss as WT mice (**Figure 3A**). In addition, lung remodeling factors MMP-9 and TIMP-1 were similarly increased comparing BLM-treated WT versus *Ifnar1*$^{-/-}$ mice, while *Sting*$^{-/-}$ mice displayed higher expressions (**Figures 3B, C**). *Ifnar1*$^{-/-}$ mice did not display enhanced lung cell influx (**Figure 3D**) and lung fibrosis as shown by representative lung histology (**Figure 3E**) and Ascroft fibrosis score (**Figure 3F**) and the expression of the extracellular matrix protein fibronectin (*Fn1*) (**Figure 3G**). Together, these results suggest that STING is protective against BLM-induced fibrosis in a type I IFN-independent manner. Since IL-17A is a major pro-fibrotic cytokine (27) and in line with a recent study showing that STING-mediated protection relies of IL-17A modulation (28), we analyzed IL-17A production by CD4^{+} T lymphocytes using flow cytometry (**Supplementary Figures 2A, B**). We show no difference in terms of frequencies (**Figure 3H**) or

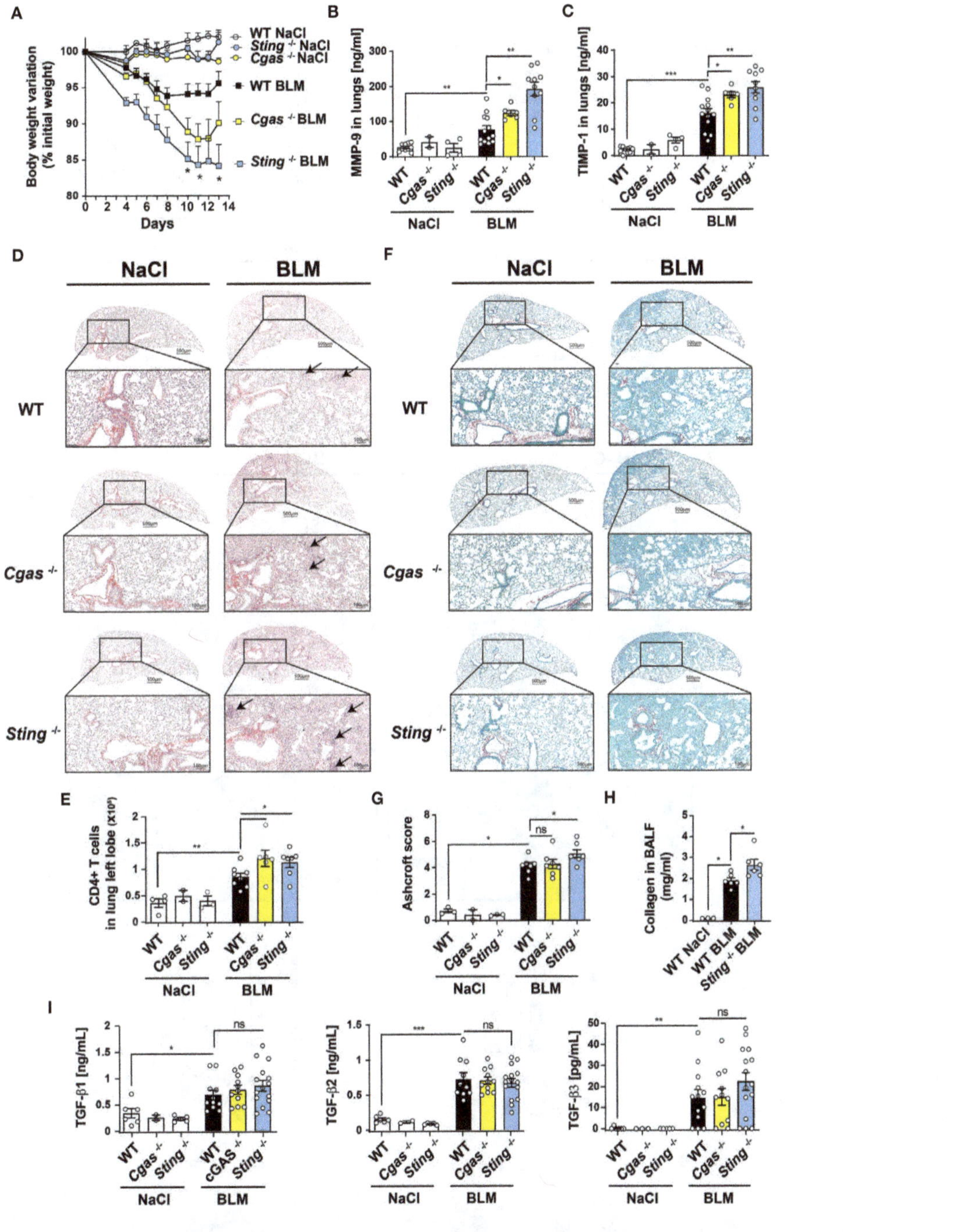

FIGURE 2 | Increased fibrosis in absence of STING. WT, *Cgas*$^{-/-}$ and *Sting*$^{-/-}$ mice were treated with NaCl or BLM (3 mg/kg intranasally) and BALF and lungs were collected after 14 days. **(A)** Body weight evolution. Asterisks depict p < 0.05 comparing BLM-treated WT and *Sting*$^{-/-}$ groups at indicated time points **(B)** MMP-9 and **(C)** TIMP-1 levels in the lungs measured by ELISA. **(D)** Lung micrographs stained by Hematoxylin and Eosin (H&E). **(E)** CD4^{+} T lymphocyte numbers in the lung left lobe. **(F)** Lung micrographs stained by Red Sirius/Fast Green highlighting collagen fibers. **(G)** Fibrosis score using Ashcroft modified scale. **(H)** BALF collagen content measured by Sircol assay. **(I)** TGF-β1-3 in the lungs measured by multiplex assay. Data are representative of 2-3 independent experiments, showed as mean ± SEM, ns: non-significant; *p < 0.05; **p < 0.01; ***p < 0.001.

total numbers (**Figure 3I**) of IL-17^{+} CD4^{+} T cells comparing WT and *Sting*$^{-/-}$ mice. Unexpectedly, *Ifnar1*$^{-/-}$ CD4^{+} T lymphocytes displayed lower frequency of IL-17+ cells in the lungs. Having excluded a major role for type I IFN and IL-17A to explain STING-dependent protection, we next investigated a potential role for IL-28 (type III IFN) (15–17). Interestingly, we show that BLM induces IL-28 in the lungs and that its production partially depends on STING (**Supplementary Figures 3A–C**).

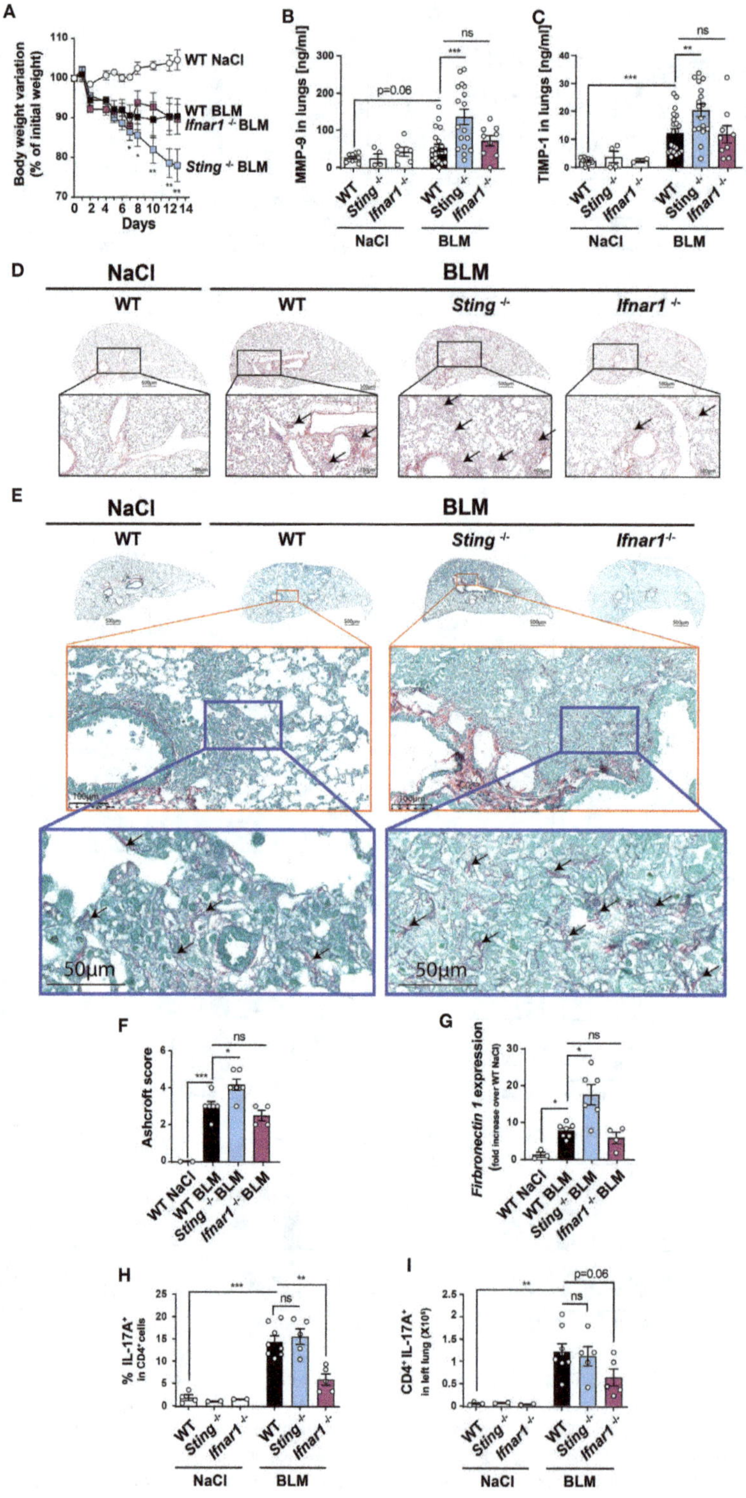

FIGURE 3 | STING deficiency leads to increased fibrosis independently of type I IFN signaling. WT, *Sting*$^{-/-}$, and type I Interferon receptor deficient (*Ifnar1*$^{-/-}$) mice were treated with NaCl or BLM (3 mg/kg intranasally), and BALF and lungs were collected after 14 days. **(A)** Body weight evolution. Asterisks depict $p < 0.05$ comparing BLM-treated WT and *Sting*$^{-/-}$ groups. **(B)** MMP-9 and **(C)** TIMP-1 levels in the lungs measured by ELISA. Lung micrographs stained by **(D)** Hematoxylin and Eosin (H&E) (black arrows show cell foci) and **(E)** Red Sirius/Fast Green highlighting collagen fibers. Higher magnification are depicted using red and blue rectangles and black arrows show collagen deposition. **(F)** Fibrosis score using Ashcroft modified scale. **(G)** Lung *fibronectin 1* gene expression by RT qPCR. **(H)** Frequencies and **(I)** total numbers of lung CD4^{+} IL-17^{+} T cells assessed by flow cytometry. Data are representative of 2-3 independent experiments, showed as mean ± SEM, ns: non-significant $^{*}p < 0.05$; $^{**}p < 0.01$; $^{***}p < 0.001$.

STING Deficiency Affects Neutrophil Numbers and Function

The fibrotic stage of the pathology is accompanied by the recruitment of adaptive immune cells. As expected, at this time point the main BALF cell populations in WT mice are $CD4^+$ and $CD8^+$ T lymphocytes as well as B lymphocytes, and the proportion of neutrophils is low (**Figures 4A, B**). In contrast, neutrophils remained high in BALF and lungs of STING-deficient mice (**Figures 4B–E** and **Supplementary Figures 4A, B**). We performed kinetic studies and found that BALF neutrophils persisted by days 8–14 post-BLM treatment (**Figure 4F**), suggesting prolonged inflammation. In addition to increased numbers in the BALF, lung STING-deficient neutrophils (**Supplementary Figure 4B**) display reduced MHC-II (I-A/I-E) upregulation following BLM treatment as compared to their WT counterparts (**Figures 4G, H**). In contrast, STING-deficient neutrophils show a strong upregulation of arginase-1 expression (**Figures 4I, J**), suggesting that STING controls neutrophil persistence and function.

DISCUSSION

STING has been identified in 2008 as an endoplasmic reticulum receptor that induces innate immune responses (29) and is currently a hot topic in several fields including cancer immunotherapy (30), vaccines (31) and autoimmunity (32, 33). Depending on the microenvironment and responsive cell types, enhancing STING signaling pathway might favor antitumor activity for instance by promoting IFN-β-dependent T cell priming (34). On the other hand, constitutive self-DNA-mediated sustained STING activation induces tolerance breakdown and autoimmunity (32, 33).

There are several STING allelic variants in the general population (35) and STING-associated vasculopathy with onset in infancy (SAVI) is an autoinflammatory disease caused by gain-of-function mutations in *TMEM173* (36, 37). Affected children display constitutive STING activation leading to increased *IFNB1* transcription and even higher transcripts levels upon cGAMP stimulation, whereas other pro-inflammatory gene levels such as interleukin-1 (*IL1*), interleukin-6 (*IL6*), and tumor necrosis factor (*TNF*) remain unaffected (36). In addition to cutaneous vasculopathy, a major feature of SAVI is interstitial lung disease (38). Of note, the STING knock-in mouse strain (V154M) corresponding to a recurrent mutation in SAVI patients exhibit a severe combined immunodeficiency disease (SCID) phenotype (39).

Here, we employed the classical murine model of idiopathic pulmonary fibrosis (IPF) induced by BLM administration in the airways. We show that BLM induces a strong increase of cell-free self-DNA in the airways, which can act as a danger signal by triggering DNA sensing pathways to activate innate immune responses (40) and notably in the lungs (11). However, the mechanisms by which self-DNA becomes accessible for intracellular DNA sensors remain uncertain. Several context-dependent pathways have been reported, such as IgG- or HMGB1-bound DNA internalization following interaction with FcγRIIa or receptor for advanced glycation end products (RAGE), respectively (41). The antimicrobial peptide LL37 was shown to transport extracellular DNA into the cytoplasm of human primary monocytes triggering STING activation (42).

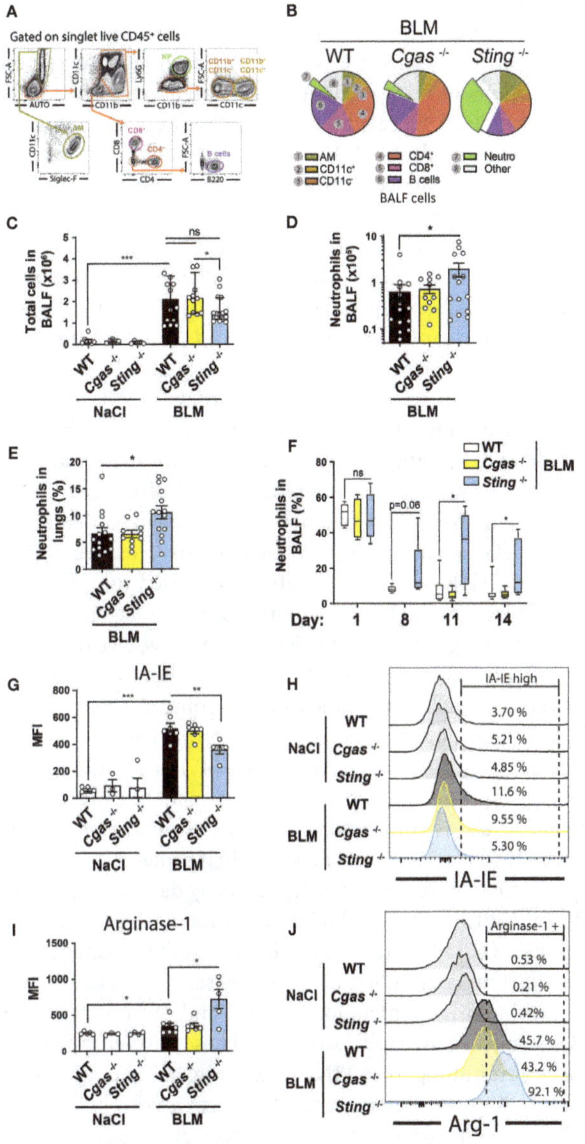

FIGURE 4 | STING deficiency leads to dysregulated neutrophils. WT, *Cgas*$^{-/-}$ and *Sting*$^{-/-}$ mice were treated with NaCl or BLM (3 mg/kg intranasally) and BALF and lungs were collected after 14 days. **(A)** Flow cytometry gating strategy used to identify **(B)** BALF cell populations. Cells are gated on singlets, live, $CD45^+$ events. NP: Neutrophils; AM: Alveolar macrophages. Total BALF cell numbers **(C)**, neutrophil **(D)** BALF total numbers and **(E)** lung percentages. **(F)** Kinetic of BALF neutrophil frequencies at indicated time points. MHC-II (I-A/I-E) **(G, H)** and arginase-1 (Arg-1) **(I, J)** Mean Fluorescence Intensity (MFI) assessed by flow cytometry. Data are representative of two to three independent experiments, showed as mean ± SEM, $^*p < 0.05$; $^{***}p < 0.001$.

IL-10-family member IL-26 binds to genomic, mtDNA or neutrophil extracellular traps (NETS) DNA and traffic them into the cytosol of human myeloid cells activating STING (43). Further investigations are required to decipher the respective contributions of nuclear DNA versus mtDNA in activating the STING pathway. Elevated plasma mtDNA copy numbers in IPF patients predicts death (44); however, it remains unsure whether mtDNA is a mere marker or whether it actually modulates pathology.

Investigating sensors involved in self-DNA recognition, our results indicate that the cGAS/STING pathway does not seem to play a major role in the early airway inflammatory response, as we did not observe major changes in terms of canonical markers such as neutrophil recruitment and remodeling factors production comparing WT versus cGAS or STING deficient mice. In contrast, our data show that STING-dependent responses are important during the fibrotic stage of the disease. First, lung cGAS and STING expressions are increased both at gene and protein levels. Interestingly, Mb21d1 (encoding for cGAS) gene expression but not cGAS protein is decreased in STING deficient animals suggesting potential cross regulation. In addition, STING deficiency leads to increased lung fibrosis, as characterized by higher histological score, collagen deposition and remodeling factors expression. A protective role of STING in IPF patients has been reported recently. Authors show that blood mononuclear cells from patients undergoing acute exacerbation display significantly reduced STING protein levels correlating with decreased partial oxygen pressure (45). In addition, patients showing clinical improvement post-treatment had higher STING protein levels as compared to patients with worsen condition (45). STING has also been shown to elicit protective responses in experimental autoimmune encephalitis by dampening effector T cell infiltration and inducing dominant T cell regulatory response (46). On the other hand, STING contributes to pathology in a number of other disease settings, including silica-induced lung inflammation (47) and carbon-tetrachloride (CCl4)-induced liver fibrosis (48). These discrepancies might reflect fine-tuning of STING signaling as well as potential differences in the kinetics and cell subsets involved.

We sought to determine STING-dependent signaling pathway mediating protection in the context of lung fibrosis and first addressed the role of type I IFN. Interestingly, our results show that STING-dependent effect does not rely on type I IFN signaling as mice deficient for its receptor do not display exacerbated pathology. While type I IFN induction is a major consequence of STING activation, several publications demonstrated that this cytokine does not directly contribute to STING-dependent effect in a number of situations. For instance, STING-associated lung disease due to a gain of function mutation in the protein (N153S) is T cell dependent but does not require IRF3/IRF7 or IFNAR (49). Similarly, SCID phenotype in STING V154M mice occurs similarly when type I IFN signaling is absent (39). STING-associated vasculopathy also develops independently of IRF3 in mice (50). Besides type I IFN induction, several publications showed STING-dependent type III IFN induction (IL-28/IL-29) in the context of viral infection (16) and exogenous DNA (17) or di-GMP mucosal adjuvant (15) stimulations. Interestingly, a SAVI patient presented increased plasma IL-29 expression (51). Here, we show that BLM triggers IL-28 and that its production is decreased in STING-deficient mice as compared to their WT relatives. Type III IFN was shown to suppress neutrophil response either by directly limiting its influx in a collagen-induced arthritis model (52) or by primarily modifying neutrophil effector functions *via* posttranslational modifications in the gut (53). Follow-up experiments are needed to delineate the exact contribution of type III interferons in experimental lung fibrosis. Another possibility to explain a protective role of STING was its potential action on IL-17A production, a potent pro-fibrotic cytokine (27). Indeed, STING deficiency was reported to enhance Th17 polarization and IL-17A production therefore promoted pancreatic inflammation and fibrosis (28). However, in our model IL-17A production by $CD4^+$ T cells was not increased in STING deficient mice as compared to their WT relatives. In our experimental setup, we found that while mice deficient for type I IFN signaling did not show altered fibrosis, their lung $CD4^+$ T lymphocytes display lower frequencies of IL-$17A^+$ cells. In addition, our data indicate that cGAS deficiency does not fully mirror STING deficiency phenotype, as BLM-treated *Cgas*$^{-/-}$ mice displayed increased expression of the fibrosis-associated remodeling factors MMP-9 and TIMP-1 as compared to WT animals but intermediate weight loss and similar Ashcroft histological score. These results suggest an intricate role of cGAS in the development of experimental lung fibrosis and that other DNA sensors might be involved such as DDX41 or IFI16 (13, 54, 55). Interestingly, it was recently shown that etoposide-induced DNA damage leads to cGAS-independent STING activation (56), while on the other hand cGAS protects hepatocytes by triggering autophagy independently of STING in mouse models of ischemia-reperfusion (57).

We report that STING deficiency leads to sustained BALF and lung neutrophil infiltration following BLM administration. Additional experiments are required to determine whether prolonged BALF and lungs neutrophil presence in the context of STING deficiency reflects different tissue lifespan and/or recurrent neutrophils recruitment. Airway neutrophilia has been associated with early mortality in IPF (58) and concentrations of the neutrophil chemoattractant CXCL8 are increased in IPF patients (59). Interestingly, we show that lung neutrophils from STING deficient mice exhibit higher levels of arginase-1. L-arginine catabolism by iNOS and arginase is related to cytotoxicity and tissue repair and classically associated with pro- versus anti-inflammatory functions of macrophages, respectively (60, 61). Interestingly, L-arginine levels in the lungs of BLM-treated mice decrease due to increased arginase-1 expression and the addition of an arginase inhibitor limits TGF-β-induced collagen production by fibroblasts (62). It remains to be investigated whether neutrophil-derived arginase-1 can influence fibroblast function. In addition, we also report lower MHC II levels on STING-deficient lung neutrophils. Neutrophil are able to perform MHC-II-mediated antigen presentation to $CD4^+$ T cells (63) and recent literature reviewed regulatory roles of neutrophils in adaptive immunity (64). However, the exact meaning of reduced MHC-II expression on STING-deficient neutrophils following BLM treatment is unclear, potentially reflecting altered T cell activation properties. As a whole, our data show an unexpected regulatory function of STING to limit BLM-induced pulmonary fibrosis associated with neutrophilic inflammation regulation.

ETHICS STATEMENT

The animal study was reviewed and approved by Ethics Committee for Animal Experimentation of CNRS Campus Orleans (CCO) 2015-1087 and APAFIS#19361.

AUTHOR CONTRIBUTIONS

FS, CS, NL-Q, MM, MN, SH-M, FG, AG, and NR performed experiments and/or analyzed data. NR and IC conceived and directed the project with assistance from AG, MB, and BR. NR and IC wrote the manuscript. All authors had the opportunity to discuss the results and comment on the manuscript. All authors contributed to the article and approved the submitted version.

ACKNOWLEDGMENTS

The authors thank Nathalie Froux, Mathilde Fravat and all technicians from our specific pathogen-free animal facility at CNRS (TAAM UPS44, Orleans, France) for breeding and animal care. We thank Valérie Quesniaux for support and helpful discussions.

SUPPLEMENTARY MATERIAL

SUPPLEMENTARY FIGURE 1 | WT, *Cgas*$^{-/-}$ and *Sting*$^{-/-}$ mice were treated with NaCl or BLM (7 mg/kg intranasally) and BALF and lungs were collected at 24 h. **(A)** BALF cell-free dsDNA content. BALF **(B)** total numbers and **(C)** neutrophil frequencies. KC/CXCL-1 **(D)**, MMP-9 **(E)** and TIMP-1 **(F)** levels in the lungs measured by ELISA. Data are a pool of two to three independent experiments showed as mean ± SEM, ns: non-significant; $^{***}p < 0.001$.

SUPPLEMENTARY FIGURE 2 | WT, *Sting*$^{-/-}$ and *Ifnar1*$^{-/-}$ mice were treated with NaCl or BLM (3 mg/kg intranasally) and lungs cells were collected after 14 days and incubated for 5 h at 37°C in presence of BFA. **(A)** Gating strategy employed to delineate lung IL-17A^{+} CD4^{+} T lymphocytes. **(B)** Representative flow cytometry plots. Data are representative of 2 independent experiments.

SUPPLEMENTARY FIGURE 3 | WT, *Cgas*$^{-/-}$, *Sting*$^{-/-}$ and *Ifnar1*$^{-/-}$ mice were treated with NaCl or BLM (3 mg/kg intranasally) and lungs were collected after 14 days. **(A)** IL-28 content in the lungs measured by ELISA and **(B)** by Western-Blotting with **(C)** semi-quantitative band analysis. Data are representative of 2 independent experiments showed as mean ± SEM, ns: non-significant; $^{*}p < 0.05$

SUPPLEMENTARY FIGURE 4 | Gating strategy used to delineate neutrophil populations **(A)** in the BALF and **(B)** in the lungs by flow cytometry.

REFERENCES

1. King TEJr, Pardo A, Selman M. Idiopathic pulmonary fibrosis. *Lancet* (2011) 378:1949–61. doi: 10.1016/S0140-6736(11)60052-4
2. Richeldi L, Collard HR, Jones MG. Idiopathic pulmonary fibrosis. *Lancet* (2017) 389:1941–52. doi: 10.1016/S0140-6736(17)30866-8
3. Martinez FJ, Collard HR, Pardo A, Raghu G, Richeldi L, Selman M, et al. Idiopathic pulmonary fibrosis. *Nat Rev Dis Primers* (2017) 3:17074. doi: 10.1038/nrdp.2017.74
4. Strieter RM, Mehrad B. New mechanisms of pulmonary fibrosis. *Chest* (2009) 136:1364–70. doi: 10.1378/chest.09-0510
5. Wynn TA, Ramalingam TR. Mechanisms of fibrosis: therapeutic translation for fibrotic disease. *Nat Med* (2012) 18:1028–40. doi: 10.1038/nm.2807
6. Ellson CD, Dunmore R, Hogaboam CM, Sleeman MA, Murray LA. Danger-associated molecular patterns and danger signals in idiopathic pulmonary fibrosis. *Am J Respir Cell Mol Biol* (2014) 51:163–8. doi: 10.1165/rcmb.2013-0366TR
7. Riteau N, Gasse P, Fauconnier L, Gombault A, Couegnat M, Fick L, et al. Extracellular ATP is a danger signal activating P2X7 receptor in lung inflammation and fibrosis. *Am J Respir Crit Care Med* (2010) 182:774–83. doi: 10.1164/rccm.201003-0359OC
8. Gasse P, Riteau N, Charron S, Girre S, Fick L, Petrilli V, et al. Uric acid is a danger signal activating NALP3 inflammasome in lung injury inflammation and fibrosis. *Am J Respir Crit Care Med* (2009) 179:903–13. doi: 10.1164/rccm.200808-1274OC
9. Akira S, Uematsu S, Takeuchi O. Pathogen recognition and innate immunity. *Cell* (2006) 124:783–801. doi: 10.1016/j.cell.2006.02.015
10. Ahn J, Barber GN. Self-DNA, STING-dependent signaling and the origins of autoinflammatory disease. *Curr Opin Immunol* (2014) 31:121–6. doi: 10.1016/j.coi.2014.10.009
11. Benmerzoug S, Ryffel B, Togbe D, Quesniaux VFJ. Self-DNA Sensing in Lung Inflammatory Diseases. *Trends Immunol* (2019) 40:719–34. doi: 10.1016/j.it.2019.06.001
12. Jonsson KL, Laustsen A, Krapp C, Skipper KA, Thavachelvam K, Hotter D, et al. IFI16 is required for DNA sensing in human macrophages by promoting production and function of cGAMP. *Nat Commun* (2017) 8:14391. doi: 10.1038/ncomms14391
13. Parvatiyar K, Zhang Z, Teles RM, Ouyang S, Jiang Y, Iyer SS, et al. The helicase DDX41 recognizes the bacterial secondary messengers cyclic di-GMP and cyclic di-AMP to activate a type I interferon immune response. *Nat Immunol* (2012) 13:1155–61. doi: 10.1038/ni.2460
14. Barber GN. STING: infection, inflammation and cancer. *Nat Rev Immunol* (2015) 15:760–70. doi: 10.1038/nri3921
15. Blaauboer SM, Mansouri S, Tucker HR, Wang HL, Gabrielle VD, Jin L. The mucosal adjuvant cyclic di-GMP enhances antigen uptake and selectively activates pinocytosis-efficient cells in vivo. *Elife* (2015) 4:e06670. doi: 10.7554/eLife.06670
16. Kim JA, Park SK, Seo SW, Lee CH, Shin OS. STING Is Involved in Antiviral Immune Response against VZV Infection via the Induction of Type I and III IFN Pathways. *J Invest Dermatol* (2017) 137:2101–9. doi: 10.1016/j.jid.2017.03.041
17. Sui H, Zhou M, Imamichi H, Jiao X, Sherman BT, Lane HC, et al. STING is an essential mediator of the Ku70-mediated production of IFN-lambda1 in response to exogenous DNA. *Sci Signal* (2017) 10(488). doi: 10.1126/scisignal.aah5054
18. Lazear HM, Nice TJ, Diamond MS. Interferon-lambda: Immune Functions at Barrier Surfaces and Beyond. *Immunity* (2015) 43:15–28. doi: 10.1016/j.immuni.2015.07.001
19. Zanoni I, Granucci F, Broggi A. Interferon (IFN)-lambda Takes the Helm: Immunomodulatory Roles of Type III IFNs. *Front Immunol* (2017) 8:1661. doi: 10.3389/fimmu.2017.01661
20. West AP, Shadel GS. Mitochondrial DNA in innate immune responses and inflammatory pathology. *Nat Rev Immunol* (2017) 17:363–75. doi: 10.1038/nri.2017.21
21. Ablasser A, Hertrich C, Wassermann R, Hornung V. Nucleic acid driven sterile inflammation. *Clin Immunol* (2013) 147:207–15. doi: 10.1016/j.clim.2013.01.003
22. Liu T, De Los Santos FG, Phan SH. The Bleomycin Model of Pulmonary Fibrosis. *Methods Mol Biol* (2017) 1627:27–42.

23. Ahn J, Gutman D, Saijo S, Barber GN. STING manifests self DNA-dependent inflammatory disease. *Proc Natl Acad Sci U States America* (2012) 109:19386–91. doi: 10.1073/pnas.1215006109
24. Li XD, Wu J, Gao D, Wang H, Sun L, Chen ZJ. Pivotal roles of cGAS-cGAMP signaling in antiviral defense and immune adjuvant effects. *Science* (2013) 341:1390–4. doi: 10.1126/science.1244040
25. Muller U, Steinhoff U, Reis LF, Hemmi S, Pavlovic J, Zinkernagel RM, et al. Functional role ofand type II interferons in antiviral defense. *Science* (1994) 264:1918–21. doi: 10.1126/science.8009221
26. Hubner RH, Gitter W, El Mokhtari NE, Mathiak M, Both M, Bolte H, et al. Standardized quantification of pulmonary fibrosis in histological samples. *Biotechniques* (2008) 44:507–11, 514-507. doi: 10.2144/000112729
27. Gasse P, Riteau N, Vacher R, Michel ML, Fautrel A, di Padova F, et al. IL-1 and IL-23 mediate early IL-17A production in pulmonary inflammation leading to late fibrosis. *PloS One* (2011) 6:e23185. doi: 10.1371/journal.pone.0023185
28. Zhao Q, Manohar M, Wei Y, Pandol SJ, Habtezion A. STING signalling protects against chronic pancreatitis by modulating Th17 response. *Gut* (2019) 68(10):1827–37. doi: 10.1136/gutjnl-2018-317098
29. Ishikawa H, Barber GN. STING is an endoplasmic reticulum adaptor that facilitates innate immune signalling. *Nature* (2008) 455:674–8. doi: 10.1038/nature07317
30. Iurescia S, Fioretti D, Rinaldi M. Targeting Cytosolic Nucleic Acid-Sensing Pathways for Cancer Immunotherapies. *Front Immunol* (2018) 9:711. doi: 10.3389/fimmu.2018.00711
31. Wu JJ, Zhao L, Hu HG, Li WH, Li YM. Agonists and inhibitors of the STING pathway: Potential agents for immunotherapy. *Medicinal Res Rev* (2019) 40 (3):1117–41. doi: 10.1002/med.21649
32. Paludan SR, Bowie AG. Immune sensing of DNA. *Immunity* (2013) 38:870–80. doi: 10.1016/j.immuni.2013.05.004
33. Pelka K, Shibata T, Miyake K, Latz E. Nucleic acid-sensing TLRs and autoimmunity: novel insights from structural and cell biology. *Immunol Rev* (2016) 269:60–75. doi: 10.1111/imr.12375
34. Falahat R, Perez-Villarroel P, Mailloux AW, Zhu G, Pilon-Thomas S, Barber GN, et al. STING Signaling in Melanoma Cells Shapes Antigenicity and Can Promote Antitumor T-cell Activity. *Cancer Immunol Res* (2019) 7:1837–48. doi: 10.1158/2326-6066.CIR-19-0229
35. Yi G, Brendel VP, Shu C, Li P, Palanathan S, Cheng Kao C. Single nucleotide polymorphisms of human STING can affect innate immune response to cyclic dinucleotides. *PloS One* (2013) 8:e77846. doi: 10.1371/journal.pone.0077846
36. Liu Y, Jesus AA, Marrero B, Yang D, Ramsey SE, Sanchez GAM, et al. Activated STING in a vascular and pulmonary syndrome. *N Engl J Med* (2014) 371:507–18. doi: 10.1056/NEJMoa1312625
37. Jeremiah N, Neven B, Gentili M, Callebaut I, Maschalidi S, Stolzenberg MC, et al. Inherited STING-activating mutation underlies a familial inflammatory syndrome with lupus-like manifestations. *J Clin Invest* (2014) 124:5516–20. doi: 10.1172/JCI79100
38. Clarke SL, Pellowe EJ, de Jesus AA, Goldbach-Mansky R, Hilliard TN, Ramanan AV. Interstitial Lung Disease Caused by STING-associated Vasculopathy with Onset in Infancy. *Am J Respir Crit Care Med* (2016) 194:639–42. doi: 10.1164/rccm.201510-2102LE
39. Bouis D, Kirstetter P, Arbogast F, Lamon D, Delgado V, Jung S, et al. Severe combined immunodeficiency in stimulator of interferon genes (STING) V154M/wild-type mice. *J Allergy Clin Immunol* (2019) 143:712–25.e715. doi: 10.1016/j.jaci.2018.04.034
40. Wu J, Chen ZJ. Innate immune sensing and signaling of cytosolic nucleic acids. *Annu Rev Immunol* (2014) 32:461–88. doi: 10.1146/annurev-immunol-032713-120156
41. Porat A, Giat E, Kowal C, He M, Son M, Latz E, et al. DNA-Mediated Interferon Signature Induction by SLE Serum Occurs in Monocytes Through Two Pathways: A Mechanism to Inhibit Both Pathways. *Front Immunol* (2018) 9:2824. doi: 10.3389/fimmu.2018.02824
42. Chamilos G, Gregorio J, Meller S, Lande R, Kontoyiannis DP, Modlin RL, et al. Cytosolic sensing of extracellular self-DNA transported into monocytes by the antimicrobial peptide LL37. *Blood* (2012) 120:3699–707. doi: 10.1182/blood-2012-01-401364
43. Poli C, Augusto JF, Dauve J, Adam C, Preisser L, Larochette V, et al. IL-26 Confers Proinflammatory Properties to Extracellular DNA. *J Immunol* (2017) 198:3650–61. doi: 10.4049/jimmunol.1600594
44. Ryu C, Sun H, Gulati M, Herazo-Maya JD, Chen Y, Osafo-Addo A, et al. Extracellular Mitochondrial DNA Is Generated by Fibroblasts and Predicts Death in Idiopathic Pulmonary Fibrosis. *Am J Respir Crit Care Med* (2017) 196:1571–81. doi: 10.1164/rccm.201612-2480OC
45. Qiu H, Weng D, Chen T, Shen L, Chen SS, Wei YR, et al. Stimulator of Interferon Genes Deficiency in Acute Exacerbation of Idiopathic Pulmonary Fibrosis. *Front Immunol* (2017) 8:1756. doi: 10.3389/fimmu.2017.01756
46. Lemos H, Huang L, Chandler PR, Mohamed E, Souza GR, Li L, et al. Activation of the STING adaptor attenuates experimental autoimmune encephalitis. *J Immunol* (2014) 192:5571–8. doi: 10.4049/jimmunol.1303258
47. Benmerzoug S, Rose S, Bounab B, Gosset D, Duneau L, Chenuet P, et al. STING-dependent sensing of self-DNA drives silica-induced lung inflammation. *Nat Commun* (2018) 9:5226. doi: 10.1038/s41467-018-07425-1
48. Iracheta-Vellve A, Petrasek J, Gyongyosi B, Satishchandran A, Lowe P, Kodys K, et al. Endoplasmic Reticulum Stress-induced Hepatocellular Death Pathways Mediate Liver Injury and Fibrosis via Stimulator of Interferon Genes. *J Biol Chem* (2016) 291:26794–805. doi: 10.1074/jbc.M116.736991
49. Luksch H, Stinson WA, Platt DJ, Qian W, Kalugotla G, Miner CA, et al. STING-associated lung disease in mice relies on T cells but not type I interferon. *J Allergy Clin Immunol* (2019) 144(1):254–66.e8. doi: 10.1016/j.jaci.2019.01.044
50. Warner JD, Irizarry-Caro RA, Bennion BG, Ai TL, Smith AM, Miner CA, et al. STING-associated vasculopathy develops independently of IRF3 in mice. *J Exp Med* (2017) 214:3279–92. doi: 10.1084/jem.20171351
51. Gul E, Sayar EH, Gungor B, Eroglu FK, Surucu N, Keles S, et al. Type I IFN-related NETosis in ataxia telangiectasia and Artemis deficiency. *J Allergy Clin Immunol* (2018) 142:246–57. doi: 10.1016/j.jaci.2017.10.030
52. Blazek K, Eames HL, Weiss M, Byrne AJ, Perocheau D, Pease JE, et al. IFN-lambda resolves inflammation via suppression of neutrophil infiltration and IL-1beta production. *J Exp Med* (2015) 212:845–53. doi: 10.1084/jem.20140995
53. Broggi A, Tan Y, Granucci F, Zanoni I. IFN-lambda suppresses intestinal inflammation by non-translational regulation of neutrophil function. *Nat Immunol* (2017) 18:1084–93. doi: 10.1038/ni.3821
54. Lee KG, Kim SS, Kui L, Voon DC, Mauduit M, Bist P, et al. Bruton's tyrosine kinase phosphorylates DDX41 and activates its binding of dsDNA and STING to initiate type 1 interferon response. *Cell Rep* (2015) 10:1055–65. doi: 10.1016/j.celrep.2015.01.039
55. Parvatiyar K, Zhang Z , Teles RM , Ouyang S, Jiang Y, Iyer SS, et al. The helicase DDX41 recognizes the bacterial secondary messengers cyclic di-GMP and cyclic di-AMP to activate a type I interferon immune response. *Nat Immunol* 13:1155-61.
56. Dunphy GSM, Flannery JF, Almine DJ, Connolly C, Paulus KL, Jønsson MR, et al. Non-canonical Activation of the DNA Sensing Adaptor STING by ATM and IFI16 Mediates NF-κB Signaling after Nuclear DNA Damage. *Mol Cell* (2018) 71:745–60.e745.
57. Lei Z, Deng M, Yi Z, Sun Q, Shapiro R. A, Xu H, Li T, et al. cGAS-mediated autophagy protects the liver from ischemia-reperfusion injury independently of STING. *Am J Physiol Gastrointest Liver Physiol* (2018) 314:G655–67.
58. Kinder BW, Brown KK, Schwarz MII, Ix JH, Kervitsky A, King TEJr. Baseline BAL neutrophilia predicts early mortality in idiopathic pulmonary fibrosis. *Chest* (2008) 133:226–32. doi: 10.1378/chest.07-1948
59. Xaubet A, Agusti C, Luburich P, Barbera JA, Carrion M, Ayuso MC, et al. Interleukin-8 expression in bronchoalveolar lavage cells in the evaluation of alveolitis in idiopathic pulmonary fibrosis. *Respir Med* (1998) 92:338–44. doi: 10.1016/S0954-6111(98)90118-4
60. Gieseck RL3, Wilson MS, Wynn TA. Type 2 immunity in tissue repair and fibrosis. *Nat Rev Immunol* (2018) 18:62–76. doi: 10.1038/nri.2017.90
61. Wynn TA, Vannella KM. Macrophages in Tissue Repair, Regeneration, and Fibrosis. *Immunity* (2016) 44:450–62. doi: 10.1016/j.immuni.2016.02.015
62. Kitowska K, Zakrzewicz D, Königshoff M, Chrobak I, Grimminger F, Seeger W, et al. Functional role and species-specific contribution of arginases in pulmonary fibrosis. *Am J Physiol Lung Cell Mol Physiol* (2008) 294:L34–45. doi: 10.1152/ajplung.00007.2007
63. Vono M, Lin A, Norrby-Teglund A, Koup RA, Liang F, Loré K. Neutrophils acquire the capacity for antigen presentation to memory CD4(+) T cells in vitro and ex vivo. *Blood* (2017) 129:1991–2001. doi: 10.1182/blood-2016-10-744441
64. Li Y, Wang W, Yang F, Xu Y, Feng C, Zhao Y. The regulatory roles of neutrophils in adaptive immunity. *Cell Communication Signal: CCS* (2019) 17:147. doi: 10.1186/s12964-019-0471-y

20

Alterations to the Lung Microbiome in Idiopathic Pulmonary Fibrosis Patients

Xunliang Tong[1†], Fei Su[2†], Xiaomao Xu[1], Hongtao Xu[3], Ting Yang[4,5], Qixia Xu[6], Huaping Dai[4,5], Kewu Huang[7], Lihui Zou[8], Wenna Zhang[1], Surui Pei[9], Fei Xiao[2,8], Yanming Li[1] and Chen Wang[4,5,10*]*

[1] Department of Respiratory and Critical Care Medicine, National Center of Gerontology, Beijing Hospital, Beijing, China, [2] Clinical Biobank, National Center of Gerontology, Beijing Hospital, Beijing, China, [3] Department of Laboratory Medicine, Beijing Hospital, Beijing, China, [4] National Clinical Research Center for Respiratory Diseases, Center for Respiratory Diseases, China-Japan Friendship Hospital, Peking University Health Science Center, Beijing, China, [5] Department of Pulmonary and Critical Care Medicine, China-Japan Friendship Hospital, Peking University Health Science Center, Beijing, China, [6] Department of Respiratory and Critical Care Medicine, Bengbu University Affiliated Hospital, Bengbu, China, [7] Department of Respiratory and Critical Care Medicine, Beijing Chao-Yang Hospital, Capital Medical University and Beijing Institute of Respiratory Medicine, Beijing, China, [8] The Key Laboratory of Geriatrics, National Center of Gerontology, Beijing Hospital, Beijing, China, [9] Annoroad Gene Technology (Beijing) Co., Ltd., Beijing, China, [10] National Clinical Research Center for Respiratory Diseases, Peking Union Medical College, Chinese Academy of Medical Sciences, Beijing, China

***Correspondence:**
Yanming Li
liyanming2632@bjhmoh.cn
Chen Wang
wangchen66366@163.com

†These authors have contributed equally to this work

Lung microbiome ecosystem homeostasis in idiopathic pulmonary fibrosis (IPF) remains uncharacterized. The aims of this study were to identify unique microbial signatures of the lung microbiome and analyze microbial gene function in IPF patients. DNA isolated from BALF samples was obtained for high-throughput gene sequencing. Microbial metagenomic data were used for principal component analysis (PCA) and analyzed at different taxonomic levels. Shotgun metagenomic data were annotated using the KEGG database and were analyzed for functional and metabolic pathways. In this study, 17 IPF patients and 38 healthy subjects (smokers and non-smokers) were recruited. For the PCA, the first and the second principal component explained 16.3 and 13.4% of the overall variability, respectively. The β diversity of microbiome was reduced in the IPF group. Signature of IPF's microbes was enriched of *Streptococcus*, *Pseudobutyrivibrio, and Anaerorhabdus.* The translocation of lung microbiome was shown that 32.84% of them were from oral. After analysis of gene function, ABC transporter systems, biofilm formation, and two-component regulatory system were enriched in IPF patients' microbiome. Here we shown the microbiology characteristics in IPF patients. The microbiome may participate in altering internal conditions and involving in generating antibiotic resistance in IPF patients.

Keywords: idiopathic pulmonary fibrosis, bronchoalveolar lavage fluid, microbiota, antibiotic resistant gene, virulence factor

INTRODUCTION

Idiopathic pulmonary fibrosis (IPF) is a progressive, fatal disease without a known cause (Molyneaux et al., 2014). IPF is increasing in prevalence and has a median survival of 3 years after diagnosis; the life expectancy for IPF patients is worse than those of some cancers (Maher et al., 2007; Ley et al., 2011; Navaratnam et al., 2011; Molyneaux et al., 2014). Because microorganisms may disturb the internal environment of the lower airway and cause lung damage, it is crucial to determine the precise composition of the lung microbiota and predict associated gene functions to understand IPF (Han et al., 2014; O'dwyer et al., 2016).

Traditional microbiological culture-based methods do not provide a complete profile of the microbiota in the lower respiratory tract (Garg et al., 2017; Ubags and Marsland, 2017). In contrast, culture-independent approaches, primarily based on gene sequencing, better describe the wide diversity of the microbial inhabitants of the lung microbiota and are able to identify significant differences between healthy subjects and patients with various respiratory diseases (Turnbaugh et al., 2007; Huse et al., 2012; Dickson and Huffnagle, 2015; O'dwyer et al., 2016).

Bronchoalveolar lavage fluid (BALF) samples obtained from the lower respiratory tract are used for routine diagnostic procedures. BALF sampling is suitable for the identification of a distinct microbiome in the lower respiratory tract (Zemanick et al., 2017). The bronchi harbor a specific microbiome associated with healthy individuals as well as a microbiome specific to pulmonary fibrosis patients (Charlson et al., 2011; Zimmermann et al., 2015). In addition, some studies have identified differences in the microbiomes of the upper respiratory tracts of smokers vs. non-smokers (Morris et al., 2013; Faner et al., 2017). Smoking may directly affect the composition of the respiratory microbiome, leading to changes or shifts in microbial community structure (Charlson et al., 2010; Sapkota et al., 2010; Lee et al., 2012). However, few studies have examined differences in the microbiomes of the lower respiratory tract in smokers vs. non-smokers (Garmendia et al., 2012; Morris et al., 2013).

In our current study, we broadly characterized the BALF-associated microbial communities in IPF patients and healthy individuals, including smokers and non-smokers. Additionally, we compared the lung microbiome with other local microbial communities, including those of the upper airway tract (the oropharynx) and gut. We attempted to assess the usefulness of shotgun metagenomics applied directly to DNA extracted from BALF samples to characterize the lung microbiomes in IPF and healthy patients and to reveal the role of the microbiome in IPF pathophysiology.

METHODS

Study Design

A diagnosis of IPF was made after multidisciplinary consultations. Only individuals diagnosed according to the international guidelines of the American Thoracic Society (ATS) and the European Respiratory Society (ERS) were subsequently included in this study (Travis et al., 2013). Healthy control subjects included non-smokers and smokers with normal lung function. Exclusion criteria included: (a) a history of self-reported upper or lower respiratory tract infection in the previous 3 months; (b) antibiotic use in the previous 3 months; (c) acute IPF exacerbation; and (d) other respiratory disorders. Written informed consent was obtained from all subjects, and the study was approved by the Institutional Review Board and Ethics Committee of Beijing Hospital (Beijing, China). The workflow of this research is shown in **Supplementary Figure 1**.

Bronchoscopy

Fiberoptic bronchoscopies with bronchoalveolar lavage (BAL) were performed according to ATS guidelines via the oropharyngeal route in accordance with a standard operating procedure, during which 20 ml of normal saline was instilled into a designated segment of the lobe showed in **Figure 1A** (Busse et al., 2005). After specimen collection, an aliquot of unfiltered and unprocessed BAL was immediately placed on ice and then frozen at −80°C for further analysis.

DNA Extraction

DNA was extracted from 3.0 ml of each original BALF sample using a QIAamp DNA Microbiome Kit (catalog 51704, Qiagen, Hilden, Germany) in strict accordance with the manufacturer's instructions. The DNA concentration was measured using a Qubit® 2.0 Fluorimeter (Life Technologies, Invitrogen, USA).

DNA Library Construction and Sequencing

DNA libraries were constructed using an Illumina TruSeq DNA kit according to the manufacturer's instructions. The same Illumina workflows were used to perform cluster generation, template hybridization, isothermal amplification, linearization, blocking, denaturation and hybridization of the sequencing primers. We performed paired-end sequencing on 2 × 100 base pairs (bp) or single-end sequencing on 100 bp. The base-calling pipeline was used to process raw fluorescent images and to call sequences. Reads that mapped to the human genome (hg19) were removed from each sample with BWA MEM using the default parameter (Li and Durbin, 2009). For quality control, we employed Trimmomatic (version 0.36) with the following criteria: (a) scan the read with a 4-base-wide sliding window, cutting when the average quality per base drops below 15; (b) drop reads below 50 bases in length; and (c) remove leading/tailing low quality ($Q < 13$). This produced an average of 8.5 gigabases (Gb) of high-quality sequences for each sample, resulting in a total of 470 Gb of sequence data (**Supplementary Table 1**). The reads were assembled into contigs for all samples using the assembly software IDBA (version 1.1.1) (Peng et al., 2012). IDBA was applied for Illumina short read assembly with the parameters "–pre_correction –mink 30 –maxk 120 –step 10." Then, we removed ambiguous bases from the assembled scaffolds and discarded scaffolds with lengths less than 500 bp. Finally, 73% of the total reads were used to generate 88,761 contigs without ambiguous bases (minimum length of 500 bp). These contigs had a total length of 210,670,314 bp, an average N50 length of 4,151 bp and ranged from 503 to 620,529 bp.

Construction of a Non-redundant Microbiome Gene Set

To predict microbial genes from the assembly, we applied the methodology used in the MetaHIT human gene catalog study (Qin et al., 2010). MetaGeneMark (MetaGeneMark_v1.mod) was used to predict the open reading frames (ORFs) in contigs

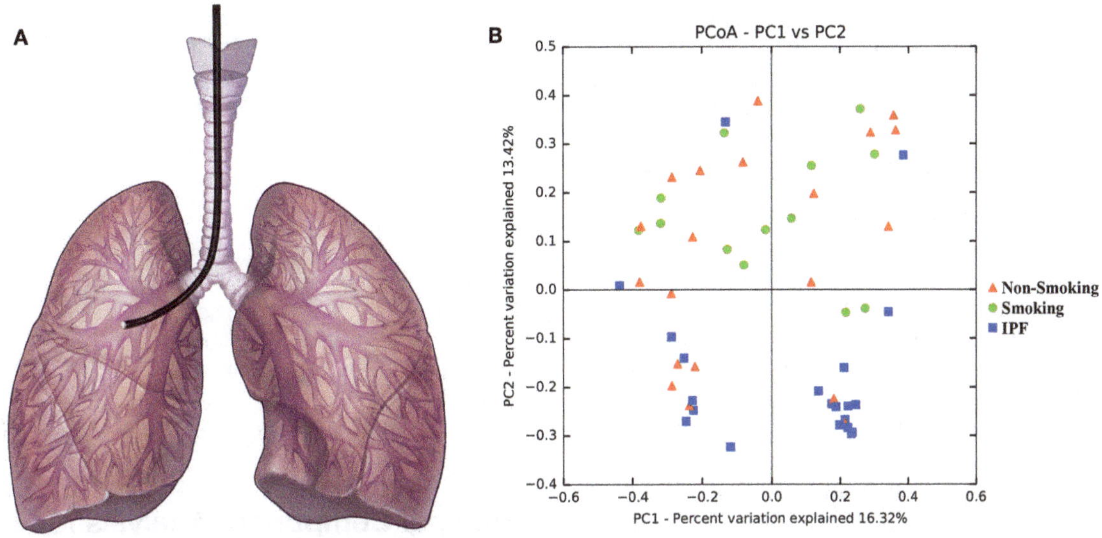

FIGURE 1 | Principal component analysis with BALF samples from IPF patients and health subjects. **(A)** Diagram of the bronchoscopy performance. **(B)** Principal component analysis with BALF samples from IPF patients and health subjects (including smokers and non-smokers) was performed based on the taxonomic profiles at species level. Different colors of points were represented for different groups: the blue points represent BALF samples from IPF group, the green points represent BALF samples from smoking control subjects, and the red points represent BALF samples from non-smoking control subjects. BALF samples from IPF patients were with an apparent clustering pattern of microbial composition compared with smoking control subjects, but no significant distribution pattern with the non-smoking control subjects.

without ambiguous bases (Zhu et al., 2010). The program predicted 250,268 ORFs using a 100-bp cut-off. The total length of the predicted ORFs was 183,986,409 bp, representing 87.3% of the total contig length. Among these ORFs, 142,871 (57.1%) were complete genes, while 107,397 (42.9%) were incomplete without a start or stop codon. A non-redundant "gene set" was established by removing redundant ORFs, defined as those sharing 95% identity with VSEARCH (Rognes et al., 2016). Then, genes from the HMP and HOMD databases (Dewhirst et al., 2010) were merged as a non-redundant reference gene set for gene-source analysis.

Organism Abundance Profiling

We followed the approach described in previous study to perform organism abundance profiling (Qin et al., 2014). BWA was applied to align paired-end clean reads against reference genomes using default parameters. Reads with alignments on the same reference genomes were assigned into the following two groups: reads having alignments with only one genome were identified as unique reads (U), and reads having alignments with more than one genome were identified as multiple reads (M).

For species S, if its abundance was Ab (S), and if it potentially aligned with U unique reads and M multiple reads, the following formulae were used:

$$\text{Ab}\,(\text{S}) = Ab\,(U) + Ab\,(M)$$
$$\text{Ab}\,(\text{U}) = U/l$$
$$\text{Ab}\,(\text{M}) = (\sum_{i=l}^{M} Co * \{M\})/l$$

Shannon diversity index (H) at the species level was calculated as the following, with p_i denoting the proportion in group k.

$$H = -\sum_{i=1}^{k} p_i \log(p_i)$$

Gene Abundance Profiling

Gene abundance was determined using a method similar to RPKM (reads per kilobases per million reads) used to quantify gene expression based on RNA sequencing data. In brief, high-quality original Illumina reads from each sample were aligned with a reference gene set using BWA. For each gene, G_i, the number of read pairs that aligned to it divided by the length of the gene was calculated as Num_G_i, and the relative abundance, RNum_G_i, of each gene in each sample (n genes) was computed using the following formula:

$$\text{RNum}_{\text{Gi}} = Num\_Gi/\sum_{i=1}^{n} Num\_Gi$$

Gene Function Classification and Ortholog Group Abundance Profiling

Protein sequences of the predicted genes were searched using BLASTp (Altschul et al., 1990) against the EggNOG 4.5 database (Huerta-Cepas et al., 2016) (**Supplementary Table 3**) and the KEGG gene database(Kanehisa et al., 2017) with the parameters "-num_descriptions 10,000, -*e*-value 1e-5." Genes that had alignments with a score slightly higher than 60 were assigned into one or more eggnog or KEGG ortholog groups. We used the methods introduced in previous study (Li et al., 2014) to calculate the abundances of KEGG ortholog groups; additionally, we added the abundances of proteins assigned into the same KEGG ortholog groups as abundances of KEGG ortholog groups, and KEGG ortholog group profiles were generated.

Quantification of Antibiotic Resistance Genes and Virulence Factors

Antibiotic resistance genes (ARGs) were annotated using the ARDB (Liu and Pop, 2009) database with BLASTp (*e*-value $< 1 \times 10^{-5}$). Then, antibiotic resistance gene abundance was determined as mentioned above. We used the Wilcoxon rank sum test to determine significantly different abundances between conditions. Virulence factors (VFs) were analyzed using a similar strategy. In brief, all VFs were identified using the VFDB database (Chen et al., 2016) with BLASTp (*e*-value $< 1 \times 10^{-5}$). Gene abundances and related statistical analysis were followed the ARGs' method.

Multivariate Analysis

To analyze the beta diversity of various groups based on the Bray-Curtis dissimilarity, ANOSIM was performed to detect significant dissimilarity or similarity in community composition among different groups (IPF/smoking/non-smoking). Pairwise comparisons were performed in ANOSIM, and pairwise *P*-values were obtained to assess significant differences in community composition between any two groups.

Statistical Analysis

PCA was analyzed using QIIME (Version 1.9.1) (Caporaso et al., 2010). Differential gene abundance and KEGG modules were tested with the Wilcoxon rank-sum test. One-way ANOVA test was performed and *P*-values were corrected for multiple testing with the Benjamin & Hochberg method using R software Version 3.1.1 (http://www.r-project.org/).

Availability of Data

The data set supporting the results of this article has been deposited in the NCBI Short Read Archive database under BioProject accession code PRJNA387212.

RESULTS

Patients Characteristics

In total, 17 IPF patients (IPF group) and 38 healthy control subjects (control group, including 23 non-smokers and 15 smokers) were included according to the inclusion criteria. The demographic data for these subjects are summarized in **Table 1**. IPF groups were slightly older than healthy subjects (IPF group vs. control group: [62.71 ± 7.90] years vs. [61.28 ± 9.37] years). As expected, IPF patients exhibited reduced forced expiratory volume in 1 one second (FEV1) and forced vital capacity (FVC) compared with those of healthy subjects. Total lung volume (TLC), residual lung volume (VR), lung diffusing capacity (DLCO) and the transfer coefficient (KCO) were sharply reduced in the IPF group, shown in **Table 1**.

TABLE 1 | Patient characteristics.

	Healthy control ($n = 38$)	IPF patients ($n = 17$)
Age, years	62.71 ± 7.90	61.28 ± 9.37
Gender (M/F)	24/14	11/6
Smoker (Never/current), n	23/15	11/6
Pack-year	14 ± 6	48 ± 32
FEV1% pred	110 ± 10	68 ± 17
FVC% pred	115 ± 14	66 ± 16
FEV1/FVC%	82 ± 5	77 ± 12
TLC, %pred	nd	65 ± 13
RV, %pred	nd	65 ± 30
DLCO% pred	nd	34 ± 12
KCO% pred	nd	54 ± 14

Principal Component Analysis for Microbiome

To identify any differences in the organismal structure of the lung microbiota, principal component anlaysis was performed based on taxonomic profiles at the species level (**Figure 1B**). Different colored points represent different groups: the blue points represent BALF samples from the IPF group, the green points represent BALF samples from smoking control subjects, and the red points represent BALF samples from non-smoking control subjects. The first principal component explained 16.32% of the overall variability among different groups, whereas the second principal component explained 13.42% of variability. As shown in **Figure 1B**, an apparent microbial composition clustering pattern was identified for IPF patients and smoking control subjects. Conversely, non-smoking control subjects, which are marked in red, exhibited no significant distribution pattern.

Microbial Community Structure of BALF

Sequencing reads (average number: 7,242,099) were aligned against 3,096 reference genomes from the National Center for Biotechnology Information and the HMP reference sequence, which contains 131 archaeal strains comprising 97 species, 326 lower eukaryotes comprising 326 species, 3,683 viral strains comprising 1,420 species, and 1,751 bacterial strains comprising 1,253 species (**Supplementary Table 1**). Relative abundances at the phylum, class, order, family, genus, and species levels were compared between the IPF group and control group. Intrinsic differences in lung microbiota composition are shown in **Figure 2** and **Supplementary Table 2**. Species with a median relative abundance larger than 0.01% of the total abundance in either the control group or the IPF group were included for comparison. Furthermore, we imported taxonomic data into QIIME for comparison. At the phylum level, *Firmicutes* (ANOVA, *P*-value = 0.02) and *Fusobacterium* (ANOVA, *P*-value = 0.04) dominated the BALF microbial communities in both groups (**Figure 2**). Compared to the control group, the IPF group had lower levels of *Bacteroidetes* (ANOVA, *P*-value = 0.03) but higher levels of *Proteobacteria* (ANOVA, *P*-value = 0.004) and *Fusobacteria* (ANOVA, *P*-value = 0.022). At the genus

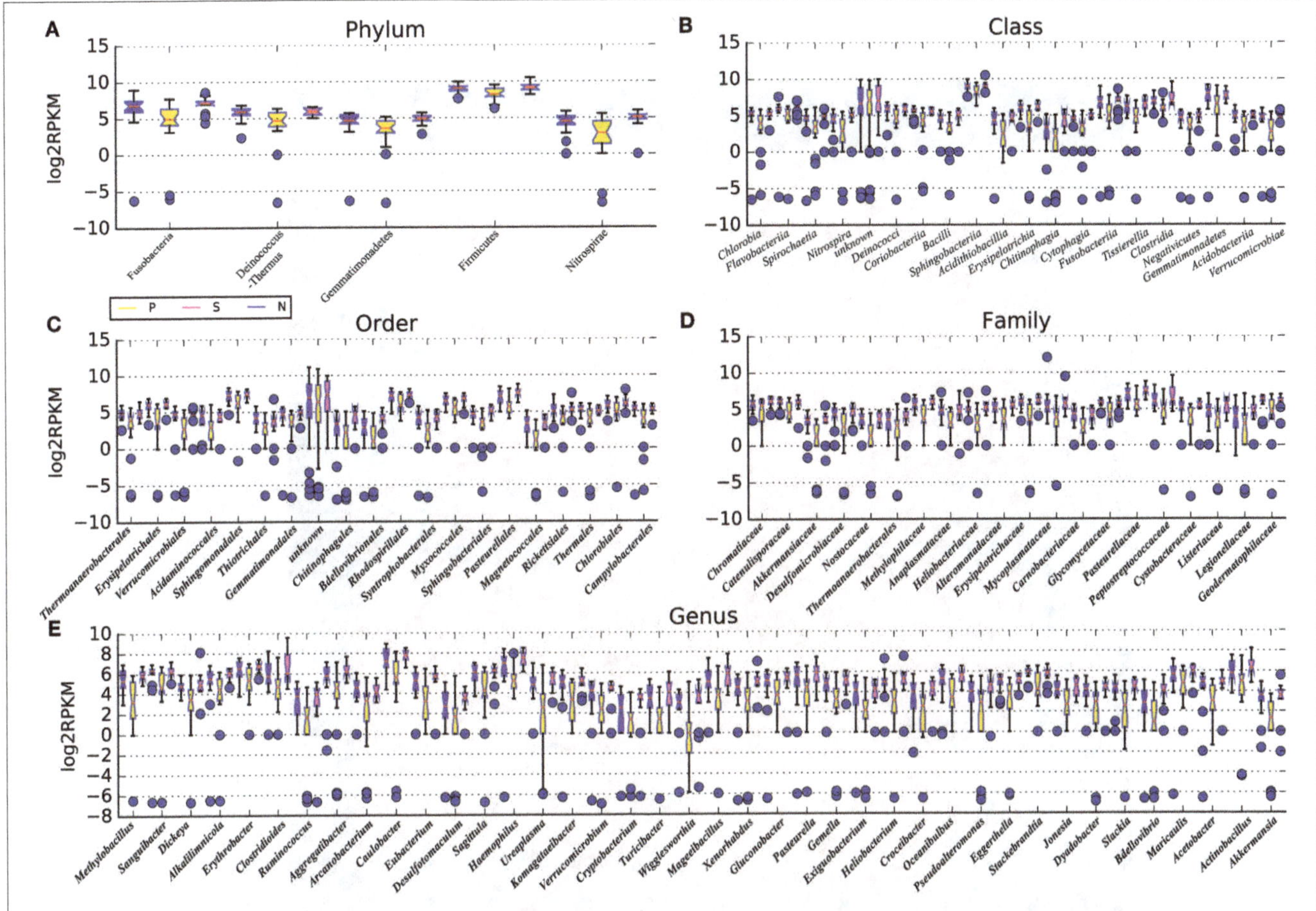

FIGURE 2 | Microbiota composition of BALF samples in IPF and healthy subjects. The microbiota in IPF patients and healthy subjects (including smokers and non-smokers) were shown at the phylum **(A)**, class **(B)**, order **(C)**, family **(D)**, and genus **(E)** levels. Species with a median relative abundance larger than 0.01% of the total abundance in either the control group or the IPF group were included for comparison. P stands for IPF group, N stands for non-smoking normal subjects, S stands for smoking normal subjects. All results are presented as the median, the 25–75 % percentiles and the variation range; results for IPF group (P) are presented as yellow boxes, smoking control subjects (S) are marked with pink boxes and non-smoking control subjects (N) are marked with violet boxes. Blue dots represent the abnormal observations at the corresponding taxonomic levels.

level (**Figure 2E**), *Bacteroides* was the dominant phylotype in both groups but was significantly decreased in the IPF group. Similar to previous studies (Morris et al., 2014), *Streptococcus*, representing 23.0 % of total reads, was the most common genus in subjects with IPF, followed by *Pseudobutyrivibrio*, *Anaerorhabdus*, *Campylobacter*, and *Blautia*, all of which were enriched in the IPF group. In contrast, *Sutterella*, *Coprococcus*, *Parasutterella*, *Paludibacter* and *Dorea* were dominant in the healthy group. The microbial communities of subjects with IPF were by contrast less diverse (Shannon diversity index, 2.81 ± 0.08 vs. 4.01 ± 0.10; $P = 0.004$) than the healthy subjects.

Biodiversity Analysis of BALF Samples

To measure the diversity of the BALF communities in IPF patients and healthy subjects (including smokers and non-smokers), we employed various methods, such as Adonis and ANOSIM of QIIME, to evaluate differences (beta-diversity) in the lung microbiota among the groups. BALF biodiversity was significantly reduced (*P*-value = 0.01) in the IPF group compared with that in the smoking/non-smoking groups according to the ADONIS results. A similar grouping pattern was identified based on the Bray-Curtis matrix using hclust2 (**Figure 3**). We identified the following two groups that were differentiated based on combinations of sex, age, and condition: Group 1, opportunistic pathogenic bacteria primarily derived from the skin and mouth, according to study of Blauwkamp (Blauwkamp et al., 2019); and Group 2, bacteria derived from the gut. These two groups were similar to those identified by ANOSIM. Mantel tests of the vegan package revealed the significant correlation of community structure with a *P*-value = 0.001 (Mantel Statistic R: 0.3057).

Crosstalk of BALF Microbiom to the Oral and Gut Microbiomes

To explore the origins of the lung microbiome, we constructed a reference gene catalog based on the HOMD and HMP (https://portal.hmpdacc.org) databases. We compared annotated genes with the reference database to determine functional gene sources. According to our results, the majority of genes were shared,

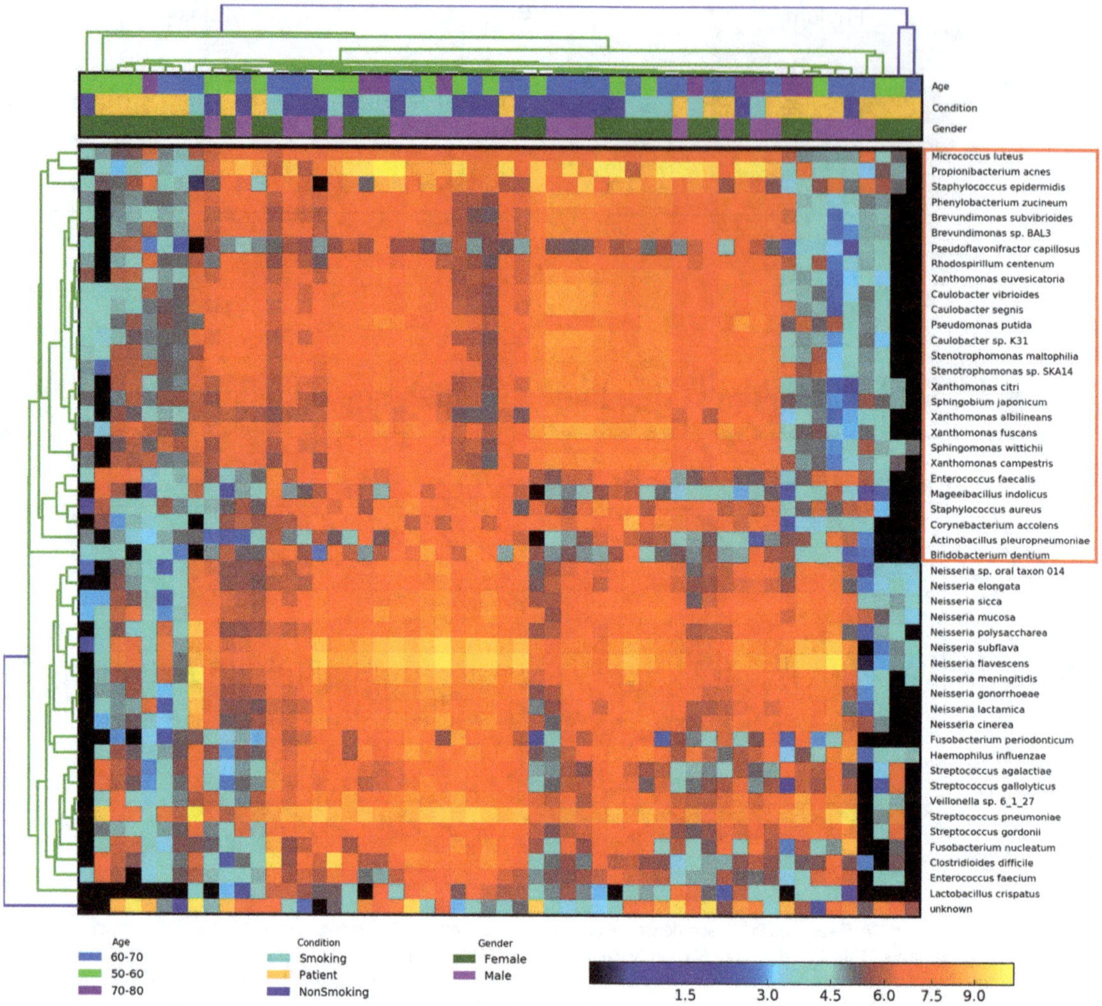

FIGURE 3 | Heatmap of the normalized abundances of all BALF samples. A similar grouping pattern on the combinations of the gender, age, and condition was also identified by Bray-Curtis matrix using the hclust2 and Mantel tests. The significant correlated of community structure of two groups was revealed (*P*-value = 0.01). The species in the red box are group 1, opportunistic pathogenic bacteria primarily derived from the skin and mouth, as mentioned above. The rest species are group 2, which is mainly from gut. Heatmap is color-coded based on the normalized abundance of species, from black (lower abundance) to red (higher abundance).

32.84% genes were derived from oral, and 1.32% genes were derived from the gut, as determined by V search (see the Methods section for details) and the results were shown in **Figure 4A**. We also analyzed the crosstalk of the different enriched genes between smoking group and IPF group: 38% of them were from oral and rest of them were unique in BALF (**Figure 4B**). None of the different enriched genes were from gut.

Functional Analysis of the Lung Microbiome

To identify functional differences in the BALF microbiome between control subjects (including smokers and non-smokers) and IPF patients, shotgun metagenomics data were annotated using the KEGG and eggNOG database and analyzed for functional and metabolic pathways (**Supplementary Tables 3, 4**). A total of 2,707 KOs were identified either in healthy controls or IPF samples. We further mapped these KOs to KEGG modules and pathways and calculated the adjusted *P*-value for the hypergeometric distribution. In particular, ABC transporter systems, the two-component regulatory system, biofilm formation, methane metabolism, aromatic compound degradation, amino acid biosynthesis (including alanine, tyrosine, valine and leucine), vitamin biosynthesis, biotin metabolism, and amino sugar and nucleotide sugar metabolism were enriched in the IPF group (**Supplementary Figure 2**). Among these pathways, the ABC transporter system, which imports amino acids, represented the majority of the enriched genes in the IPF group (**Supplementary Figure 3**). Multidrug efflux genes, which contribute to drug resistance, were enriched in the IPF group. According to ARDB databases, antibiotic resistant genes (ARG) was checked and 48 different types of ARGs was identified, which showed in **Supplementary Table 5**. The relative abundance of identified ARGs in IPF group and healthy control groups (smoking and non-smoking) was shown

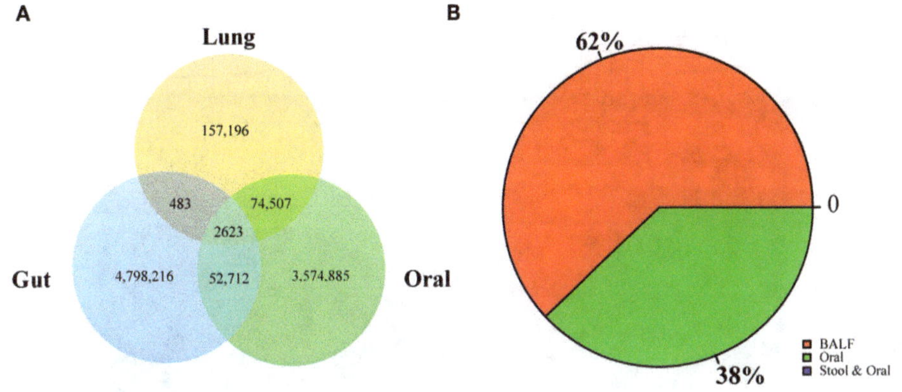

FIGURE 4 | Crosstalk of BALF's microbiome to oral and gut microbiome. **(A)** The origin lung microbiome was explored by comparison with HOMD and HMP databases. The genes rescore was shown: 32.84% genes were from oral and 1.32% genes were from the gut, as determined by the Vsearch. **(B)** Crosstalk of the different enriched genes were analyzed in this research: 38% of them were from oral and rest of them were unique in BALF.

in **Figure 5**. Compared with microbial genes from healthy control subjects, genes from IPF group were enriched of ARGS (5/10), including *tet*40, *acr*R, *evg*A, *tol*C, *mdt*O, with significantly abundance changes. These ARGs identified in IPF group are related to multidrug efflux, suggesting that the multidrug efflux pumps maybe the primary mechanism for bacteria to extrude antibiotics and other materials (**Figure 5A**). At the same time, virulence genes were also detected in this research showed in **Supplementary Table 6** and the relative abundance of each group was showed in **Figure 6**.

DISCUSSION

The Human Microbiome Project was launched in 2007 to study the microbial inhabitants of the human body and the microbes that live on human mucosal surfaces with the understanding that human biology may partially depend on interactions with these microorganisms (Turnbaugh et al., 2007). Because the human lung was believed to be sterile, it was not included in the original Human Microbiome Project. However, a growing number of studies have revealed the presence of microbial communities in the lungs. Next generation sequencing technology has dramatically improved lung microbiome identification in healthy subjects and in patients with chronic airway diseases, but humanized genomic DNA contamination remains a major technical challenge (Corless et al., 2000; Zoetendal et al., 2006; Salonen et al., 2010; Wu et al., 2010). As shown in our previous study, the use of pure microbial DNA avoids humanized genomic pollution and facilitates investigation of the lung microbiota (Wen et al., 2016).

In our current study, bacteria and virus microbial genes discriminated between IPF patient BALF and the BALF of healthy individuals with a high specificity; for example, *Acinetobacter* and *Neisseria* were identified at the genus level. The most common pathogenic bacteria in the IPF group were *Acinetobacter* and *Neisseria* (at the genus level), and the most common pathogenic viruses were microvirus, simplex virus and varicella virus. The same results had been reported with an increased bacterial load and decreased microbial diversity in BAL samples from IPF patients (Morris et al., 2014). At the same time, there are clear differences in the IPF BAL microbiome (increase in *Neisseria, Streptococcus* and some other species) compared to healthy subjects, which was also proven in our study. The bacterial load affects survival in these patients whereas retrospective analysis of the lung microbiome in BAL samples from the COMET-cohort suggested that presence of specific *Streptococcus* operational taxonomic units (OTU) or *Staphylococcus* OTU was associated with worse outcomes of IPF. These studies were showed the differential microbiome and specific microbial genes changes in BALF isolated from IPF patients, which suggested microbiota-targeted biomarkers may be potential tools for disease diagnosis and predicting prognosis. Biodiversity analysis revealed greater microbiome diversity associated with better lung function in the control group; conversely, the IPF group demonstrated decreased microbial diversity in terms of bacterial gene richness. Analysis of BALF microbiome revealed the appearance of common oral and gut inhabitants in BALF. Notably, shifts in the bacterial make-up of the BALF were associated with the human gut and oral microbiotas. In the IPF group, the majority of inhabitants were derived from the oral microbiome, suggesting they shifted from the mouth and throat. Comparison of BALF microbial genes to oral and gut microbiomes demonstrated that majority genes were from oral source, which hint the potential mechanism of oral aspiration as a risk factor in pathogenesis of IPF.

This study provides an opportunity to identify the bacterial functions required for a bacterium to thrive in the context of the BALF from IPF group and healthy subjects. To identify the functions of the BALF genome, gene length and copy number were normalized, and the relative frequencies of different functions were deduced based on the number of genes recruited to different EggNOG clusters. ABC transporter systems, the two-component regulatory system, biofilm formation, amino acid and vitamin biosynthesis, and central carbon metabolism were enriched in the IPF group. Not surprisingly,

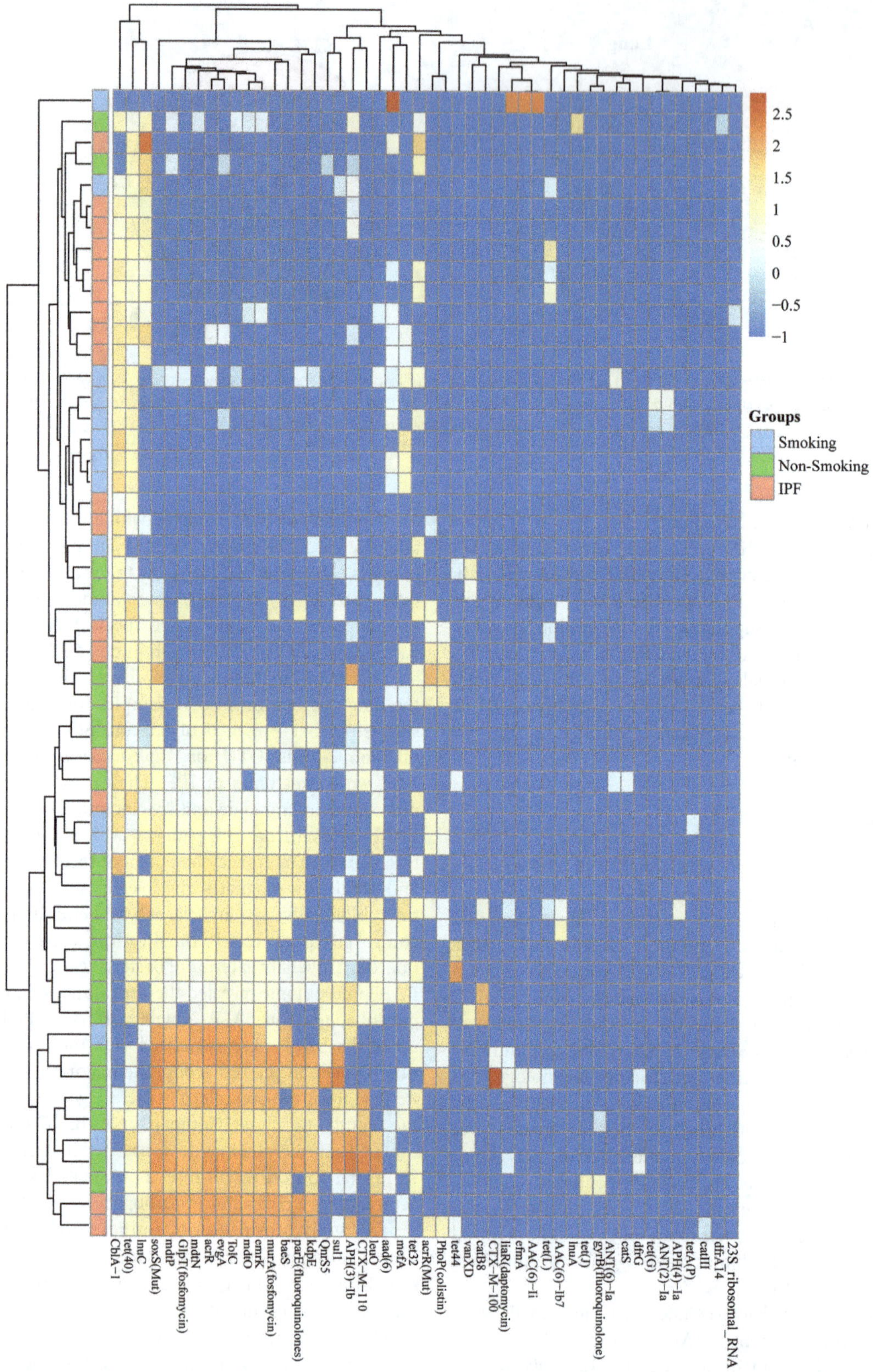

FIGURE 5 | Abundances of antibiotic resistant genes from BALF samples. Each column corresponds to an individual BALF's sample from IPF group (pink color) and healthy control group (smoking: blue color; non-smoking: green color) showed on the left side. The types of antibiotic resistant genes were indicated in the boxes at the bottom. Each row corresponds to a specific abundance of antibiotic resistant genes based on different colors according to different abundance folds.

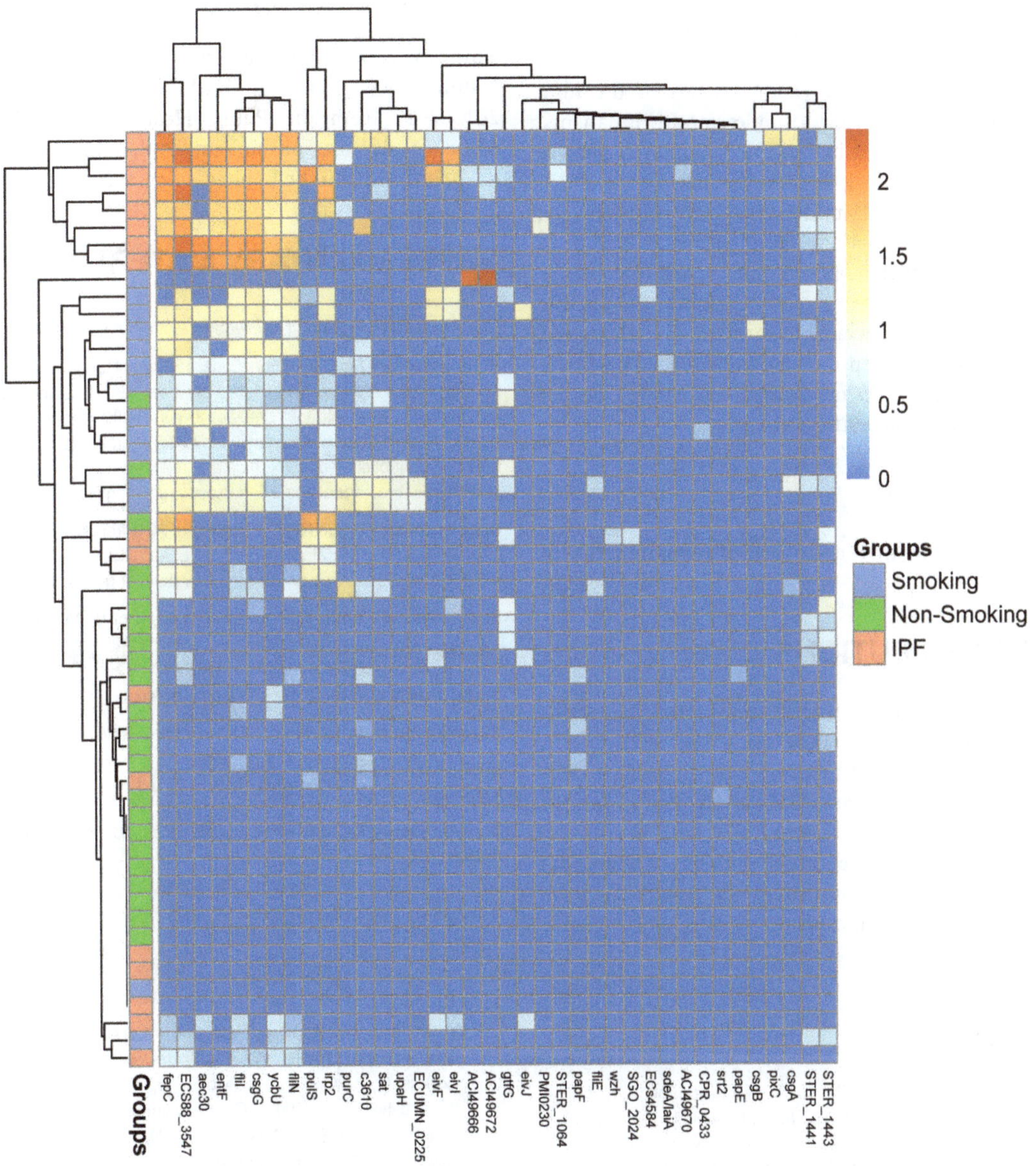

FIGURE 6 | Abundances of virulence genes from BALF samples. Each column corresponds to an individual BALF's sample from IPF group (pink color) and healthy control group (smoking: blue color; non-smoking: green color) showed on the left side. The types of virulence factors were indicated in the boxes at the bottom. Each row corresponds to a specific abundance of virulence genes based on different colors according to different abundance folds.

projection of the range clusters in KEGG metabolic pathways provided highly explicit directions associated with antimicrobial resistance. Antimicrobial resistance is a natural response of bacteria to antibiotic exposure (Sherrard et al., 2014). Antimicrobial resistance may be intrinsic to a bacterium, arise from spontaneous genetic mutations, or be associated with horizontal gene transfer (Sherrard et al., 2014). The enrichment of ABC transporters and biofilm formation signals indicates the presence of major antimicrobial resistance pathways in the IPF lung.

ABC transporter systems play a large variety of biological roles in processes such as translation, elongation, and DNA repair. In some antibiotic-producing or drug-resistant bacteria, particularly Gram-negative bacteria, ABC systems are responsible for the active efflux of drugs and other harmful compounds across the cell envelope (Seeger and Van Veen, 2009). Relative abundance of multidrug efflux genes were increased in IPF group compared with healthy controls which listed in this research. Furthermore, the virulence factors also evaluated in this research and showed significant differences between IPF group and control group. Biofilm formation is a feature of chronic airway infection. Bacteria growing in biofilms are embedded in a matrix of exopolymeric substances and are much more resistant to antibiotics than organisms growing planktonically (Stewart and Costerton, 2001; Wu et al., 2015). Together, these findings emphasize antimicrobial resistance as a primary function of the BALF ecosystem.

Our descriptions of the major characteristics of the lung microbiome provide a holistic view to understand IPF patients. In our study, intrinsic changes in the microbiome emphasize the production of strong antimicrobial resistance by the BALF ecosystem, which is important to understand pathophysiological processes. The interesting modules and pathways found in this project suggest the BALF microbiome in IPF patients is related to antibiotic resistance. Therefore, more therapeutic options for IPF may become available through the adaptation of lung environments or the identification of beneficial probiotic microorganisms. Further studies in this area will lead to a deeper understanding of bacterial life in the BALF.

ETHICS STATEMENT

Institutional Review Board and Ethics Committee of Beijing Hospital.

AUTHOR CONTRIBUTIONS

CW, YL, FX, and XT designed the study, interpreted the results, and drafted the manuscript. FS and SP analyzed the data. HD, TY, XX, QX, and KH made substantial contributions to the experimental protocol. HX, LZ, and WZ participated in sample preparation and DNA extraction. CW, YL, XT, and FS critically revised the manuscript for intellectual content. All authors participated in discussing and interpreting the results and gave final approval for manuscript submission.

ACKNOWLEDGMENTS

This project was supported by grant 81400037 from the National Natural Science Foundation of China, grants 2015SQ00301 and 201302017 from the Public Health Special Research of the Ministry of Health of the People's Republic of China, and grant BJ-2016-039 from the Beijing Hospital Nova Project.

SUPPLEMENTARY MATERIAL

Supplementary Figure 1 | The workflow of this research was shown in this figure.

Supplementary Figure 2 | Functional analysis of lung microbiome. The shotgun metagenomics data were annotated using the KEGG databases and analyzed at the functional and metabolic pathway levels. The KOs to KEGG modules and pathways were mapped to identify the BALF microbial functional differences between control subjects. The blue and red lines denote the enriched KEGG pathways in the control and IPF subjects, representatively.

Supplementary Figure 3 | Enrichment of ABC transporter systems based on the knowledge of KEGG database. The red boxes stand for the enriched genes in BALF samples. The blue boxes stand for the rest genes from KEGG database.

Supplementary Table 1 | Sequencing statistic of all BALF samples.

Supplementary Table 2 | Taxonomy composition at different levels.

Supplementary Table 3 | KEGG functional enrichment analysis.

Supplementary Table 4 | EggNOG functional enrichment analysis.

Supplementary Table 5 | Antibiotic resistant genes abundance comparison between different conditions.

Supplementary Table 6 | Virulence genes abundance comparison between different conditions.

REFERENCES

1. Altschul, S. F., Gish, W., Miller, W., Myers, E. W., and Lipman, D. J. (1990). Basic local alignment search tool. *J. Mol. Biol.* 215, 403–410. doi: 10.1016/S0022-2836(05)80360-2
2. Blauwkamp, T. A., Thair, S., Rosen, M. J., Blair, L., Lindner, M. S., Vilfan, I. D., et al. (2019). Analytical and clinical validation of a microbial cell- free DNA sequencing test for infectious disease. *Nat. Microbiol.* 4, 663–674. doi: 10.1038/s41564-018-0349-6
3. Busse, W. W., Wanner, A., Adams, K., Reynolds, H. Y., Castro, M., Chowdhury, B., et al. (2005). Investigative bronchoprovocation and bronchoscopy in airway diseases. *Am. J. Respir. Crit. Care Med.* 172, 807–816. doi: 10.1164/rccm.200407-966WS
4. Caporaso, J. G., Kuczynski, J., Stombaugh, J., Bittinger, K., Bushman, D., Costello, E. K., et al. (2010). QIIME allows analysis of high- throughput community sequencing data. *Nat. Methods* 7, 335–336. doi: 10.1038/nmeth.f.303
5. Charlson, E. S., Bittinger, K., Haas, A. R., Fitzgerald, A. S., Frank, I., Yadav, A., et al. (2011). Topographical continuity of bacterial populations in the healthy human respiratory tract. *Am. J. Respir. Crit. Care Med.* 184, 957–963. doi: 10.1164/rccm.201104-0655OC
6. Charlson, E. S., Chen, J., Custers-Allen, R., Bittinger, K., Li, H., Sinha, R., et al. (2010). Disordered microbial communities in the upper respiratory tract of cigarette smokers. *PLoS ONE* 5:e15216. doi: 10.1371/journal.pone.0015216
7. Chen, L., Zheng, D., Liu, B., Yang, J., and Jin, Q. (2016). VFDB 2016: hierarchical and refined dataset for big data analysis–10 years on. *Nucleic Acids Res.* 44, D694–D697. doi: 10.1093/nar/gkv1239
8. Corless, C. E., Guiver, M., Borrow, R., Edwards-Jones, V., Kaczmarski, E. B., and Fox, A. J. (2000). Contamination and sensitivity issues with a real-time universal 16S rRNA PCR. *J. Clin. Microbiol.* 38, 1747–1752.
9. Dewhirst, F. E., Chen, T., Izard, J., Paster, B. J., Tanner, A. C., Yu, W. H., et al. (2010). The human oral microbiome. *J. Bacteriol.* 192, 5002–5017. doi: 10.1128/JB.00542-10
10. Dickson, R. P., and Huffnagle, G. B. (2015). The lung microbiome: new principles for respiratory bacteriology in health and disease. *PLoS Pathog.* 11:e1004923. doi: 10.1371/journal.ppat.1004923
11. Faner, R., Sibila, O., Agusti, A., Bernasconi, E., Chalmers, J. D., Huffnagle, B., et al. (2017). The microbiome in respiratory medicine: current challenges and future perspectives. *Eur. Respir. J.* 49:1602086. doi: 10.1183/13993003.02086-2016
12. Garg, N., Wang, M., Hyde, E., Da Silva, R. R., Melnik, A. V., Protsyuk, I., et al. (2017). Three-dimensional microbiome and metabolome cartography of a diseased human lung. *Cell Host Microbe.* 22, 705–716.e704. doi: 10.1016/j.chom.2017.10.001
13. Garmendia, J., Morey, P., and Bengoechea, J. A. (2012). Impact of cigarette smoke exposure on host-bacterial pathogen interactions. *Eur. Respir. J.* 39, 467–477. doi: 10.1183/09031936.00061911
14. Han, M. K., Zhou, Y., Murray, S., Tayob, N., Noth, I., Lama, V. N., et al. (2014). Lung microbiome and disease progression in idiopathic pulmonary fibrosis: an analysis of the COMET study. *Lancet Respir. Med.* 2, 548–556. doi: 10.1016/S2213-2600(14) 70069-4

15. Huerta-Cepas, J., Szklarczyk, D., Forslund, K., Cook, H., Heller, D., Walter, M. C., et al. (2016). eggNOG 4.5: a hierarchical orthology framework with improved functional annotations for eukaryotic, prokaryotic and viral sequences. *Nucleic Acids Res.* 44, D286–293. doi: 10.1093/nar/gkv1248
16. Huse, S. M., Ye, Y., Zhou, Y., and Fodor, A. A. (2012). A core human microbiome as viewed through 16S rRNA sequence clusters. *PLoS ONE* 7:e34242. doi: 10.1371/journal.pone.0034242
17. Kanehisa, M., Furumichi, M., Tanabe, M., Sato, Y., and Morishima, K. (2017). KEGG: new perspectives on genomes, pathways, diseases and drugs. *Nucleic Acids Res.* 45, D353–D361. doi: 10.1093/nar/gkw1092
18. Lee, J., Taneja, V., and Vassallo, R. (2012). Cigarette smoking and inflammation: cellular and molecular mechanisms. *J. Dent. Res.* 91, 142–149. doi: 10.1177/0022034511421200
19. Ley, B., Collard, H. R., and King, T. E. Jr. (2011). Clinical course and prediction of survival in idiopathic pulmonary fibrosis. *Am. J. Respir. Crit. Care Med.* 183, 431–440. doi: 10.1164/rccm.201006-0894CI
20. Li, H., and Durbin, R. (2009). Fast and accurate short read alignment with burrows-wheeler transform. *Bioinformatics* 25, 1754–1760. doi: 10.1093/bioinformatics/btp324
21. Li, J., Jia, H., Cai, X., Zhong, H., Feng, Q., Sunagawa, S., et al. (2014). An integrated catalog of reference genes in the human gut microbiome. *Nat. Biotechnol.* 32, 834–841. doi: 10.1038/nbt.2942
22. Liu, B., and Pop, M. (2009). ARDB–antibiotic resistance genes database. *Nucleic Acids Res.* 37, D443–D447. doi: 10.1093/nar/gkn656
23. Maher, T. M., Wells, A. U., and Laurent, G. J. (2007). Idiopathic pulmonary fibrosis: multiple causes and multiple mechanisms? *Eur. Respir. J.* 30, 835–839. doi: 10.1183/09031936.00069307
24. Molyneaux, P. L., Cox, M. J., Willis-Owen, S. A., Mallia, P., Russell, K. E., Russell, A. M., et al. (2014). The role of bacteria in the pathogenesis and progression of idiopathic pulmonary fibrosis. *Am. J. Respir. Crit. Care Med.* 190, 906–913. doi: 10.1164/rccm.201403-0541OC
25. Morris, A., Beck, J. M., Schloss, P. D., Campbell, T. B., Crothers, K., Curtis, J. L., et al. (2013). Comparison of the respiratory microbiome in healthy nonsmokers and smokers. *Am. J. Respir. Crit. Care Med.* 187, 1067–1075. doi: 10.1164/rccm.201210-1913OC
26. Morris, A., Gibson, K., and Collman, R. G. (2014). The lung microbiome in idiopathic pulmonary fibrosis. what does it mean and what should we do about it? *Am. J. Respir. Crit. Care Med.* 190, 850–852. doi: 10.1164/rccm.201409-1626ED
27. Navaratnam, V., Fleming, K. M., West, J., Smith, C. J., Jenkins, R. G., Fogarty, A., et al. (2011). The rising incidence of idiopathic pulmonary fibrosis in the U.K. *Thorax* 66, 462–467. doi: 10.1136/thx.2010.148031
28. O'dwyer, D. N., Dickson, R. P., and Moore, B. B. (2016). The lung microbiome, immunity, and the pathogenesis of chronic lung disease. *J. Immunol.* 196, 4839–4847. doi: 10.4049/jimmunol.1600279
29. Peng, Y., Leung, H. C., Yiu, S. M., and Chin, F. Y. (2012). IDBA-UD: a de novo assembler for single-cell and metagenomic sequencing data with highly uneven depth. *Bioinformatics* 28, 1420–1428. doi: 10.1093/bioinformatics/bts174
30. Qin, J., Li, R., Raes, J., Arumugam, M., Burgdorf, K. S., Manichanh, C., et al. (2010). A human gut microbial gene catalogue established by metagenomic sequencing. *Nature* 464, 59–65. doi: 10.1038/nature08821
31. Qin, N., Yang, F., Li, A., Prifti, E., Chen, Y., Shao, L., et al. (2014). Alterations of the human gut microbiome in liver cirrhosis. *Nature* 513, 59–64. doi: 10.1038/nature13568
32. Rognes, T., Flouri, T., Nichols, B., Quince, C., and Mahe, F. (2016). VSEARCH: a versatile open source tool for metagenomics. *PeerJ* 4:e2584. doi: 10.7717/peerj.2584
33. Salonen, A., Nikkila, J., Jalanka-Tuovinen, J., Immonen, O., Rajilic-Stojanovic, M., Kekkonen, R. A., et al. (2010). Comparative analysis of fecal DNA extraction methods with phylogenetic microarray: effective recovery of bacterial and archaeal DNA using mechanical cell lysis. *J. Microbiol. Methods* 81, 127–134. doi: 10.1016/j.mimet.2010.02.007
34. Sapkota, A. R., Berger, S., and Vogel, T. M. (2010). Human pathogens abundant in the bacterial metagenome of cigarettes. *Environ. Health Perspect.* 118, 351–356. doi: 10.1289/ehp.0901201
35. Seeger, M. A., and Van Veen, H. W. (2009). Molecular basis of multidrug transport by ABC transporters. *Biochim. Biophys. Acta* 1794, 725–737. doi: 10.1016/j.bbapap.2008.12.004
36. Sherrard, L. J., Tunney, M. M., and Elborn, J. S. (2014). Antimicrobial resistance in the respiratory microbiota of people with cystic fibrosis. *Lancet* 384, 703–713. doi: 10.1016/S0140-6736(14)61137-5
37. Stewart, P. S., and Costerton, J. W. (2001). Antibiotic resistance of bacteria in biofilms. *Lancet* 358, 135–138. doi: 10.1016/S0140-6736(01)05321-1
38. Travis, W. D., Costabel, U., H ansell, D. M., King, T. E. Jr., Lynch, D. A., Nicholson, A. G., et al. (2013). An official american thoracic society/european respiratory society statement: update of the international multidisciplinary classification of the idiopathic interstitial pneumonias. *Am. J. Respir. Crit. Care Med.* 188, 733–748. doi: 10.1164/rccm.201308-1483ST
39. Turnbaugh, P. J., Ley, R. E., Hamady, M., Fraser-Liggett, C. M., Knight, R., and Gordon, J. I. (2007). The human microbiome project. *Nature* 449, 804–810. doi: 10.1038/nature06244
40. Ubags, N. D. J., and Marsland, B. J. (2017). Mechanistic insight into the function of the microbiome in lung diseases. *Eur. Respir. J.* 50:1602467. doi: 10.1183/13993003.02467-2016
41. Wen, Y., Xiao, F., Wang, C., and Wang, Z. (2016). The impact of different methods of DNA extraction on microbial community measures of BALF samples based on metagenomic data. *Am. J. Transl. Res.* 8, 1412–1425.
42. Wu, G. D., Lewis, J. D., Hoffmann, C., Chen, Y. Y., Knight, R., Bittinger, K., et al. (2010). Sampling and pyrosequencing methods for characterizing bacterial communities in the human gut using 16S sequence tags. *BMC Microbiol.* 10:206. doi: 10.1186/1471-2180-10-206
43. Wu, H., Moser, C., Wang, H. Z., Hoiby, N., and Song, Z. J. (2015). Strategies for combating bacterial biofilm infections. *Int. J. Oral Sci.* 7, 1–7. doi: 10.1038/ijos.2014.65
44. Zemanick, E. T., Wagner, B. D., Robertson, C. E., Ahrens, R. C., Chmiel, J. F., Clancy, J. P., et al. (2017). Airway microbiota across age and disease spectrum in cystic fibrosis. *Eur. Respir. J.* 50:1700832. doi: 10.1183/13993003.0083 2-2017
45. Zhu, W., Lomsadze, A., and Borodovsky, M. (2010). Ab initio gene identification in metagenomic sequences. *Nucleic Acids Res.* 38:e132. doi: 10.1093/nar/gkq275
46. Zimmermann, A., Zissel, G., Muller-Quernheim, J., Hofmann, S., Schreiber, S., and Fischer, A. (2015). Are bronchoalveolar lavages a good source for microbial profiling? differences between throat and bronchoalveolar lavage microbiomes. *J. Med. Microbiol.* 64, 948–951. doi: 10.1099/jmm.0.000112
47. Zoetendal, E. G., Heilig, H. G., Klaassens, E. S., Booijink, C. C., Kleerebezem, M., Smidt, H., et al. (2006). Isolation of DNA from bacterial samples of the human gastrointestinal tract. *Nat. Protoc.* 1, 870–873. doi: 10.1038/nprot.2006.142

21

Catalpol Protects Against Pulmonary Fibrosis Through Inhibiting TGF-β1/Smad3 and Wnt/β-Catenin Signaling Pathways

Fan Yang[1], Zhen-feng Hou[2], Hao-yue Zhu[1], Xiao-xuan Chen[1], Wan-yang Li[3], Ren-shuang Cao[1], Yu-xuan Li[4], Ru Chen[5] and Wei Zhang[6]**

[1]College of Traditional Chinese Medicine, Shandong University of Traditional Chinese Medicine, Jinan, China, [2]College of Life Sciences, Shandong Normal University, Jinan, China, [3]School of Public Health, Xiangya Medical College, Central South University, Changsha, China, [4]Second School of Clinical Medicine, Beijing University of Chinese Medicine, Beijing, China, [5]Biomedical Research Institute of Fudan University, Shanghai, China, [6]Department of Pulmonary Diseases, Affiliated Hospital of Shandong University of Traditional Chinese Medicine, Jinan, China

***Correspondence:**
Wan-Yang Li
liwanyang@csu.edu.cn
Wei Zhang
hxzjss@163.com

Idiopathic pulmonary fibrosis (IPF) is a fatal lung disease characterized by fibroblast proliferation and extracellular matrix remodeling; however, the molecular mechanisms underlying its occurrence and development are not yet fully understood. Despite it having a variety of beneficial pharmacological activities, the effects of catalpol (CAT), which is extracted from *Rehmannia glutinosa*, in IPF are not known. In this study, the differentially expressed genes, proteins, and pathways of IPF in the Gene Expression Omnibus database were analyzed, and CAT was molecularly docked with the corresponding key proteins to screen its pharmacological targets, which were then verified using an animal model. The results show that collagen metabolism imbalance, inflammatory response, and epithelial-mesenchymal transition (EMT) are the core processes in IPF, and the TGF-β1/Smad3 and Wnt/β-catenin pathways are the key signaling pathways for the development of pulmonary fibrosis. Our results also suggest that CAT binds to TGF-βR1, Smad3, Wnt3a, and GSK-3β through hydrogen bonds, van der Waals bonds, and other interactions to downregulate the expression and phosphorylation of Smad3, Wnt3a, GSK-3β, and β-catenin, inhibit the expression of cytokines, and reduce the degree of oxidative stress in lung tissue. Furthermore, CAT can inhibit the EMT process and collagen remodeling by downregulating fibrotic biomarkers and promoting the expression of epithelial cadherin. This study elucidates several key processes and signaling pathways involved in the development of IPF, and suggests the potential value of CAT in the treatment of IPF.

Keywords: catalpol, idiopathic pulmonary fibrosis, epithelial-mesenchymal transition, Smad3, Wnt3a

---

Abbreviations: BALF, bronchoalveolar lavage fluid; BLM, Bleomycin; CAT, Catalpol; DAVID, The database for Annotation, Visualization and Integrated Discovery; DEGs, differentially expressed genes; ECM, extracellular matrix; EMT: epithelial-mesenchymal transition; GEO, Gene Expression Omnibus database; ILDs, interstitial lung diseases; IPF, idiopathic pulmonary fibrosis; KEGG, Kyoto Encyclopedia of Genes and Genomes; PF, pulmonary fibrosis; PFD, Pirfenidone; PPI, protein-protein interaction.

INTRODUCTION

Pulmonary fibrosis (PF), which usually manifests at the end stages of various interstitial lung diseases, is characterized by alveolar epithelial cell damage and abnormal deposition of extracellular matrix (ECM) (Herrera et al., 2018). There are a variety of causes of PF—idiopathic pulmonary fibrosis (IPF) is a form of an unexplained and severe PF with a 5-years survival rate of less than 30% (Nalysnyk et al., 2012). Currently, the only drugs recommended for the treatment of mild-to-moderate IPF are pirfenidone (PFD) and nintedanib, both of which, however, fail to prolong the survival of patients (Ogura et al., 2015; Jo et al., 2016). Moreover, PFD has several side effects, such as gastrointestinal reactions, rash, and photosensitivity (Cottin and Maher, 2015). Thus, there is an urgent need for the development of new drugs for IPF.

Bioinformatics utilizes sequence comparison and cluster analysis methods to extract biological information using technologies such as GeneChip, which enables more comprehensive and systematic study of disease pathology. With the development of high-throughput microarray and sequencing technologies in recent years, it has become possible to investigate the gene expression profiles of IPF and the corresponding changes in PF tissue and key genes. Moreover, the differentially expressed gene (DEG) data obtained in this manner has in many cases enabled the successful screening of potential drugs by the docking of small molecular compounds with the corresponding proteins.

Rehmannia glutinosa is a traditional Chinese herb that has been widely used for the treatment of circulatory diseases for thousands of years (Li and Kan, 2017; Xu et al., 2017). Catalpol (CAT), a compound extracted from *R. glutinosa*, is known to have anti-inflammatory, anti-epithelial-mesenchymal transition (EMT), anti-oxidative, anti-apoptoti, and anti-angiogenesis properties, and to have favorable pharmacological effects in patients with asthma (Chen et al., 2017), lung cancer, glomerulonephritis, and colon cancer (Zhu et al.,2017b; Yang et al., 2020). In recent years, studies have focused on the protective effects of R. glutinosa extract, represented by CAT, on nerve cells and kidney cells. The mechanism of action is to target SIRT1 and Wnt/β-catenin signaling pathways, stabilize cytoskeleton and enhance autophagy (Chen et al., 2019; Liu et al., 2019; Zhang et al., 2019; Zhou et al., 2019; Cheng et al., 2020; Wang et al., 2020). However, its effects on IPF remain unknown. In order to investigate the effect of CAT on IPF, we screened the Gene Expression Omnibus (GEO) database for DEGs in IPF and investigated the important signaling pathways and proteins involved in the development of IPF. We also used molecular docking to virtually screen proteins expressed by the DEGs and estimate the theoretical stability of their binding to CAT. Furthermore, we established a rat IPF model to verify the efficacy of CAT against IPF and explore its mechanisms of action.

MATERIALS AND METHODS

Microarray Data

The following gene expression profile datasets were obtained from the GEO database (https://www.ncbi.nlm.nih) (Rosas et al., 2008; Meltzer et al., 2011; DePianto et al., 2015): GSE10667 (platform: GPL4133 Agilent-014850 Whole Human Genome Microarray 4 × 44K G4112F), obtained using a total of 31 IPF and 15 normal specimens; GSE24206 (platform: GPL570 Affymetrix Human Genome U133 Plus 2.0 Array), obtained using 17 IPF and six normal specimens; and GSE53845 (platform: GPL6480 Agilent-014850 Whole Human Genome Microarray 4 × 44K G4112F), obtained using 40 IPF and eight normal specimens.

Data Processing

GEO2R allows users to compare different sample groups in the GEO series and to screen genes that are differentially expressed under different experimental conditions. GEO2R compares original submitter-supplied processed data tables using the GEOquery and limma (Linear Models for Microarray Analysis) R packages from the Bioconductor project. The GEOquery R package parses GEO data into R data structures that can be used by other R packages. The limma R package has emerged as one of the most widely used statistical tools for identifying DEGs. We used the GEO2R online software to analyze the microarray data provided by the original submitter and identify DEGs with recognition thresholds set to false discovery rate (FDR) < 0.05 and $|\log 2$ fold change $(FC)| > 1$. The upregulated and downregulated genes were analyzed, and volcano maps of the three datasets were drawn. We then selected the DEGs present in two or three datasets as the total differential genes, which exceeded 600 in number. Venn diagrams were drawn for upregulated and downregulated genes. Finally, hierarchical cluster analysis was performed on DEGs, with heat maps drawn for the three chips using the heatmap package.

Gene Ontology and Pathway Enrichment Analysis

DAVID (http://david.abcc.ncifcrf.gov/) is an online gene function annotation tool that provides information regarding the biological significance of a large number of genes (Huang et al., 2007). The GO analysis provided by DAVID for researchers includes the cellular components (CC), molecular functions (MF), and biological processes (BP) categories (Gene Ontology, 2006). We used this database for annotation, data analysis, and visualization. In addition, we performed a Kyoto Encyclopedia of Genes and Genomes (KEGG) pathway function enrichment analysis on the DEGs described above (Kanehisa and Goto, 2000). $p < 0.05$ was considered statistically significant.

Protein-Protein-Interaction Network Construction and Module Analysis

PPI analysis can be used to directly explain the molecular mechanism underlying key protein interactions. In this study, we used the STRING database to construct PPI networks for all upregulated and downregulated proteins (Missiuro et al., 2009). Then, we utilized Cytoscape for visualization and the MCODE plug-in for subset analysis (Barabasi et al., 2011).

Molecular Docking

Based on the differential expression results of the above genes and proteins and information from the pathway enrichment analysis, core proteins were selected for forward molecular docking with CAT. CAT molecular structure data were obtained from the PubChem website (https://pubchem.ncbi.nlm.nih.gov/) (Kim et al., 2019) and protein crystal structure data from the RCSB website (http://www.rcsb.org/) (Berman et al., 2003). We used Discovery Studio 2016 (DS) for creating the 2D and 3D effect pictures and for the molecular docking calculations. DS was used to extract the ligands with crystal structure of protein. After exposing active sites, excluding crystalized water, hydrogens, and side chain residues, the CHARMm force field and Momany-Rone charge were added. The docking file of the active region was then obtained using default parameters. Docking files for crystal structures without ligand were automatically generated using default parameters. Using the DS CDOCKER module, the possible multiple conformations, interaction energies and main action sites of CAT to target protein docking were obtained. Molecular docking results can indicate the mechanism of action of CAT on IPF and guide the selection of related detection indicators in subsequent animal experiments.

Antibodies and Reagents

CAT (purity: 98.3%, HPLC) was purchased from Shanghai Yuanye Bio-Technology Co., Ltd. (L20N8Y48597), bleomycin (BLM) from Cool Chemical Technology Co., Ltd. Beijing (S656455V), and PFD from Beijing Continent Pharmaceutical Co., Ltd. (190806). The Masson tricolor staining kit (G1006-100), hematoxylin-eosin (HE) staining kit (GP1031), reactive oxygen species (ROS) test kit (2019-07), detection kits for hydroxyproline (HYP) (201900711), aspartate aminotransferase (AST) (20190712), alanine aminotransferase (ALT) (20190711), malondialdehyde (MDA) (20190830), superoxide dismutase (SOD) (20191125), and the bicinchoninic acid (BCA) method total protein quantification kit (20190711) were all purchased from Nanjing Jiancheng Bioengineering Research Institute. Rabbit anti-Wnt3a antibody (BS-1700r), rabbit anti-phosphorylated-Smad3 antibody (bs-19452r), and rabbit anti-Smad3 antibody (BS-3484r) were purchased from Biosynthesis Biotechnology Inc. Beijing, China. Rabbit anti-α-SMA antibody (GB11044), rabbit anti-matrix metalloprotease (MMP)-7 antibody (A0695), rabbit anti-COL1A1 antibody (GB11022-3), rabbit anti-COL3A1 antibody (GB13023-2), rabbit anti-β-catenin antibody (GB12015), rabbit anti-GSK-3β antibody (GB11099), rabbit anti-E-cadherin (E-cad) antibody (GB13083), and HRP-labeled goat anti-rabbit IgG antibodies (GB23303) were purchased from Wuhan Servicebio Technology Co., Ltd. The rat TGF-β1 enzyme-linked immunosorbent assay (ELISA) kit (E04019240) was purchased from Cusabio Biotech Co., Ltd. Wuhan. Rabbit anti-anti-β-actin antibody (AC026), rabbit anti-phosphorylated-GSK3β antibody (AP0039), and rabbit anti-phosphorylated-β-catenin antibody (AP0979) were obtained from ABclonal Biotechnology Co., Ltd. Wuhan. Rat IL-6 (CSB-E04640r), IL-1β (CSB-E08055r), and TNF-α (CSB-E11987r) ELISA kits were purchased from Wuhan Huamei Bioengineering Co., Ltd.

Animal Grouping and Modeling

The study protocol was approved by the Research Ethics Committee of the Affiliated Hospital of Shandong University of Traditional Chinese Medicine (Approval No. AWE-2019-046) and followed the National Institutes of Health Guide for the Care and Use of Laboratory Animals (NIH Publications No. 8023, revised 1978). Male Sprague Dawley rats (180–220 g, SPF grade) purchased from Jinan Pengyue Experimental Animal Breeding Co., Ltd. (Certificate No. SCXK [Lu]2014-0007, Jinan, China) were maintained under 12-h light/12-h darkness conditions with free access to feed and water. After 7 days of adaptive breeding, the rats were randomly divided into six groups (6 in each group): 1) saline (NS) group; 2) BLM + NS group; 3) BLM + CAT (10 mg/kg/d) group; 4) BLM + CAT (20 mg/kg/d) group; 5) BLM + CAT (40 mg/kg/d) group; and 6) BLM + PFD (150 mg/kg/d) group. A single intratracheal instillation of BLM (5 mg/kg) was used to induce PF in rats. After the modeling, rats in the CAT groups were injected intraperitoneally with the corresponding concentration of drugs, while rats in the PFD group were administered PFD intragastrically; all animals were sacrificed 28 days later. Rat blood from the abdominal aorta was centrifuged at 5,000 rpm for 10 min at 4°C, and the serum was stored at -80°C. Lung tissues were also collected and weighed. Lung index was calculated as lung weight (g)/(body weight (g) × 100%. The whole lung was lavaged three times using 2 ml of physiological saline, and bronchoalveolar lavage fluid (BALF) was then collected. Some of the lung tissue was placed in 4% paraformaldehyde, with the rest frozen in liquid nitrogen and stored at −80°C for further examination.

Morphological and Histological Analysis

Lung tissues fixed using 4% paraformaldehyde for 48 h were embedded in paraffin and sectioned (thickness, 5 μm). The slices were stained with HE and Masson trichrome for the evaluation of lung tissue pathological changes and then imaged at a magnification of ×200 using an optical microscope. According to the Szapiel scoring standard and Ashcroft scoring standard, the degree of alveolitis and PF were scored, respectively (Szapiel et al., 1979; Ashcroft et al., 1988).

Measurement of HYP, MDA, and ROS Levels and SOD, ALT, and AST Activity

Lung tissues were ground in cold physiological saline to obtain a 10% homogenate, which was centrifuged at 3,500 rpm for 10 min at 4°C, and the supernatant was retained for the assessing HYP, MDA, and ROS levels and SOD activity. Serum samples were used to detect ALT and AST activity according to the corresponding kit instructions.

ELISA

BALF and serum were prepared for ELISA, and the appropriate kits were used to assess the TNF-α, IL-1β, and IL-6 levels in rat BALF and TGF-β1 level in serum samples.

Western Blotting

Lung tissues were harvested, washed with cold PBS and lysed with PIRA lysis buffer containing protease and phosphatase inhibitor and phenylmethylsulphonyl fluoride for 30 min on ice and then

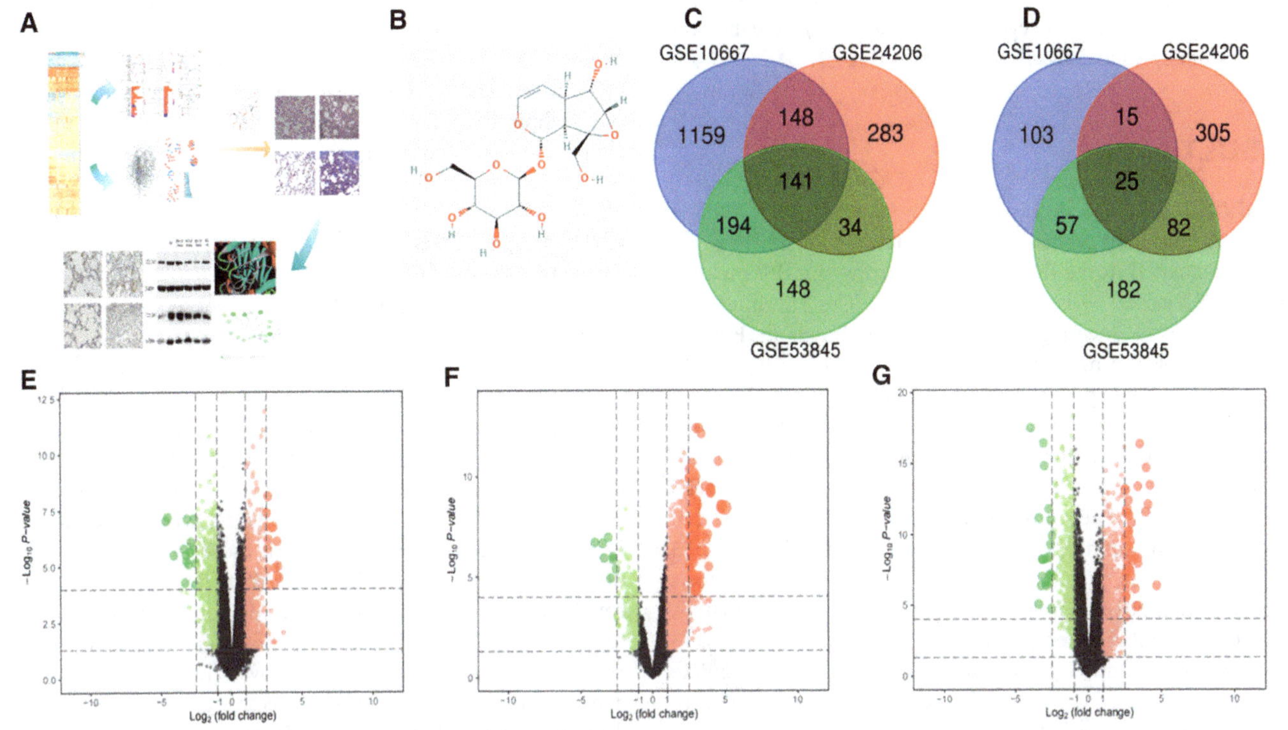

FIGURE 1 | In this study, we screened the GEO database for DEGs in IPF to find the key signaling pathways and proteins in the occurrence and development of this disease. Next, molecular docking was used to virtually screen the DEG proteins and estimate the theoretical stability of their binding to CAT. Furthermore, a rat IPF model was established to verify the effect of CAT on the key signaling pathways in IPF and to explore its mechanism of action **(A)**. The chemical structure of CAT **(B)**. Upregulated genes in the datasets **(C)**. Downregulated genes in the datasets **(D)**. **(E–G)** are the volcano maps and heat maps of the highly expressed genes and the low expressed genes in the data sets GSE24206, GSE10667, and GSE53845. In the volcano map, green represents down-regulated genes and red represents up-regulated genes; in the heat map, blue represents down-regulated genes, and red represents up-regulated genes between IPF samples and normal samples. $p < 0.01$ and FC > 1 were considered as cut-off values.

were centrifuged at 12,000 g for 15 min at 4°C; thereafter, proteins were extracted from the lung tissue lysates and the BCA protein detection kit was used to measure the protein concentrations according to the instructions provided. Equal amounts of protein were separated by sodium dodecyl sulfate-polyacrylamide gel electrophoresis and transferred onto polyvinylidene fluoride membranes. After blocking with 5% (wt/vol) nonfat milk in Tris-buffered saline Tween-20 at room temperature, the membranes were incubated with primary antibodies against α-SMA (diluted 1:2000), COL1A1 (diluted 1:1,000), COL3A1 (diluted 1:750), *p*-Smad3 (diluted 1:750), Smad3 (diluted 1:1,000), Wnt3a (diluted 1:1,000), p-β-catenin (diluted 1:1,000), β-catenin (diluted 1:1,200), *p*-GSK-3β (diluted 1: 1,000), or GSK-3β (diluted 1:1,000) overnight at 4°C. After washing four times with TBST, they were incubated with goat anti-rabbit secondary antibody for 1.5 h at room temperature and then washed again four times with TBST. The protein bands on the membrane were then visualized using an enhanced chemiluminescence reagent. Band intensities were quantified using ImageJ.

Immunohistochemical Analysis

After dewaxing, the lung slices were subjected to antigen recovery in citrate buffer under microwave heating. The slices were cooled down to room temperature, blocked with 3% bovine serum albumin for 30 min, and then incubated with the following primary antibodies overnight at 4°C as appropriate: rabbit anti-α-SMA antibody (diluted 1:1,000), anti-COL1A1 antibody (diluted 1:1,000), anti-COL3A1 antibody (diluted 1:200), anti-Smad3 antibody (diluted 1:200), anti-Wnt3a antibody (diluted 1: 250), anti-β-catenin antibody (diluted 1:200), anti-GSK-3βantibody (diluted 1:600), anti-E-cad antibody (diluted 1: 400), and anti-MMP-7 antibody (diluted 1:100). The slices were then washed with phosphate-buffered saline (PBS) and incubated with goat anti-rabbit secondary antibody (diluted 1: 200) at 37°C for 50 min. After rinsing with PBS, the slices were stained with diaminobenzidine and counterstained with hematoxylin. The average optical density was measured using ImageJ.

Statistical Analysis

Data are represented as mean ± standard deviation (SD). Differences between the groups were evaluated using one-way analysis of variance followed by the least significant difference (LSD) post hoc test. A value of $p < 0.05$ was considered statistically significant. IBM SPSS Statistics 19.0 (IBM SPSS

Software, NY, United States) and GraphPad Prism Version 8.0 (GraphPad Software, San Diego, CA, United States) were used for statistical analyses and figure preparation.

RESULTS

Analysis of DEGs in IPF

The study flow chart is shown in **Figure 1A**. A total of 517 genes were upregulated in the three data sets during the IPF process, while 179 genes were downregulated. The numbers of upregulated and downregulated genes are shown in **Figures 1C,D**. The volcano map and heat map of 141 high expression genes and 25 low expression genes in GSE24206 are shown in **Figure 1E**. Among all up- or downregulated genes, the top five with the most significant changes in differential expression were ZMAT, CRIP, PSD, FNDC1 (upregulated), and BTNL8 (downregulated). Their functions are mainly related to cell cycle regulation and EMT. For example, ZMAT is a p53 target gene that regulates the cell cycle and apoptosis (Bersani et al., 2014). FNDC1 is ubiquitous in the cell matrix, and related membrane receptors and enzymes can mediate Cx43 phosphorylation and G protein signal transduction to regulate cell permeability and apoptosis (Sato et al., 2009). GSK-3β is an important signal transduction molecule in the Wnt/β-catenin signaling pathway, and CRIP1 promotes EMT through zinc-induced *p*-GSK-3β in colorectal cancer (He et al., 2019). The downregulation of BTNL8 expression is related to excessive inflammation and destruction of epithelial tissue integrity (Mayassi et al., 2019). The DEGs in GSE10667 and GSE53845 are shown in **Figures 1F,G** and **Supplementary Figures S1-S6**.

GO Function Enrichment Analysis, KEGG Pathway Analysis, and PPI Network Analysis

GO analysis confirmed that the DEGs in IPF mainly coded for proteins involved in the ECM environment and the collagen metabolism process (**Figures 2A,B**), which was also evidenced by the CC and MF enrichment analyses. The BP analysis suggested that the humoral immune response of IPF patients is unbalanced and is characterized by the high expression of inflammatory mediators. Correspondingly, KEGG analysis (**Figures 2C,D**) showed high confidence in the protein degradation and synthesis process and the interaction between cytokines and receptors. It has been reported that the Wnt signaling pathway is activated in IPF, and the regulation of EMT by it is an important biological process in IPF. The TGF-β signaling pathway is a key pathway for M2 macrophages to induce EMT (Zhu et al., 2017a; Ko et al., 2019) and can also promote the development of IPF by altering the 3'-UTR of target mRNAs. The key signal transduction molecules in the two signaling pathways are shown in **Figure 2E,F**. An IPF-related PPI network (**Figure 3A**) was constructed based on the STRING database. The ranking of the top 30 key proteins is shown in **Figure 3E** and **Supplementary Table S1**. The top five pivot proteins were IL-6, COL1A1, CXCL12, COL1A2, and IGF1 (PPI enrichment *p*-value:< 1.0e-16). MCODE module analysis (**Figures 3B–D**) showed that chemokine signal transduction, cell cycle and proteasome, and collagen and vascular remodeling were the main functions of the three important core modules, suggesting that the expression of the MMP family was upregulated.

CAT Improves BLM-Induced PF

The 2D structure of CAT (PubChem CID: 91520, CAS No. 2415-24-9) is shown in **Figure 1B**. PF was successfully induced by intratracheal instillation of BLM (5 mg/kg) in rats. HE staining confirmed that the structure of rat lung tissues in the BLM group was disordered, with alveolar wall thickening, infiltration of a large number of inflammatory cells in the alveolar and the interstitial cavities, and the disappearance of some alveoli. All rats survived until the samples were collected. In the three days after modeling, the weight of all rats decreased, after which it gradually increased. Compared with those in the NS group, all rats administered BLM had different degrees of wheezing, coughing, and bradykinesia, and Masson trichrome staining revealed extensive collagen deposition (**Figures 4A–D**). However, CAT significantly improved lung tissue structural damage caused by BLM. The protective effect of the 40 mg/kg dose was better than that of 150 mg/kg PFD, and the lung coefficient was significantly reduced in a dose-dependent manner (**Figure 4E**). HYP is the main component of collagen, and TGF-β1 can induce fibroblasts to synthesize a large amount of collagen. After treatment with CAT at doses of 10–40 mg/kg, HYP levels in the lung tissues of rats with lung fibrosis and TGF-β1 levels in the serum were reduced compared to those in the BLM group (**Figures 4F,G**). There was no significant difference between the 40 mg/kg CAT group and 150 mg/kg PFD groups, and no impairment of liver functions was observed (**Figures 4H,I**). E-cad and α-SMA are considered biomarkers of epithelial cells and myofibroblasts, respectively. During EMT, the expression of E-cad decreases, while the expression of α-SMA increases significantly. In addition, the EMT process in lung tissues is accompanied by collagen deposition and the activation of MMPs in the ECM. As shown in **Figures 5A–D**, the WB results demonstrated increased expression of α-SMA, COL1A1, and COL3A1 in the BLM group, which was also evidenced by immunohistochemistry (**Figure 5E**). However, CAT dramatically reversed the upregulation of these proteins and attenuated the expression of MMP-7 and the downregulation of E-cad (**Supplementary Figure S7**), with a better effect than that of 150 mg/kg PFD. These results suggest that CAT may be alleviating PF by inhibiting the EMT process to reduce ECM deposition.

CAT Alleviates PF by Inhibiting the TGF-β1/Smad3 and Wnt/β-Catenin Signaling Pathways

In order to determine the mechanism of action of CAT in IPF, we used molecular docking technology to dock key proteins from the PPI network analysis and KEGG pathway analysis with CAT. The

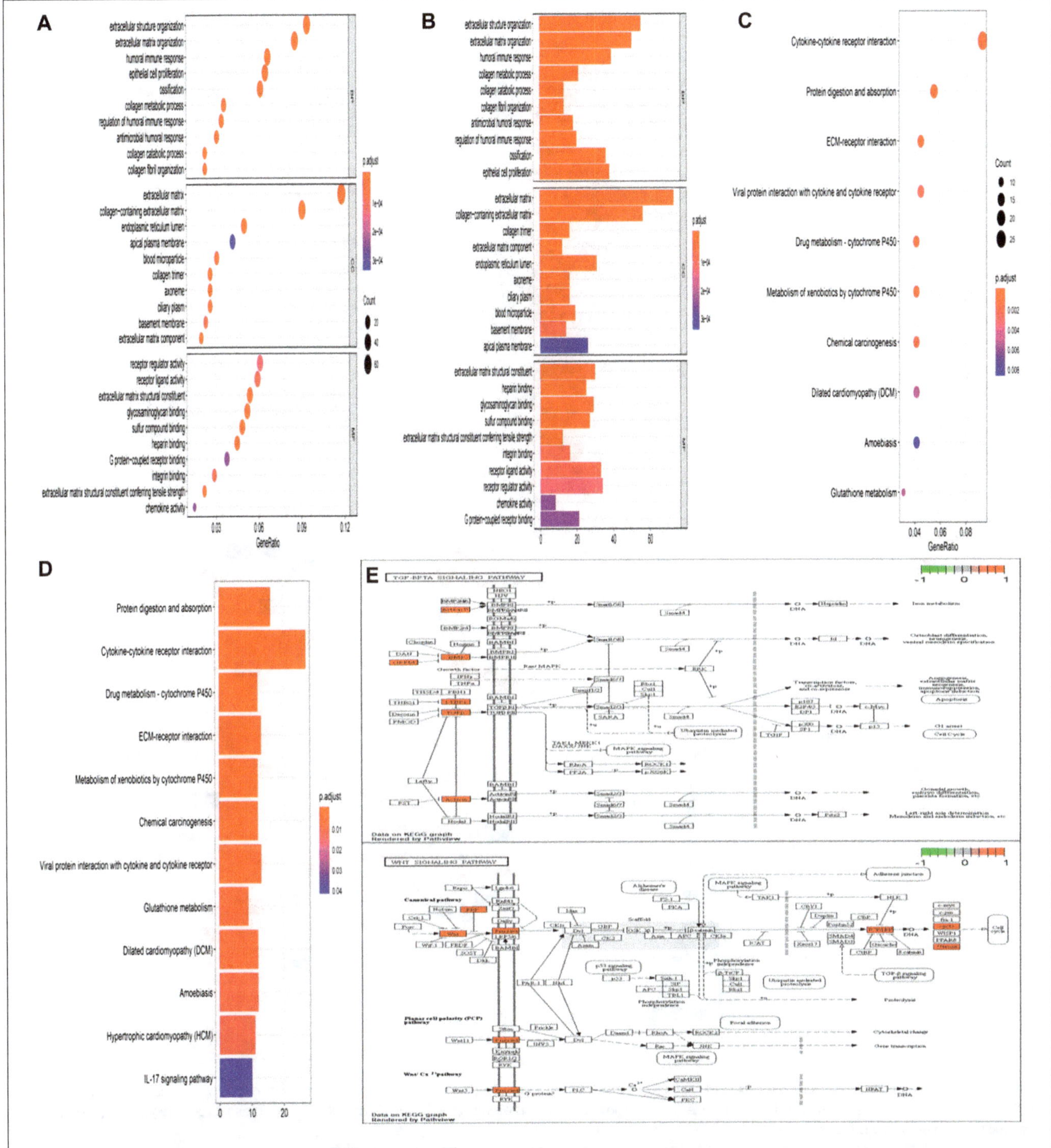

FIGURE 2 | GO function enrichment analysis and KEGG pathway analysis. Bubble chart of enrichment analysis results of GO function **(A)**. Histogram of enrichment analysis results of GO function **(B)**. Bubble chart of KEGG pathway enrichment analysis results **(C)**. Histogram of KEGG pathway enrichment analysis results **(D)**. The key target of the TGF-β/Smad signaling pathway in IPF **(E)**. The key target of the Wnt signaling pathway in IPF **(F)**.

CDOCKER results revealed that CAT can be docked effectively with Wnt3a (PDB code: 4A0P), Smad3 (PDB code: 1U7F), GSK-3β (PDB code: 4J1R), and TGF-βR1 (PDB code: 6B8Y) (binding energies: 57.42 kcal/mol, 48.22 kcal/mol, 36.10 kcal/mol, and 23.75 kcal/mol, respectively). CAT forms an alkyl interaction with residue ILE1023 of Wnt3a; Van der Waals bonds with residues VAL1194, PRO974, ASP1022, VAL1063, CA1360, ALA1108, LEU1109, PHE1153, and SER1111; hydrogen bonds

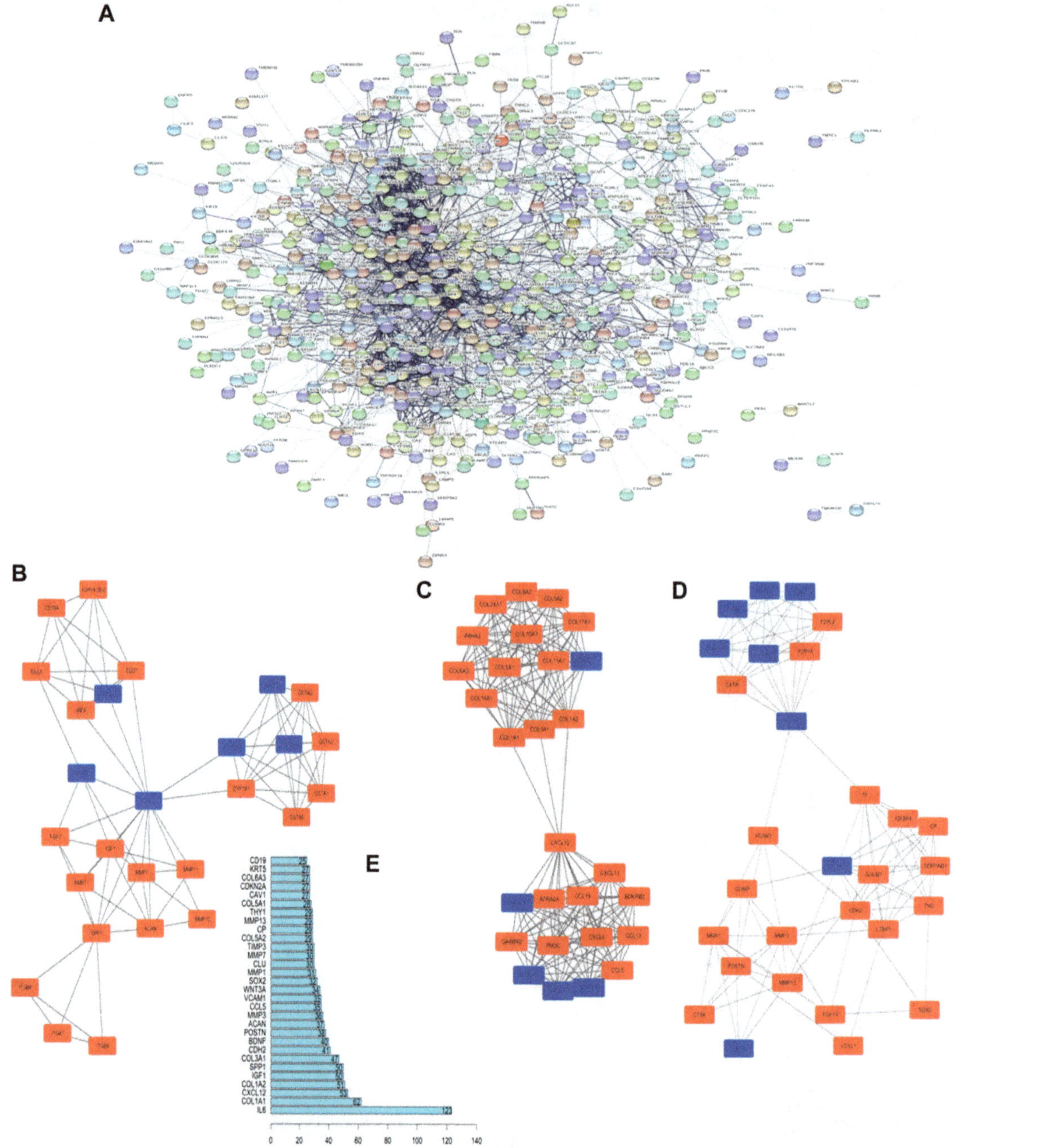

FIGURE 3 | Key proteins and interactions in IPF. **(A)** PPI network of differentially expressed proteins in IPF. This network consists of 572 nodes and 2,432 edges. **(B–D)** The three important core modules in MCODE module analysis. The red square represents upregulation and the blue block represents downregulation. **(E)** Ranking of correlation degree of key proteins.

with residues VAL1152, THR1151, ASP971, SER1020, and ILE1021; and carbon-hydrogen bonds with residues HIS1192, PRO1066, VAL1064, ALA1193, CL1355, LYS1195, ASP1110. It forms alkyl interactions with residue ARG243 of Smad3; van der Waals bonds with residues GLN242, VAL277, ASN278, TYR238, ASN276, GLY245, VAL244, GLU246, and THR247; hydrogen bonds with residues ARG243, ASN241, GLU337, and GLY245; and carbon-hydrogen bonds with residues VAL244, and SER275.

It forms van der Waals bonds with residues ASN186, ASP200, ILE217, ARG223, ARG220, and TYR221 of GSK-3β; hydrogen bonds with residues ARG220, LYS183, and SER219; and carbon-hydrogen bonds with residues SER203, ASP181, and CYS218. It forms alkyl interactions with residues ALA399 and VAL383 of TGF-βR1; van der Waals bonds with residues HIS331, ALA330, SER395, ILE388, MET390, HIS371, ASN370, VAL373, GLY374, MET379, ALA380, LYS376, LYS335, ASP333, TYR402, and

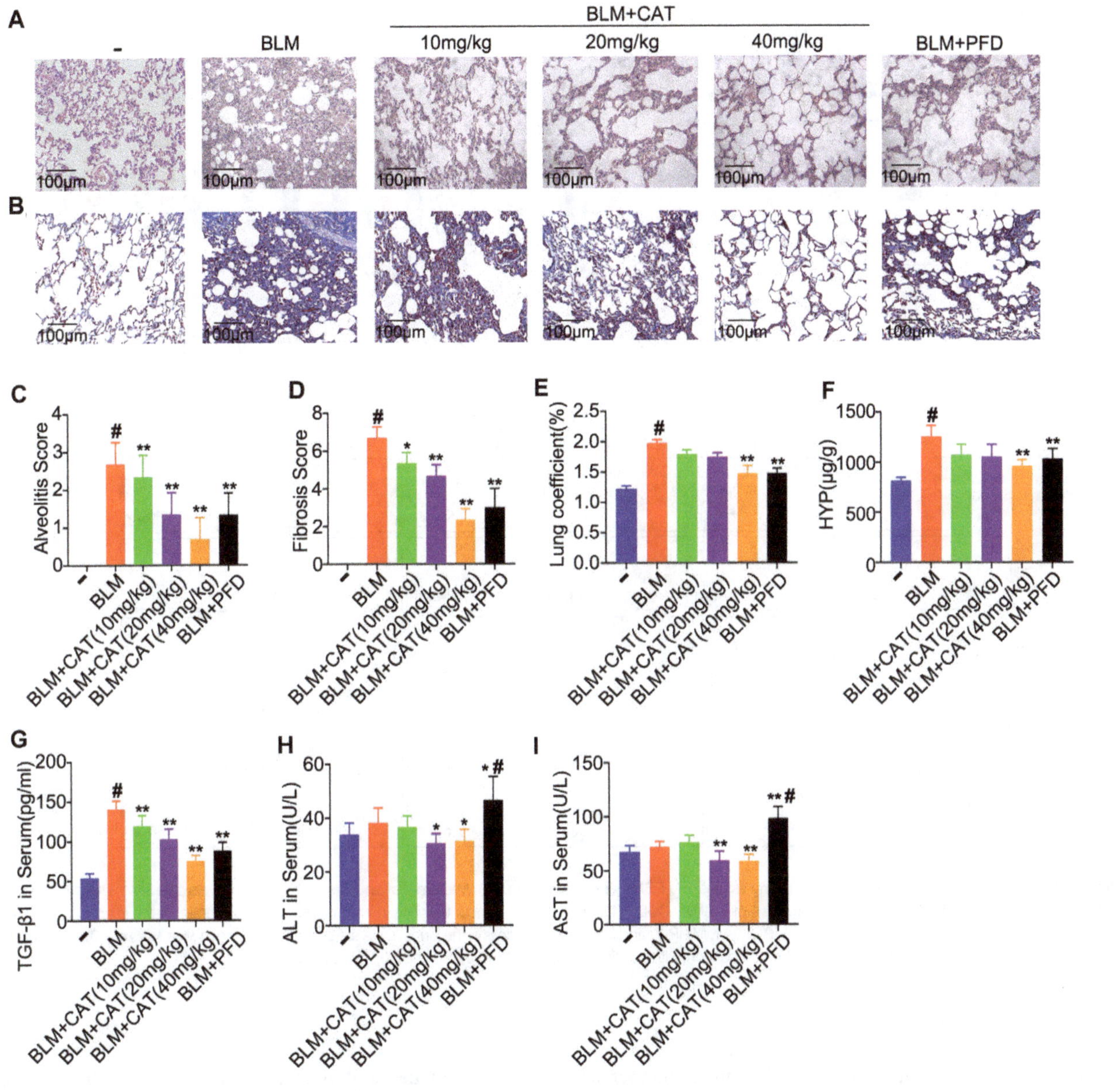

FIGURE 4 | The protective effects of CAT on BLM-induced PF in rats. **(A)** Photomicrographs of HE-stained lung sections. **(B)** Photomicrographs of Masson Trichrome stained lung sections. **(C)** Alveolitis score of each group. **(D)** Statistics of pulmonary fibrosis area in each group. **(E)** Measurement of lung coefficient in each group. **(F)** Determination of HYP level in lung tissues of each group. **(G)** Determination of serum TGF-β1 levels of each group. **(H)** Determination of serum ALT levels of each group. **(I)** Determination of serum AST levels of each group. Data are presented as the means ± SD (n = 3 or 6), # represents a comparison with the control group, * represents a comparison with the BLM group. #$p < 0.01$; *$p < 0.05$; **$p < 0.01$.

ALA403; hydrogen bonds with residues LEU334, ASP400, ARG372, ARG332, and THR375; and carbon-hydrogen bonds with residues TYR378 and PHE396 (**Figures 6A–D**). After BLM (5 mg/kg) successfully established the PF rat model, the expression of Smad3, Wnt3a, β-catenin, and GSK-3β were all upregulated in the BLM group ($p < 0.01$). After PFD and different doses of CAT were administered, the expression of Smad3, Wnt3a, β-catenin, and GSK-3β decreased in a dose-dependent manner ($p < 0.05$) (**Figure 6E**). The immunohistochemistry results also reflected this (**Figure 6F**). It was found that BLM induced the phosphorylation of β-catenin, GSK-3β, and Smad3 in the rat model, while p-β-catenin, *p*-GSK-3β, and *p*-Smad3 levels were significantly downregulated by CAT at doses of 20 mg/kg and 40 mg/kg (**Supplementary Figure S8**). PFD downregulated p-β-catenin and *p*-Smad3 levels, but had no significant effect on *p*-GSK-3β level. In conclusion, the TGF-β1/Smad3 and Wnt/β-catenin signaling pathways were activated in the lung tissue of rats with PF. CAT downregulated the expression of Wnt3a,

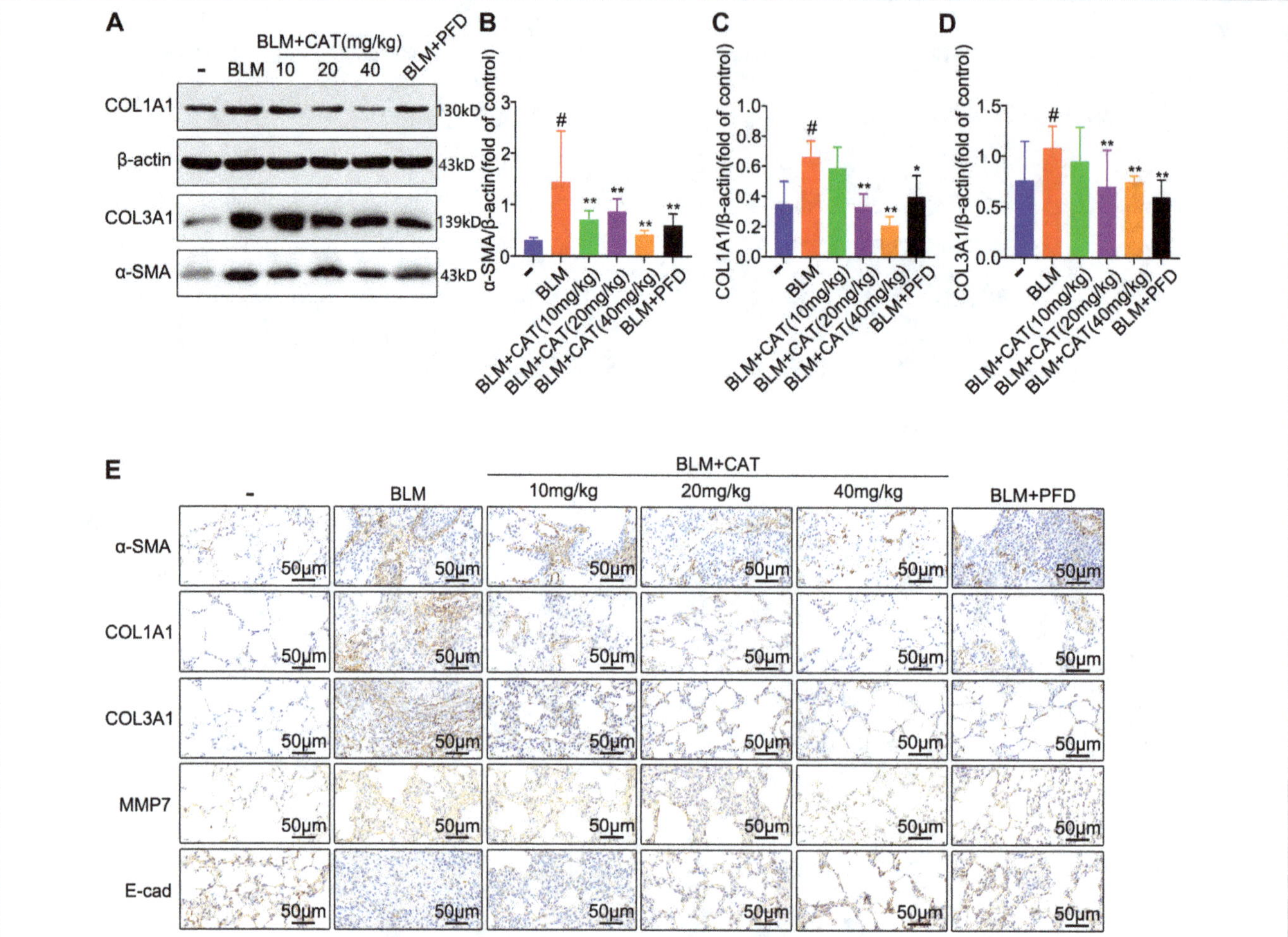

FIGURE 5 | CAT attenuates BLM-induced EMT in lung tissues and ECM deposition *in vivo*. **(A)** Western blot analysis of the protein levels of α-SMA, COL1A1, and COL3A1 in lung tissues. **(B–D)** Densitometric analysis of α-SMA, COL1A1, and COL3A1 band intensities in immunoblots, using β-actin as the internal reference. **(E)** Immunohistochemical staining of α-SMA, COL1A1, COL3A1, MMP-7, and E-cad positive cells in the lungs. Data are presented as the means ± SD (n = 3), # represents a comparison with the control group, * represents a comparison with the BLM group. #$p < 0.01$; *$p < 0.05$; **$p < 0.01$.

β-catenin, GSK-3β, and Smad3 in a dose-dependent manner, and inhibited the phosphorylation of β-catenin, GSK-3β, and Smad3.

CAT Reduces Oxidative Stress and Inflammation in Lung Tissue of Rats With PF

TNF-α induces activation of the NF-κB signaling pathway and exacerbates PF caused by BLM(Hou et al., 2018). To verify the anti-inflammatory and anti-oxidant effects of CAT, we used ELISA to detect the relevant biomarkers. As expected, 28 days after successful modeling, the levels of inflammatory mediators and oxidative stress markers in the lung tissue of rats in the BLM group were increased, while CAT reduced the levels of IL-1β (**Figure 7A**), TNF-α (**Figure 7B**), IL-6 (**Figure 7C**), MDA (**Figure 7D**), and ROS (**Figure 7E**) and increased the activity of SOD (**Figure 7F**) in the lung tissues of IPF rats. The CAT and PFD at 40 mg/kg were significantly different from BLM groups. In summary, CAT can downregulate the expression of cytokines in lung tissues and reduce the level of oxidative stress, thus alleviating BLM-induced PF in rats.

DISCUSSION

IPF is an irreversible, progressive, and fatal lung disease with a poor prognosis that often occurs during acute exacerbation (Border and Noble, 1994; Lopez et al., 2009). Since the molecular mechanisms underlying the occurrence and development of PF are not fully understood, the treatments approved so far are limited to those effective against mild-to-moderate IPF(Mora et al., 2017). The pathogenesis of IPF involves a variety of processes, such as inflammation, oxidative stress, and fibrosis. In this study, we discovered that 141 upregulated genes and 25 downregulated genes were common between the three IPF data sets analyzed. GO analysis of the DEGs revealed that they were mainly involved in humoral

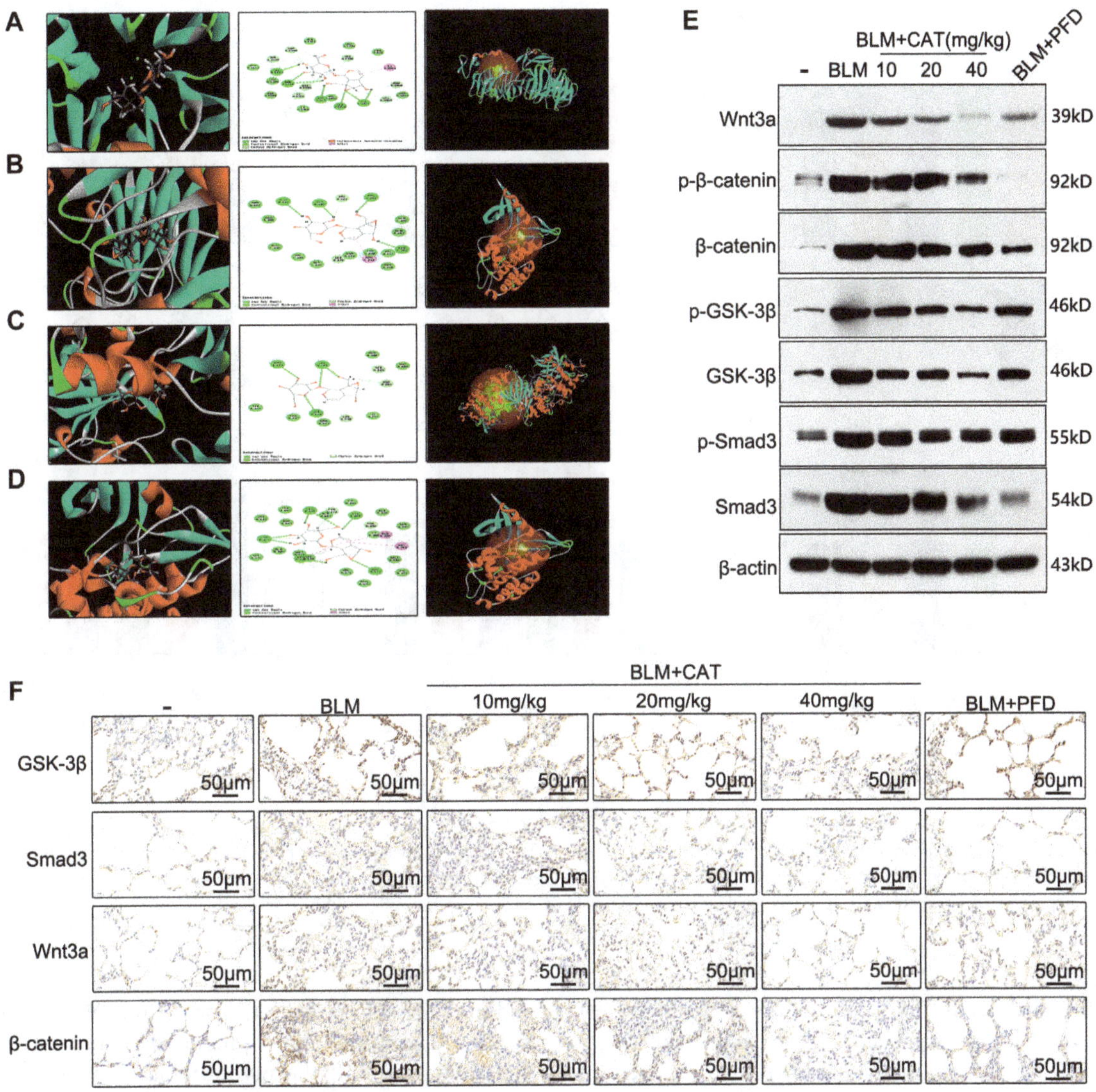

FIGURE 6 | CAT alleviates PF by inhibiting the TGF-β1/Smad3 and Wnt/β-catenin signaling pathways. The docking conformation and main active site of CAT and Wnt3a **(A)**, Smad3 **(B)**, GSK-3β **(C)**, and TGF-βR1 **(D)**. **(E)** WB analysis of the protein levels of Wnt3a, p-β-catenin, β-catenin, *p*-GSK-3β, GSK-3β, *p*-Smad3, and Smad3 in lung tissues. **(F)** Immunohistochemical staining of Wnt3a, Smad3, GSK-3β, and β-catenin positive cells in the lungs. Data are presented as the means ± SD (n = 3), # represents a comparison with the control group, * represents a comparison with the BLM group. #$p < 0.01$; *$p < 0.05$; **$p < 0.01$.

immunity, collagen metabolism, epithelial cell proliferation, mesenchymal development, and cell matrix adhesion, which is consistent with the strong inflammatory response and the imbalance of collagen metabolism observed in IPF (Xin et al., 2019). KEGG pathway enrichment analysis showed significant enrichment in protein degradation and absorption, cytokine-cytokine receptor interaction, and ECM-receptor interaction, all of which are areas most current studies on IPF are focused on (Du et al., 2019). Although hypoxia is a significant pathological feature of PF (Senavirathna et al., 2018)—for example, the nuclear HIF-1α protein is involved in hypoxia-induced EMT (Senavirathna et al., 2018)—several key protein targets for cellular hypoxia as well as oxidative stress did not appear in the PPI results. Correspondingly, the support for the GO analysis and KEGG pathway enrichment analysis is not high. Although the reasons for these differences are not clear, we suggested that researchers should re-examine the importance of the known key signaling pathways and biological processes in the development of IPF.

Traditional Chinese medicine is a potential source of treatments for PF (Li and Kan, 2017). We performed molecular docking of CAT, the active constituent of *Rehmannia glutinosa*, with several key protein targets suggested by the PPI and KEGG enrichment analyses and found that CAT has high binding to several components of the TGF-β1/Smad3 and Wnt/β-catenin pathways. TGF-β1 is a key protein among the many factors and cytokines that regulate PF (Border and Noble, 1994). It can induce

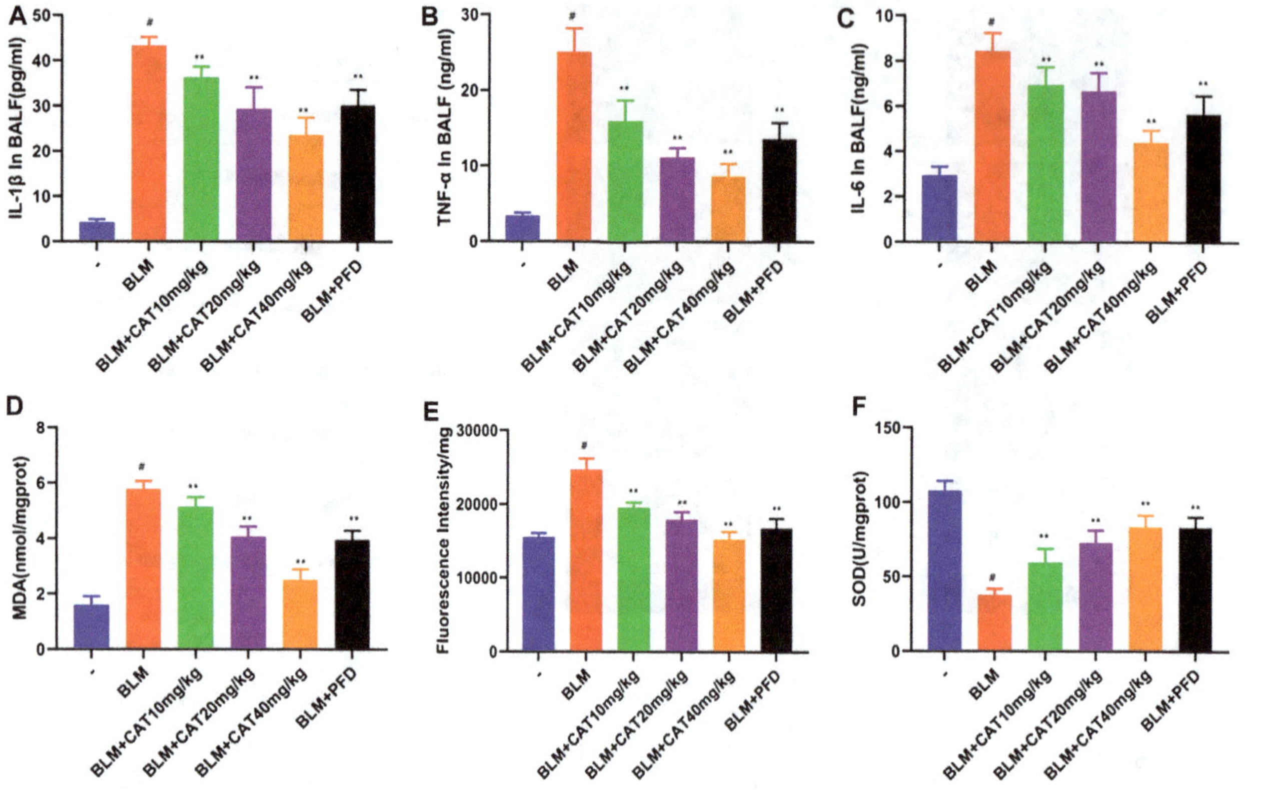

FIGURE 7 | CAT reduces oxidative stress and inflammation in lung tissue of rats with PF. **(A)** Determination of IL-1β levels in BALF of each group. **(B)** Determination of TNF-α levels in BALF of each group. **(C)** Determination of IL-6 levels in BALF of each group. **(D)** Determination of MDA levels in lung tissue of each group. **(E)** Determination of ROS levels in lung tissue of each group. **(F)** Determination of SOD levels in lung tissue of each group. Data are presented as the means ± SD (n = 6); # represents a comparison with the control group, * represents a comparison with the BLM group. #$p < 0.01$; *$p < 0.05$; **$p < 0.01$.

alveolar epithelial cells to acquire the phenotype of mesenchymal cells, which become the main source of fibroblasts and myofibroblasts and lead to ECM deposition (Song et al., 2013). This process, as a typical EMT, is a very important mechanism of PF (Piera-Velazquez et al., 2011), and had a high score in GO analysis and KEGG pathway enrichment analysis. Specifically, TGF-β1 interacts with fibroblast surface receptors and phosphorylates Smad proteins, which form Smad3/4 complexes. These enter the nucleus and bind to the promoter regions of fibrogenic genes, such as those for type I collagen, fibronectin, and α-SMA, to activate downstream target gene transcription (Santibanez et al., 2011). However, although TGF-βR1-mediated receptor-activated Smad proteins are most closely related with the occurrence of PF(Ask et al., 2008) and can participate in the regulation of EMT through multiple pathways, the Wnt/β-catenin signaling pathway is even more critical for mediating EMT. It is a key pathway regulating cell proliferation and differentiation, with β-catenin as its major signal transduction molecule. Trauma and other stimuli activate the expression and secretion of the Wnt protein, which leads to the inhibition of β-catenin phosphorylation (Li et al., 1999). Once a certain amount of free β-catenin accumulates, it enters the nucleus and activates target gene transcription (Nusse and Clevers, 2017). The epithelial phenotypic marker E-cad is downregulated and the myofibroblast markers α-SMA and type I collagen are upregulated in PF (Qu et al., 2015; Lacy et al., 2018), and the high expression of α-SMA is associated with a lower survival rate in patients with PF. As targets gene for β-catenin activation, the expression of MMPs accelerates the degradation of ECM. MMPs are the main rate-limiting enzymes that regulate ECM metabolism. MMP-7, which is able to activate other proteases while degrading ECM components such as cell-associated Fas ligands and E-cad, plays a key role in regulating various cell processes such as matrix remodeling, apoptosis, and EMT (Zhou et al., 2017). Wnt/β-catenin signaling pathway is a key factor in the regulation of MMP-7 *in vivo*. The activation of β-catenin promotes the expression of MMP-7 (He et al., 2012; Zuo and Liu, 2018). Thus, it can be seen that the Wnt/β-catenin pathway plays a significant role in the process of PF.

In recent years, several studies have shown that there is crosstalk between the TGF-β/Smad3 and Wnt/β-catenin signaling pathways. Axin and GSK-3β in the Wnt/β-catenin pathway can affect TGF-β signaling by controlling the stability of Smad3 (Guo et al.,2008), while Smad3-mediated regulation enhances the stability of β-catenin and promotes the activation of downstream target genes (Zhang et al., 2010). In addition, p-β-catenin/p-Smad2 complexes were also found in the lung tissues of patients with PF (Kim et al., 2009), while Wnt3a/β-catenin/GSK-3β were mainly localized in alveolar and bronchial epithelial cells (Konigshoff et al., 2008). Therefore, targeting the TGF-β1/Smad3 and Wnt/β-catenin signaling pathways is an effective strategy for regulating EMT and inhibiting the progression of PF. *In vivo* experiments showed that the TGF-β/Smad3 and Wnt/β-catenin pathways were activated in a rat model of PF (Henderson et al., 2010; Kim et al., 2011), which was consistent with previous studies. Molecular docking, WB, and immunohistochemistry experiments confirmed that CAT can bind to Wnt3a, Smad3, GSK-3β, and TGF-βR1. Furthermore, by inhibiting the activation of the TGF-β/Smad3 and Wnt/β-catenin pathways, CAT reduced the secretion of key signal transduction molecules such as Smad3, Wnt3a, GSK3β, and β-catenin, and also reduced the expression of α-SMA, COL1A1, COL3A1, and MMP7, effectively inhibited EMT, ECM deposition, and lung structural remodeling and reduced the downregulation of the epithelial phenotype marker E-cad. This demonstrates that CAT can maintain the balance of ECM degradation in the local lung microenvironment, which is of great significance for improving outcomes in PF.

As IPF occurs, fibroblasts and myofibroblasts proliferate extensively in fibroblast foci. Factors such as CXCL12 are released by damaged alveolar epithelial cells and cause CXC chemokine type 4 receptor-positive circulating fibroblasts to enter the lungs, expanding the fibroblast pool (Andersson-Sjoland et al., 2008; Mehrad et al., 2009). At the same time, alveolar epithelial cells entering the phenotypic state associated with aging produce and release a large number of cytokines such as TNF-α. Moreover, high inflammatory levels also cause local fibroblasts to migrate and hyperproliferate, and oxidative stress can also lead to the release of pro-inflammatory factors such as IL-1β, which plays an important role in the pathogenesis of IPF (Kliment et al., 2009). Oxidative stress is essentially the imbalance between oxidation and reduction caused by excessive generation of ROS in the body (Kala et al., 2017). SOD is an important antioxidant enzyme that maintains the dynamic balance between free radical generation and removal (He et al., 2016). BLM can cause alveolar epithelial cells and macrophages to produce a large amount of ROS, resulting in lipid peroxidation in biofilms, while MDA can reflect the degree of cell damage by reflecting lipid peroxidation (Teixeira et al., 2008; Yu et al., 2016). This study revealed that oxidative stress and inflammation levels were elevated in rats with PF, which is consistent with previous findings (Xin et al., 2019). With reference to the results of the bioinformatics analysis, *in vivo* experiments confirmed that CAT could increase the activity of SOD in rat lung tissues and decrease the levels of MDA, IL-6, IL-1β, TNF-α, and ROS, suggesting that CAT may inhibit the development of PF by reducing the levels of inflammation and oxidative stress. Although our results prove that CAT has a potential therapeutic effect on BLM-induced pulmonary fibrosis in rats, the more detailed mechanism of action is still unclear. For example, how does CAT inhibit β-catenin activation/phosphorylation in the Wnt signaling pathway? One possible explanation is that CAT blocks the interaction between Wnt3a and β-catenin. In addition, if we use primary human embryonic lung fibroblasts for *in vitro* experiments, our findings will be more meaningful.

CONCLUSION

In summary, the results of this study suggest that the collagen metabolism imbalance, inflammatory responses, and EMT activation are the core processes of IPF, and that the TGF-β1/Smad3 and Wnt/β-catenin signaling pathways and related signal transduction molecules are key targets for the treatment of IPF. The ability of CAT to protect against lung fibrosis induced by BLM in rats was reported for the first time. This mechanism is related to the downregulation of Smad3, Wnt3a, GSK-3β, and β-catenin as well as the phosphorylation of Smad3, GSK-3β, and β-catenin. This study also provided new insights into the potential value of CAT for the treatment of IPF. Considering that CAT did not harm the liver during this study and that there have been previous studies on CAT in combination with other compounds to reduce drug-induced hepatitis, further research should focus on clinically evaluating the effectiveness and side-effects of CAT in patients with PF.

ETHICS STATEMENT

The animal study was reviewed and approved by Research Ethics Committee of the Affiliated Hospital of Shandong University of Traditional Chinese Medicine.

AUTHOR CONTRIBUTIONS

FY, WZ, and WL conceived and designed the experiments; ZH, HZ, and XC performed the experiments; RC, YL contributed reagents/materials/analysis tools; FY and RC analyzed the data and wrote the paper. All authors have read and agreed to the published version of the manuscript.

REFERENCES

1. Andersson-Sjöland, A., de Alba, C. G., Nihlberg, K., Becerril, C., Ramírez, R., Pardo, A., et al. (2008). Fibrocytes are a potential source of lung fibroblasts in idiopathic pulmonary fibrosis. *Int. J. Biochem. Cell Biol.* 40, 2129–2140. doi:10. 1016/j.biocel.2008.02.012
2. Ashcroft, T., Simpson, J. M., and Timbrell, V. (1988). Simple method of estimating severity of pulmonary fibrosis on a numerical scale. *J. Clin. Pathol.* 41, 467–470. doi:10.1136/jcp.41.4.467
3. Ask, K., Bonniaud, P., Maass, K., Eickelberg, O., Margetts, P. J., Warburton, D., et al. (2008). Progressive pulmonary fibrosis is mediated by TGF-beta isoform 1 but not TGF-beta3. *Int. J. Biochem. Cell Biol.* 40, 484–495. doi:10.1016/j.biocel. 2007.08.016

4. Barabási, A. L., Gulbahce, N., and Loscalzo, J. (2011). Network medicine: a network-based approach to human disease. *Nat. Rev. Genet.* 12, 56–68. doi:10.1038/nrg2918
5. Berman, H., Henrick, K., and Nakamura, H. (2003). Announcing the worldwide protein data bank. *Nat. Struct. Biol.* 10, 980. doi:10.1038/nsb1203-980
6. Bersani, C., Xu, L. D., Vilborg, A., Lui, W. O., and Wiman, K. G. (2014). Wig-1 regulates cell cycle arrest and cell death through the p53 targets FAS and 14-3- 3σ. *Oncogene* 33, 4407–4417. doi:10.1038/onc.2013.594
7. Border, W. A., and Noble, N. A. (1994). Transforming growth factor beta in tissue fibrosis. *N. Engl. J. Med.* 331, 1286–1292. doi:10.1056/NEJM199411103311907
8. Chen, Y., Liu, Q., Shan, Z., Mi, W., Zhao, Y., Li, M., et al. (2019). Catalpol ameliorates podocyte injury by stabilizing cytoskeleton and enhancing autophagy in diabetic nephropathy. *Front. Pharmacol.* 10, 1477. doi:10.3389/fphar.2019.01477
9. Chen, Y., Zhang, Y., Xu, M., Luan, J., Piao, S., Chi, S., et al. (2017). Catalpol alleviates ovalbumin-induced asthma in mice: reduced eosinophil infiltration in the lung. *Int. Immunopharm.* 43, 140–146. doi:10.1016/j.intimp.2016.12.011
10. Cheng, X., Zhang, Q., Li, Z., Dong, C., Jiang, S., Sun, Y. A., et al. (2020). Determination of behavior of catalpol hexapropionate in simulated gastric conditions by UPLC-ESI-HRMS. *Sci. Rep.* 10, 11185. doi:10.1038/s41598-020- 68056-5
11. Cottin, V., and Maher, T. (2015). Long-term clinical and real-world experience with pirfenidone in the treatment of idiopathic pulmonary fibrosis. *Eur. Respir. Rev.* 24, 58–64. doi:10.1183/09059180.00011514
12. DePianto, D. J., Chandriani, S., Abbas, A. R., Jia, G., N'Diaye, E. N., Caplazi, P., et al. (2015). Heterogeneous gene expression signatures correspond to distinct lung pathologies and biomarkers of disease severity in idiopathic pulmonary fibrosis. *Thorax* 70, 48–56. doi:10.1136/thoraxjnl-2013-204596
13. Du, M. Y., Duan, J. X., Zhang, C. Y., Yang, H. H., Guan, X. X., Zhong, W. J., et al. (2019). Psoralen attenuates bleomycin-induced pulmonary fibrosis in mice through inhibiting myofibroblast activation and collagen deposition. *Cell Biol. Int.* doi:10.1002/cbin.11205
14. Gene Ontology, C. (2006). The gene Ontology (GO) project in 2006. *Nucleic Acids Res.* 34, D322–D326. doi:10.1093/nar/gkj021
15. Guo, X., Ramirez, A., Waddell, D. S., Li, Z., Liu, X., and Wang, X. F. (2008). Axin and GSK3- control Smad3 protein stability and modulate TGF-signaling. *Genes Dev.* 22, 106–120. doi:10.1101/gad.1590908
16. He, C., Larson-Casey, J. L., Gu, L., Ryan, A. J., Murthy, S., and Carter, A. B. (2016). Cu,Zn-Superoxide dismutase-mediated redox regulation of jumonji domain containing 3 modulates macrophage polarization and pulmonary fibrosis. *Am. J. Respir. Cell Mol. Biol.* 55, 58–71. doi:10.1165/rcmb.2015-0183OC
17. He, G., Zhu, H., Yao, Y., Chai, H., Wang, Y., Zhao, W., et al. (2019). Cysteine-rich intestinal protein 1 silencing alleviates the migration and invasive capability enhancement induced by excessive zinc supplementation in colorectal cancer cells. *Am J Transl Res* 11, 3578–3588.
18. He, W., Tan, R. J., Li, Y., Wang, D., Nie, J., Hou, F. F., et al. (2012). Matrix metalloproteinase-7 as a surrogate marker predicts renal Wnt/β-catenin activity in CKD. *J. Am. Soc. Nephrol.* 23, 294–304. doi:10.1681/ASN.2011050490
19. Henderson, W. R., Jr., Chi, E. Y., Ye, X., Nguyen, C., Tien, Y. T., Zhou, B., et al. (2010). Inhibition of Wnt/beta-catenin/CREB binding protein (CBP) signaling reverses pulmonary fibrosis. *Proc. Natl. Acad. Sci. U.S.A.* 107, 14309–14314. doi:10.1073/pnas.1001520107
20. Herrera, J., Henke, C. A., and Bitterman, P. B. (2018). Extracellular matrix as a driver of progressive fibrosis. *J. Clin. Invest.* 128, 45–53. doi:10.1172/ jci93557
21. Hou, J., Ma, T., Cao, H., Chen, Y., Wang, C., Chen, X., et al. (2018). TNF-α-induced NF-κB activation promotes myofibroblast differentiation of LR-MSCs and exacerbates bleomycin-induced pulmonary fibrosis. *J. Cell. Physiol.* 233, 2409–2419. doi:10.1002/jcp.26112
22. Huang, D. W., Sherman, B. T., Tan, Q., Kir, J., Liu, D., Bryant, D., et al. (2007). DAVID Bioinformatics Resources: expanded annotation database and novel algorithms to better extract biology from large gene lists. *Nucleic Acids Res.* 35, W169–W175. doi:10.1093/nar/gkm415
23. Jo, H. E., Randhawa, S., Corte, T. J., and Moodley, Y. (2016). Idiopathic pulmonary fibrosis and the elderly: diagnosis and management considerations. *Drugs Aging* 33, 321–334. doi:10.1007/s40266-016-0366-1
24. Kala, M., Shaikh, M. V., and Nivsarkar, M. (2017). Equilibrium between anti-oxidants and reactive oxygen species: a requisite for oocyte development and maturation. *Reprod. Med. Biol.* 16, 28–35. doi:10.1002/rmb2.12013
25. Kanehisa, M., and Goto, S. (2000). KEGG: kyoto encyclopedia of genes and genomes. *Nucleic Acids Res.* 28, 27–30. doi:10.1093/nar/28.1.27
26. Kim, K. K., Wei, Y., Szekeres, C., Kugler, M. C., Wolters, P. J., Hill, M. L., et al. (2009). Epithelial cell alpha3beta1 integrin links beta-catenin and Smad signaling to promote myofi broblast formation and pulmonary fibrosis. *J. Clin. Invest.* 119, 213–224. doi:10.1172/JCI36940
27. Kim, S., Chen, J., Cheng, T., Gindulyte, A., He, J., He, S., et al. (2019). PubChem 2019 update: improved access to chemical data. *Nucleic Acids Res.* 47, D1102–D1109. doi:10.1093/nar/gky1033
28. Kim, T. H., Kim, S. H., Seo, J. Y., Chung, H., Kwak, H. J., Lee, S. K., et al. (2011). Blockade of the Wnt/β-catenin pathway attenuates bleomycin-induced pulmonary fibrosis. *Tohoku J. Exp. Med.* 223, 45–54. doi:10.1620/tjem. 223.45
29. Kliment, C. R., Englert, J. M., Gochuico, B. R., Yu, G., Kaminski, N., Rosas, I., et al. (2009). Oxidative stres s alters syndecan-1 distribution in lungs with pulmonary fibrosis. *J. Biol. Chem.* 284, 3537–3545. doi:10.1074/jbc.M807001200
30. Ko, J., Mills, T., Huang, J., Chen, N. Y., Mertens, T. C. J., Collum, S. D., et al. (2019). Transforming growth factor β1 alters the 3'-UTR of mRNA to promote lung fibrosis. *J. Biol. Chem.* 294, 15781–15794. doi:10.1074/jbc.RA119.009148
31. Königshoff, M., Balsara, N., Pfaff, E. M., Kramer, M., Chrobak, I., Seeger, W., et al. (2008). Functional Wnt signaling is increased in idiopathic pulmonary fibrosis. *PloS One* 3, e2142. doi:10.1371/journal.pone.0002142
32. Lacy, S. H., Epa, A. P., Pollock, S. J., Woeller, C. F., Thatcher, T. H., Phipps, R. P., et al. (2018). Activated human Tlymphocytes inhibit TGFβ-induced fibroblast to myofibroblast differentiation via prostaglandins D2 and E2. *Am. J. Physiol. Lung Cell Mol. Physiol.* 314, L569–L582. doi:10.1152/ajplung.00565.2016
33. Li, L., Yuan, H., Weaver, C. D., Mao, J., Farr, G. H., 3rd, Sussman, D. J., et al. (1999). Axin and Frat1 interact with dvl and GSK, bridging Dvl to GSK in Wnt- mediated regulation of LEF-1. *EMBO J.* 18, 4233–4240. doi:10.1093/emboj/18. 15.4233
34. Li, L. C., and Kan, L. D. (2017). Traditional Chinese medicine for pulmonary fibrosis therapy: progress and future prospects. *J. Ethnopharmacol.* 198, 45–63. doi:10.1016/j.jep.2016.12.042
35. Liu, D., Chen, L., Zhao, H., Vaziri, N. D., Ma, S. C., and Zhao, Y. Y. (2019). Small molecules from natural products targeting the Wnt/β-catenin pathway as a therapeutic strategy. *Biomed. Pharmacother.* 117, 108990. doi:10.1016/j.biopha. 2019.108990
36. Lopez, A. D., Avasarala, S., Grewal, S., Murali, A. K., and London, L. (2009). Differential role of the Fas/Fas ligand apoptotic pathway in inflammation and lung fibrosis associated with reovirus 1/L-induced bronchiolitis obliterans organizing pneumonia and acute respiratory distress syndrome. *J. Immunol.* 183, 8244–8257. doi:10.4049/jimmunol.0901958
37. Mayassi, T., Ladell, K., Gudjonson, H., McLaren, J. E., Shaw, D. G., Tran, M. T., et al. (2019). Chronic inflammation permanently reshapes tissue-resident immunity in celiac disease. *Cell* 176, 967–e19. doi:10.1016/j.cell.2018.12.039
38. Mehrad, B., Burdick, M. D., and Strieter, R. M. (2009). Fibrocyte CXCR4 regulation as a therapeutic target in pulmonary fibrosis. *Int. J. Biochem. Cell Biol.* 41, 1708–1718. doi:10.1016/j.biocel.2009.02.020
39. Meltzer, E. B., Barry, W. T., D'Amico, T. A., Davis, R. D., Lin, S. S., Onaitis, M. W., et al. (2011). Bayesian probit regression model for the diagnosis of pulmonary fibrosis: proof-of-principle. *BMC Med. Genomics* 4, 70. doi:10.1186/1755-8794- 4-70
40. Missiuro, P. V., Liu, K., Zou, L., Ross, B. C., Zhao, G., Liu, J. S., et al. (2009). Information flow analysis of interactome networks. *PLoS Comput. Biol.* 5, e1000350. doi:10.1371/journal.pcbi.1000350
41. Mora, A. L., Rojas, M., Pardo, A., and Selman, M. (2017). Emerging therapies for idiopathic pulmonary fibrosis, a progressive age-related disease. *Nat. Rev. Drug Discov.* 16, 755–772. doi:10.1038/nrd.2017.170

42. Nalysnyk, L., Cid-Ruzafa, J., Rotella, P., and Esser, D. (2012). Incidence and prevalence of idiopathic pulmonary fibrosis: review of the literature. *Eur. Respir. Rev.* 21, 355–361. doi:10.1183/09059180.00002512
43. Nusse, R., and Clevers, H. (2017). Wnt/β-Catenin signaling, disease, and emerging therapeutic modalities. *Cell* 169, 985–999. doi:10.1016/j.cell.2017.05.016
44. Ogura, T., Taniguchi, H., Azuma, A., Inoue, Y., Kondoh, Y., Hasegawa, Y., et al. (2015). Safety and pharmacokinetics of nintedanib and pirfenidone in idiopathic pulmonary fibrosis. *Eur. Respir. J.* 45, 1382–1392. doi:10.1183/09031936.00198013
45. Piera-Velazquez, S., Li, Z., and Jimenez, S. A. (2011). Role of endothelial-mesenchymal transition (EndoMT) in the pathogenesis of fibrotic disorders. *Am. J. Pathol.* 179, 1074–1080. doi:10.1016/j.ajpath.2011.06.001
46. Qu, Y., Zhang, L., Kang, Z., Jiang, W., and Lv, C. (2015). Ponatinib ameliorates pulmonary fibrosis by suppressing TGF-β1/Smad3 pathway. *Pulm. Pharmacol. Therapeut.* 34, 1–7. doi:10.1016/j.pupt.2015.07.004
47. Rosas, I. O., Richards, T. J., Konishi, K., Zhang, Y., Gibson, K., Lokshin, A. E., et al. (2008). MMP1 and MMP7 as potential peripheral blood biomarkers in idiopathic pulmonary fibrosis. *PLoS Med.* 5, e93. doi:10.1371/journal.pmed.0050093
48. Santibañez, J. F., Quintanilla, M., and Bernabeu, C. (2011). TGF-β/TGF-β receptor system and its role in physiological and pathological conditions. *Clin. Sci.* 121, 233–251. doi:10.1042/CS20110086
49. Sato, M., Jiao, Q., Honda, T., Kurotani, R., Toyota, E., Okumura, S., et al. (2009). Activator of G protein signaling 8 (AGS8) is required for hypoxia-induced apoptosis of cardiomyocytes: role of G betagamma and connexin 43 (CX43). *J. Biol. Chem.* 284, 31431–31440. doi:10.1074/jbc.M109.014068
50. Senavirathna, L. K., Huang, C., Yang, X., Munteanu, M. C., Sathiaseelan, R., Xu, D., et al. (2018). Hypoxia induces pulmonary fibroblast proliferation through NFAT signaling. *Sci. Rep.* 8, 2709. doi:10.1038/s41598-018-21073-x
51. Song, X., Liu, W., Xie, S., Wang, M., Cao, G., Mao, C., et al. (2013). All-transretinoic acid ameliorates bleomycin-induced lung fibrosis by downregulating the TGF- β1/Smad3 signaling pathway in rats. *Lab. Invest.* 93, 1219–1231. doi:10.1038/ labinvest.2013.108
52. Szapiel, S. V., Elson, N. A., Fulmer, J. D., Hunninghake, G. W., and Crystal, R. G. (1979). Bleomycin-induced interstitial pulmon ary disease in the nude, athymic mouse. *Am. Rev. Respir. Dis.* 120, 893–899. doi:10.1164/arrd.1979.120.4.893
53. Teixeira, K. C., Soares, F. S., Rocha, L. G. C., Silveira, P. C. L., Silva, L. A., Valença, S. S., et al. (2008). Attenuation of bleomycin-induced lung injury and oxidative stress by N-acetylcysteine plus deferoxamine. *Pulm. Pharmacol. Ther.* 21, 309–316. doi:10.1016/j.pupt.2007.07.006
54. Wang, H., Xu, X., Yin, Y., Yu, S., Ren, H., Xue, Q., et al. (2020). Catalpol protects vascular structure and promotes angiogenesis in cerebral ischemic rats by targeting HIF-1α/VEGF. *Phytomedicine* 78, 153300. doi:10.1016/j.phymed. 2020.153300
55. Xin, X., Yao, D., Zhang, K., Han, S., Liu, D., Wang, H., et al. (2019). Protective effects of Rosavin on bleomycin-induced pulmonary fibrosis via suppressing fibrotic and inflammatory signaling pathways in mice. *Biomed. Pharmacother.* 115, 108870. doi:10.1016/j.biopha.2019.108870
56. Xu, L., Zhang, W., Zeng, L., and Jin, J. O. (2017). Rehmannia glutinosa polysaccharide induced an anti-cancer effect by activating natural killer cells. *Int. J. Biol. Macromol.* 105, 680–685. doi:10.1016/j.ijbiomac.2017.07.090
57. Yang, C., Shi, Z., You, L., Du, Y., Ni, J., and Yan, D. (2020). Neuroprotective effect of catalpol via anti-oxidative, anti-inflammatory, and anti-apoptotic mechanisms. *Front. Pharmacol.* 11, 690. doi:10.3389/fphar.2020.00690
58. Yu, W. N., Sun, L. F., and Yang, H. (2016). Inhibitory effects of astragaloside IV on bleomycin-induced pulmonary fibrosis in rats *via* attenuation of oxidative stress and inflammation. *Inflammation* 39, 1835–1841. doi:10.1007/s10753-016-0420-5
59. Zhang, J., Bi, R., Meng, Q., Wang, C., Huo, X., Liu, Z., et al. (2019). Catalpol alleviates adriamycin-induced nephropathy by activating the SIRT1 signalling pathway *in vivo* and *in vitro*. *Br. J. Pharmacol.* 176, 4558–4573. doi:10.1111/ bph.14822
60. Zhang, M., Wang, M., Tan, X., Li, T. F., Zhang, Y. E., and Chen, D. (2010). Smad3 prevents beta-catenin degradation and facilitates beta-catenin nuclear translocation in chondrocytes. *J. Biol. Chem.* 285, 8703–8710. doi:10.1074/jbc.M109.093526
61. Zhou, D., Tian, Y., Sun, L., Zhou, L., Xiao, L., Tan, R. J., et al. (2017). Matrix metalloproteinase-7 is a urinary biomarker and pathogenic mediator of kidney fibrosis. *J. Am. Soc. Nephrol.* 28, 598–611. doi:10.1681/ASN.2016030354
62. Zhou, X. D., Shi, D. D., and Zhang, Z. J. (2019). Ameliorative effects of Radix rehmanniae extract on the anxiety- and depression-like symptoms in ovariectomized mice: a behavioral and molecular study. *Phytomedicine* 63, 153012. doi:10.1016/j.phymed.2019.153012
63. Zhu, L., Fu, X., Chen, X., Han, X., and Dong, P. (2017a). M2 macrophages induce EMT through the TGF-β/Smad2 signaling pathway. *Cell Biol. Int.* 41, 960–968. doi:10.1002/cbin.10788
64. Zhu, P., Wu, Y., Yang, A., Fu, X., Mao, M., and Liu, Z. (2017b). Catalpol suppressed proliferation, growth and invasion of CT26 colon cancer by inhibiting inflammation and tumor angiogenesis. *Biomed. Pharmacother.* 95, 68–76. doi:10.1016/j.biopha.2017.08.049
65. Zuo, Y., and Liu, Y. (2018). New insights into the role and mechanism of Wnt/ β-catenin signalling in kidney fibrosis. *Nephrology* 23 (Suppl. 4), 38–43. doi:10. 1111/nep.13472

22

Fisetin Alleviated Bleomycin-Induced Pulmonary Fibrosis Partly by Rescuing Alveolar Epithelial Cells from Senescence

*Li Zhang, Xiang Tong, Jizhen Huang, Man Wu, Shijie Zhang, Dongguang Wang, SiTong Liu and Hong Fan **

Department of Respiratory and Critical Care Medicine, West China Hospital/West China School of Medicine, Chengdu, China

Correspondence:
Hong Fan
fanhongfan@qq.com

Idiopathic pulmonary fibrosis is an aging-associated disease, satisfactory therapies are not yet available. Accelerated senescence of alveolar epithelial cells plays an important part in Idiopathic pulmonary fibrosis pathogenesis. Fisetin (FIS) is a natural non-toxic flavonoid, which has many pharmacological functions. However, the role of FIS in pulmonary fibrosis has not been established. In this study, we found that FIS treatment apparently alleviated BLM-induced weight loss, inflammatory cells infiltration, inflammatory factors expression, collagen deposition and alveolar epithelial cell senescence, along with AMPK activation and the down regulation of NF-κB and TGF-β/Smad3 *in vivo*. *In vitro*, FIS administration significantly inhibited the senescence of alveolar epithelial cells and senescence-associated secretory phenotype, followed by reduced transdifferentiation of fibroblasts to myofibroblasts as well as collagen deposition in fibroblasts, which was blocked by an AMPK inhibitor, Compound C. Together, these results suggest that FIS can alleviate the development of BLM-induced pulmonary fibrosis, which is related to the inhibition of TGF-β/Smad3 signaling and the reduction of alveolar epithelium cell senescence by regulating AMPK/NF-κB signaling pathway. FIS may be a promising candidate for patients with pulmonary fibrosis.

Keywords: fisetin, pulmonary fibrosis, cellular senescence, senescence-associated secretory phenotype, AMP-activated protein kinase

INTRODUCTION

Idiopathic pulmonary fibrosis (IPF) is a chronic, progressive lung disease, which is characterized by the aberrant accumulation of extracellular matrix (ECM) in the lung parenchyma and deterioration of lung function (Richeldi et al., 2017). Both clinical observations and epidemiological investigations indicate that IPF is an aging-associated disease, since IPF occurs primarily in middle-aged and elderly people (median age at diagnosis is around 65 years), and the incidence rises remarkably with advancing age (Richeldi et al., 2017; Tian et al., 2019). More importantly, all nine primary markers of aging have been found to participate in the pathogenesis of IPF (López-Otín et al., 2013; Meiners et al., 2015). Several scholars even use the term "senescence-associated pulmonary fibrosis" to describe the phenomenon (Chen et al., 2020).

Cellular senescence is pivotal for phenotype of aging (Meiners et al., 2015). The characteristics of senescent cells include growth arrest, enlarged cell morphology, elevated activity of SA-β-Gal as well as increased expression of cell cycle inhibitors, such as p16 and p21 (Kuwano et al., 2016).

Dysfunctional re-epithelialisation, following repetitive micro-injury, initiates the process of pulmonary fibrosis (PF). Increasing evidences have implicated that accelerated senescence of alveolar epithelial cells, a main cause of epithelial dysfunction, plays an important role in IPF pathogenesis (Kuwano et al., 2016; Lehmann et al., 2017). Senescent alveolar epithelial cells not only lose the ability of regeneration and repair, but also exert deleterious effects on neighboring cells by secreting a variety of proinflammatory cytokines, pro-fibrosis factors, growth factors, matrix metalloproteinases and chemokines, described as senescence-associated secretory phenotype (SASP) (Salminen et al., 2012).

Fisetin (FIS), a natural non-toxic flavonoid, is present in various plants, fruits and vegetables. Previous researches have demonstrated that FIS has anti-inflammatory (Huang et al., 2018), anti-fibrosis, anti-oxidant (Hussain et al., 2019) and anti-aging properties (Yousefzadeh et al., 2018). FIS supplementation can prevent or alleviate hepatic and myocardial fibrosis by inhibiting the expression of fibrosis-related genes and inactivating TGF-β1/Smad3 signaling (Liu et al., 2019; Choi et al., 2020; Hu et al., 2020). Senolytic drugs, dasatinib and quercetin (D + Q), can attenuate experimental PF via selective depletion of senescent alveolar epithelial cells (Lehmann et al., 2017). More encouragingly, a recent first-in-human open-label clinical trial has suggested that short-term administration of D + Q could improve the physical dysfunction in IPF patients (Justice et al., 2019). Both FIS and quercetin belong to the flavonoid class, and FIS exhibits stronger senotherapeutic activity in cultured cells than quercetin, and can extend lifespan in mice (Yousefzadeh et al., 2018). These traits remind us that FIS may have protective effect in PF. However, the role of FIS in PF has not been elucidated.

AMP-activated kinase (AMPK), a dominant regulator of energy metabolism, not only controls the aging process, but also regulates the development of lung fibrosis (Salminen and Kaarniranta, 2012; Jiang et al., 2017). Currently, AMPK is viewed as a potential therapeutic target for PF. Bleomycin (BLM)-induced PF is the most frequently used animal model. Treatment with BLM can also induce alveolar epithelial cell senescence *in vitro* and *in vivo* (Aoshiba et al., 2003; Qiu et al., 2019). In this study, BLM was used to reproduce PF in mice and induce alveolar epithelial cell senescence to investigate the effect and mechanism of FIS in experimental PF.

MATERIALS AND METHODS

Chemicals and Reagents

FIS (purity over 98%), Compound C (CC) and BLM were purchased from Selleck (Houston, United States). Hydroxyproline (HYP) Assay Kit was obtained from Nanjing Jiancheng Bio-Engineering Institute (Nanjing, China). Antibodies against GAPDH, AMPK, phospho-AMPK (p-AMPK), Smad3, phospho-Smad3 (p-Smad3), p65, and phospho-P65 were provided by Cell Signal Technology, Inc. (Massachusetts, United States). Antibodies against β-actin, TGF-β and alpha-smooth muscle actin (α-SMA) were purchased from Proteintech Group, Inc. (Wuhan, China). Antibodies against Collagen 1, p21 and p16 were gained from Abcam Technology Inc (Cambridge, United Kingdom).

Animals

Male C57BL/6J mice (25 ± 2 g), 8–10 weeks of age, were supplied by GemPharmatech Co. Ltd. (Jiangsu, China). All animals for this experiment were fed with standard diet and water at libitum and housed in a temperature-controlled room at 23 ± 2 °C and 50–60% humidity (12 h light/dark cycle) for 1 week before the experiments. All animals received care in accordance with the recommendations of the National Institutes of Health Guide for Care and Use of Laboratory Animals, and the experiment scheme was approved by the Committee on the Ethics of Animal Experiments of Sichuan University.

Mouse Model of Bleomycin-Induced Pulmonary Fibrosis

The animal model of BLM-induced pulmonary fibrosis was performed as described previously (Aoshiba et al., 2013). In brief, 70 mice were randomly divided into four groups. Control (CON) group: mice were given intra-tracheal administration of 50 μl of saline at day 0; FIS group: the saline-instilled mice were intragastrically administered with 100 mg/kg of FIS (suspended in 150 μl of 0.5% carboxy methyl cellulose sodium) starting at day 7 and treated once every other day for 3 weeks (Yousefzadeh et al., 2018); BLM group: mice were given intra-tracheal instillation of 50 μl of bleomycin (2.5 mg/kg); BLM + FIS group: On day 7 after BLM treatment, mice were orally administered with FIS once every other day for 3 weeks. On day 28, mice were euthanized by intraperitoneal injection of excessive pentobarbital sodium.

Broncho-Alveolar Lavage Fluid Collection

The BALF was harvested according to previously described (Wang et al., 2018). Briefly, the right lung was lavaged with 0.5 ml of iced phosphate-buffered saline (PBS) for three times, and fluid recovery is about 80% per time. The BALF were centrifuged at 1,000 g for 5 min, and then the supernatant was collected and stored at −80 °C.

Histological Analysis and Immunohistochemistry

The left lung tissues were fixed with 4% formalin, embedded in paraffin. Histological sections (6 μm) were stained with hematoxylin-eosin (HE) and Masson's trichrome staining. According to previous literature, the dimensions of inflammation and pulmonary fibrosis were evaluated quantitatively (Szapiel et al., 1979). Immunohistochemistry was used to investigate the expression of p21. Paraffin-embedded lung sections were dewaxed with xylene, and endogenous peroxidase was removed with 3% H_2O_2. Antigen retrieval was performed by heating tissue sections, and non-specific binding sites were blocked with 5% BSA for 20 min. The primary anti-p21 antibody (1:200) was incubated at 4°C overnight, and the second antibody was incubated at room temperature for 1 h. Color was visualized via incubation with diaminobenzidine.

Hydroxyproline Assay

HYP content in lung tissues was determined by using a test kit according to the manufacturers' instructions. About 30 mg of tissue samples were mixed with 1 ml of hydrolysase, placed in 60°C boiling water bath for about 20 min. After centrifugation of the supernatant at 3,500 rpm/min for 10 min, the absorbance at 550 nm was determined. HYP content was expressed as μg/mg.

Cell Culture

A549 and human embryonic lung fibroblast (HELF) cells were purchased from American Type Culture Collection (Rockville, MD, United States). These cells were cultured in DMEM (Hyclone, United States) supplemented with 10% FBS (ZETA, United States) and 1× solution of penicillin-streptomycin (Hyclone) at 37°C in a humidified 5% CO_2 atmosphere.

To build the model of alveolar epithelial cell senescence and select the optimal concentration of BLM, A549 cells were stimulated with different doses of BLM for 3 days (Qiu et al., 2019). Next, we observed the roles of FIS and AMPK in alveolar epithelial cell senescence. Before BLM (5 μg/ml) was added to induce cell senescence, A549 cells in six-well plate were pretreated with or without 10 μM Compound C (CC, an inhibitor of AMPK) for 1 h (Liu et al., 2018). Subsequently, cells grew in the presence or absence of FIS (10 μM) for 3 days (Yousefzadeh et al., 2018).

In order to mimic SASP and observe its effects on epithelial-mesenchymal crosstalk, we used A549-derived conditioned mediums to further culture HELF cells. After treating with or without 5 μg/ml of BLM and 10 μM FIS for 3 days, the culture supernatants of A549 cells were replaced by fresh culture mediums without BLM, and A549 cells were cultured for another 2 days. Normal A549-derived conditioned mediums (N-CM), BLM-induced A549-derived conditioned mediums (B-CM) as well as BLM and FIS co-stimulated A549-derived conditioned mediums (BF-CM) were collected to analyze cytokines and further culture HELF cells with one half of concentration for 3 days. The protein expressions of collagen 1 and α-SMA in HELF cells were detected to reflect the fibrotic response.

Senescence-Associated β-Galactosidase Staining

SA-β-Gal staining was performed by using the senescence β-Galactosidase staining kit (Beyotime, Shanghai, China) as previously described (Tian et al., 2019). Frozen lung tissue sections and cell samples were fixed with 4% formaldehyde for 10–15 min at room temperature, washed three times with PBS for 5 min each time, and then placed in freshly prepared staining solution overnight at 37°C. To better show lung structure, the tissue sections were further stained with eosin. SA-β-Gal-positive cells (bluish green color) were counted in three random microscopic fields and expressed as % of total cells.

TABLE 1 | Primers for quantitative real-time (qRT)-PCR.

Primer name	Sequence (5' to 3')
Mouse p16-F	ATCTGGAGCAGCATGGAGTC
Mouse p16-R	TCGAATCTGCACCGTAGTTG
Mouse p21-F	CCTGGTGATGTCCGACCTG
Mouse p21-R	CCATGAGCGCATCGCAATC
Mouse collagen I-F	CTGTCTGCTTCCTGTAAACT
Mouse collagen I-R	TCCATGTGAAATTGTCTCCC
Mouse α-SMA-F	TCAGGGAGTAATGGTTGGAATG
Mouse α-SMA-R	CCAGAGTCCAGCACAATACCAG
Mouse β-actin-F	CACTCTTCCAGCCTTCCTTCC
Mouse β-actin-R	AGGTCTTTGCGGATGTCCAC

Western Blot Analysis

Lung tissues or cells were collected and lysed in ice-cold RIPA lysis buffer containing fresh protease and phosphatase inhibitor cocktails (MedChemExpress, United States). Protein samples were separated on 10% or 12.5% SDS-PAGE gels, and then transferred to methanol-activated PVDF membranes (Merck Millipore, Germany). After 1 h blocking with 5% nonfat milk, these membranes were incubated with primary antibodies overnight at 4°C. After membranes were washed three times, the corresponding secondary antibody was added for incubation at room temperature for 1–2 h. Protein expression was visualized using ECL (GE Healthcare, United Kingdom), and band intensities were measured using ImageJ software 6.0.

Real-Time Quantitative Polymerase Chain Reaction Assay

Total RNA was extracted from lung tissues using TRIzol reagent (Invitrogen Life Technologies, United States), reverse-transcribed to complementary DNA (cDNA) using ReverTra Ace qPCR RT Master Mix with gDNA Remover (Toyobo, Japan). Relative gene expression was quantified using iTaq Universal SYBR Green Supermix (Bio-Rad, United States). **Table 1** shows the primer sequences, relative gene expression levels were normalized to β-actin and calculated using the $2^{-\Delta\Delta Ct}$ method.

Enzyme-Linked Immunosorbent Assay Detection

The levels of IL-1β, IL-6, TGF-β, MMP-9, and TNF-α in BALF and culture mediums were detected by ELISA assay following the manufacturer's instructions (NeoBioscience, Shenzhen, China).

Statistical Analysis

Statistical analyses were performed using GraphPad Prism version 6.0 (GraphPad software, United States). All the original data were showed as mean ± SD. One-way analysis of variance and repeated-measures analysis of variance followed by the Tukey's multiple comparison test were used for comparisons of multiple groups. The survival curve of each group was drawn using the Kaplan-Meier method. Values of $p < 0.05$ were considered statistically significant.

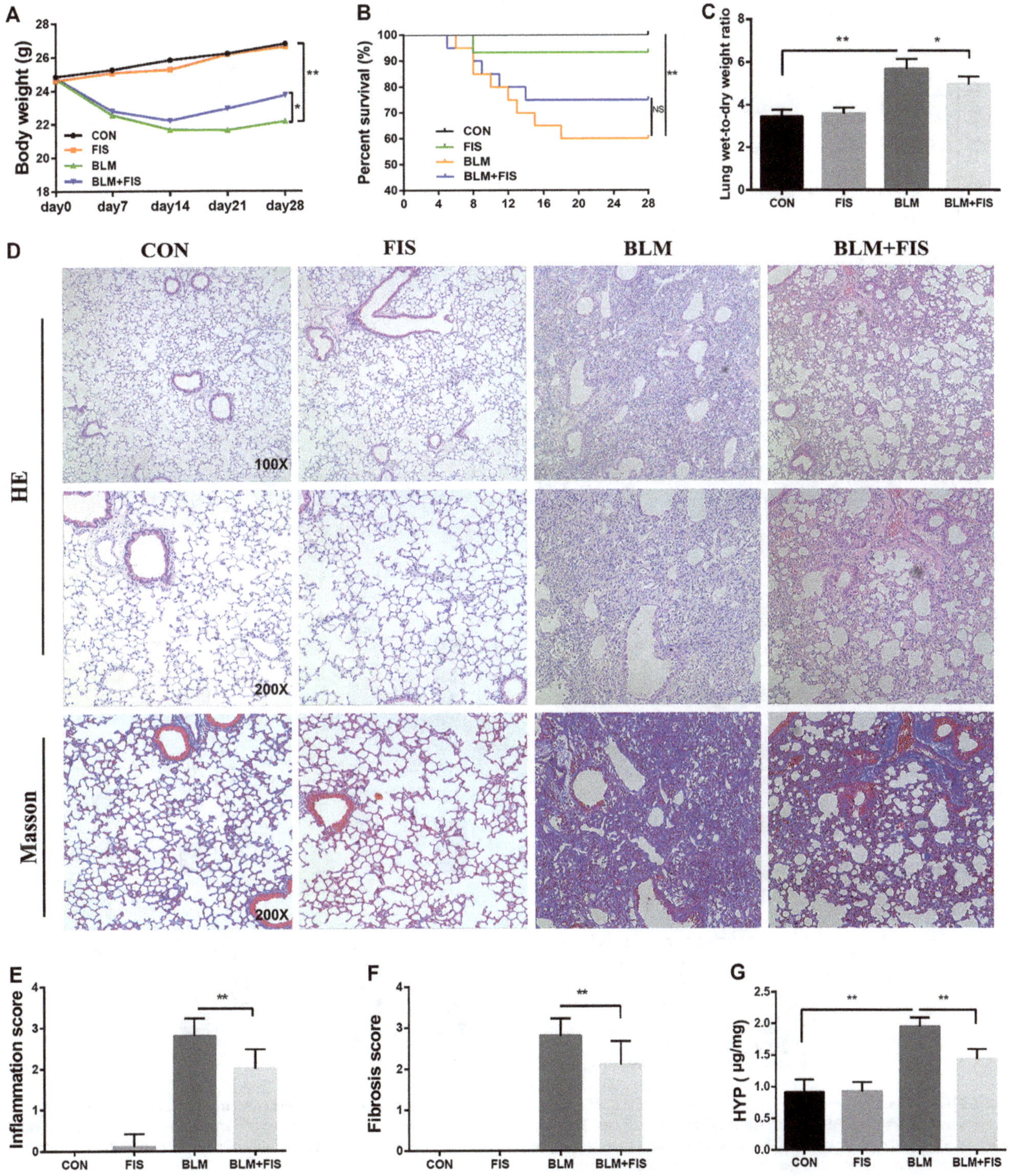

FIGURE 1 | Fisetin (FIS) alleviated bleomycin (BLM)-induced pulmonary fibrosis in mice. On day 7 after BLM treatment (2.5 mg/kg), mice were intragastrically administered with FIS (100 mg/kg) once every other day for 3 weeks. Mouse lungs were collected on day 28 after BLM treatment. The body weight **(A)**, survival rate **(B)**, lung wet-to-dry weight ratio **(C)**, and hydroxyproline content **(G)** in lungs were determined. The representative images of HE-stained (×100 and ×200 magnification) and Masson's trichrome-stained (×200 magnification) lung sections in mice **(D)** and comparisons of the inflammation score **(E)** and fibrosis score **(F)** between the experimental groups were shown. Data were presented as the means ± SD. $^{*}p < 0.05$, $^{**}p < 0.01$. NS, non-significant.

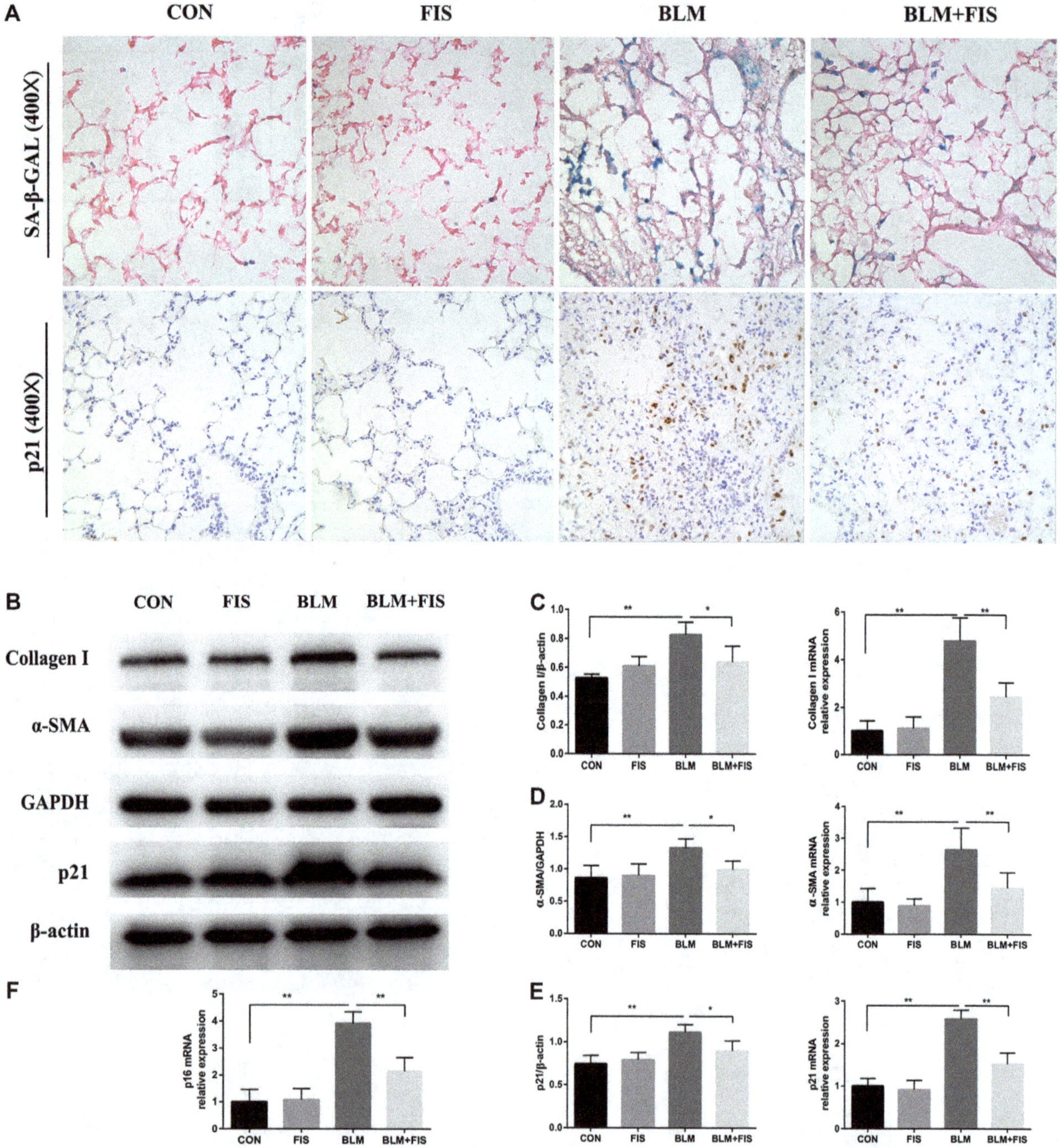

FIGURE 2 | FIS reduced the senescent cell burden and attenuated fibrotic marker in fibrotic lung tissue of mice. One week after 2.5 mg/kg of BLM treatment, mice were orally administered with FIS (100 mg/kg) once every other day for 3 weeks. Representative images of SA-β-Gal staining and immunohistochemistry for p21 were displayed under ×400 magnification **(A)**. Protein and gene expression of collagen 1 **(B, C)**, α-SMA **(B, D)** and p21 **(B, E)** as well as p16 mRNA level **(F)** were detected using Western blot and quantitative real-time (qRT)-PCR. Data were expressed as mean ± SD ($n \geq 3$). * $p < 0.05$, ** $p < 0.01$.

RESULTS

Fisetin Alleviated Bleomycin-Induced Pulmonary Fibrosis in Mice

After intra-tracheal instillation of BLM, significant weight loss, survival rate reduction and increased wet/dry weight ratio of lung were noticed (**Figures 1A–C**). The seventh day after BLM administration is considered to be the beginning of the fibrotic phase (Li et al., 2019), FIS was intragastrically administered at day 7 for 21 days. BLM-induced weight loss and the increase in the wet/dry weight ratio were attenuated by FIS administration. There was no significant difference in the survival rate between the BLM group and BLM + FIS group, but a trend was revealed that FIS treatment would improve the survival rate of mice (**Figure 1B**).

In terms of histopathology, no significant pathological alteration in lung architecture was observed in the CON and FIS group. However, HE staining showed obvious morphologic changes of lung in the BLM group, including thickening of alveolar septum, alveolar structure destruction, and heavy inflammatory cell infiltration in alveolar space and pulmonary interstitium (**Figure 1D**). In addition, the lung tissues of BLM treated mice also displayed an increase in collagen deposition, which was evident from the increase of blue fiber bundles in Masson-stained lung sections (**Figure 1D**). As expected, treatment with FIS markedly reduced inflammatory cell infiltration, interstitial thickness and collagen deposition. In accordance with these observations, there was a statistically significant increase in the inflammation and fibrosis scores in the BLM group, while protection of FIS on lung microstructure was clearly reflected in the lower scores in the BLM + FIS group (**Figures 1E,F**).

Massive collagen secreted by myofibroblasts is the major source of ECM, while α-SMA is a biomarker protein of myofibroblasts (Li et al., 2019). HYP is one of the main components of collagen. As shown in **Figures 2B–D**, FIS administration obviously reduced the expressions of collagen 1 and α-SMA both at mRNA and protein levels as well as HYP content (**Figure 1G**) in lung tissues, suggesting that FIS suppressed transdifferentiation of fibroblasts to myofibroblasts and therefore decreased accumulation of collagen. Taken together, these data indicate that FIS can effectively alleviate the development of BLM-induced PF.

Fisetin Attenuated Bleomycin-Induced Alveolar Epithelial Cell Senescence and Inflammatory Responses *in Vivo*

Prior studies have shown that BLM treatment can effectively induce cellular senescence in alveolar epithelial cells (Aoshiba et al., 2003). Cyclin-dependent kinase inhibitors p16 and p21, as well as SA-β-Gal activity are often used to confirm the appearance of senescence (Aoshiba et al., 2013; Qiu et al., 2019). As shown in **Figure 2**, both p16 and p21 gene expressions were apparently up-regulated in BLM-induced fibrotic mouse lungs, p21 protein was also significantly increased compared with the control group. Unfortunately, due to lacking of an ideal p16 antibody for mice (Demaria et al., 2014; Lehmann et al., 2017), we could not analyze p16 on protein level. In addition, using immunohistochemical staining, we found that the positive staining of p21 was mainly located in lung structural cells that morphologically resembled alveolar epithelial cells in BLM-induced mice (**Figure 2A**). Subsequently, we evaluated SA-β-Gal activity, a widely used indicator for detecting senescent cells, which will be dyed bluish green color. As previous findings demonstrated, an increase in the number of blue-green stained senescent cells was observed in fibrotic lung tissues, whereas that was barely seen in normal lungs (**Figure 2A**). However, both the strong SA-β-gal positive staining and the elevated expression of p21 and p16 induced by BLM were significantly alleviated by treatment with FIS compared to the BLM group.

To further explore the effects of FIS on inflammatory reaction, several common cytokines were analyzed by ELISA, which have also been suggested to be part of the SASP (Aoshiba et al., 2013; Qiu et al., 2019). In **Figure 3**, the levels of pro-inflammatory cytokines (IL-1β, IL-6, TNF-α), profibrogenic cytokine (TGF-β) and metalloproteinase-9 (MMP-9) in the BALF of BLM-induced mice were significantly higher than those in healthy mice. In contrast, intervention with FIS dramatically decreased the release of these cytokines, except for MMP-9. Together, these results indicate that FIS can attenuate BLM-induced alveolar epithelial cells senescence and inflammatory responses *in vivo*.

Fisetin Inhibited Transforming Growth Factor-β/Smad3 Signaling and Regulated the Activity of AMP-Activated Protein Kinase and Nuclear Factor-κB in Pulmonary Fibrosis in Mice

TGF-β/Smad3 signaling plays a critical role in the development of pulmonary fibrosis. The phosphorylation of Smad3 was used to reflect Smad3 activity. As shown in **Figures 3A,B**, compared with the CON and FIS group, the protein levels of TGF-β and phospho-Smad3 (p-Smad3) were significantly increased in the BLM group. However, the increase was effectively reduced in the BLM + FIS group.

The activity of AMPK were evaluated by measuring the phosphorylation of Thr172 of AMPK. As illustrated in **Figure 3**, the levels of phosphorylated AMPK (p-AMPK) were obviously lower in the BLM group as compared to the CON and FIS group. However, FIS evidently increased the expression of p-AMPK thus to enhance AMPK activity in lungs compared with the BLM group.

Similarly, we detected the phosphorylation levels of p65 component of NF-κB to reflect NF-κB activity. Elevated levels of phospho-p65 (p-p65) were detected in the BLM group as compared to the CON and FIS group, while p-p65 protein levels in the BLM + FIS group were obviously lower than that in the BLM group (**Figures 3A,B**). These results suggest that FIS can suppress TGF-β/Smad3 signaling and regulate the activity of AMPK and NF-κB.

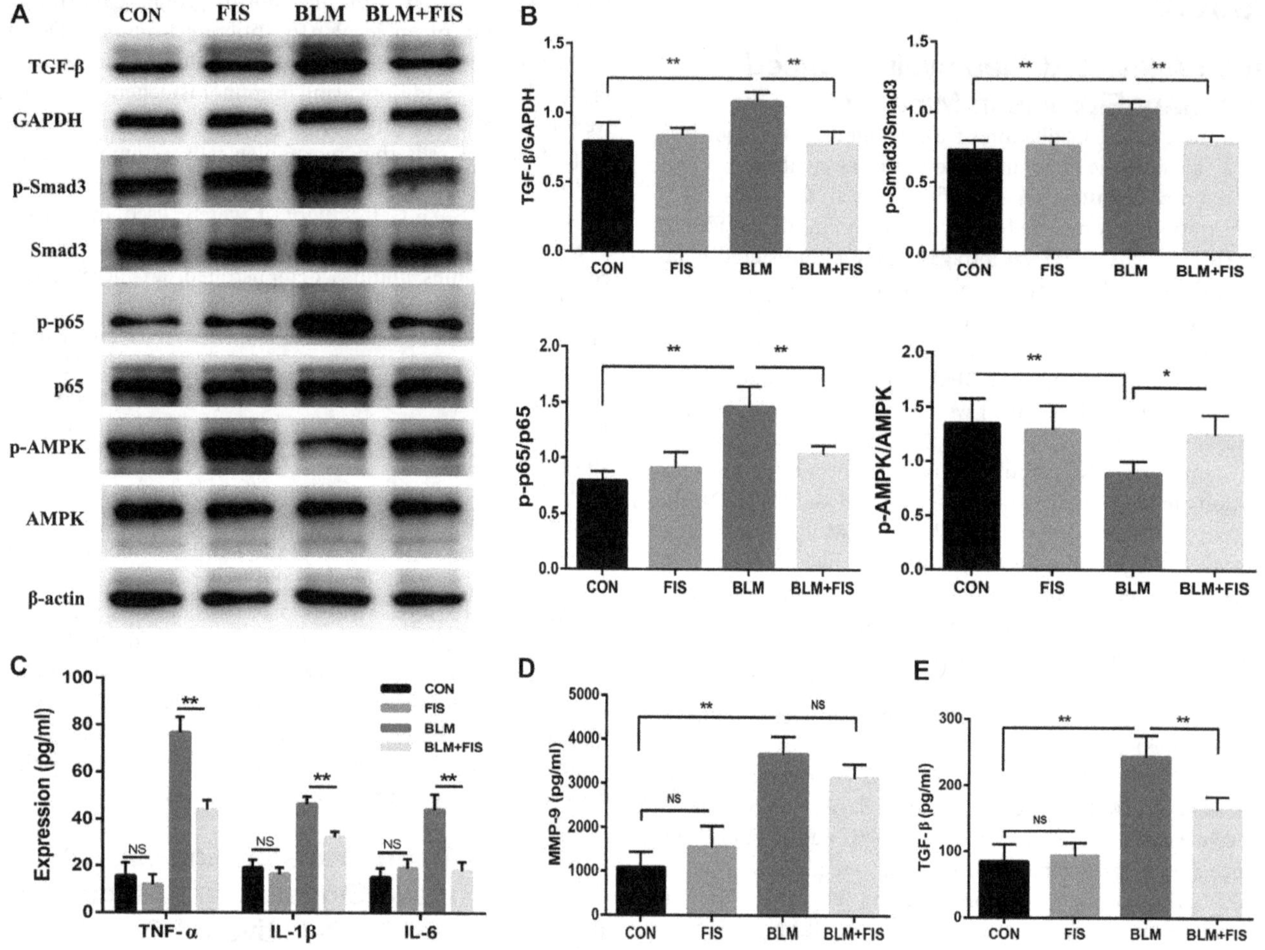

FIGURE 3 | FIS regulated the activity of AMPK and NF-κB and inflammatory responses in BLM-induced mice. One week after 2.5 mg/kg of BLM treatment, mice were orally administered with FIS (100 mg/kg) once every other day for 3 weeks. Protein expressions of TGF-β, p-Smad3/Smad3, p-AMPK/AMPK and p-p65/p65 in lung tissue were detected by Western blotting analysis **(A, B)**. The levels of IL-1β, IL-6, TGF-β, MMP-9 and TNF-α in BALF were detected by ELISA assay. Data were expressed as mean ± SD ($n \geq 3$). $^{*}p < 0.05$, $^{**}p < 0.01$. NS, non-significant.

Fisetin Relieved Bleomycin-Mediated Alveolar Epithelial Cell Senescence via AMP-Activated Protein Kinase/Nuclear Factor-κB Signaling Pathway *in Vitro*

Refer to previous literatures (Aoshiba et al., 2003; Qiu et al., 2019; Tian et al., 2019), we used BLM to build a cellular senescence model. Different concentrations of BLM were used to stimulate A549 cells for 3 days. Treatment of A549 cells with BLM caused a dose-dependent increase in protein expression of p21 (**Figure 4C**), and this increase paralleled with a distinct, flat, and enlarged cell morphology (**Figure 4A**). Meanwhile, with the increase of BLM concentration, the SA-β-Gal activity was also up-regulated. However, there was no significant change between 5 and 10 μg/ml of BLM (**Figure 4B**). Therefore, the following experiments were continued with 5 μg/ml of BLM.

Further study found that the activity of SA-β-Gal in BLM-induced senescent A549 cells was remarkably increased as compared to the CON and FIS group, while FIS prevented this change (**Figures 5A,B**). Consistent with the results of *in vivo* experiments, the decreased protein expressions of p-AMPK and increased protein levels of p-p65 were detected in BLM-induced senescent A549 cells (**Figure 5D**), which were obviously improved by FIS, whereas such changes were reversed by AMPK inhibitor Compound C (CC). Similarly, FIS notably inhibited p21 and p16 protein expressions, which were partially blocked by CC (**Figure 5C**). These findings confirme that FIS can effectively relieve alveolar epithelial cell senescence partly through activating AMPK and inhibiting NF-κB activity.

Fisetin Ameliorated Senescence-Associated Secretory Phenotype From Senescent Alveolar Epithelial Cells and Reduced Collagen Deposition in Fibroblasts

Several widely-used cytokines, IL-1β, TNF-α, IL-6 and TGF-β were detected to reflect SASP from A549 cells in this study

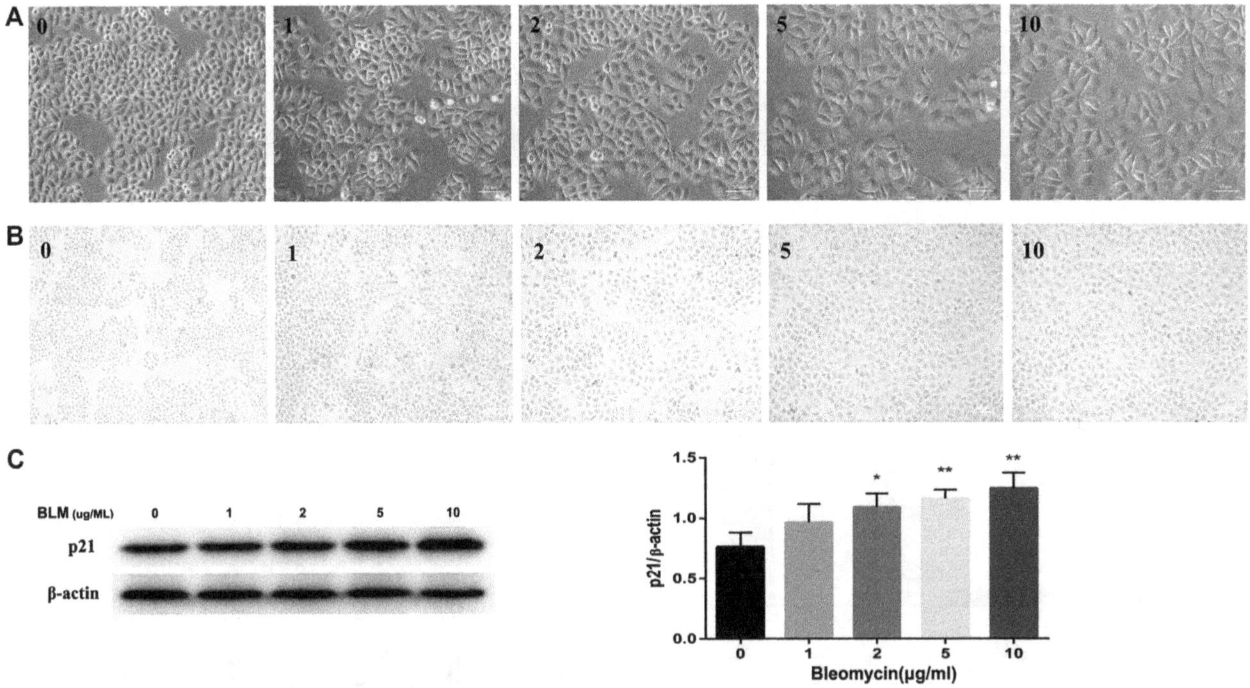

FIGURE 4 | BLM induced senescence in A549 cells in a dose-dependent manner. A549 cells were stimulated with different doses of BLM for 3 days. Morphology of A549 cells treated with 0–10 μg/ml of BLM was observed under ×200 magnification **(A)**. SA-β-Gal staining was shown under ×100 magnification **(B)**. P21 protein expression was detected by Western blotting analysis **(C)**. * $p < 0.05$ and ** $p < 0.01$ is significantly different from the control.

(Aoshiba et al., 2013; Tian et al., 2019). In **Figure 6A**, the levels of IL-1β, TNF-α, TGF-β, and IL-6 in the BLM-induced A549-derived conditioned mediums (B-CM) were higher than those in the normal A549-derived conditioned mediums (N-CM). All the above inflammatory cytokines, except for TNF-α, were significantly ameliorated in the BLM and FIS co-stimulated A549-derived conditioned mediums (BF-CM). As shown in **Figures 6B–D**, exposure of HELF cells to conditioned mediums for 3 days, increased protein expressions of collagen 1 and α-SMA were detected in B-CM stimulated HELF cells as compared to N-CM cultured HELF cells, whereas BF-CM obviously decreased the protein expressions of collagen 1 and α-SMA in HELF cells as compared to B-CM. These results suggest that FIS can ameliorate SASP from senescent alveolar epithelial cells, and therefore reduce transdifferentiation of fibroblasts to myofibroblasts as well as collagen deposition in fibroblasts.

DISCUSSION

PF is a serious threat to human health, however, for many patients, effective treatment options are still lacking. Therefore, novel therapeutic strategies are urgently required. FIS is a dietary flavonoid, the average daily intake of naturally occurring FIS in Japan is about 0.4 mg/day (Kimira et al., 1998; Arai et al., 2000). Mounting evidence has indicated that FIS has potential to prevent or treat a variety of chronic diseases by acting as an anti-inflammatory, anti-oxidant, anti-aging and anti-fibrotic agent (Pal et al., 2016; Choi et al., 2020). However, the role of FIS in PF remains unclear.

In the present study, FIS treatment significantly improved BLM-induced weight loss and lung pathological changes in mice. Additionally, FIS notably decreased the levels of collagen 1 and α-SMA as well as HYP contents in fibrotic lung tissues, indicating that FIS reduced the accumulation of ECM. TGF-β/Smads signaling appears to be critical in pulmonary fibrosis, and Smad3's key role in TGF-β-induced deposition of ECM has been widely recognized (Dobaczewski et al., 2010). In this study, we also confirmed that FIS remarkably inhibited the expression of TGF-β and Smad3 phosphorylation in the BLM-induced PF. Although FIS did not demonstrate survival benefits, it showed a trend in favour of a reduction in mortality. These results suggest that FIS has protective effect on PF. Previous studies have shown that FIS supplementation prevents hepatic fibrosis by suppressing the gene expressions of COL1, MMP2, MMP3, and MMP9 and collagen accumulation (Choi et al., 2020). FIS treatment markedly reduces the expression of fibrosis-related genes and inhibits myocardial fibrosis by inactivating TGF-β/Smads signaling (Liu et al., 2019; Hu et al., 2020). More importantly, no side effects of FIS have been reported, even when given at high doses (Maher, 2015).

IPF is an aging-associated disease. In general, the number of senescent cells increases with age, however, cellular senescence is not a universal property in aged tissues, and senescence is not exactly equivalent to aging (Kuwano et al., 2016). In the lung, approximately 6.7% and 19% of senescent cells are detected in

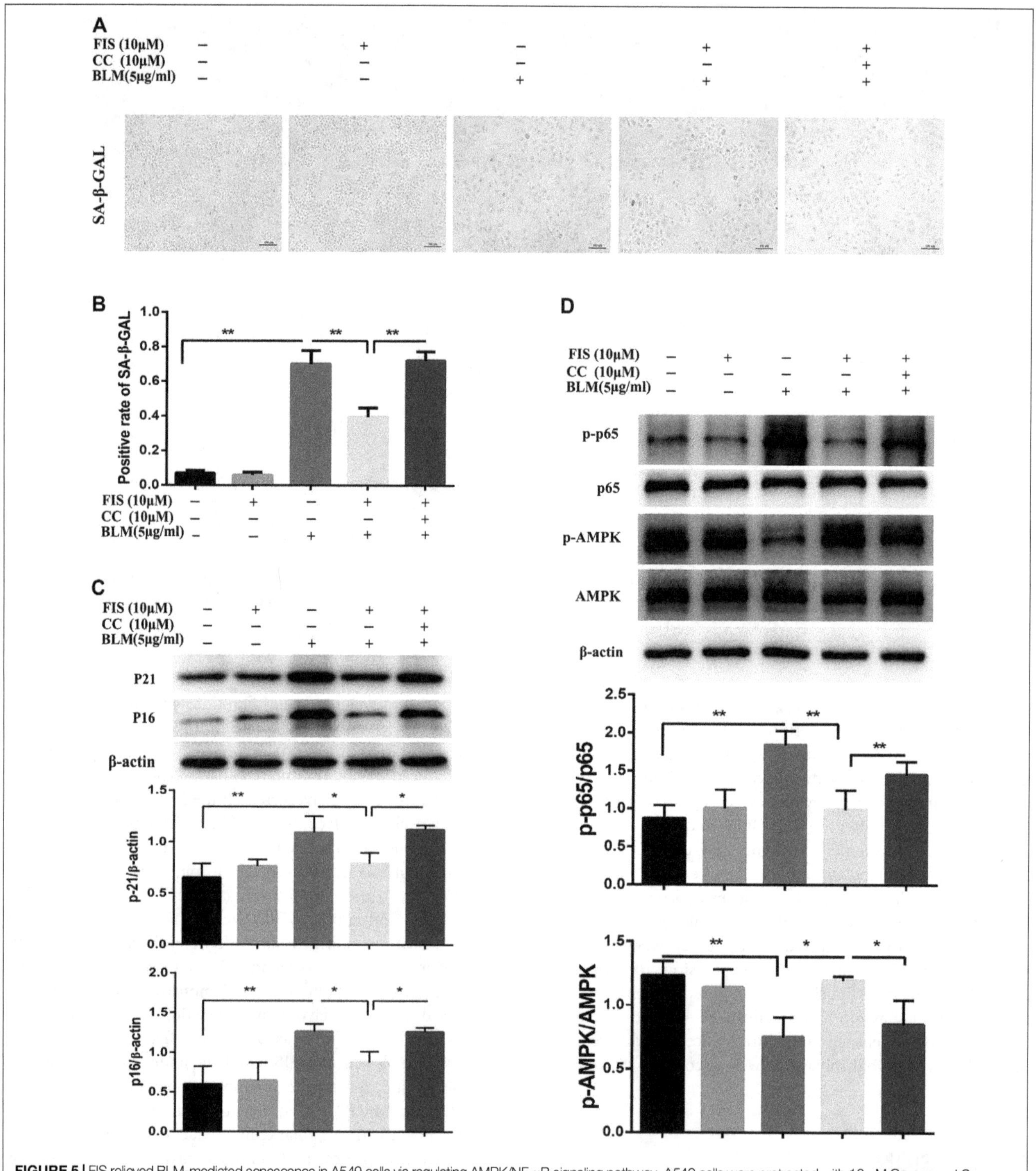

FIGURE 5 | FIS relieved BLM-mediated senescence in A549 cells via regulating AMPK/NF-κB signaling pathway. A549 cells were pretreated with 10 μM Compound C (CC) and subsequently incubated with/without BLM (5 μg/ml), FIS (10 μM) for 3 days. SA-β-Gal staining was shown under ×100 magnification **(A, B)**. Protein expressions of p16, p21, p-AMPK/AMPK and p-p65/P65 were detected by Western blotting analysis **(C, D)**. Data were shown as mean ± SD ($n \geq 3$). $^{*}p < 0.05$, $^{**}p < 0.01$.

young and old mice, respectively; however, there are no obvious differences in the eye, skeletal muscle and heart (Wang et al., 2018). Accelerated cellular senescence is now considered as an important driving mechanism for IPF (Minagawa et al., 2011; Kuwano et al., 2016; Barnes et al., 2019). Although increased senescence has been identified in both alveolar epithelial cells and

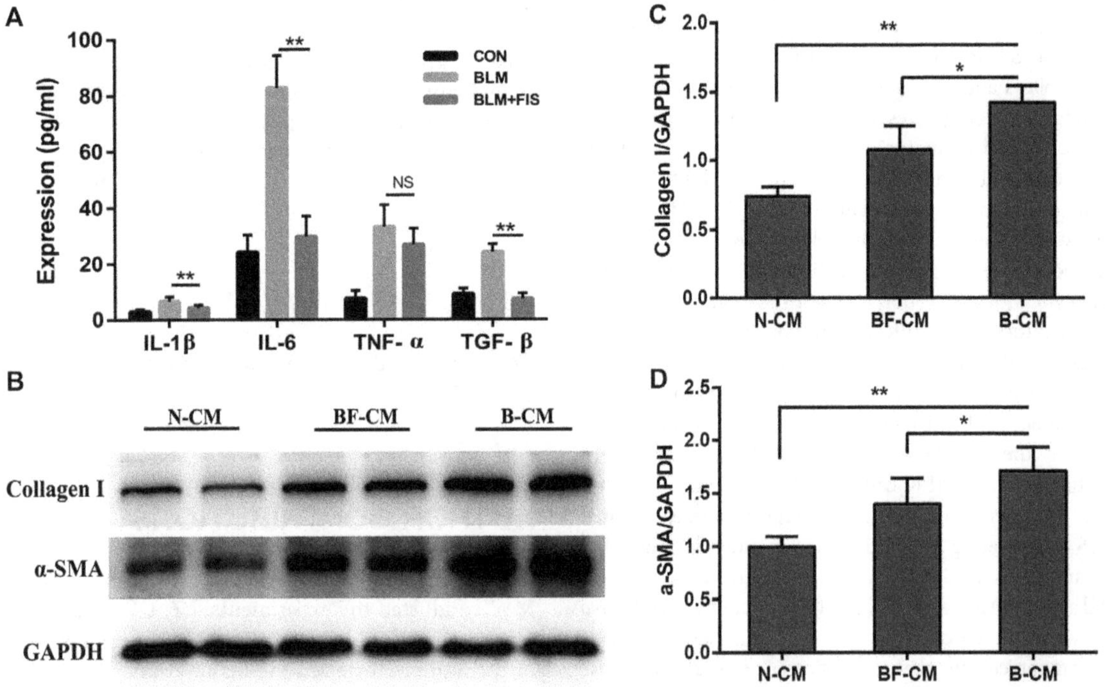

FIGURE 6 | FIS ameliorated SASP from senescent A549 cells and reduced collagen deposition in HELF cells. After treatment with or without 5 μg/ml of BLM and 10 μM FIS for 3 days, the culture supernatants of A549 cells were replaced by fresh culture mediums, and A549 cells were cultured for another 2 days. A549-derived conditioned mediums were collected to analyze cytokines and further culture HELF cells with one half of concentration for 3 days. The levels of IL-1β, IL-6, TGF-β, and TNF-α in conditioned mediums were detected by ELISA assay **(A)**. Protein expressions of collagen I and α-SMA in HELF cells were detected by Western blotting analysis **(B–D)**. N-CM, Normal A549-derived conditioned mediums. B-CM, BLM-induced A549-derived conditioned mediums. BF-CM, BLM and FIS co-stimulated A549-derived conditioned mediums. Data were expressed as mean ± SD ($n \geq 3$). $^{*}p < 0.05$, $^{**}p < 0.01$. NS, non-significant.

fibroblasts in the lung tissues of IPF patients, alveolar epithelial cells are the major target of BLM-induced senescence in mice, while fibroblasts are not affected to a great extent (Aoshiba et al., 2013; Lehmann et al., 2017). Interestingly, the role of senescent fibroblasts in PF is conflicting, since both an anti-fibrotic role (Cui et al., 2017) and a detrimental role (Schafer et al., 2017) have been reported. However, almost all reports indicate that senescent alveolar epithelium cells, as a major senescent cell type in IPF, are detrimental in PF patients (Lehmann et al., 2017; Tian et al., 2019).

Although A549 cells are a lung cancer cell lines, their response to BLM-induced senescence is not significantly different from that of normal alveolar epithelial cells (Aoshiba et al., 2003). Besides, primary alveolar epithelial cells are difficult to obtain and maintain *in vitro*. Therefore, A549 cells were used as an alveolar epithelial cell model in this study. In line with previous studies (Aoshiba et al., 2003; Tian et al., 2019), increased senescence was found in alveolar epithelium cells of murine fibrotic lungs and cultured A549 cells treated with BLM, while FIS administration apparently reduced senescent cell burden along with decreased fibrotic markers. Therefore, the anti-fibrotic effects of FIS is at least partly related to its senolytic activity. It's not surprising, quercetin, a flavonoid family member, has shown anti-fibrotic effect by reducing senescent cell burden in PF, while FIS has more stronger senotherapeutic activity than quercetin (Yousefzadeh et al., 2018; Hohmann et al., 2019).

Different from apoptotic cells, senescent epithelial cells have metabolic activity and may secrete multiple growth factors, cytokines, and proteases, known as SASP, leading to low-grade chronic inflammation, which further initiates senescence and abnormal epithelial cell-fibroblast interactions, promotes the transformation of fibroblasts into myofibroblasts and considerable ECM accumulation (Aoshiba et al., 2013; Tian et al., 2019). Multiple inflammatory cytokines in the supernatant of senescent fibrotic alveolar epithelial cells were up regulated 1.5 times by analysis using mass spectrometry proteomics (Lehmann et al., 2017). FIS can inhibit the release of various inflammatory cytokines, such as IL-1β, TNF-α, IL-6 and NF-κB, which are also considered to be SASP components (Gupta et al., 2014). As expected, FIS treatment obviously decreased levels of inflammatory cytokines (TNF-α, IL-6 and IL-1β) and pro-fibrosis factor (TGF-β) in the BLAF of BLM-induced mice, exerted its anti-inflammatory effect.

As we all know, one important anti-fibrosis pathway is to effectively inhibit the synthesis of collagen or increase its degradation. Collagen, mainly secreted by myofibroblasts, is the most important part of ECM, while α-SMA is a specific biomarker of fibroblast to myofibroblast transdifferentiation (Yang J. Y. et al., 2019). *In vitro* study, we also found that FIS suppressed the secretion of inflammatory cytokines by senescent alveolar epithelium cells, followed by reduced transdifferentiation of fibroblasts to myofibroblasts and collagen deposition in fibroblasts. These results suggest that FIS treatment can improve aberrant inflammatory microenvironment by reducing alveolar epithelial cell senescence and accompanying SASP, which is beneficial to maintain normal function of fibroblasts and reduce ECM accumulation.

Energy metabolism regulates tissue repair and remodeling responses. As a pivotal regulator of energy metabolism, AMPK plays important roles in the process of aging and fibrogenesis (Salminen and Kaarniranta, 2012; Jiang et al., 2017). The lack of AMPK activity with aging can provoke many age-associated diseases, including IPF. AMPK activation is significantly decreased in regions of active fibrosis of IPF patients and mouse model. The activators of AMPK can inhibit the expression of α-SMA, collagen and fibronectin in fibroblasts stimulated with TGF-β, and reverse established lung fibrosis in an AMPK-dependent manner in BLM-induced mice (Rangarajan et al., 2018). NF-κB is the primary regulator of the appearance of SASP, the activation of AMPK can inhibit NF-κB signaling and inflammation (Salminen et al., 2011). Some reports have established the role of FIS in regulating AMPK/NF-κB signaling pathways (Liu et al., 2019; Yang W. et al., 2019). Consistently, our results revealed that FIS could activate AMPK and inhibit NF-κB activity both *in vivo* and *in vitro*, whereas such changes were partly blocked by AMPK inhibitor, accompanied by elevated senescence markers. These results indicate that AMPK/NF-κB signal pathway is involved in the anti-aging and fibrotic effects of FIS in PF.

CONCLUSION

Taken together, FIS can alleviate the development of BLM-induced pulmonary fibrosis, which is related to the inhibition of TGF-β/Smad3 signaling and the reduction of alveolar epithelium cell senescence by regulating AMPK/NF-κB signaling pathway. FIS may be a promising candidate for patients with PF.

ETHICS STATEMENT

The animal study was reviewed and approved by the Committee on the Ethics of Animal Experiments of Sichuan University.

AUTHOR CONTRIBUTIONS

LZ, XT, JH, and HF conceived the experiment, LZ, JH, XT, and MW conducted the experiments, LZ, DW, and SZ analyzed the results, and LZ and SL contributed to the manuscript writing. All of the authors reviewed the manuscript.

REFERENCES

1. Aoshiba, K., Tsuji, T., Kameyama, S., Itoh, M., Semba, S., Yamaguchi, K., et al. (2013). Senescence-associated secretory phenotype in a mouse model of bleomycin-induced lung injury. *Exp. Toxicol. Pathol.* 65 (7–8), 1053–1062. doi:10.1016/j.etp.2013.04.001
2. Aoshiba, K., Tsuji, T., and Nagai, A. (2003). Bleomycin induces cellular senescence in alveolar epithelial cells. *Eur. Respir. J.* 22 (3), 436–443. doi:10.1183/09031936. 03.00011903
3. Arai, Y., Watanabe, S., Kimira, M., Shimoi, K., Mochizuki, R., and Kinae, N. (2000). Dietary intakes of flavonols, flavones and isoflavones by Japanese women and the inverse correlation between quercetin intake and plasma LDL cholesterol concentration. *J. Nutr.* 130 (9), 2243–2250. doi:10.1093/jn/130.9.2243
4. Barnes, P. J., Baker, J., and Donnelly, L. E. (2019). Cellular senescence as a mechanism and target in chronic lung diseases. *Am. J. Respir. Crit. Care Med.* 200 (5), 556–564. doi:10.1164/rccm.201810-1975TR
5. Chen, H., Chen, H., Liang, J., Gu, X., Zhou, J., Xie, C., et al. (2020). TGF-β1/IL-11/MEK/ERK signaling mediates senescence-associated pulmonary fibrosis in a stress-induced premature senescence model of Bmi-1 deficiency. *Exp. Mol. Med.* 52 (1), 130–151. doi:10.1038/s12276-019-0371-7
6. Choi, M. S., Choi, J. -Y., and Kwon, E. Y. (2020). Fisetin alleviates hepatic and adipocyte fibrosis and insulin resistance in diet-induced obese mice. *J. Med. Food* 23, 1019–1032. doi:10.1089/jmf.2019.4619
7. Cui, H., Ge, J., Xie, N., Banerjee, S., Zhou, Y., Antony, V. B., et al. (2017). miR-34a inhibits lung fibrosis by inducing lung fibroblast senescence. *Am. J. Respir. Cell Mol. Biol.* 56 (2), 168–178. doi:10.1165/rcmb.2016-0163OC
8. Demaria, M., Ohtani, N., Youssef, S. A., Rodier, F., and Toussain, W. (2014). An essential role for senescent cells in optimal wound healing through secretion of PDGF-AA. *Dev. Cell* 31 (6), 722–733. doi:10.1016/j.devcel. 2014.11.012
9. Dobaczewski, M., Bujak, M., Li, N., Gonzalez-Quesada, C., Mendoza, L. H., Wang, X.-F., et al. (2010). Smad3 signaling critically regulates fibroblast phenotype and function in healing myocardial infarction. *Circ. Res.* 107, 418–428. doi:10.1161/ CIRCRESAHA.109.216101
10. Gupta, S. C., Tyagi, A. K., Deshmukh-Taskar, P., Hinojosa, M., Prasad, S., and Aggarwal, B. B. (2014). Downregulation of tumor necrosis factor and other proinflammatory biomarkers by polyphenols. *Arch. Biochem. Biophys.* 559, 91–99. doi:10.1016/j.abb.2014.06.006
11. Hohmann, M. S., Habiel, D. M., Coelho, A. L., Verri, W. A., and Hogaboam, C. M. (2019). Quercetin enhances ligand-induced apoptosis in senescent idiopathic pulmonary fibrosis fibroblasts and reduces lung fibrosis in vivo. *Am. J. Respir. Cell Mol. Biol.* 60 (1), 28–40. doi:10.1165/rcmb.2017-0289OC
12. Hu, L. F., Feng, J., Dai, X., Sun, Y., Xiong, M., Lai, L., et al. (2020). Oral flavonoid fisetin treatment protects against prolonged high-fat-diet-induced cardiac dysfunction by regulation of multicombined signaling. *J. Nutr. Biochem.* 77, 108253. doi:10.1016/j.jnutbio.2019.108253
13. Huang, W., Li, M.-L., Xia, M.-Y., and Shao, J.-Y. (2018). Fisetin-treatment alleviates airway inflammation through inhbition of MyD88/NF-κB signaling pathway. *Int. J. Mol. Med.* 42 (1), 208–218. doi:10.3892/ijmm.2018.3582
14. Hussain, T., Al-Attas, O. S., Alamery, S., Ahmed, M., Odeibat, H. A. M., et al. (2019). The plant flavonoid, fisetin alleviates cigarette smoke-induced oxidative stress, and inflammation in Wistar rat lungs. *J. Food Biochem.* 43 (8), e12962. doi:10.1111/jfbc.12962
15. Jiang, S., Li, T., Yang, Z., Yi, W., Di, S., Sun, Y., et al. (2017). AMPK orchestrates an elaborate cascade protecting tissue from fibrosis and aging. *Ageing Res. Rev.* 38, 18–27. doi:10.1016/j.arr.2017.07.001
16. Justice, J. N., Nambiar, A. M., Tchkonia, T., LeBrasseur, N. K., Pascual, R., Hashmi, S. K., et al., (2019). Senolytics in idiopathic pulmonary fibrosis: results from a first-in-human, open-label, pilot study. *EBiomedicine* 40, 554–563. doi:10.1016/ j.ebiom.2018.12.052
17. Kimira, M., Arai, Y., Shimoi, K., and Watanabe, S. (1998). Japanese intake of flavonoids and isoflavonoids from foods. *J. Epidemiol.* 8 (3), 168–175. doi:10. 2188/jea.8.168
18. Kuwano, K., Araya, J., Hara, H., Minagawa, S., Takasaka, N., Ito, S., et al. (2016). Cellular senescence and autophagy in the pathogenesis of chronic obstructive pulmonary disease (COPD) and idiopathic pulmonary fibrosis (IPF). *Respir Investig.* 54 (6), 397–406. doi:10.1016/j.resinv.2016.03.010

19. Lehmann, M., Korfei, M., Mutze, K., Klee, S., Skronska-Wasek, W., Alsafadi, H. N., et al. (2017). Senolytic drugs target alveolar epithelial cell function and attenuate experimental lung fibrosis *ex vivo*. *Eur. Respir. J.* 50 (2), 1602367. doi:10.1183/ 13993003.02367
20. Li, R.S., Xu, G.-h., Cao, J., Liu, B., Xie, H.-f., Ishii, Y., et al. (2019). Alpha-mangostin ameliorates bleomycin-induced pulmonary fibrosis in mice partly through activating adenosine 5'-monophosphate-activated protein kinase. *Front. Pharmacol.* 10, 1305. doi:10.3389/fphar.2019.01305
21. Liu, B., Tu, Y., He, W., Liu, Y., Wu, W., Fang, Q., et al. (2018). Hyperoside attenuates renal aging and injury induced by D-galactose via inhibiting AMPK- ULK1 signaling-mediated autophagy. *Aging (Albany NY)* 10 (12), 4197–4212. doi:10.18632/aging.101723
22. Liu, L., Gan, S., Li, B., Ge, X., Yu, H., Zhou, H., et al. (2019). Fisetin alleviates atrial inflammation, remodeling, and vulnerability to atrial fibrillation after myocardial infarction. *Int. Heart J.* 60, 1398–1406. doi:10.1536/ihj. 19-131
23. López-Otín, C., Blasco, M. A., Partridge, L., Serrano, M., Kroemer, G., et al. (2013). The hallmarks of aging. *Cell* 153 (6), 1194–1217. doi:10.1016/j.cell.2013.05.039 Maher, P. (2015). How fisetin reduces the impact of age and disease on CNS function. *Front. Biosci.* 7, 58–82. doi:10.2741/s425
24. Meiners, S., Eickelberg, O., and Königshoff, M. (2015). Hallmarks of the ageing lung. *Eur. Respir. J.* 45 (3), 807–827. doi:10.1183/09031936.00186914
25. Minagawa, S., Araya, J., Numata, T., Nojiri, S., Hara, H., and Yumino, Y., (2011). Accelerated epithelial cell senescence in IPF and the inhibitory role of SIRT6 in TGF-β-induced senescence of human bronchial epithelial cells. *Am. J. Physiol. Lung Cell Mol. Physiol.* 300 (3), L391–L401. doi:10.1152/ajplung.00097.2010
26. Pal, H. C., Pearlman, R. L., and Afaq, F. (2016). Fisetin and its role in chronic diseases. *Adv. Exp. Med. Biol.* 928, 213–244. doi:10.1007/978-3-319-41334-1_10
27. Qiu, T., Tian, Y., Gao, Y., Ma, M., Li, H., Liu, X., et al. (2019). PTEN loss regulates alveolar epithelial cell senescence in pulmonary fibrosis depending on Akt activation. *Aging (Albany NY)* 11 (18), 7492–7509. doi:10.18632/aging.102262
28. Rangarajan, S., Bone, N. B., Zmijewska, A. A., Park, D. W., Bernard, K., et al. (2018). Metformin reverses established lung fibrosis in a bleomycin model. *Nat. Med.* 24 (8), 1121–1127. doi:10.1038/s41591-018-0087-6
29. Richeldi, L., Collard, H. R., and Jones, M. G. (2017). Idiopathic pulmonary fibrosis. *Lancet* 389 (10082), 1941–1952. doi:10.1016/S0140-6736(17)30866-8
30. Salminen, A., Hyttinen, J. M., and Kaarniranta, K. (2011). AMP-activated protein kinase inhibits NF-κB signaling and inflammation: impact on healthspan and lifespan. *J. Mol. Med.* 89 (7), 667–676. doi:10.1007/ s00109-011-0748-0
31. Salminen, A., and Kaarniranta, K. (2012). AMP-activated protein kinase (AMPK) controls the aging process via an integrated signaling network. *Ageing Res. Rev.* 11 (2), 230–241. doi:10.1016/j.arr.2011.12.005
32. Salminen, A., Kauppinen, A., and Kaarniranta, K. (2012). Emerging role of NF-κB signaling in the induction of senescence-associated secretory phenotype (SASP). *Cell. Signal.* 24 (4), 835–845. doi:10.1016/j.cellsig.2011.12.006
33. Schafer, M. J., White, T. A., Iijima, K., Haak, A. J., Ligresti, G., Atkinson, E. J., et al. (2017). Cellular senescence mediates fibrotic pulmonary disease. *Nat. Commun.* 8, 14532. doi:10.1038/ncomms14532
34. Szapiel, S. V., Elson, N. A., Fulmer, J. D., Hunninghake, G. W., Crystal, R. G., et al. (1979). Bleomycin-induced interstitial pulmonary disease in the nude, athymic mouse. *Am. Rev. Respir. Dis.* 120 (4), 893–899. doi:10.1164/arrd.1979.120.4.893
35. Tian, Y., Li, H., Qiu, T., Dai, J., Zhang, Y., Chen, J., et al. (2019). Loss of PTEN induces lung fibrosis via alveolar epithelial cell senescence depending on NF-κB activation. *Aging Cell* 18 (1), e12858. doi:10.1111/acel.12858
36. Wang, C., Jurk, D., Maddick, M., Nelson, G., Martin-Ruiz, C., and von Zglinicki, T. (2009). DNA damage response and cellular senescence in tissues of aging mice. *Aging Cell* 8 (3), 311–323. doi:10.1111/j.1474-9726.2009.00481.x
37. Wang, H., Yang, T., Wang, T., Hao, N., Shen, Y., Wu, Y., et al. (2018). Phloretin attenuates mucus hypersecretion and airway inflammation induced by cigarette smoke. *Int. Immunopharm.* 55, 112–119. doi:10. 1016/j.intimp.2017.12.009
38. Yang, J. Y., Tao, L.-j., Liu, B., You, X.-y., Zhang, C.-f., Xie, H.-f., et al. (2019). Wedelolactone attenuates pulmonary fibrosis partly through activating AMPK and regulating raf-MAPKs signaling pathway. *Front. Pharmacol.* 10, 151. doi:10.3389/fphar.2019.00151
39. Yang, W., Tian, Z.-K., Yang, H.-X., Feng, Z.-J., Sun, J.-M., Jiang, H., et al. (2019). Fisetin improves lead-induced neuroinflammation, apoptosis and synaptic dysfunction in mice associated with the AMPK/SIRT1 and autophagy pathway. *Food Chem. Toxicol.* 134 (110824), 17.
40. Yousefzadeh, M. J., Zhu, Y., McGowan, S. J., Angelini, L., Fuhrmann-Stroissnigg, H., Xu, M., et al. (2018). Fisetin is a senotherapeutic that extends health and lifespan. *EBioMedicine* 36, 18–28. doi:10.1016/j.ebiom.2018.09.015

Permissions

All chapters in this book were first published by Frontiers; hereby published with permission under the Creative Commons Attribution License or equivalent. Every chapter published in this book has been scrutinized by our experts. Their significance has been extensively debated. The topics covered herein carry significant findings which will fuel the growth of the discipline. They may even be implemented as practical applications or may be referred to as a beginning point for another development.

The contributors of this book come from diverse backgrounds, making this book a truly international effort. This book will bring forth new frontiers with its revolutionizing research information and detailed analysis of the nascent developments around the world.

We would like to thank all the contributing authors for lending their expertise to make the book truly unique. They have played a crucial role in the development of this book. Without their invaluable contributions this book wouldn't have been possible. They have made vital efforts to compile up to date information on the varied aspects of this subject to make this book a valuable addition to the collection of many professionals and students.

This book was conceptualized with the vision of imparting up-to-date information and advanced data in this field. To ensure the same, a matchless editorial board was set up. Every individual on the board went through rigorous rounds of assessment to prove their worth. After which they invested a large part of their time researching and compiling the most relevant data for our readers.

The editorial board has been involved in producing this book since its inception. They have spent rigorous hours researching and exploring the diverse topics which have resulted in the successful publishing of this book. They have passed on their knowledge of decades through this book. To expedite this challenging task, the publisher supported the team at every step. A small team of assistant editors was also appointed to further simplify the editing procedure and attain best results for the readers.

Apart from the editorial board, the designing team has also invested a significant amount of their time in understanding the subject and creating the most relevant covers. They scrutinized every image to scout for the most suitable representation of the subject and create an appropriate cover for the book.

The publishing team has been an ardent support to the editorial, designing and production team. Their endless efforts to recruit the best for this project, has resulted in the accomplishment of this book. They are a veteran in the field of academics and their pool of knowledge is as vast as their experience in printing. Their expertise and guidance has proved useful at every step. Their uncompromising quality standards have made this book an exceptional effort. Their encouragement from time to time has been an inspiration for everyone.

The publisher and the editorial board hope that this book will prove to be a valuable piece of knowledge for researchers, students, practitioners and scholars across the globe.

List of Contributors

Thomas Planté-Bordeneuve
Pôle de pneumologie, O.R.L. et dermatologie, Institut de Recherche Expérimentale et Clinique, Université catholique de Louvain, Bruxelles, Belgium

Charles Pilette and Antoine Froidure
Pôle de pneumologie, O.R.L. et dermatologie, Institut de Recherche Expérimentale et Clinique, Université catholique de Louvain, Bruxelles, Belgium
Service de pneumologie, Cliniques universitaires Saint-Luc, Bruxelles, Belgium

Argyrios Tzouvelekis
First Academic Respiratory Department, Sotiria General Hospital for Thoracic Diseases, University of Athens, Athens, Greece
Division of Immunology, Alexander Fleming Biomedical Sciences Research Center, Athens, Greece

Demosthenes Bouros and Theodoros Karampitsakos
First Academic Respiratory Department, Sotiria General Hospital for Thoracic Diseases, University of Athens, Athens, Greece

Rebecca Toonkel
Department of Medicine, Florida International University Herbert Wertheim College of Medicine, Miami, FL, United States

Kantha Medapalli
Department of Medicine, Florida International University Herbert Wertheim College of Medicine, Miami, FL, United States
Department of Surgery, University of Miami Miller School of Medicine, Miami, FL, United States

Vasilis Aidinis
Division of Immunology, Alexander Fleming Biomedical Sciences Research Center, Athens, Greece
Department of Surgery, University of Miami Miller School of Medicine, Miami, FL, United States

Marilyn K. Glassberg
Department of Surgery, University of Miami Miller School of Medicine, Miami, FL, United States
Department of Medicine, University of Miami Miller School of Medicine, Miami, FL, United States

Yuqiong Wang
Peking University China-Japan Friendship School of Clinical Medicine, Beijing, China
Department of Pulmonary and Critical Care Medicine, Center of Respiratory Medicine, National Center for Respiratory Medicine, China-Japan Friendship Hospital, Beijing China

Xiaoyan Zhang, Yingying Feng, Yunxia Zhang, Bin Xing, Ting Sun, Qingyuan Zhan and Ye Tian
Department of Pulmonary and Critical Care Medicine, Center of Respiratory Medicine, National Center for Respiratory Medicine, China-Japan Friendship Hospital, Beijing China

Ling Zhao
Department of Pathology, China-Japan Friendship Hospital, Beijing, China

Hanbo Yang
Department of Rheumatology, China-Japan Friendship Hospital, Beijing, China

Wenlin Guo
China-Japan Union Hospital of Jilin University, Changchun, China

François Huaux
Louvain Centre for Toxicology and Applied Pharmacology (LTAP), Institut de Recherche Experimentale et Clinique (IREC), Université Catholique de Louvain, Brussels, Belgium

Ilianna Barbayianni, Ioanna Ninou and Vassilis Aidinis
Division of Immunology, Biomedical Sciences Research Center Alexander Fleming, Athens, Greece

Hui Xu, Jie Weng, Mengying Xie and Zhiliang Zhou
Department of General Practice, The Second Affiliated Hospital of Wenzhou Medical University, Wenzhou, China

Jingwen Yang
Department of Geriatric Medicine, The First Affiliated Hospital of Wenzhou Medical University, Wenzhou, China

Mengyun Tu
Department of Clinical Laboratory, Hangzhou TCM Hospital Affiliated to Zhejiang Chinese Medical University, Hangzhou, China

Peisen Zhou
Department of Emergency Medicine, The Second Affiliated Hospital of Wenzhou Medical University, Wenzhou, China

Liang Wang
Department of Public Health, Robbins College of Health and Human Sciences, Baylor University, Waco, TX, United States

Chan Chen
Department of Geriatric Medicine, The First Affiliated Hospital of Wenzhou Medical University, Wenzhou, China
Institute of Bioscaffold Transplantation and Immunology, School of Basic Medical Sciences, Wenzhou Medical University, Wenzhou, China

Zhiyi Wang
Department of General Practice, The Second Affiliated Hospital of Wenzhou Medical University, Wenzhou, China
Institute of Hypoxia Medicine, School of Basic Medical Sciences, Wenzhou Medical University, Wenzhou, China

Chiel van Geffen
Department of Experimental and Clinical Pharmacology and Pharmacogenomics, University Hospital Tübingen, Tübingen, Germany

Markus Quante
Department of General, Visceral and Transplant Surgery, University Hospital Tübingen, Tübingen, Germany

Astrid Deißler
Department of Experimental and Clinical Pharmacology and Pharmacogenomics, University Hospital Tübingen, Tübingen, Germany
Department of General, Visceral and Transplant Surgery, University Hospital Tübingen, Tübingen, Germany

Harald Renz
Institute of Laboratory Medicine and Pathobiochemistry, Molecular Diagnostics, Philipps University of Marburg, Marburg, Germany
Universities of Giessen and Marburg Lung Center, German Center for Lung Research (DZL), Marburg, Germany

Dominik Hartl
Department of Pediatrics I, Eberhard Karls University of Tübingen, Tübingen, Germany
Dominik Hartl, Novartis Institutes for BioMedical Research, Basel, Switzerland

Saeed Kolahian
Department of Experimental and Clinical Pharmacology and Pharmacogenomics, University Hospital Tübingen, Tübingen, Germany
Institute of Laboratory Medicine and Pathobiochemistry, Molecular Diagnostics, Philipps University of Marburg, Marburg, Germany
Universities of Giessen and Marburg Lung Center, German Center for Lung Research (DZL), Marburg, Germany

Paolo Spagnolo
Respiratory Disease Unit, Department of Cardiac, Thoracic and Vascular Sciences, University of Padova, Padova, Italy

Argyris Tzouvelekis
Division of Immunology, Biomedical Sciences Research Center "Alexander Fleming", Athens, Greece

Francesco Bonella
Interstitial and Rare Lung Disease Unit, Ruhrlandklinik, University of Duisburg-Essen, Essen, Germany

Jiali Min, Qiao Li, Suosi Liu, Qianrong Wang, Min Yin, Yan Zhang and Shanshan Liu
National Clinical Research Center for Metabolic Diseases, Key Laboratory of Diabetes Immunology, Ministry of Education, Department of Metabolism and Endocrinology, The Second Xiangya Hospital of Central South University, Changsha, China

Jun Yan
Beijing Institute of Brain Disorders, Capital Medical University, Beijing, China

Bing Cui
State Key Laboratory of Bioactive Substance and Function of Natural Medicines, Institute of Materia Medica, Chinese Academy of Medical Sciences and Peking Union Medical College, Beijing, China

Xinyu Li, Quyan Zhang and Yinghe Ding
Transplantation Center, The 3rd Xiangya Hospital, Central South University, Changsha, China
Xiangya School of Medicine, Central South University, Changsha, China

Haozheng Cai
Transplantation Center, The 3rd Xiangya Hospital, Central South University, Changsha, China

Yufeng Cai
School of Life Science, Central South University, Changsha, China

Quan Zhuang
Transplantation Center, The 3rd Xiangya Hospital, Central South University, Changsha, China
Research Center of National Health Ministry on Transplantation Medicine, Changsha, China

Justin M. Oldham
Department of Medicine, Division of Pulmonary, Critical Care and Sleep Medicine, University of California at Davis, Davis, CA, United States

Harold R. Collard
Department of Medicine, Division of Pulmonary and Critical Care Medicine, University of California at San Francisco, San Francisco, CA, United States

Yuanying Wang, Ziyun Guo, Ruimin Ma, Jingwei Wang and Yali Fan
Clinical Center for Interstitial Lung Diseases, Beijing Institute of Respiratory Medicine, Beijing Chaoyang Hospital, Capital Medical University, Beijing, China

Na Wu and Qiao Ye
Clinical Center for Interstitial Lung Diseases, Beijing Institute of Respiratory Medicine, Beijing Chaoyang Hospital, Capital Medical University, Beijing, China
Department of Occupational Medicine and Toxicology, Beijing Chaoyang Hospital, Capital Medical University, Beijing, China

Hope Steele
Division of Immunobiology, Cincinnati Children's Hospital Medical Center, Cincinnati, OH, United States

Kacey Sachen, Andrew J. McKnight and Rachel Soloff
Kyowa Kirin Pharmaceutical Research, Inc., La Jolla, CA, United States

Rana Herro
Division of Immunobiology, Cincinnati Children's Hospital Medical Center, Cincinnati, OH, United States
Department of Pediatrics, University of Cincinnati, Cincinnati, OH, United States

Amarpreet Kaur
Department of Medicine, University of Colorado Denver School of Medicine, Aurora, CO, United States

Susan K. Mathai and David A. Schwartz
Department of Medicine, Division of Pulmonary Sciences and Critical Care Medicine, University of Colorado Denver School of Medicine, Aurora, CO, United States

Eliza Tsitoura, Eirini Vasarmidi, Semeli Mastrodemou, Nikos Tzanakis and Katerina M. Antoniou
Laboratory of Molecular and Cellular Pneumonology, Department of Respiratory Medicine, School of Medicine, University of Crete, Heraklion, Greece

Athina Trachalaki
Laboratory of Molecular and Cellular Pneumonology, Department of Respiratory Medicine, School of Medicine, University of Crete, Heraklion, Greece
Interstitial Lung Disease Unit, Royal Brompton and Harefield Hospital National Health Service (NHS) Foundation Trust, Imperial College, London, United Kingdom

George A. Margaritopoulos, Maria Kokosi, Elizabeth Renzoni and Athol U. Wells
Interstitial Lung Disease Unit, Royal Brompton and Harefield Hospital National Health Service (NHS) Foundation Trust, Imperial College, London, United Kingdom

Dionysios Fanidis and Apostolos Galaris
Division of Immunology, Alexander Fleming Biomedical Sciences Research Centre, Athens, Greece

Omkar Desai, Julia Winkler, Maksym Minasyan and Erica L. Herzog
Section of Pulmonary, Critical Care and Sleep Medicine, Department of Internal Medicine, Yale School of Medicine, New Haven, CT, United States

Marialuisa Bocchino and Ludovica Capitelli
Respiratory Medicine Division, Department of Clinical Medicine and Surgery, Federico II University, Naples, Italy

Serena Zanotta and Domenico Galati
Hematology–Oncology and Stem Cell Transplantation Unit, Department of Hematology and Developmental Therapeutics, Istituto Nazionale Tumori-IRCCS-Fondazione G. Pascale, Naples, Italy

Catharina C. Moor, Peter Heukels, Mirjam Kool and Marlies S. Wijsenbeek
Department of Respiratory Medicine, Erasmus Medical Center, University Hospital Rotterdam, Rotterdam, Netherlands

Florence Savigny, Corinne Schricke, Norinne Lacerda-Queiroz, Mélanie Meda, Mégane Nascimento, Sarah Huot-Marchand, Felipe Da Gama Monteiro, Bernhard Ryffel, Aurélie Gombault, Marc Le Bert, Isabelle Couillin and Nicolas Riteau
Experimental and Molecular Immunology and Neurogenetics Laboratory (INEM), CNRS Orleans (UMR7355) and University of Orleans, Orleans, France

Xunliang Tong, Yanming Li Wenna Zhang and Xiaomao Xu
Department of Respiratory and Critical Care Medicine, National Center of Gerontology, Beijing Hospital, Beijing, China

Fei Su
Clinical Biobank, National Center of Gerontology, Beijing Hospital, Beijing, China

Hongtao Xu
Department of Laboratory Medicine, Beijing Hospital, Beijing, China

Ting Yang and Huaping Dai
National Clinical Research Center for Respiratory Diseases, Center for Respiratory Diseases, China-Japan Friendship Hospital, Peking University Health Science Center, Beijing, China
Department of Pulmonary and Critical Care Medicine, China-Japan Friendship Hospital, Peking University Health Science Center, Beijing, China

Qixia Xu
Department of Respiratory and Critical Care Medicine, Bengbu University Affiliated Hospital, Bengbu, China

Kewu Huang
Department of Respiratory and Critical Care Medicine, Beijing Chao-Yang Hospital, Capital Medical University and Beijing Institute of Respiratory Medicine, Beijing, China

Lihui Zou
The Key Laboratory of Geriatrics, National Center of Gerontology, Beijing Hospital, Beijing, China

Fei Xiao
Clinical Biobank, National Center of Gerontology, Beijing Hospital, Beijing, China
The Key Laboratory of Geriatrics, National Center of Gerontology, Beijing Hospital, Beijing, China

Surui Pei
Annoroad Gene Technology (Beijing) Co., Ltd., Beijing, China

Chen Wang
National Clinical Research Center for Respiratory Diseases, Center for Respiratory Diseases, China-Japan Friendship Hospital, Peking University Health Science Center, Beijing, China
Department of Pulmonary and Critical Care Medicine, China-Japan Friendship Hospital, Peking University Health Science Center, Beijing, China
National Clinical Research Center for Respiratory Diseases, Peking Union Medical College, Chinese Academy of Medical Sciences, Beijing, China

Fan Yang, Hao-yue Zhu, Xiao-xuan Chen and Ren-shuang Cao
College of Traditional Chinese Medicine, Shandong University of Traditional Chinese Medicine, Jinan, China

Zhen-feng Hou
College of Life Sciences, Shandong Normal University, Jinan, China

Wan-yang Li
School of Public Health, Xiangya Medical College, Central South University, Changsha, China

Yu-xuan Li
Second School of Clinical Medicine, Beijing University of Chinese Medicine, Beijing, China

Ru Chen
Biomedical Research Institute of Fudan University, Shanghai, China

Wei Zhang
Department of Pulmonary Diseases, Affiliated Hospital of Shandong University of Traditional Chinese Medicine, Jinan, China

Li Zhang, Xiang Tong, Jizhen Huang, Man Wu, Shijie Zhang, Dongguang Wang, SiTong Liu and Hong Fan
Department of Respiratory and Critical Care Medicine, West China Hospital/West China School of Medicine, Chengdu, China

Index

www.ingramcontent.com/pod-product-compliance
Lightning Source LLC
LaVergne TN
LVHW082126200926
848484LV00008B/2008